A
Handbook
of
Treatment

A Handbook of Treatment

Edited by
H. W. PROCTOR &
P. S. BYRNE

MTP

Published by

MTP Press Ltd
St. Leonard's House
Lancaster, England

Copyright © 1976 MTP Press Ltd
Softcover reprint of the hardcover 1st edition 1976

ISBN-13: 978-94-011-5909-8   e-ISBN-13: 978-94-011-5907-4
DOI: 10.1007/978-94-011-5907-4

Contents

Contributors

P. Amlot — *Department of Medicine, Guy's Hospital Medical School, London.*

P. Barkhan — *Consultant Haematologist, Guy's Hospital Medical School, London.*

R. D. Bradley — *Consultant in Clinical Physiology, St. Thomas's Hospital, London.*

W. I. Cranston — *Professor of Medicine, St. Thomas's Hospital Medical School, London.*

D. N. Croft — *Consultant Physician, St. Thomas's Hospital, London.*

D. C. Deuchar — *Physician to the Cardiac Department, Guy's Hospital, London.*

J. M. Evanson — *Professor of Medicine, University Hospital of South Manchester.*

P. Fells — *Honorary Consultant Surgeon, Institute of Ophthalmology, Moorfields Eye Hospital, London.*

J. L. Fluker — *Consultant in Charge, Department of Genitourinary Medicine, Charing Cross Hospital Group, London; Senior Lecturer, Institute of Obstetrics and Gynaecology, and Honorary Consultant, Hammersmith Hospital, London.*

P. I. Folb — *Professor of Clinical Pharmacology, University of Capetown.*

J. Fry — *General Practitioner, Beckenham, Kent.*

G. I. C. Ingram — *Professor of Experimental Haematology and Consultant Haematologist, Department of Haematology, St. Thomas's Hospital Medical School, London.*

N. F. Jones — *Consultant Physician, St. Thomas's Hospital, London.*

W. R. Keatinge — *Professor of Physiology, London Hospital Medical College, London.*

R. K. Knight — *Physician, Guy's Hospital, London.*

D. R. London — *Consultant Endocrinologist, Queen Elizabeth Hospital, Birmingham.*

B. H. McGibbon — *Senior Lecturer in Haematology and Consultant Haematologist, St. Thomas's Hospital Medical School.*

M. N. Maisey — *Department of Endocrinology, Guy's Hospital, London.*

J. A. Mathews — *Consultant Physician, Department of Rheumatology and Physician, St. Thomas's Hospital, London.*

P. F. D. Naylor — *Titular Professor of Dermatology, University of London, Consultant Dermatologist and Adviser in Clinical Studies, St. Thomas's Hospital, London.*

P. J. R. Nichols — *Consultant Physician in Rehabilitation, The Nuffield Orthopaedic Centre, Headington, Oxford.*

M. D. O'Brien — *Department of Neurology, Guy's Hospital, London.*

C. S. Ogg — *Renal Physician, Guy's Hospital, London.*

R. L. Parsons	*Department of Clinical Pharmacology, Guy's Hospital Medical School, London.*
M. Potts	*Medical Director, Population Services International, 500 Chesham House, 150 Regent Street, London.*
A. J. Ralston	*Consultant Physician, Department of Medicine, Withington Hospital, West Didsbury, Manchester.*
W. G. Reeves	*Consultant Immunologist, Nottingham City Hospital.*
R. W. Ross Russell	*Consultant Neurologist, St. Thomas's Hospital and The National Hospital for Nervous Diseases, London.*
H. A. K. Rowland	*Senior Lecturer in Clinical Tropical Medicine, London School of Hygiene and Tropical Medicine; and First Assistant, Medical Unit, Hospital for Tropical Diseases, London.*
K. B. Saunders	*Senior Medical Registrar, St. Thomas's Hospital, London.*
G. L. Scott	*Senior Lecturer in Haematology and Consultant Haematologist, Department of Haematology, St. Thomas's Hospital Medical School, London.*
S. J. G. Semple	*Professor of Medicine, Middlesex Hospital, London.*
M. C. Stone	*Research Associate, Clinical Research Unit, Leigh, Lancashire.*
F. M. Sullivan	*Department of Pharmacology, Guy's Hospital Medical School, London.*
J. C. Taylor	*Senior Lecturer in Medicine and Honorary Consultant Physician, St. Thomas's Hospital, London.*
J. R. Trounce	*Professor of Clinical Pharmacology, Guy's Hospital Medical School, London.*
J. R. Wall	*Department of Medicine, Guy's Hospital Medical School, London.*
G. Wetherley-Main	*Professor of Haematology and Consultant Haematologist, Department of Haematology, St. Thomas's Hospital Medical School, London.*
J. M. A. Whitehouse	*Senior Lecturer and Honorary Consultant Physician, Department of Medical Oncology, St. Bartholomew's Hospital, London.*
E. Wilkes	*Professor of Community Care and General Practice, Sheffield University.*
F. Wilson	*Consultant Anaesthetist, Pain Relief Clinic, Lancaster District, Lancashire Area Health Authority, Lancaster.*
A. J. Wing	*Consultant Physician, St. Thomas's Hospital, London.*

Foreword

This book attempts to provide we general physicians with a conveniently sized work for daily reference. It deals with an area of medical practice which is rapidly changing. For that reason regular updating with new material will need to be considered.

The book does not profess to be encyclopaedic. In order to keep the size of the book within bounds, there are no sections devoted solely to psychological medicine or to paediatrics, but the book does deal with the more common diseases as revealed by morbidity studies.

The main section of the book—A—is concerned with these commoner diseases and is set out in conventional fashion. It is in two parts; the one dealing with therapeutics, the other with clinical pharmacology. The second section—B—reviews therapy in some selected areas. Cancer, pain and terminal care, contraception, and hyperlipoproteinaemias. It also contains pieces on common emergencies, home renal dialysis and tropical diseases in non-tropical countries.

The creation of 'pain clinics', and the possibilities for the treatment of intractable pain are innovations calculated to be more widely used as we become more aware of their value. The field of rehabilitation is one of which we general physicians are on less familiar ground. To say that by us it is a neglected field is perhaps not too strong a statement.

The section on Drugs concentrates on the practical side of drug administration and hence the stress is on the incompatibilities, side effects and contraindications, with less on the pure science. In those relatively few conditions where a 'drug of choice' appears to exist it may be indicated, otherwise alternatives are discussed. The rationale for the choice of therapy is outlined.

New therapies are often complicated, as for example, the sequential 'cocktails' provided for the sufferers from leukaemia, and not always known to us in general practice. We may be faced with patients who are undergoing therapy at home which was initiated in hospital. We must know what is being administered and why, and be able to recognise the complications or the patient's needs which we may be the first as the doctor to have to face.

Each of us should be able to produce a rationale for our therapy of an individual patient. This is well recognised by the Americans in whose Speciality Board examinations there often appears an oral section on 'Defence of Therapy'. In so many conditions there exists a range of choice, usually indicating that no prescriptive solution is either available or agreed for that particular problem. A case may then be made for a personal particular choice, but it has to be made rationally and take into account the circumstances of the individual patient for whom we are prescribing. It must not reflect a fashion nor a whimsy nor the persuasive efforts of the marketing 'reps'.

The old couplet: 'Be not the first by whom the new is tried, nor yet the last to set the old aside' has still great valid force. It is better to use a small, personal, well tried pharmacopoeia than to undertake a series of wide-ranging uncontrolled experiments through the National Formulary and MIMS. The editors, as experienced dispensing general practitioners, know also that a more sordid yet practical factor, that of cost, reinforces this important point.

It is a fact that it is difficult for most of us to make a critical evaluation of the papers advanced by the 'reps' in support of their product. Often the writers are unknown to us, generalisations are made from small numbers, and advanced statistics are beyond us. We may place some deserved reliance on the several review articles which appear in our plethora of postgraduate journals, yet this does not relieve us of the responsibility for being critical. It is our critical faculty which might well prompt us to practice on the ground rules of the old couplet. It is our critical faculty which we need to sharpen.

One way to do this is by using our own clinical records. Most experienced general practitioners have achieved over the years a series of clinical impressions. Many of these are potentially valuable, but it is rare for them to be supported by hard objective evidence. Regular examination of our clinical records, comparing clinical outcomes in the short and long term with the provided therapy is a well tried method of critical evaluation which we in general practice do not use as we could.

A book 'Treatment or Diagnosis' edited by the late Michael Balint has salutary lessons for us all. It is a study by experienced general practitioners of their long term prescribing. Many patients were discovered to have been taking, or to have been receiving, prescriptions for the same drugs for many years. Excluding such necessities as insulin or digitalis in the appropriate condition, the majority of the prescriptions were for a variety of tranquillisers and other preparations for emotional disorders which had never been well defined. It was found that although little rationale appeared to exist for their continuance, any attempt to stop the exhibition of these drugs led to immediate and hostile patient reaction. For us the lesson would appear to lie in more careful consideration of the need to commence drug therapy. If indeed it is thought necessary to prescribe, frequent review of the situation is required. In many instances it can prove effective to prescribe for and discuss with the patient, a specific 'limited period' course of therapy. The editors must confess that their examination of their own practice at one time revealed that they conformed to the pattern demonstrated by Balint and his co-workers.

The post-war plethora of new drugs has required the neologism of 'iatrogenic disease'. By their own clinical observations reported to the Medicines Commission, general practitioners have made valuable contributions to the knowledge of the side effects of drugs. While the Commission requires much specific evidence on new drugs prior to their being marketed, it may not be until a new drug has been widely used that some side effects may come to light. Chloramphenicol and thalidomide were two examples. Again the advice of the old couplet is valuable.

Much has been written and debated about the use of placebos. We all use them if only in a limited fashion. Yet it seems important to make one or two points about placebos. Firstly, we must be aware that the substance prescribed is calculated by us to be a placebo. It seems that many prescriptions may come under the heading of placebo when they are believed by the prescriber to be of therapeutic value. Secondly, they should be cheap, and thirdly, they should be inert. The use of pharmacologically active preparations in derisory small dosage as placebos seems to be unjustifiable. Thus calcium lactate even in multi-coloured variations of tablets might fit with these requirements. Vitamin B_{12} does not. It is cheap enough but could have unfortunate effects if stopped when the patient had commenced to suffer from pernicious anaemia. If a 'bottle' seems appropriate Inf Gent. Co. would be acceptable whereas an expensive, elegant but useless perparation of hypophosphites (with or without an alcoholic base) would not.

One less appreciated valid use of the placebo could be described as 'buying time'. It represents the modest reinforcement of the well-tried clinical ploy of masterly inactivity as a means of permitting our observation of the development of a clinical problem.

In essence the use of the placebo is a confidence trick, but it is the patient who has to achieve the confidence. We must never con ourselves.

One fundamental point is to be made about the exhibition of drugs to the elderly. There is too much of it. There is little rationale to be observed in an enthusiastic attack on 'hypertension' measured by a high systolic pressure in an eighty-year-old person. Drugs prescribed for the elderly should be well known to the prescriber, as few as possible in number, with the simplest possible dosage schedules. Perhaps the safest method of procedure is not to start therapy at all except with clear cut clinical indication.

So often medical journals have engaged in the useful abstraction of a series of 'Favourite Prescriptions'. Most of us have a set of personal preferences. One or two each perhaps from the cornucopia of antihistamines, pencillins, hormones, diuretics, tranquillisers, etc. Where there is no concensus drug of choice we are then prescribing from the base of experienced clinical observation. From the large number of people known to any one of we general practitioners we have each only a few close and trusted friends. The same might well apply to our prescribing.

In any publication of multi-anthorship there is the problem of differing styles. The editors have made no attempt to achieve an overall uniformity. It seems to them an impertinence to tamper with an external expression of the personality of their distinguished colleagues.

H. W. PROCTOR
P. S. BYRNE

Section A

A Guide to
Modern Treatment

Therapy of
Common
Diseases

Edited by W. I. Cranston

Contents

1

THE GASTROINTESTINAL TRACT

D. N. CROFT

ESOPHAGUS

Hiatus hernia

Asymptomatic hiatus hernia is common and requires no treatment. Regurgitation of bitter gastric juice into the mouth occurs and is particularly related to bending, stooping and lying flat. Patients should be advised to avoid these positions. They should sleep propped up with pillows or with the head of the bed raised. In babies, specially constructed cradles are used. Reflux esophagitis occurs when the acidic gastric contents repeatedly bathe the lower esophagus and it is this that causes heartburn. It can be prevented by advice on posture, but if the symptom persists and is troublesome, the patient should be treated with regular doses of alkalis. These are best given as a mixture after meals and as tablets 1–2 hourly between meals. Proprietary preparations such as Gaviscon produce a floating viscous gel in the stomach which is claimed to block reflux of gastric contents into the stomach. Such preparations appear to be symptomatically effective in patients who have not responded to simple alkali treatment. Patients with symptoms from hiatus hernia are commonly obese and are often improved by being put on a reducing diet and losing weight. Smoking has been shown to cause relaxation of the lower esophageal sphincter and reflux. Patients with reflux esophagitis should stop smoking. There is recent evidence to show that metoclopramide 10 mg t.d.s. is more effective than a placebo in relieving heartburn and flatulent dyspepsia. This may be because of its ability to increase the tone of the lower esophageal sphincter. Its value in clinical practice requires further evaluation.

Persistent reflux esophagitis leads to an inflammatory narrowing of the lower esophagus and this results in dysphagia. The narrowing is initially due to edema and at this stage dysphagia is reversible by medical measures outlined above. At a later date a true fibrous stricture forms and surgical intervention will have to be considered. Whether or not this is necessary will depend on various clinical factors – such as the age and general health of the patient. If surgery is contraindicated patients may be kept relatively well by the medical measures outlined above and, if necessary, by mincing their food and avoiding solids that are prone to stick.

The surgical treatment of hiatus hernia is not generally satisfactory. This is probably because the surgeon cannot repair the dysfunctioning lower esophageal sphincter, despite successful replacement of the stomach below the diaphragm. Surgery should therefore only be considered if medical treatment has been rigorously instituted and shown to be unsuccessful, or if a fibrous stricture has formed. If it is undertaken its success is largely determined by the interest and expertise of the surgeon.

Achalasia

Achalasia is a neuromuscular disorder of the esophagus which causes dysphagia, esophageal regurgitation and esophageal pain. These symptoms are best treated by a Heller's operation if a surgeon experienced in the operation is available. The operation consists in cutting the muscular layers of the lower two inches of the esophagus. This allows food to pass through the previously narrow segment. Reflux esophagitis may occur following the operation and will require treatment as indicated above. In some centres the muscle fibres of the lower esophagus are forcibly split by inflating a balloon (e.g. Mosher bag), placed in the lumen of the gastro-esophageal junction under X-ray control. In experienced hands the procedure is successful and it has the advantage of avoiding a major surgical operation. It is usually done without general anaesthetic and is painful. If a Heller's operation is contraindicated, because of age or infirmity, it is sometimes possible to manage the patient with repeated dilatations with bougies. These patients will also have to mince their food.

Scleroderma (diffuse systemic sclerosis)

Scleroderma commonly affects the lower two-thirds of the esophagus. It causes progressive narrowing of the lumen and dysphagia. In this condition dysphagia is best treated by repeated dilations with a bougie, which the patient can be taught to pass once or twice a day if necessary. Surgical resection of the stricture is contraindicated as the esophageal wall is usually too diseased for satisfactory anastomosis to be achieved.

Diffuse esophageal spasm

Diffuse esophageal spasm is a neuromuscular disorder of the esophagus in which the organ goes into intermittent episodes of spasm. It commonly presents with episodes of severe retrosternal pain that may mimic cardiac pain. The pain is not usually sufficiently frequent or troublesome to require a major surgical procedure, but, in selected cases, successful results have been achieved by esophageal myotomy. In this operation the muscle coats are split over a long length of the esophagus.

Belching

It is a normal physiological event for the lower esophageal sphincter to relax from time to time and to allow gastric gas to pass into the esophagus. This can be promoted by carminatives such as peppermint, which cause relaxation of the sphincter. Once in the esophagus the gas is usually expelled quietly. Noisy belching requires constriction of voluntary muscle and is thus under conscious control. This should be pointed out to patients who complain of noisy belching, and they should also be told not to swallow air. In a rare condition termed 'speaking esophagus syndrome' the patient appears unable to prevent the noise which may be a considerable embarrassment to her.

STOMACH

Gastritis

Acute gastritis is a transient response of the stomach to ingestion of insulting substances. The gastric mucosa has remarkable recuperative abilities and therefore, although the mucosa can be shown to sustain damage from, for instance, a few soluble aspirin tablets, no significant clinical effect ensues. However ingestion of a large dose of gastric irritant, such as staphylococcal endotoxin, corrosive poison or a bottle of whisky, will have significant clinical effects: vomiting, diarrhea and, on occasion, gastrointestinal bleeding. An acute episode such as this is usually self-limiting within a few hours, but

may require intravenous saline if loss of fluids is excessive. Repeated ingestion of alcohol causes early morning nausea and vomiting of mucus-rich fluid. This is best treated by reducing intake of alcohol but, if this is not possible, the patient should be advised to drink plenty of fluids and to use alkalis liberally. Because of the risk of precipitating gastric bleeding he should be advised not to take preparations that contain aspirin—even those that are advertised for 'hangovers'.

Haemorrhagic (erosive) gastritis is a common cause of acute gastrointestinal bleeding and it accounts for about one quarter of the cases of haematemesis and melaena admitted to hospital in Great Britain. It is usually precipitated by aspirin, although other factors (alcohol, antirheumatic drugs, stress, malnutrition) are important in its pathogenesis. Patients who have had an aspirin-induced acute bleed should be advised, if possible, to avoid this drug. There are now available preparations of aspirin that cause significantly less gastrointestinal bleeding (enteric coated aspirin, benorylate) than soluble aspirin, and these preparations can be tried in patients who require salicylate therapy but who have gastric problems with the commonly available formulations.

Atrophic gastritis is common in persons over 50, particularly if they smoke, or drink alcohol. It does not cause pain and there is no specific treatment for it. Patients with atrophic gastritis develop iron deficiency or frank gastric bleeding, and this will require appropriate treatment. Complete gastric atrophy in certain individuals leads to vitamin B_{12} deficiency and pernicious anaemia. This will require appropriate investigaton and treatment with injections of vitamin B_{12}.

Peptic ulcer

The common sites for peptic ulcers are the duodenum and stomach but they may also occur in the lower esophagus, jejunum and in a Meckel's diverticulum. The management of gastric and duodenal ulcers that are causing pain as a predominant symptom and haematemesis and melaena will be discussed in this section.

Gastric ulcer

It is usually possible to decide on radiological or gastroscopic criteria that an ulcer in the stomach is benign, but it is important in terms of management to appreciate that malignancy is always a possibility. Gastroscopy with biopsy using flexible fibre optic endoscopes may help in selected cases. Benign gastric ulcers can, by appropriate medical management, be made to heal and it should be the aim of the physician to see that this occurs within 3 months. Failure to do this is an indication for surgery. Two-fifths of the chronic gastric ulcers that heal, recur within 2 years and these should be treated surgically. *Removal of provoking factors.* Alcohol, aspirin, indomethacin and phenylbutazone are known to damage gastric mucosa and can cause gastric ulcers. Patients should be advised to avoid these substances. Those with chronic rheumatic disorders who require continuous administration of aspirin may be given this drug enteric coated or as benorylate, which are preparations that do not harm the stomach. There is no proof that small doses of steroids (i.e. prednisone 5–20 mg/day) are harmful to the human stomach. Larger doses are. Smoking has been shown to delay healing of gastric ulcers and patients should therefore refrain from, or at least reduce, their tobacco consumption. Chronic diseases such as rheumatoid arthritis, cirrhosis and bronchitis and emphysema may well predispose to gastric ulceration. Patients' general health should be improved as much as possible by appropriate treatment of coexisting disease.

Alkalis. Frequent doses of alkalis are of known value in the treatment of pain due to gastric ulcers. They have not however been proved to heal ulcers. They should be given regularly—hourly or even half-hourly if necessary—either as mixtures or in tablet form. Out patients may find it convenient to take mixtures at meal times and to carry alkali tablets to suck in the intervals. Milk may be taken in lieu of alkalis between meals. Magnesium trisilicate causes diarrhea in some patients and if this is troublesome, aluminium hydroxide, which tends to be constipating, can be used. The laxative effect of magnesium trisilicate is an advantage to bedbound patients.

Bed rest. Hospitalisation and bed rest has been shown to improve the healing rate of gastric ulcers. It is common clinical experience that acute exacerbations of peptic ulcer settle within a week of the patient being admitted. Most gastric ulcers heal satisfactorily with conventional outpatient treatment, but if the ulcer is very large or does no heal, in-patient treatment is indicated. Out-patients should be advised to get as much rest as possible and it may be necessary for them to have a period off work in order to do so.

Ulcer healing drugs. Carbenoxolone has been shown to enhance the rate of healing of gastric ulcers in out-patients. In fact it is the only drug that has been shown to do so. Unfortunately it has undesirable side effects—fluid and salt retention and occasionally hypokalaemia. These effects are commoner with larger doses of carbenoxolone. Patients are at risk of being precipitated into cardiac failure and this is a particular problem in the elderly who should be seen weekly for weighing and blood pressure. Weight gain of 4 pounds (2.0 kg) is an indication to start a thiazide diuretic and Slow-K. Spironolactone should not be used because it prevents ulcer healing. In view of these problems carbenoxolone should only be used on those patients who have failed to respond satisfactorily to the conservative regime outlined above. Deglycyrrhizinated liquorice has been shown to heal gastric ulcers without causing edema or cardiac failure. Although more clinical trials are required, this preparation does appear to have advantages over carbenoxolone. Gefarnate is another drug without significant side-effects that needs further evaluation.

Anticholinergics. These only produce a significant reduction in gastric acidity if given in sufficient amount to cause other unpleasant effects such as dry mouth, bladder dysfunction and blurred vision. As the symptoms of gastric ulcers can usually be controlled with regular meals and frequent ingestion of milk or alkalis, there is no indication to use anti-cholinergics.

Sedatives and tranquillizers. These may be required for patients with insomnia or anxiety states. There is evidence that they reduce gastric acid secretion precipitated by emotion and thus they may help to heal gastric ulcers.

'Bland' diets. There is no evidence that 'bland' (uninteresting) diets improve the healing of gastric ulcers. Individual patients discover that particular foods upset them, and they should avoid these items. Patients should be advised to have meals at regular intervals and to have snacks or milk and biscuits between their main meals. Milk has a good buffering capacity and should be taken liberally during exacerbations of pain. Rigid 'bland' foods are of no proven value. Patients should be advised to eat foods that suit them and that they like.

Duodenal ulcer

The essential of treating dyspepsia due to duodenal ulceration is to control the symptoms. It is not usually possible to show by radiology that the ulcer has healed. If fibre-optic endoscopy is available for diagnosis and follow-up more acceptable assessment of therapeutic regimes will be obtained. The symptoms can usually be controlled satisfactorily by frequent administration of alkalis and milk, regular meals, bed rest and hospitalisation if necessary. 'Bland' diets are not indicated. Carbenoxolone or similar drugs have not been proved to be effective for duodenal ulceration. If the pain persists and disrupts the patient's life, surgery should be advised.

Surgery for peptic ulcers

Perforation, possibility of carcinoma, and recurrent bleeding are absolute indications for surgery for gastric ulcers. Pyloric obstruction, perforation and repeated bleeding are absolute indications in the case of duodenal ulcers. Patients with repeated and incapacitating pain from gastric and duodenal ulcers may require surgery but the criteria for this decision will depend on many factors. In general it is best to operate on gastric ulcers if they fail to heal or if they recur after successful healing. For duodenal ulcers the decision about surgery depends mainly on an assessment of the patient's symptoms rather than the barium meal appearances. If the patient's life, and particularly his work, is being seriously disturbed by pain from the ulcer an operation should be advised. In general, gastric surgery for peptic ulcers is very satisfactory and patients are relieved of distressing symptoms.

Haematemesis and melaena

There are approximately 28 000 acute upper gastrointestinal bleeds admitted to hospital in the UK each year. Approximately one quarter of these are precipitated by aspirin and occur from acute erosions. Patients with haematemesis and melaena should be asked about recent ingestion of aspirin and alcohol for, if they have, it is probable that surgical intervention will not be required. A history of taking indomethacin, phenylbutazone or corticosteroids will suggest bleeding from a drug induced chronic gastric ulcer.

A haematemesis indicates that the patient has lost one third of his blood volume (or 1.5–2.0 litres) and the size of the haematemesis is an indication of the amount of blood lost. Patients with melaena lose less than one quarter of the blood volume (or 1 litre or less). These facts are more useful in assessing the volume of blood loss than the pulse rate or blood pressure. A haemoglobin of less than 11.2 g indicates a bleed of more than 2–2.5 litres (half the blood volume).

On admission patients require blood transfusion if they have lost 1.5 litres or more of blood volume. Central venous pressure measurement is the most accurate method of measuring transfusion requirements. If the patient is shocked and requires large amounts of blood the metabolic acidosis should be corrected with intravenous sodium bicarbonate. A barium meal within 24 hours of admission is valuable in detecting large ulcers, cancer, etc., that may require surgical treatment. Gastroscopy has enthusiastic advocates but can be very difficult in the presence of blood in the stomach. If bleeding continues for more than 48 hours requiring more than 10 pints (5 litres) of blood, the patient should be referred for surgical treatment. A rebleed after admission is a further indication for surgery. The following factors are known to be associated with bleeding again after admission:

> large initial bleed, admission following haematemesis rather than melaena, presence of esophageal varices, presence of gastric ulcer.

Age, sex and ABO blood group are not related. If the patient has not bled for 48 hours he is unlikely to bleed again in the near future.

Selective angiography can define the site of a large gastrointestinal bleed and has been combined with infusion of vasopressin, (in order to lower mesenteric blood flow), in an attempt to stop the bleeding. This technique is at present being evaluated.

SMALL INTESTINE

Celiac syndrome

Celiac syndrome is the adult equivalent of celiac disease. It is malabsorption due to a primary abnormality of the small intestinal mucosa ('flat' mucosa). At least 75% of adults with celiac syndrome respond dramatically to gluten withdrawal. A gluten-free diet imposes restrictions and inconvenience on the patient but there are two reasons for insisting that the patient should stick to it, even when clinically improved. Firstly, because he is likely to relapse if gluten is reintroduced. Secondly, because it is becoming increasingly appreciated that the celiac mucosa is pre-malignant, and there is some evidence that gluten withdrawal reduces the risk of malignancy. Patients who respond well to gluten withdrawal do not require any other medicaments once their body stores of vitamins, iron, etc., have been repleted. A gluten-free wheat starch, bread, biscuits, and pasta, are prescribable under the National Health Service in the UK on an EC10. The Coeliac Society, (PO Box No T81, London NW2 2QY, England), a patients' association, can advise and help those with this condition. A book giving useful recipes and advice on cooking with gluten-free flour has been published.

During active phases of the disease patients may have deficiency of folic acid, iron, vitamin K, vitamin D and calcium, and hypoproteinaemia. These substances should not be replaced before a firm diagnosis has been made by small intestinal biopsy. For 3 months after starting a gluten-free diet, replacements of appropriate substances should be given. In the case of iron, vitamin K and vitamin D the drugs should be given initially by injection. Iron, folic acid and calcium should also be given by mouth. After 3 months patients do not require supplements if they have responded well to gluten withdrawal. They should however be kept under continuous observation.

A proportion—perhaps one quarter—of patients do not respond to gluten withdrawal. In these, and also in patients who are severely ill, prednisone 10–20 mg thrice daily for 2 weeks, and reducing slowly to a maintenance dose of 5–15 mg/day should be given. Some patients are dramatically improved by this. The few that are not may have coexisting pancreatic failure which may need appropriate treatment. A course of antibiotics (e.g. tetracycline 250 mg four times daily for 2 weeks) is sometimes worth trying in these individuals, as there is evidence that the small gut may become infected with pathogenic bacteria.

Other causes of malabsorption

Excess fat in the stool (steatorrhea) is a common feature of many systemic disorders. For instance steatorrhea may occur in diabetes, thyrotoxicosis, Addison's disease, cirrhosis and superior mesenteric artery occlusion. Treatment of the primary disorder (e.g. thyrotoxicosis or Addison's disease) will often reverse the disorder. In this section only intestinal causes of malabsorption will be considered and mainly those that have a precise and definite method of therapy.

Post-gastric surgery. Any operation for peptic ulceration (vagotomy, pyloroplasty, partial gastrectomy) may cause steatorrhea. In most patients this is of no significance and can only be detected by biochemical measurement of stool fat. Patients who have had gastric surgery are at risk of developing clinically significant malabsorption, particularly those who have had a partial gastrectomy. Weight loss or failure to gain weight, may be due to malabsorption, although in many patients it is due to inadequate intake of calories.

Iron deficiency anaemia is also common after gastric surgery. Women in their reproductive years are at particular risk and should be treated with parenteral and oral iron. Folic acid deficiency may cause megaloblastic anaemia and is usually due to inadequate diet. Megaloblastic anaemia due to Vitamin B_{12} deficiency results from inadequate secretion of intrinsic factor from the gastric remnant. This will require treatment with injections of vitamin B_{12} (500 μg monthly). Osteomalacia occurs due to vitamin D malabsorption and loss of calcium in the stools. This requires treatment with injections of vitamin D (20 000–40 000 u weekly), until the bone lesions have healed. Calcium lactate in effervescent form should be given in a dose of 15 g thrice daily.

The question of preventing overt iron deficiency and osteomalacia by prophylactic treatment with oral iron and oral calcium and vitamin D is a much disputed topic. In the writer's opinion these drugs should not be used prophylactically on patients who are clinically well. Patients who have had gastric operations should be seen annually so that they can be weighed and have haemoglobin estimations.

Short small intestine. Occasionally patients who have had intestinal surgery are left with an inadequate length of small intestine. These patients have to be carefully assessed to see that they do not have blind loops. Considerable improvement can be effected by the use of a low fat diet.

Bacterial invasion of the small intestine. Bacteria invade the small intestine if there is a stagnant segment of the gut. Blind loops of small intestine may result from gastrointestinal surgery. These should be corrected surgically. If this is not possible broad spectrum antibiotics may be used (i.e. tetracycline 250 mg three or four times a day). Fistulae between segments of intestine may occur from Crohn's disease, carcinomas or after surgery and if possible these should be corrected surgically. Jejunal diverticulosis occurs in the elderly and is a not uncommon cause of diarrhea, steatorrhea and occasionally vitamin B_{12} deficiency. Intermittent courses of oral tetracycline (250 mg thrice daily for 5–10 days) will control the symptoms in many of these patients and should be tried before subjecting the patient to surgery. It is often useful in these patients to give them a supply of the antibiotic and to advise them to take them for 5 days at the first sign of recurrence of diarrhea. Scleroderma (diffuse systemic sclerosis) may affect the small intestine which dilates and becomes stagnant. Steatorrhea can be improved in these patients by antibiotics. *Giardiasis.* Infestation of the small intestine with *Giardia lamblia* causes diarrhea and steatorrhea with malabsorption. It is diagnosed by finding the organism in stools or the aspirate from the small intestine. It is treated with mepacrine 100 mg three times daily for 1 week or metronidazole 200 mg three times daily for 1 week. Two or more courses may be required to eliminate the infection and if the infection is not eradicated larger doses of mepacrine can be used.

Whipple's disease is a rare disorder affecting the small intestinal mucosa and having a characteristic histological appearance. It is probable that it is caused by a bacterial infection, but specific organisms have not been cultured. Patients with this condition are improved or cured by treatment with tetracycline 250 mg q.d.s. for 18 months. Unless the antibiotic is continued for this length of time relapse will occur.

Worms

Most of the population of the world is infested with worms. Clinical symptoms usually depend on the number of worms present, and from the therapeutic point of view it is often more important to reduce the level of infestation rather than to attempt to completely eradicate the worm. In the Western world, however, the presence of any worms in the stools are regarded with horror and patients demand that they be removed.

Threadworms. Enterobius vermicularis infestation is the most common form of helminthiasis in temperate climates. The adult worms live in the caecum and neighbouring intestine. At night the female, loaded with eggs, migrates to the rectum and anus. Movement of the worms around the anus causes intense itching which wakes the child at night. The eggs are liberated from the anus and readily reinfest the child or are spread to others in the family. The crux of treatment is to treat the child and also the rest of the family who are likely to have asymptomatic infestation.

Piperazine hydrochloride or citrate may be given in tablets or syrup. The whole family should be given 0.5 g three times a day for 1 week. After an interval of 1 week the course should be repeated. An alternative treatment is viprynium embonate tablets (50 mg) or suspension (viprynium 10 mg/ml). It may be given in a single dose but nausea or vomiting occasionally results. It is important to inform the parents that the stools will be turned red by this drug.

Roundworms. (Ascaris lumbricoides). Adult worms in the small bowel may occasionally cause intestinal symptoms. Very heavy infestation may cause intestinal colic or obstruction and migration of the larvae through the lungs may cause a bronchitis-like illness. Often infestation with ascaris is only appreciated when the worm is seen in the stool. Piperazine is a useful drug in the treatment of this condition. In a single dose of 4.0 g in tablet or elixir it is usually effective. Pripsen is a preparation of piperazine with senna purgative which may be used in adults or children. A single dose of 5 g bephenium hydroxynaphthoate is also a convenient treatment for ascariasis.

Tapeworm. Taenia saginata is the beef tapeworm. It is acquired by ingesting the larvae in beef. After the head emerges from the cysticercus it attaches itself to the mucosa of the human small intestine. The worm grows and sheds the terminal segments which appear in the stools. It does not usually cause symptoms or have undesirable effects, but patients naturally wish to be rid of it if they notice the segments in the stools. *Taenia solium* is the pork tapeworm which develops similarly but is not indigenous in the UK. It can occasionally become disseminated throughout the body and give rise to cysticercosis. When this occurs the larvae may lodge in muscles and brain where they give rise to epilepsy which will require treatment with anticonvulsants.

Extract of male fern is effective in dispelling the adult worms from the gastrointestinal tract of man but has been supplanted by other more convenient remedies. Mepacrine can be used but requires a purgative such as magnesium sulphate on the day before treatment. The following morning 1 g of mepacrine is given in 100 mg divided doses over an hour. The drug is given in this way in order to prevent nausea and vomiting. Two hours later the patient is given another purge of magnesium sulphate. There is little to recommend the common practice of looking in the stool for the head of the worm, which is an extremely unpleasant procedure and which in any case does not ensure that another worm has not been left behind. The patients should instead be asked to report for another course of treatment if the segments reappear in their stools.

Niclosamide 2 g in a single dose or dichlorophen 6 g on two successive days may be used for the expulsion of tapeworms. Using these drugs no starvation or purgation are necessary. The theoretical risk of autoinfection of the host with *T. solium* infections is not borne out by practical experience. Patients should be re-examined 3 months after treatment and if no further segments are passed a cure can be presumed.

Hookworms. Ancylostoma duodenale infestation is common in the Middle and Far East and Europe. *Necator americanus* is found in the New World and tropical Africa. Heavy infestation causes significant bleeding and leads to chronic iron deficiency anaemia. The object of treatment is to reduce the load of infestation rather than to eliminate the worm completely. This is conveniently done with bephenium hydroxynaphthoate 5 g in a single dose. Some clinicians would advise that this can be given twice after a single dose of tetrachlorethylene (0.1 ml/kg) given on an empty stomach. Pyrantel pamoate (single dose 10 mg/kg body weight) is also effective. In patients with anaemia oral iron should be given, and folic acid if there is evidence of malabsorption.

Crohn's disease

Crohn's disease affects predominantly the terminal small intestine but may involve any section of the gastrointestinal tract from mouth to anus. Crohn's colitis is becoming increasingly recognised and its treatment will be considered in the section dealing with colitis. In its usual form in the small intestine, the disease is a protracted one with relapses and remissions. Both medical measures and surgical intervention are valuable in its management, so close co-operation is necessary between physician and surgeon. There is a form of acute localised small intestinal Crohn's disease, often indistinguishable from acute appendicitis, which has a good prognosis. In one series 70% of patients had no recurrence after 5 years.
Medical measures. During acute exacerbations of the disease with pain, diarrhea, steatorrhea, fever and weight loss, patients will require admission to hospital. Bed rest is beneficial during these phases of the disease. Diarrhea should be controlled with codeine phosphate or Lomotil (diphenoxylate hydrochloride and atropine sulphate). Cholestyramine is occasionally effective in stopping diarrhea due to the cathartic effect of unabsorbed bile acids on the colon. Patients are commonly anaemic due to gastrointestinal bleeding and this should be corrected by parenteral iron or, if necessary, blood transfusion. Other deficiencies may be present because of malabsorption. Vitamin B_{12} deficiency occurs when there is a considerable involvement of the ileum and should be treated by monthly injections of 500 μg of this vitamin. Hypoproteinaemia is due to loss of protein from the gut and requires a high protein diet. Weight loss may be helped by a diet containing medium chain triglycerides (MCT) rather than ordinary fats. MCT are more readily absorbed by diseased mucosa. MCT are obtained as an oil which may be used instead of fat for cooking and preparing food. A dietician's advice is required.

Corticosteroids are valuable in suppressing the inflammatory features of the disease. Prednisone should be given in doses of 45 mg/day for 2 weeks and then slowly reduced to a maintenance dose of 10–20 mg/day. They are particularly valuable in acute types of the disease when large portions of the small intestine are involved. There is some evidence that prednisone given on alternate days is as effective and avoids undesirable side effects. Some physicians prefer Inj ACTH (20 units/day for 2 weeks) for inpatients at the onset of treatment. Azathioprine (2 mg/kg/day) has been successfully used to induce remission in Crohn's disease. There is not adequate controlled data to assess its role in the management of this condition and it should only be used with caution under expert supervision. Antibiotics do not usually help patients with Crohn's disease, but they are occasionally dramatically successful if the small intestine is infected through fistula formation or blind loops. Tetracycline 250 mg four times daily for 10 days is recommended.
Surgical measures. Surgery is required if there is intestinal obstruction or fistulae small intestine and large bowel or bladder. It is also useful in patients with chronic illness, pain or debility due to a localised mass. Surgery may also be required for perianal abscess and anal fistula which commonly occur in this disorder. There is a high rate of recurrence (50–90%) after surgery. The current trend is to resect the main segment of diseased gut but to be as conservative as possible. By-pass operations are felt, at present, to be less satisfactory. After surgery some believe there is a good case for putting the patient on long term steroids (prednisone 15 mg/day) as there is some evidence that this may reduce the recurrence rate.

There are many therapeutic possibilities for patients with Crohn's disease and it is uncommon not to be able to improve them even in the face of severe relapse.

LARGE BOWEL

Proctitis

This is inflammation of the rectal mucosa without involvement of the colon. It may be caused by gonococcal infection in which case it will require treatment with a single injection of 300 000 u of procaine penicillin, kanamycin or co-trimoxazole—see p. 71. Lymphogranuloma venereum causes proctitis that is usually associated with rectal stricture, fistula formation and inguinal lymphadenopathy. Tetracycline (2.0 g daily for at least 10 days) may prevent stricture formation in the early stages of this disease.

Non-specific proctitis is a condition analogous to ulcerative colitis but confined to the rectal mucosa. This is the commonest form of proctitis in the UK. Although a proportion of patients ultimately develop true ulcerative colitis, in many the disease remains localised to the rectum and in some it becomes quiescent after appropriate treatment. The symptoms of tenesmus and discharge of blood and mucus can often be considerably improved by the use of prednisolone (5 mg) suppositories. These should be given morning and night for 3 months and, if the symptoms are controlled and sigmoidoscopic appearance improved at the end of this, the frequency of administration should be gradually reduced over the succeeding 3 months. If the symptoms persist or become worse, ulcerative colitis should be suspected.

Ulcerative colitis

Patients with ulcerative colitis require the help and understanding of a sympathetic physician. Some physicians claim dramatic cures by unravelling the psychological background of the patients, but most rely on drugs. Tenesmus and frequent rectal discharge can often be improved by prednisolone suppositories twice daily which are worth trying initially. Even in its mild form the disease usually requires more energetic measures and it is advisable to admit the patient to hospital for a period of bed rest and assessment. Total withdrawal of milk and milk products is occassionally successful even in severe attacks. Persistent diarrhea is an indication for prednisolone retention enemeta (20 mg prednisolone in 100 ml isotonic buffered solution), and while the patient is in hospital he can be taught to administer these himself. They should be given twice daily while in hospital but once the patient has been discharged it is preferable, if possible, for him to have them only at night just before retiring to bed. After instillation he should lie in bed for half an hour and should be encouraged to retain the enema for as long as possible. Sulphasalazine has been shown to reduce the incidence of relapse once a remission has been induced. It has no place in the treatment of the acute episode which can be better controlled by systemic steroids (see below). There is a good case for giving sulphasalazine (1.0 g twice daily for 1 year), after a remission has been induced. Most patients can tolerate this dose but those that develop nausea and vomiting should be given 0.5 g twice daily.

So far only mild attacks of ulcerative colitis have been considered. Patients may present initially with a severe 'fulminating' attack, or at any time a patient with a mild form may have a severe attack. These attacks require much more energetic measures for the patients are severely ill, dehydrated, anaemic and toxic. General measures include correction of fluid balance, administration of electrolytes—particularly potassium—and blood transfusion. Local corticosteroids in the form of prednisolone enemata may be tried. It is these patients that usually require systemic steroids. If the patient is having intravenous therapy hydrocortisone hemisuccinate sodium 200–300 mg/day can be given in the drip. Otherwise oral prednisone (60 mg/day) can be used. Some physicians believe that a remission is more likely to be induced if ACTH is used and they recommend an initial dose of 80 u day. There are some data to indicate that this clinical impression is valid. Immunosuppressives have been used with apparent success and are at present under trial. At present their use should be confined to centres where their effectiveness can be properly evaluated. If the patient is severely ill an intravenous broad spectrum antibiotic such as ampicillin can be given after blood cultures have been taken. It is best to avoid oral antibiotics such as sulphonamides and tetracycline as these can provoke colitis. Anaemia is, in acute attacks, best treated by blood transfusion and body iron stores can be subsequently replenished by a course of parenteral iron. Lomotil (diphenoxylate hydrochloride and atropine sulphate) and codeine phosphate are usually useless in controlling the diarrhea of severe attacks.

Surgical Measures. Total proctocolectomy and ileostomy cures ulcerative colitis. It is however a major surgical procedure with a significant mortality. It also leaves the patient with an ileostomy. The Ileostomy Society of Great Britain and Ireland (The Drive, Fuzzy Drive, Kempshot, Basingstoke, Hants.), advises such patients. The few patients who have the rectum spared of disease can be treated with total colectomy and ileorectal anastomosis. There is a tendency to advise early surgery as an elective procedure as the prognosis is worse in acute attacks and in patients over the age of sixty. Definite indications for surgery include:

(a) Toxic megacolon and failure to induce a remission in an acute fulminating episode of ulcerative colitis.

(b) Persistent illness and debility in patients with the chronic form of the disease.

(c) Risk of carcinoma occurring in a colitic colon. If there is total involvement of the colon with the disease in a young patient who started with an acute attack, and if the patient has had the condition for 10 years there are strong grounds for recommending proctocolectomy because of the high risk of carcinoma.

Diverticular disease

Diverticular disease is a condition of disordered motility due to inadequate bulk in the stool. Patients with uncomplicated diverticular disease (diverticulosis) have abdominal discomfort and altered bowel habits. The nature of the condition should be explained to them and they should be advised to keep their bowel actions regular by means of bran or similar bulk forming foods. They should take enough bran to keep their stools to the consistency of toothpaste. Remarkable symptomatic improvement commonly occurs as a result of this simple regime. Medicament such as methyl cellulose or sterculia, 1 teaspoonful daily, may also be required. The amount of these substances should be increased until the patients are having daily actions. Acute episodes of constipation can be treated wth standardized senna extract, or dioctyl sodium sulphosuccinate. Stronger purgatives, colonic lavage and enemata are dangerous and should not be used. Low residue diet has no place in the management of the condition and these patients should be advised to avoid medicaments containing codeine. *Diverticulitis.* Diverticulitis causes persistent left iliac fossa pain, tenderness, fever and malaise. It may progress to pericolic abscess. The patient should be treated in hospital. Initially no solid food should be allowed and fluids given orally, or intravenously. A broad spectrum antibiotic such as tetracycline is given by mouth, or if there is vomiting, intravenously. Pethidine, but not morphia, should be used to relieve the pain. Most cases of diverticulitis will respond to this regime and once the episode has subsided the patient should be advised to adhere to the medical regime described for diverticulosis. If the symptoms persist or become recurrent an operation may be necessary. Most surgeons advise resection but recently sigmoid myotomy has been used with apparent success. Vesicocolic fistula is not uncommon in this condition and requires surgical treatment.

Chronic constipation

In a recent survey of bowel habit in a healthy population 98% of 1500 people had between 3 bowel actions per day and 3 bowel actions per week. On this evidence the authors suggested that, in terms of frequency constipation be defined as less than 3 bowel actions per week.

Although, according to these criteria, only 1% of subjects were constipated 20% took laxatives. It is clear that in healthy individuals there is considerable variations in the frequency of bowel action, and as long as an individual is having regular actions it is of no importance that he is having them only 3 or 4 times a week. The sensible management of ambulant healthy individuals who have occasional episodes of constipation is to increase the bulk of the stool by adding bran to the diet. Aperients may be required for 1–2 weeks only.

The old, infirm and bedridden are a considerable problem in regard to constipation and in them more energetic measures are required. In this group, in addition to bran and medicaments that increase the bulk of the stool, aperients may be required. Senokot (standardised senna extract) can be given regularly in order to prevent severe constipation and faecal impaction. Senokot granules (1–2 teaspoonsfuls every night) are recommended.

LIVER

Infective hepatitis

This is usually a mild illness from which the patient makes a spontaneous and complete recovery within a few weeks. During the prodromal phase anorexia and fever occur before the patient is noticeably jaundiced, and hepatitis may not be suspected. During this phase the patient should be kept in bed and antipyretics should be used. There is some evidence that excessive physical exertion at the onset of the illness may cause fulminating hepatitis, so patients should be discouraged from taking strenuous exercise in order to 'work off' their symptoms. It is also a mistake to drink alcohol during the prodromal phase of hepatitis, but, as most patients lose their taste for alcohol early in the illness, this is not usually a clinical problem. Once the jaundice appears the patient often begins to feel better. He should be kept in bed while he is feeling ill and has a fever. The jaundice may take a few weeks to go and during this time he can be up and about, but he should not return to work until it has gone. If available, liver function tests will influence the management, and persistently abnormal biochemistry will result in a more cautious attitude. Once the patient has recovered he should be advised to avoid alcohol for 6 months. γ-Globulin or human normal immunoglobulin (HNI) protects effectively against virus A (infective) hepatitis for about 6 months. It should be offered to high risk contacts of cases of infective hepatitis. Whether HNI protects against virus B (serum or Australia antigen positive) hepatitis is at present uncertain.

A typical case of infective hepatitis occurring in a local epidemic is not difficult to diagnose correctly. It is important in any patient with jaundice to consider the differential diagnoses such as:

serum hepatitis (Hepatitis B antigen positive, hypodermic needles, tattooing, blood trans-fusions),

drug induced hepatitis (monoamine oxidase in-hibitors, halothane, chlorpromazine, anabolic steroids, oral contraceptives),

Gilbert's disease (recurrent jaundice without bile in the urine and with normal liver function tests),

ascending cholangitis (usually older patients with abdominal pain and fever),

cirrhosis,

alcoholic hepatitis and

chronic active hepatitis.

Most cases of jaundice can be diagnosed by the history, clinical examination and liver function tests but a few cases will require admission to hospital for further investigation.

Acute liver failure

This is usually the result of infective hepatitis, the majority of cases being Australia antigen negative. Other causes include overdose with paracetamol, amino oxidase inhibitors and halothane anaesthesia. It carries a poor prognosis and in cases in which jaundice is progressive the condition is best treated at centres with a special interest in the subject. Treatments include the standard measures for portal systemic encephalo-pathy (see below), heparin to prevent intravas-cular coagulation, and corticosteroids. Patients should be admitted to hospital immediately where the treatment for hepatic failure will be instituted. Exchange transfusion is successful in getting some of these patients out of coma, and in some centres is thought to be the treatment of choice for this condition. The view is not universally held and it is doubtful if exchange transfusion is justified, for it is expensive in terms of blood and has not been proved to be of value. Pro-cedures such as perfusing the patient's blood through a recently removed pig's liver can also improve the patient, but it has no effect on the progress of the hepatitis within the liver. Liver transplant has a place in selected cases.

Active chronic hepatitis ('lupoid' hepatitis)

This condition often starts with an illness indis-tinguishable from infective hepatitis. However the illness persists, liver function tests remain abnormal, and the patient has recurrent bouts of jaundice and ill health. Further investigations show that the immunoglobulins are disturbed, LE cells may be found in the blood. Some of these patients appear to go through an active phase of active chronic hepatitis and then make a clinically satisfactory recovery. Others have intermittent jaundice and ill health over months or years. Other organs may be involved during this illness including the joints and lungs. Liver biopsy is useful in the management of this con-dition and the histological appearance of chronic aggressive hepatitis is an indication to use corti-costeroids. Prednisone 10–15 mg/day improves the patients symptomatically and also the prognosis, at least in the succeeding 4 years. Azathioprine (1–2 mg/kg body weight) has been used in addition to corticosteroids without proven benefit. Present evidence suggests that low dose cortico-steroids is indicated for chronic aggressive hepatitis and that it should be continued until all evidence of activity of the disease has dis-appeared.

Primary biliary cirrhosis

This is a condition that occurs in middle-aged women and is another form of diffuse hepatic disorder with an autoimmune background. An important clinical feature of this condition is itching due to failure of the liver to excrete bile salts. Jaundice is often mild or absent at the onset. The itching can be considerably improved in these patients with cholestyramine hydroch-loride 1 g four times daily which prevents the re-absorption of bile salts from the gut. Steatorrhea occurs with failure to absorb vitamin A and vitamin D. This may lead to osteomalacia. Patients should therefore have monthly injections of 100 000 u vitamin D and 10 mg vitamin K. Oral calcium (Calcium Sandoz) 6 tablets per day should also be given. Corticosteroids do not stop the pro-gression of the disease. Azathioprine may help and is under trial. The disease tends to be progressive ending in cirrhosis and requiring treatment for the complications of that condition.

Cirrhosis

Treating the cause. In most patients with cirrhosis the pathological changes in the liver are irrevers-ible. However, in cirrhosis due to alcoholism and in haemochromatosis some improvement within the liver can be expected from appropriate treat-ment. Treatment of alcoholism is perhaps the most effective step in the management of the patient with alcoholic cirrhosis. The problems in stopping the individual drinking are considerable but, if the patient does stop, the prognosis is improved. Haemochromatosis is a rare cause of cirrhosis and one that is not uncommonly associated with alcoholism. Reduction of total body iron by repeated bleeding has been shown to reverse the cirrhotic process within the liver. In Wilson's disease (hepatolenticular degeneration) cirrhosis is due to copper overload. Methods of reducing body copper stores are successful. *Haematemesis and melaena.* Esophageal varices are an important cause of acute gastrointestinal bleeding associated with cirrhosis. However varices are by no means the only cause of bleeding in cirrhotic patients, particularly in the alcoholics. Chronic peptic ulcers are not uncommon in these patients, and multiple gastric erosions also occur. It is important to diagnose in each patient the precise cause of the bleeding as this will affect the management of the case.

Prophylactic porta-caval anastomosis reduces the incidence of death from bleeding varices. Patients need to be carefully selected for this procedure, for those with poor hepatic function develop portal systemic encephalopathy and hepatic failure. The group that appear to do best after prophylactic porta-caval shunt are young patients that have cryptogenic (post hepatitis) cirrhosis and good hepatic function, as assessed by liver function tests and serum albumin level. It is doubtful if the overall prognosis is improved.

The initial treatment of active bleeding varices should be blood replacement and pitressin. The latter is given intravenously in a dose of 20 u in 100 ml normal saline in 10 minutes. Side effects are pallor, abdominal colic and bowel evacuation. Pitressin reduces splanchnic and hepatic blood flow and thus allows the bleeding sites in the varix to become occluded. Local perfusion of pitressin into the superior mesenteric artery has been used to control bleeding. Unfortunately rebleeding is not uncommon. Esophageal tamponade using a Sengstaken tube is a cumbersome and dangerous procedure which should not be used except by experienced physicians. Its only place would now appear to be in halting catastrophic haemorrhage while preparing for emergency surgery. Emergency surgery should be advised if the patient rebleeds, particularly if there is an experienced surgeon available. Apart from dealing with varices and portal hypertension the surgeon is able to deal with bleeding from an undiagnosed chronic peptic ulcer or erosion. *Portal systemic encephalopathy (PSE).* Hepatic precoma occurs when ammonia and amines ab-

sorbed from the gut have not been adequately detoxicated by the liver. These substances reach the brain and cause clouding of consciousness, neurological defects and coma. Failure of detoxication occurs both because of liver cell failure and because the absorbed materials from the gut are shunted past the liver via varices or portacaval anastomoses. Hepatic precoma is particularly likely to occur after a gastrointestinal bleed when there is protein in the gut, if the patient is constipated, has intercurrent infection, or electrolyte disturbance. There are four measures that reverse this process:

1. Removal of protein from the gut lumen by enemata and aperients.
2. Neomycin 1 g four times daily (to reduce bacteria which break down the proteins).
3. Reduce protein intake by placing the patient on a restricted protein diet.
4. Lactulose has been introduced for the treatment of PSE. This substance is metabolised by bacteria and converted to lactic acid which is thought to trap ammonia in the large bowel and remove it in the stools. It appears to be a useful measure in the management. The initial dose is 25–50 ml syrup three times daily which can be increased to 150 ml or more per day.

Edema and ascites. Ascites in cirrhosis is usually due to a combination of raised intra-hepatic pressure and reduced serum albumin in the blood. It is generally a mistake to treat it by paracentesis which will remove a large quantity of protein from the body. Rapid paracentesis can induce acute hepatic failure and should always be avoided. The patient should be treated by sodium restriction, diuretics and potassium chloride. Spironolactone 25 mg q.d.s. is of particular value. A double ended porta-caval shunt in which both ends of the cut portal vein are anastomosed to the inferior vena cava, has been used in an attempt to reduce the intra-hepatic pressure. Although it is often successful in reducing ascites the patient may be made worse because of portal systemic encephalopathy. Once edema and electrolyte disturbances, and renal failure develop in decompensated cirrhosis the prognosis is grave.

Amoebic hepatitis and amoebic abscess

Chloroquine is concentrated 500 times by the liver and is the drug of first choice for hepatic amoebiasis. It is usual to give 1 g by mouth daily for 2 days followed by 0.5 g daily for 19 days. If after 4 days there is no clinical improvement emetine hydrochloride, which is also concentrated in the liver, should be given. It is given by subcutaneous injection 60 mg daily for 10 days. Needle aspiration may be required to hasten resolution if an abscess is present, and open drainage may be required if there is secondary infection. Metronidazole 400 mg three times daily for 5 days has resulted in 90% cure rate without drainage. Twice this dose of metronidazole is required for amoebic dysentery.

GALL BLADDER

Biliary colic

The pain of biliary colic is sufficiently severe to require potent analgesics. Morphia and pethidine are effective but both have the theoretical disadvantage that they cause spasm of smooth muscle. It is doubtful if this is relevant in relation to the disturbed motility of the duct caused by impaction of a biliary stone. Antispasmodics such as atropine (0.5 mg) or propantheline (15 mg) may be given 20 minutes before morphia or pethidine in order to prevent spasm. The new analgesics phenazocine and pentazocine are said not to affect smooth muscle and may be drugs of choice for biliary colic. Cholecystectomy is still the treatment of choice for removal of gall stone. Gall stone dissolution with chenodeoxycholic acid has been achieved and is under investigation at a few centres.

Acute cholecystitis

Acute cholecystitis is usually treated conservatively initially but early in the course of the disease it is possible to perform acute cholecystectomy. Some surgeons prefer to manage the condition by immediate cholecystectomy. The orthodox management is to treat the patient with bed rest, fluids, restricted diet and antibiotics. Tetracycline, ampicillin or sulphadimidine may be used and are usually effective. Once the attack has subsided the patient should have biliary tract radiology followed by elective cholecystectomy 2–3 months later.

Ascending cholangitis

In ascending cholangitis there is recurring fever (Charcot's intermittent fever), rigors, jaundice, abdominal pain and leucocytosis. There are three main causes: gall stone impacted in the common bile duct, stricture of the common bile duct and following surgical implantation of common bile duct into the upper small intestine. If the cause is a stone or stricture, symptoms will continue until the obstruction has been corrected surgically. The object of medical treatment of these patients should be to get them in as good condition as possible for surgery. The offending organism may be isolated by blood culture and the patient should then be given antibiotics. Patients who have had biliary tract surgery with reimplantation of the common bile duct (such as those who have had radical surgery for carcinoma of ampulla of Vater), may have recurrent attacks of ascending cholangitis which will require repeated courses of antibiotics. It is always worth performing an intravenous or percutaneous transhepatic cholangiogram to see if a stricture is present. This should be removed surgically. If the cause cannot be corrected surgically prophylactic antibiotics may be used in order to prevent organisms from invading the common bile duct.

HICCOUGH

Hiccough is spasmodic contraction of the diaphragm with simultaneous contracture of the glottis. It is commonly due to irritation of the stomach by alcohol, over-eating, and highly spiced foods. Simple measures such as holding the breath, pulling the tongue, inducing sneezing by tickling the nose, sodium bicarbonate (0.6–1.2 g in water) or a carminative or 'gripe water' relieve most cases. Persistent hiccough is usually due to diaphragm irritation from peritonitis, paralytic ileus, subphrenic abscess, intra-hepatic abscess, cholangitis and pancreatitis. It also occurs in uraemia and encephalitis. Occasionally hiccough lasting a few days occurs for no obvious cause and epidemics of hiccough have been described. If hiccough is due to paralytic ileus gastric intubation may relieve it by releasing gas from the descended stomach. In other cases, treatment of the cause (i.e. uraemia, subphrenic abscess), will stop the spasms. Injections of hyoscine, chlorpromazine or morphia will relieve hiccough in some cases. If it persists and the patient is becoming exhausted he should be admitted to hospital. Crushing one or both phrenic nerves and causing temporary diaphragmatic paralysis may be required in severe cases.

PANCREAS

Acute pancreatitis

This condition usually presents as an acute abdominal emergency with severe pain, paralytic ileus and shock. Occasionally patients present without pain but with severe shock. Diagnosis can be difficult and may only be made at laparotomy. Once the diagnosis has been firmly established most clinicians manage the condition conservatively.

Pain. Pain is severe and requires potent analgesics. Morphia causes spasm of the sphincter of Oddi and is best avoided. Pethidine is therefore probably the analgesic of choice and some recommend that atropine be given with it.

Paralytic ileus. Many of these patients have some degree of paralytic ileus and it is therefore advisable to institute gastric suction. The removal of gastric acid may also inhibit a stimulus to pancreatic secretion.

Shock. During the acute phase the blood pressure may fall and this requires urgent treatment with intravenous blood and plasma. Intravenous electrolytes are needed to replace loss of intravascular fluids into the tissues. Released vasodepressive substances (i.e. kinins) may cause the low blood pressure and if hypotension persists intravenous steroids in large doses may be used. Intravenous vasopressor drugs may be used to raise the blood pressure.

Hypocalcaemia. Hypocalcaemia is a feature of acute pancreatitis and may, on occasion, cause tetany. It is due to breakdown of fat by released pancreatic lipase and the subsequent formation of calcium soaps. If the serum calcium falls or tetany occurs intravenous calcium gluconate (20 ml of 10%) should be given.

Antibiotics. Antibiotics do not influence the initial course of acute pancreatitis but should be used in an attempt to prevent the formation of abscess in the necrotic gland. Tetracycline or ampicillin should be given by mouth or intravenously.

Other measures. In severe cases other techniques have been claimed to be useful. Trasylol (a kallikrein inhibitor) has had enthusiastic supporters, but there is little evidence that it affects the outcome of acute pancreatitis in man, despite its efficiency in experimental pancreatitis in the dog. Trasylol is not recommended for this condition. Removal of pancreatic enzymes by peritoneal dialysis is worth considering. It is not advisable to use this technique unless experience and facilities are available. Total pancreatectomy has been successfully used for fulminant pancreatitis but this should only be considered if an experienced surgeon is available for the operative risks are considerable. After the initial episode the patient may develop a pancreatic abscess or pancreatic pseudocyst. This will require drainage or appropriate surgical treatment.

Relapsing pancreatitis

Relapsing pancreatitis may be caused by chronic alcoholism. Some cases are associated with gall stones. The most distressing feature of this condition is the recurring episodes of severe epigastric pain. The bizarre features of the pain may make the diagnosis difficult. The simplest investigation is a straight X-ray of the abdomen, which may reveal pancreatic calcification. Secretin tests of pancreatic function are required to unravel the more difficult cases. All cases require biliary tract radiology.

Once the diagnosis has been made the essence of management is to relieve the pain. Pancreatic surgery for relapsing painful pancreatitis is difficult and requires considerable experience. Many surgical manoeuvres have been recommended, the simplest being sphincterotomy. Some surgeons recommend localisation of the area of pancreatitis by pancreatic duct radiology at the time of surgery. They then relate the operative procedure to the radiological findings. Pancreatic drainage with removal of stones from the pancreatic duct, partial and total pancreatectomy are used to treat this condition.

Pancreatic insufficiency

Pancreatic failure may result from one attack of acute pancreatitis, or may be the end stage of recurring attacks of pancreatitis. Occasionally it develops with no preceding history of pancreatitis. Rarely it occurs in association with hyperparathyroidism, and a familial form of the condition has been described. Atrophy of the pancreas may also cause pancreatic failure, and this has been seen in severe long standing cases of celiac syndrome. In pancreatic failure both exogenous and the endogenous secretions of the pancreas are not produced and patients develop both steatorrhea and diabetes mellitus.

Pancreatic steatorrhea. The amount of fat in the stools of patients with pancreatic steatorrhea is very high—being usually more than 20 g/24 hours. The patients therefore commonly complain of diarrhea. They may notice that they pass oil in the stools. This may be noticed as an 'oil slick' floating on the surface of the water. The excretion of this large amount of fat leads to weight loss despite a good or even increased appetite. In addition to fat, the stools may have a high nitrogen content. The diarrhea and fattiness of the stools can be notably improved by placing the patient on a low fat diet. In addition the diet should be rich in protein. Pancreatic extract, such as pancreatin, can be used but it is often disappointing. It should be given with meals. A new formulation extract that has an enteric coated core of pancreatic extract and a shell of bromelains has been shown to improve fat absorption. In severe cases of pancreatic steatorrhea medium chain triglyceride (MCT) should be used instead of fat in the patient's diet. In pancreatic steatorrhea the absorption of other dietary constituents is normal and it is uncommon for these patients to develop anaemia, osteomalacia or bleeding disorders.

Pancreatic diabetes mellitus. This occurs in pancreatic insufficiency due to both pancreatitis and pancreatic atrophy. It also occurs in haemo-chromatosis. It requires insulin and diabetic control is usually not difficult.

Fibrocystic disease

This condition affects children and leads to pancreatic steatorrhea and recurrent chest infections. The principles of treating the steatorrhea are as outlined above. These children also require antibiotics for the respiratory disease.

2

RENAL DISEASE

N.F. JONES and A.J. WING

INTRODUCTION

The chapter begins with four main sections dealing with the management of the major syndromes arising in renal disease; the acute nephritic syndrome, the nephrotic syndrome, and acute and chronic renal failure. It is not possible to consider the management of renal failure without placing this in the context of dialysis as a temporary or permanent replacement of renal function, but the techniques of haemodialysis are beyond the scope of this book. Peritoneal dialysis may have to be carried out in any hospital and an outline of the technique is therefore included.

It is hoped that the fearful economic implications of providing facilities for treating terminal irreversible renal failure will stimulate a better understanding of the pathogenesis of renal diseases and eventually result in more specific and effective therapy to prevent their progression. Such measures as are at present available, are herein described.

THE MANAGEMENT OF THE ACUTE NEPHRITIC SYNDROME (ACUTE NEPHRITIS)

In its fully developed form this is an acute illness with edema, raised jugular venous pressure, haematuria, proteinuria, oliguria and often hypertension. Severe cases may be complicated by acute renal failure. There may be evidence of antecedent streptococcal infection. This syndrome may also occur in certain other diseases having in common inflammatory lesions of small blood vessels, e.g. polyarteritis nodosa, anaphylactoid (Henoch–Schonlein) purpura or systemic lupus erythematosus. These possibilities must be considered in the management of any patient with this syndrome.

General management

Treatment of any antecedent infection. A swab should be taken from the throat or any other possible site of infection. The serum antistreptolysin O (ASO) titre should also be determined. In practice many cases referred to hospital with acute nephritis have already received an antibiotic, thus reducing the chances of bacterial identification and decreasing the incidence of elevated ASO titres after streptococcal infections. It has been customary to prescribe long term oral penicillin therapy for any patient with acute nephritis in whom there is evidence or suspicion of precipitating streptococcal infection. There is, however, no proof that such long term therapy influences the course of the renal disease and it may reasonably be stopped after evidence of renal involvement has disappeared.

Bed rest. The patient should be confined to bed while edema, elevation of the jugular venous pressure, hypertension, oliguria or macroscopic haematuria persist. Microscopic haematuria may persist for many weeks and proteinuria of less than 1 g/day for many months. There is no good reason for keeping the patient in bed until these features disappear. If haematuria or proteinuria increase markedly when the patient gets up, some physicians would advise further bed rest.

Diet. Salt restriction is indicated while the jugular venous pressure remains elevated and edema or hypertension persist. The sodium intake for an adult should be less than 25 mEq/day if edema is considerable. When the patient is oliguric (urine volume less than 400 ml/day), fluid intake should not exceed 500 ml/day plus the volume of urine passed on the previous day. The adequacy of fluid restriction should be monitored by weighing the patient daily.

Protein restriction is only indicated for azotaemic patients.

Diuretics. When fluid retention is troublesome a diuretic should be given. Large doses of the more powerful diuretics, such as frusemide, may be needed to produce a satisfactory diuresis.

Management of complications

Severe hypertension. Intravenous diazoxide is a suitable drug for urgent treatment; 100 mg is given rapidly intravenously and if the resultant fall in blood pressure over the next 10 minutes or so is inadequate a further intravenous dose of 300 mg should be given. Reserpine (2.5–5.0 mg i.m.) is useful for less severe cases. Minoxidil is proving valuable in hypertension associated with severe renal disease but is not yet generally available in England. Even in the absence of symptoms antihypertensive treatment should be started if the diastolic blood pressure rises to 105–110 mmHg as serious further rises in pressure may then occur over a few hours. Alpha methyl dopa by mouth is a suitable drug for this situation.

Encephalopathy. If clouding of consciousness, focal neurological signs or fits occur, careful attention should be paid to control of hypertension and phenytoin sodium (100 mg b.d. i.m.) given. For fits or marked restlessness intravenous diazepam (2–10 mg given slowly), intravenous sodium amylobarbitone or intramuscular paraldehyde may be used.

Acute pulmonary edema. Rarely, this may require emergency treatment by venesection before dialysis can be arranged. I.v. frusemide should be given and up to 200–500 mg may be necessary. Such large doses should be given slowly. In this situation hypertension is usually severe and parenteral diazoxide may be used to control it.

Acute renal failure. When this complicates acute nephritis, it is treated as described below.

THE MANAGEMENT OF THE NEPHROTIC SYNDROME

Use of renal biopsy

Knowledge of the underlying renal lesion is necessary for correct management of the nephrotic syndrome, and a renal biopsy should be performed in any adult in whom this syndrome develops idiopathically. Renal biopsy is usually unnecessary when the nephrotic syndrome develops in a patient with long standing diabetes, established amyloidosis, or other disease likely to cause heavy proteinuria. In children the greater incidence of minimal change glomerular histology ('foot process' lesion only) which usually produces proteinuria that is highly selective, reduces the need for renal biopsy. In a child under 5 years with highly selective proteinuria it is reasonable to institute steroid therapy without renal biopsy.

Dietary and drug therapy

Treatment is aimed at ridding the patient of edema and abolishing proteinuria.

Diet. When the blood urea is normal a high protein intake of at least 2–3 g/kg bodyweight should be encouraged. This may enable a patient with prolonged heavy proteinuria to achieve positive nitrogen balance. Modern diuretic therapy usually dispels edema without strict restriction of sodium intake, but moderate salt restriction is sensible while edema persists and strict salt restriction (10–20 mEq/day) is occasionally needed when edema is resistant to therapy.

Diuretics. Mersalyl should no longer be used in the nephrotic syndrome. The thiazide diuretics, e.g. bendrofluazide 5–15 mg/day, are often effective and are cheap. Frusemide may succeed where the thiazides fail. In resistant cases large doses of frusemide, 500 mg or even more, may be needed. If the blood urea level is markedly elevated (above 100 mg/100 ml (16 mmol l^{-1}) ethacrynic acid is probably better avoided in view of the risk of deafness.

With all the above diuretics potassium supplements are usually needed, the risk of hypokalaemia during diuresis in the nephrotic syndrome being considerable, presumably due to the associated aldosteronism. In this context aldosterone antagonists, e.g. spironolactone 25 mg 4 times daily, have a role and are best used with one of the above diuretics. Triamterene and amiloride are also suitable diuretics, especially when hypokalaemia has developed, but are better avoided if the blood urea is raised and should not be used coincidently with spironolactone as dangerous hyperkalaemia may then occur. Metolazone may be effective even when resistance to other diuretics is considerable.

Albumin infusion. The intravenous infusion of salt-poor human serum albumin is expensive and its effect short-lived, the extra albumin being rapidly excreted by the kidney. Nonetheless it may occasionally permit diuretics to succeed where previously they had failed. Albumin, 1 g/kg bodyweight, is infused over several hours, a careful watch being kept on the jugular venous pressure, and the infusion slowed or stopped if the latter rises to 4 cm or more above the sternal angle.

Other plasma volume expanders, e.g. dextran, are less satisfactory but can be used in patients with diuretic resistant edema when albumin is not available. Dextran or albumin infusion is occasionally needed for the nephrotic patient with severe hypotension associated with hypovolaemia. This complication is uncommon spontaneously but may arise for instance in the patient who has been over enthusiastically treated with diuretics.

Corticosteroids. It is now generally accepted that

a trial of steroid therapy should be given to all patients with minimal glomerular changes on light microscopy ('foot process' lesion only on electron microscopy). Adult patients may respond initially only to large doses, e.g. prednisone 60 mg/day for 2–3 weeks. A smaller dose, e.g. 10–20 mg/day, may then be needed for 3–6 months to prevent or minimise proteinuria. In some patients the proteinuria returns whenever the steroid dose is reduced to this lower range. Long term steroid therapy using moderate doses, e.g. prednisone 20–40 mg/day for an adult, may then be successful but such doses carry correspondingly higher risks of serious complications. This problem is encountered most often in children and immunosuppressive drugs (see later) may prove of particular value in this group. Where steroid therapy is continued for many months or years an intermittent regime is recommended by some authorities, e.g. prednisone 20 mg/day for 4 consecutive days in each week, or on alternate days. There is however no unassailable evidence that such prolonged therapy with steroids, whether continuous or intermittent, improves the long term prognosis of patients with the minimal change lesion. The main use of steroid therapy lies in the short term treatment of those patients with 'minimal change' nephrotic syndrome who rapidly lose their proteinuria when given steroids. Such patients may not relapse for months or years and may then again respond rapidly to steroids. When relapses occur so often that steroid consumption becomes worrying immunosuppressive therapy should be considered even in the 'minimal change' group (see later).

Steroid therapy is unlikely to succeed when the nephrotic syndrome is due to membranous glomerulonephritis. It has been claimed that prolonged therapy with steroids in low doses, e.g. prednisone 10 mg/day, delays deterioration in renal function in patients with membranous glomerulonephritis but the evidence is not convincing.

When the nephrotic syndrome is caused by proliferative glomerulonephritis in adults steroid-induced remissions are uncommon, even when the proteinuria is highly selective. Some patients, especially children, do appear to benefit and a trial of steroid therapy is reasonable. There is no firm evidence that steroids affect the long term prognosis in this condition. Claims that patients with severe rapidly progressive proliferative glomerulonephritis benefit from 'cocktail' therapy with steroids, immunosuppressive drugs and anticoagulants are not substantiated.

When systemic lupus erythematosus is complicated by nephrotic syndrome steroids are usually given in high doses (see later). Steroids are not beneficial in the nephrotic syndrome associated with diabetes, amyloidosis, or renal vein thrombosis. It has been claimed that steroids may hasten the deterioration in renal function in amyloidosis and their use in this condition is best avoided.

Immunosuppressive drugs. The use of these agents in treatment of the nephrotic syndrome is based on evidence that the glomerular damage may be mediated by immunological mechanisms. There have been several reports claiming success with azathioprine or cyclophosphamide.

Encouraging results have been obtained with cyclophosphamide in children without glomerular abnormalities on light microscopy who responded to steroids initially but then either became resistant or needed an unacceptably high dose to control proteinuria. It is not yet clear whether cyclophosphamide is more effective if given in doses sufficient to cause leucopenia, or whether it is advantageous to use prednisone in combination with it.

Within the limitations imposed by these uncertainties cyclophosphamide may be given in an initial dose of 3 mg/kg/day. In an edematous child the weight to use in this calculation is the predicted mean weight for the height. Blood counts are performed 2 or 3 times each week for the first 2 or 3 weeks and weekly thereafter. This dose does not always produce leucopenia and if after 4 weeks the white count is still normal and no renal response has occurred the dose may be increased to 4 mg/kg/day, reducing to 2 or 3 mg/kg/day when leucopenia develops. Cyclophosphamide is given for a total period of 2–4 months and then withdrawn. Alopecia is common in adults with this regime, but the hair often grows again when the drug is stopped. Other side effects include chemical cystitis, nausea, vomiting and infections but these are all uncommon. Thrombocytopenia and anaemia are also uncommon but careful haematological supervision is mandatory. Cyclophosphamide may also cause suppression of gonadal function.

Dialysis

Oliguric renal failure sometimes develops in a patient with the nephrotic syndrome. Hypovolaemia with renal circulatory insufficiency must then be considered and corrected if present by expansion of the plasma volume with albumin. If renal biopsy shows only minimal abnormalities steroid therapy is given and dialysis is performed as necessary, for such patients may not only recover from the renal failure, but may subsequently enter remission from the nephrotic syndrome. When renal biopsy shows membranous or proliferative glomerulonephritis oliguric renal failure carries a very bad prognosis. However, some patients may recover useful renal function and maintenance dialysis should be given in this hope.

THE MANAGEMENT OF ACUTE RENAL FAILURE (ARF)

The prevention of ARF

The occurrence of ARF can often be anticipated and possibly prevented if the wide variety of clinical contexts in which it may occur is appreciated.

Hypovolaemia and hypotension. In the patient who is at risk of developing ARF following battle or road traffic trauma, obstetric accidents or massive losses of fluid and electrolytes, the prompt replacement of blood and fluid loss is mandatory. Rapid replacement of intravascular volume and extracellular fluid is safer if the central venous pressure (CVP) is monitored. In the management of burns the importance of fluid and electrolyte replacement must be stressed.

Septicaemia. Infection with Gram negative organisms and septic abortions require urgent treatment with appropriate antibiotics, fluids and when necessary hydrocortisone and other therapy relevant to septicaemia.

Intravascular haemolysis. When this threatens to cause ARF low molecular weight dextran up to a maximum of 300 ml intravenously is advised.

Nephrotoxins. In any case of ARF the possibility of exposure to a nephrotoxic agent must be considered. Occasionally this may lead to the use of a specific antidote, e.g. BAL in mercury poisoning.

Urinary tract obstruction. Total anuria always suggests the possibility of urinary obstruction. Anuria alternating with polyuria and a history of renal colic are further pointers towards a postrenal cause of ARF. High dose infusion IVP and radioactive renography may be helpful investigations in this context. If obstruction is diagnosed nephrostomy may be required pending definitive surgery.

Use of mannitol, diuretics and other measures. There is probably some final common pathway in the pathophysiology of acute tubular necrosis (ATN), although it is not understood. Therefore, attempts to prevent the development of ATN by interrupting the sequence of events which follow the initial precipitating factor(s) have been empirical. Paravertebral block, decapsulation of the kidneys and steroid therapy are all useless and increase the risk to the patient. Over expansion

of the extracellular fluid space and the unrestrained 'pushing of fluids' in an attempt to 'force a diuresis' are also dangerous and ineffective.

Experimental and clinical studies indicate that the use of mannitol to induce an osmotic diuresis reduces the incidence of ARF in certain situations. Therefore, mannitol (12.5–50 g) is given prophylactically during cardiopulmonary bypass, operations on the abdominal aorta and surgery on jaundiced patients. There is less good evidence that mannitol is beneficial when given after the clinical insult has occurred. Nevertheless, since 50 ml of a 25% solution of mannitol given i.v. over 3–5 minutes appears to be innocuous in the absence of circulatory overload it is probably worth a trial if ARF has been diagnosed within a matter of hours of its onset. This dose may be repeated at 3-hourly intervals to a total of 50 g unless there is any evidence of pulmonary edema or water intoxication. For similar reasons frusemide may also be tried in a dose of at least 200 mg i.v.

The early use of these measures, together with correction of the precipitating factors, may prevent the development of oliguric renal failure. A word of caution is necessary as improvement in urine flow is not invariably accompanied by restitution of normal renal function.

The management of established ARF

During the oliguric phase, the risks are those of overdehydration, hyperkalaemia, uraemia, infection and those of the precipitating condition and its complications. Management therefore consists of appropriate monitoring of the patient, the institution of dietary and specific therapeutic measures, and, as early as possible, a decision as to whether or not to dialyse the patient.

If at all possible, the patient should be weighed daily, and weight should fall by 0.2–0.8 kg/day depending on the degree of catabolism occurring. The corrected baseline weight at the time of onset of ARF is that when all blood and fluid losses have been replaced so that the blood pressure and peripheral circulation are normal and when there is no rise in venous pressure or edema. Records of fluid and electrolyte balance must be kept. A low reading thermometer should be available. An ECG affords the quickest and most relevant information about the serum potassium level. Daily (or more frequent) electrolyte, blood urea and serum creatinine estimations help to follow the anticipated metabolic changes.

Superadded infections so often jeopardise the chances of survival in these patients that there will be few in whom bacteriological investigations are not required. Infection of the urinary tract is particularly hazardous and catheterisation should therefore be carried out only if essential (e.g. fractured pelvis) or to exclude obstruction. A wet bed or inaccurate fluid output figures are preferable to the risks of infection.

Emergency treatment of hyperkalaemia is indicated by advanced ECG changes (loss of P waves, spread of QRS complex) and consists of intravenous calcium gluconate (20 ml of 10% solution) to counteract the effects of the K^+ ion, followed by intravenous dextrose (100 ml of 50% solution) with insulin (10 units). Sodium bicarbonate (e.g. 100 ml of 8.4% solution equalling 100 mEq) may be given if acidosis is present and if the sodium load is acceptable. If management is less urgent, exchange resins, preferably in the calcium phase (calcium resonium either 15 g orally up to 3 times daily or 30–60 g as a retention enema) should be given.

It has been customary to prescribe a low protein (20 g) high calorie (2000 calories if possible) diet with restricted sodium intake (less than 25 mEq) and avoidance of all foods with a high potassium content. Supplementary vitamins should be given. Fluid intake is restricted to 300–500 ml plus any measured losses per day, subject to the overriding consideration of the weight change. However, the present tendency is for this regime to become more liberalised as the use of dialysis is extended and the risks of undernutrition are appreciated. Intravenous feeding with high concentration glucose, lipids and amino acids has its risks but may be invaluable for the severely traumatised patient and for others who cannot take food by mouth.

Conservative management of ARF will result in a successful outcome when the degree of catabolism is mild and the period of renal failure is a brief one, lasting for less than a week. In these cases, especially those following obstetric accidents, it is worthwhile administering an anabolic steroid; a single dose of nandrolone decanoate 50 mg i.m. lasts for 2 weeks. Conservative management should be carried out in collaboration with the team responsible for dialysis. In patients in whom the clinical context suggests that the rate of catabolism will be high dialysis is indicated. Once it has been decided that dialysis will be required it is best to commence this early, not waiting for some arbitrary biochemical indication. Any type of dialysis is not without risk and should be performed by a team regularly providing this service. Dialysis permits a liberalisation of the diet and fluid intake, the patient is kept fitter and not confined to bed. In severely catabolic cases and in some with abdominal injuries and surgery, haemodialysis is preferred; in the majority of patients peritoneal dialysis will suffice provided the period of ARF is not too prolonged.

Frequently treatment by dialysis will have to be started in order to 'buy time' for diagnostic investigations to be performed. A renal biopsy may also be indicated at this stage. After such investigation it may become apparent that some patients presenting as ARF are, in fact, suffering from CRD. In these patients and in others with acute cortical necrosis a decision will be required as to whether to embark on a programme of maintenance haemodialysis or transplantation.

When recovery is accompanied by a diuretic phase undue losses of water and electrolytes may occur, requiring replacement with sodium and/or potassium salts and careful attention to fluid balance. Glomerular filtration rate may lag behind the recovery of urine output and dialysis may still be necessary at the start of the diuretic phase.

During the course of ARF infections require prompt antibiotic therapy. It is important to remember that the dose regimes of many antibiotics need alteration in the presence of renal failure. The importance of adequate expert nursing for patients with ARF cannot be overemphasised.

THE MANAGEMENT OF CHRONIC RENAL FAILURE (CRF)

Making the most of existing renal function

This involves titrating dietary intake against the level of renal function which remains.

Fluid and electrolytes. Urea excretion normally increases with urine flow and advantage is sometimes gained by encouraging the patient to drink sufficient water to produce a daily urinary volume of 3 litres.

If a salt or water deficit develops in a patient with CRF due to vomiting, diarrhea, or inappropriate restriction of salt and water, renal perfusion is diminished with consequent reduction in GFR.* Patients should be weighed, their blood pressure measured supine and standing and the state of hydration assessed at each outpatient visit. The importance of such monitoring cannot be overemphasised since a salt and water deficit may result in a permanent decrement in renal function.

Regular doses of exchange resins preferably in the calcium phase are sometimes needed to control hyperkalaemia.

---

*Glomerular filtration rate.

Diet. Special diets, it must be emphasised, are palliative therapy and are only used to prevent hyperkalaemia, sodium overload and the gastrointestinal symptoms associated with uraemia. In practice, it is usually necessary to restrict protein intake when the blood urea exceeds 150 mg/100 ml (25 mmol l⁻¹) or at plasma creatinine levels greater than 7.0 mg/100 ml (600 μmol l⁻¹). The Giordano–Giovannetti diet and its modifications has impressively altered the symptomatology of CRF, removing the distressing gastrointestinal symptoms and permitting life to continue, to a lower level of renal function.

However, some authorities advise a rather higher protein intake (0.5 g/kg/day). Nitrogen balance can be maintained on very low intakes of nitrogen if essential amino acids are included in the diet. The calorie intake should be as high as possible; Hycal (Beecham) and Caloreen are useful additives. Vitamin supplements should be given to all patients and iron supplements may be necessary. Patients on the Giordano–Giovannetti regime should also receive methionine 0.5 g/day.

A programme of progressive reduction of protein intake in the face of worsening renal function requires planning in the light of the rate of progression of the renal disease, and of eventual plans for maintenance haemodialysis and renal grafting. The ability of the patient to maintain dietary discipline is reflected in a plasma urea : creatinine ratio of less than 20:1 (in mg/100 ml), although it must be appreciated that this ratio is increased by other factors, e.g. fever, steroid therapy.

Dialysis. Occasional peritoneal dialysis may be required when intercurrent infections or surgery increase the rate of catabolism. Some patients, notably those with polycystic disease, do surprisingly well with monthly or even less frequent dialyses.

Treating the complications of uraemia

Gastrointestinal symptoms. Nausea and vomiting may respond to diet alone or to a period of dialysis. Symptomatic relief can be obtained with thiethylperazine, chlorpromazine or metoclopramide. Phenothiazines can also be used for the treatment of hiccough. Diarrhea for which no other cause than uraemia can be found is of grave significance: dialysis is usually required.

Peptic ulceration is common in CRF. Antacids containing magnesium should be avoided and it will often not be possible to give those containing sodium.

Acidosis. No attempt need be made to raise the serum bicarbonate level with oral alkali, with the inevitable risk of sodium overload, unless the acidosis is symptomatic, i.e. causing dyspnea and mental symptoms. Sodium bicarbonate 3–9 g/day is effective if the patient can tolerate the sodium load; if not, calcium carbonate 6–10 g/day may be used.

Cardiovascular complications. Hypertension is considered later. If digoxin is used for cardiac failure, a reduced dose is necessary in the presence of renal failure. The effects of uraemia on myocardial function are cured by dialysis. A pericardial friction rub is common in the final stages of uraemia, not infrequently developing after dialysis has been commenced. There is no treatment other than dialysis.

Anaemia. Unless there has been blood loss and consequent iron deficiency the anaemia is unresponsive to all haematinics. Transfusion is rarely necessary, but is required to replace acute blood losses and sometimes in preparation for surgery. Because of the risks of producing cardiac failure, small transfusions of packed cells are best. The correction of the anaemia of CRF by transfusion is short-lived and may suppress the patient's marrow even further. It also carries the risk of transmitting the Hepatitis B antigen and thus diminishing the acceptability of the patient for future dialysis and transplantation. Experience with dialysed patients has made it clear that a quite marked anaemia (PCV of 15—20%) is borne without undue symptoms. Claims have been made that androgenic steroids may improve the anaemia of patients receiving regular dialysis but their value is disputed and they are not without side-effects. Cobalt salts have been used but are generally considered to be unacceptably hazardous.

Haemorrhagic complications. The haemorrhagic diathesis of uraemia has a complex basis and is only corrected by adequate dialysis. However, troublesome epistaxis may occur and the use of local cautery should not then be neglected.

Renal osteodystrophy. Recent advances in understanding the pathogenesis of the bone diseases of renal failure provide theoretical grounds for predicting that control of phosphate intake during the early stages and administration of 1,25-dihydroxycholecalciferol during the latter stages of a gradually progressive renal disease would diminish the severity of osteodystrophy. However, the former manoeuvre is not often practical and the latter is not yet available.

A recalcifying regimen is indicated when the bone disease is predominantly one of defective mineralisation, *viz.* osteomalacia or rickets. Recalcification is achieved either with vitamin D or by giving calcium salts as dietary supplements or by dialysis. Vitamin D (as calciferol 20 000–500 000 units/day) may dramatically heal the bone lesions of children and adolescents; in adults it should probably be reserved for those patients with bone pain or proximal myopathy. Vitamin D enhances the risks of vascular and other soft tissue calcification, and thus of exacerbating renal damage. The calcaemic effect of vitamin D may be delayed and the dose should not be increased more often than once per month. In adults a starting dose of 50 000–100 000 units/day is recommended. This should be doubled after a month if there is no clinical or biochemical improvement.

Dietary supplements of calcium as calcium carbonate with the addition of calcium phosphate when the plasma phosphate falls result in a positive balance of calcium and phosphate. 20 g of calcium carbonate in the morning together with 5.6 g of calcium phosphate in the evening has been recommended. This has less risk than vitamin D of causing calcification of the soft tissues.

The risks of metastatic calcification are diminished if the calcium $\times$ phosphate product (when both are measured in mg/100 ml) is maintained at less than 70 (5.5 when measured in mmol l^{-1}) by the administration of aluminium hydroxide gel B.P. (60–120 ml/day), in order to bind phosphate in the gut.

In a patient receiving any of these treatments frequent estimations of plasma calcium, phosphate and alkaline phosphatase must be performed.

It is becoming apparent that subtotal parathyroidectomy is needed more frequently, and may be carried out with less operative hazard in patients who have begun regular dialysis treatment. Severe bone disease may be an indication for earlier commencement of regular dialysis.

Uraemic neuropathy. Once this complication has appeared its progression can only be arrested by adequate dialysis or transplantation and if maintenance dialysis is planned this must be commenced without delay.

Intercurrent infections. Infections of the urinary tract and other infections, e.g. pneumonia and septicaemia, are particularly likely in patients with renal failure who may also be receiving treatment with steroids and immunosuppressive drugs. Urgent therapy with an appropriate antibiotic regime (see section on the use of antibiotics in patients with renal failure) must be instituted. Dialysis may be needed to cover the period of enhanced catabolism.

Planning the transfer to maintenance haemodialysis and transplantation

It is essential that plans are made well before the patient is moribund. If eventual dialysis and transplantation are decided upon the patient may be transferred earlier if there is evidence of neuropathy, and more careful monitoring of these patients should be carried out to detect such complications. In patients on protein restriction the blood urea is a less useful parameter and it is necessary to follow the plasma creatinine also. Once the plasma creatinine has reached 15–20 mg/100 ml (1400–2000 μmol l^{-1}) a sudden disaster (pericarditis, haemorrhage, fits, etc.) is likely and it is usual to arrange for cannulation or formation of a fistula before this.

PREVENTION OF THE PROGRESSION OF CHRONIC RENAL DISEASE (CRD)

This hinges on specific treatment of the underlying renal disease and on correction of factors which accelerate the deterioration in renal function.

Glomerulonephritis

There is no conclusive evidence from controlled trials that either steroids or immunosuppressive therapy improves the prognosis of patients with progressive proliferative glomerulonephritis. Nevertheless, many units are prepared to try these agents in any patient with rapidly progressive glomerulonephritis. Claims for the value of indomethacin and of anticoagulants remain unsubstantiated.

Renal infection

In any type of renal disease, but especially in those with urinary obstruction, infection may result in a permanent decrement in renal function. Therefore bacteriological investigations and prompt therapy are important.

Urinary tract obstruction

The importance of detecting and evaluating urinary tract obstruction must be fully realised, although its surgical correction is beyond the scope of this chapter.

Nephrotoxins

Awareness of the nephropathy associated with the consumption of large quantities of analgesics, particularly phenacetin, is essential when questioning a patient with unexplained renal failure.

Enquiry must also be made about possible exposure to other nephrotoxins, e.g. lead and cadmium.

Fluid and electrolyte abnormalities

The importance of adequate hydration and electrolyte balance in patients with CRF has already been considered. Hypercalcaemia is a serious hazard and a correctable cause must be sought. Potassium deficiency also impairs renal function and must be corrected.

Hypertension

The need for an aggressive approach to anti-hypertensive therapy in patients with renal failure has become more widely recognized in the last few years. Previously it was generally believed that lowering the blood pressure in patients with advanced renal failure did little to prolong life and might even hasten death by further reducing the glomerular filtration rate (GFR). It is certainly desirable to avoid too precipitate a fall in blood pressure initially, but control of hypertension, particularly when in the malignant phase, is essential for the conservation of remaining renal function. Patients with essential hypertension in a malignant phase often present with poor renal function and may undergo periods of accelerated deterioration with very severe hypertension, florid retinopathy and rapid fall in renal function. In some patients in this group worthwhile improvements in renal function may follow control of the hypertension, and dialysis should be given when needed to allow time for healing of the arteriolar lesions. This policy should also be adopted for several weeks at least even when malignant hypertension complicates a primary renal disease such as proliferative glomerulonephritis.

There is no evidence that uraemic patients are especially prone to the side effects of any of the common anti-hypertensive drugs. Alpha-methyl dopa is a suitable drug for many patients, the required dose being judged by the blood pressure response as in non-uraemic patients. Hydralazine, guanethidine, debrisoquine, bethanidine or clonidine may be used if control cannot be obtained with alpha-methyl dopa. Diazoxide intravenously is valuable in the urgent control of severe hypertension. Minoxidil appears to be a valuable anti-hypertensive drug when renal function is poor, but is not yet generally available.

Experience with regular haemodialysis has shown the vital importance of sodium and water in the control of hypertension. Most patients on regular dialysis become normotensive without drugs when sufficient salt and water have been removed from the body. This may eventually entail loss of up to 25% of the weight at the start of dialysis.

When peritoneal dialysis is being used to control uraemia, while hypertension is treated, the removal of fluid and reduction in weight are an important part of anti-hypertensive therapy, and may rapidly lessen the need for drugs. During this phase a negative sodium balance is essential and hypernatraemia must be avoided. A dialysis solution containing 130 mEq Na/1 is suitable for this purpose (most available commercial solutions contain 141 mEq Na/l necessitating the addition of 80 ml sterile water or 5% dextrose/litre). This solution is also most appropriate for patients with hyponatremia.

The recognition of the vital importance of sodium balance in control of hypertension also has important implications for the anti-hypertensive treatment of patients whose renal function is poor but adequate to avoid the need for dialysis. If good control of the blood pressure can be achieved with drugs such patients, when free of edema, are probably best maintained in sodium balance by selecting a dietary sodium level to match their measured average daily sodium losses. An optimum weight is found for each patient at which the blood pressure is controlled. If blood pressure control cannot be achieved then negative sodium balance may be produced slowly while renal function and bodyweight are followed carefully. Frusemide is a useful diuretic to achieve this, often being effective at low levels of renal function although large doses (500 mg or more) may be needed.

ANTIBIOTICS IN PATIENTS WITH RENAL FAILURE

The doses of antibiotics must be modified when they are prescribed for a patient with renal failure. Modification depends on the relationship of blood levels to renal function and on the levels at which toxic effects may occur.

General principles

The recommended dose schedule for commonly available drugs is shown in Table 1. This table should be used when blood level estimations of antibiotics are not available, but these are desirable wherever possible as considerable individual variation is encountered at all levels of renal function.

Fear of potential toxicity (Table 2) should not

inhibit the choice of the best available antibiotic. Microscopic examination of infected material, bacteriological identification and *in vitro* sensitivity patterns should be used in making this choice.

It is always safe to give the usual loading dose of the antibiotic which is indicated. After this, if the antibiotic is one excreted through the kidney, the maintenance doses must be given less frequently to patients with renal failure than they

can be given in normal doses even in the presence of severe renal failure.

If the patient is anuric or oliguric, has a glomerular filtration rate of less than 10 ml/min, or a serum creatinine concentration of more than 8 mg/100 ml (700 μmol l^{-1}) the full modification of the dosage should be applied. If the serum creatinine is more than 2 mg/100 ml (200 μmol l^{-1}) but less than 8 mg/ 100 ml (700 μmol l^{-1}), if the blood urea is raised but the glomerular filtra-

Table 1. Recommended dose of antibiotics

		Interval between MD	
		Severe RF*	Moderate RF†
Group I			
Renal excretion	Tetracycline	avoid	avoid
Toxicity related to serum levels	Nitrofurantoin	avoid	avoid
	Amino glycosides (gentamicin, kanamycin streptomycin)	3–4 days	1–2 days
	Colistin, polymyxin B	3–4 days	1–2 days
	Vancomycin	7–14 days	3–5 days
	Cephalosporins	24 hrs	12 hrs
Group II			
Renal excretion	Co-trimoxazole	24 hrs	12 hrs
Toxicity not related to serum levels	Sulphonamides	unchanged	unchanged
	Nalidixic acid	unchanged	unchanged
	Penicillins	unchanged	unchanged
Group III			
Non-renal excretion Toxicity unaffected by renal failure	Doxycycline Chloramphenicol Fucidic acid Erythromycin Lincomycin Clindamycin Isoniazid Rifampicin	All unchanged dose schedules in renal failure. Do not achieve good urinary concentrations in renal failure.	

* Oliguria; GFR < 10 ml/min; plasma creatinine > 8 mg/100 ml (700 μmol l^{-1}).
† Plasma creatinine 3–8 mg/100 ml (300–700 μmol l^{-1}). Recovery phase of Acute Renal Failure.

MD = Maintenance dose
RF = Renal failure

would be to patients with normal renal function. The frequency of the maintenance dose depends, firstly, upon the proportion of the drugs usually removed from the blood by renal excretion, and, secondly, upon the degree of functional impairment in the individual patient. Antibiotics which are largely excreted by the kidney (e.g. streptomycin, tetracycline) have a prolonged half life in the serum of patients with renal failure and must therefore be administered less often. On the other hand, antibiotics which are excreted by extrarenal routes (e.g. chloramphenicol, erythromycin)

tion rate is more than 10 ml/min, or if the patient is in the diuretic phase of recovery from acute tubular necrosis the minor dose modification should be applied. If the glomerular filtration rate is reduced but neither the blood urea nor the serum creatinine is raised the full dose can be given.

Practical points

Combined penicillin and streptomycin. Because the excretion of these two drugs is affected unequally by renal failure, it is a dangerous combination to prescribe for any patient who may have renal disease.

Tetracycline. This antibiotic affects protein synthesis and in renal failure may cause a further elevation of the blood urea. Nausea, diarrhea and vomiting may be particularly troublesome complications of tetracycline therapy. Chelates are formed with calcium and tetany may be precipitated. Care must therefore be taken to modify the dose of tetracycline in patients with renal failure. It is preferable to use an alternative drug. Doxycycline does not share the disadvantages of other tetracyclines but does not achieve good urinary concentrations in the presence of renal failure.

Urinary infections in the presence of renal impairment. It is important to treat any infection of the urinary tract which may be causing further renal damage or may give rise to a septicaemia in a patient who already has renal failure. Unfortunately, nitrofurantoin and nalidixic acid take several days to achieve therapeutic concentrations in the urine of patients with renal failure. With high blood levels of nitrofurantoin peripheral neuropathy may occur and this drug is therefore contraindicated in this situation. Chloramphenicol is rapidly metabolised by extrarenal routes and does not reach the urine in therapeutic concentration in renal failure. Inactive metabolites accumulate in renal failure and may be responsible for the serious toxic effects of chloramphenicol. Ampicillin and cephalosporins reach the urine in good concentration even in the face of renal failure and are useful drugs for this problem. Unfortunately cephaloridine has been associated with acute tubular necrosis. This appears to be especially likely to occur if large doses are given to a patient with renal disease and if a diuretic is given at the same time. If any of the group I or group II drugs (Table 1) is chosen the dose must be modified according to the rules, and, because of the delay in renal excretion of the drug, the time taken to achieve satisfactory urinary concentrations will no longer than usual. The excretion rate of sulphadimidine is independent of glomerular filtration rate and in renal failure adequate urinary concentrations are achieved. Sulphonamides may prove especially effective when combined with trimethoprim as Co-trimoxazole.

Septicaemia with Gram negative organisms. Ampicillin is often useful in these infections. The amino glycosides, gentamicin and kanamycin in modified dosage can also be used especially if blood level estimations are available. If they are indicated potentially nephrotoxic drugs (e.g. colistin and polymyxin B) should not be withheld.

Carbenicillin is useful against pseudomonas infections and lacks toxicity. Co-trimoxazole is also useful.

Tuberculosis. The treatment of tuberculosis in uraemic patients requires an appropriate reduction in the frequency of streptomycin injections but isoniazid and rifampicin can be given in full dosage. It is probably wise to add pyridoxine to make the development of neuropathy less likely. No information is available concerning the use of thiacetazone in renal failure. Para-amino-salicylic acid (PAS) appears to be excreted solely by the kidney and its use in renal failure requires blood level estimations.

Antibiotics and dialysis. When patients are being treated by dialysis the dose of any antibiotic prescribed will require modification from the schedule given in Table 1 if it is removed appreciably by dialysis. The dialysance of drugs depends on their protein binding and other factors such as molecular size affecting transfer across the peritoneal membrane and the cellophane membranes of artificial kidneys (Table 2). For example,

Table 2. Antibiotics: Toxicity and dialysance

		Removed by dialysis
Group I		
Tetracycline	Raised blood urea, tetany	+
	D & V, nausea	−
Nitrofurantoin	Peripheral neuropathy	?
Amino glycosides	Ototoxic	+
Colistin,		
polymyxin B	Nephrotoxic, neuropathy	+
Vancomycin	Ototoxic	0
Cephalosporins	Nausea, skin rashes,	
	vaginal discharge	+ +
Group II		
Trimethoprim	Hypersensitivity	+
Sulphonamides	Hypersensitivity, rashes,	
	Stevens–Johnson syndrome,	
	nausea and vomiting	+
Nalidixic acid	Nausea, phototoxic rashes	?
Penicillins	Hypersensitivity, skin rashes	
	(especially ampicillin)	0
Group III		
Doxycycline		?
Chloramphenicol	Marrow aplasia	+
Fucidic acid	Nausea and vomiting	?
Erythromycin		?
Lincomycin		?
Clindamycin		0
Isoniazid		+
Rifampicin	Hepatocellular damage	?

cephaloridine is only loosely bound to serum proteins and is removed rapidly by dialysis; vancomycin which is a large molecule and is not removed by dialysis, persists in safe and therapeutic serum levels for 9–14 days after only a single injection of 1 g in an oliguric or anuric patient.

THE MANAGEMENT OF URINARY TRACT INFECTIONS (UTI)

Significant bacterial colonisation of the urine can only be diagnosed by quantitative cultures of a midstream specimen of urine (MSU) or by culture of urine obtained by suprapubic aspiration.

Urine culture is required not only for the diagnosis of UTI, but also for confirmation of cure and during the follow up of the patient.

An attempt should always be made to obtain a bacteriological diagnosis in an infant or child aged less than 15 or in a male adult, for in these patients a single bacteriologically proven infection is the indication for investigation, and management starts with the exclusion or correction of underlying anatomical abnormalities. In women of child-bearing age proof of bacterial infection differentiates urinary tract infection from the 'Urethral Syndrome'. In these patients investigation is indicated only if attacks recur frequently. Management is otherwise empirical, directed at the relief of symptoms and the prevention of recurrences.

Acute attack

While awaiting bacteriological identification and sensitivity reports, treatment shuold be commenced by encouraging the patient to take a high fluid intake and by prescribing the antibiotic most likely to be appropriate.

The majority of domiciliary infections are due to *E. coli* or *P. mirabilis* sensitive to most antibiotics. A week's course of sulphonamide results in sterile urine in 80–90% of these patients. If it fails to do so, the choice of a different antibiotic should be guided by sensitivity tests, but usually lies between ampicillin, nitrofurantoin, cotrimoxazole, tetracycline or cephalexin.

Infections arising in hospital are due to a wider range of organisms some of which may be resistant to many antibiotics. If symptoms necessitate treatment before the results of sensitivity testing are known, Co-trimoxazole or ampicillin should be given.

Alkalinisation of the urine enhances the effect of sulphonamides and amino glycosides. However, in patients whose renal function is not known

potassium citrate introduces the danger of hyperkalaemia, and sodium bicarbonate or citrate of sodium overload. In practice alkalinisation is rarely necessary. The urine can be rendered acid by ammonium chloride or methionine. Acidification enhances the effect of tetracycline and cycloserine and is essential for the activity of the urinary antiseptic mandelamine.

Asymptomatic bacteriuria

This is found in 5% of women at their first attendances at antenatal clinics. In this group antibiotic treatment reduces the incidence of acute pyelonephritis which is otherwise high (25–40%). The incidence is similar in non-pregnant adult females, but treatment is not indicated. The prevelance of asymptomatic bacteriuria in school girls is 1–2%. The value of investigating and treating these girls is not yet established.

Acute pyelonephritis

If there are clinical reasons for considering that the infection involves the kidneys, the antibiotic used should be one which achieves good concentrations in the blood and tissues as well as in the urine.

In domiciliary practice, where most of these infections are encountered, initial treatment with either ampicillin (which may be given intramuscularly) or trimethoprim-sulphamethoxazole is recommended.

The resistant organisms encountered in hospital frequently dictate a choice between parenteral gentamycin, kanamycin and colistin. If treatment must be started before sensitivities are available, gentamycin is probably the best choice because of its activity against *P. aeruginosa*. In patients with renal damage the dose of gentamycin and colistin must be adjusted to the level of renal failure, and it is advisable to monitor blood levels when possible. Carbenicillin is useful against infections with *P. aeruginosa*, but may need to be given in very high dosage (30–40 g/day) if renal function is good. A synergistic action with gentamycin has been described.

Recurrent UTI

In patients who have had an attack of acute pyelonephritis, relapse (same organism) and reinfection (new organism) are common. Bacteriuria recurs within 6 months in 50% of patients. Therefore, management should ideally continue with bacteriological proof of cure and follow-up to detect recurrences of bacteriuria. In this way it is hoped to detect bacteriuric recurrences and to treat them before they became symptomatic. It is not necessary to obtain such bacteriological documentation of a primary infection in a female of child bearing age, but recurrent infections should attract more attention. If there is difficulty in achieving bacteriological cure despite the isolation of an apparently sensitive organism, or if a patient has frequent relapses it suggests that there is renal involvement. Frequent re-infection raises the possibility of some anatomical abnormality in the urinary tract which makes the patient vulnerable to repeated attacks. Recurrent infections require regular bacteriological observations, possibly using the dip inocula prepared and posted to the laboratory by the patient, and the escalation of measures to prevent recurrences.

All patients with recurrent infections need radiological investigation to exclude anatomical abnormality. Some will profit from reassurance about the effect of attacks on their renal function. All should be carefully advised about maintaining a high fluid intake and about bladder emptying. If large residual bladder volumes or vesicoureteric reflux is present double or triple micturition must be practised. If attacks in the female are related to sexual intercourse, bladder emptying after intercourse is advised. The prescription of a single antibiotic tablet (co-trimoxazole, ampicillin or tetracycline) at this time has proved a useful preventive measure. Continual suppressive therapy using low dose nitrofurantoin (50 mg nightly) or co-trimoxazole (1 tablet nightly) reduces the frequency of attacks for such patients. In addition to the use of prophylactic antibiotics the patient may be given courses of antibiotics to commence as soon as symptoms recur.

SYSTEMIC DISEASES WHICH INVOLVE THE KIDNEY

This section will consider only therapy specific to the systemic disease concerned. The treatment of renal failure and the use of diuretics for edema of renal origin in these diseases follow the principles already covered in previous sections unless stated otherwise.

Systemic Lupus Erythematosus (SLE)

Specific treatment for SLE with renal involvement consists of careful avoidance of precipitating factors (e.g. sunlight and some drugs) and the use of steroids or immunosuppressive agents. Although there have been no fully controlled trials there is much evidence that steroids are beneficial in some forms of this disease. A renal biopsy provides a guide to therapy although renal func-

tion and the urinary sediment must also be considered.

If the renal biopsy is normal or shows only minor focal proliferative changes in some glomeruli without tubular or interstitial abnormalities ('lupus glomerulitis') the choice lies between no therapy and steroids in moderate doses, e.g. prednisone 10–20 mg/day. When making this decision on purely renal grounds the GFR, the extent of proteinuria, abnormalities in the urinary sediment and any trend for better or worse in these features should all be considered. There is no evidence that the risks of prolonged high dose steroid therapy are warranted for this lesion, but the patient must be kept under review.

The renal biopsy may show uniform thickening of the basement membrane affecting all glomeruli with little or no evidence of cellular proliferation. This membranous lesion appears to have a slowly progressive course but there is no evidence yet that steroid therapy retards its progress. Nephrotic syndrome may complicate this lesion and it is reasonable then to undertake a trial of steroids in high dosage (prednisone 1 mg/kg/day) for 3 or 4 weeks, thereafter reducing to a smaller dose.

The most severe lesion which biopsy may reveal is termed 'active lupus glomerulonephritis'. Cellular proliferation in the glomeruli is prominent and focal areas of basement membrane thickening are often present. Local necrosis may be seen in some glomeruli together with haematoxyphil bodies, wire loop lesions and crescents. This appearance carries a bad prognosis, particularly if the blood urea is already elevated, and steroids should be given in high doses for 4 to 6 months or longer.

The levels of complement components and of anti-DNA antibodies also appear to correlate with the activity of the inflammatory disease process. They may prove helpful guides in deciding the intensity of steroid or immunosuppressive therapy to be used but their precise role is not yet agreed.

There are reports of improvement in renal lupus following the use of nitrogen mustard, 6-mercaptopurine, azathioprine cyclophosphamide and indomethacin. Evidence is accumulating that azathioprine and cyclophosphamide are useful drugs and may be used with steroids to reduce the dose and toxicity of the latter.

Polyarteritis nodosa (PAN)

A trial of steroids in high dosage (prednisone 45–60 mg/day or more) is justified in any case of PAN with evidence of renal involvement. If hypertension or renal failure are present the chances of improvement with steroids are slender, but there is little to be lost and an occasional patient responds even when acute renal failure has developed.

There have been claims of good results with azathioprine and cyclophosphamide has also been used in Wegener's granulomatosis with encouraging results but controlled trials have not been reported.

When acute oliguric renal failure develops the outlook is very poor, but recovery of useful renal function may sometimes occur if life is preserved by dialysis for a period of a few weeks to give time for a trial of high dose steroid therapy.

Systemic sclerosis

The kidney complications of this disease rarely dominate the clinical picture until renal failure develops. This may develop acutely or insidiously. There is no evidence that steroids are beneficial and some evidence that they may accelerate the renal failure. When proteinuria alone indicates renal involvement there is again little evidence that steroids are helpful and it seems reasonable on the information available not to use them. The effect of immunosuppressive therapy in this disease is unknown. Claims for other therapeutic agents, such as vasodilator drugs and chelating agents, have not been substantiated.

Haemolytic/uraemic syndromes

This includes a number of diseases probably with different aetiologies, but having in common a microangiopathy with occlusive lesions in small blood vessels, disseminated intravascular clotting, thrombocytopenia, haemolytic anaemia and frequently renal failure. This syndrome develops most frequently in two age groups: in children, where it is often preceded by a gastrointestinal disturbance; in young adults, where it is usually called Thrombotic Thrombocytopenic Purpura (Moschowitz's Syndrome). A similar blood picture may complicate malignant hypertension, usually with renal failure, but such cases are distinguished by the sequence of events.

Steroids are usually given in large doses, but their usefulness is difficult to assess at present; in many reported cases they do not appear to have influenced the course of the disease, and one report concluded that they might be harmful. Anticoagulant therapy, usually with heparin, has been given with encouraging results. Dialysis has been used to control uraemia and subsequent improvement has been reported; although the mortality remains high when the disease is so severe. It seems reasonable at present to treat patients with this condition with heparin and dialysis as necessary. When this syndrome complicates malig-

nant hypertension urgent antihypertensive therapy is imperative.

Henoch-Schönlein purpura (Anaphylactoid purpura)

Steroids do not affect the renal lesions of this condition but may be useful in management of the extrarenal lesions. Promising reports of the use of azathioprine or cyclophosphamide have appeared, but full evaluation of these drugs is not yet possible. It should be realised that the outcome is sufficiently good in children presenting with haematuria and proteinuria, but without florid nephritic or nephrotic features to justify withholding steroids or immunosuppressive drugs.

Goodpasture's syndrome (lung purpura with nephritis)

Steroids in large doses, e.g. prednisone 60–80 mg/day, should be given. If needed early in the course of this illness dialysis should be performed to control uraemia as prolonged remissions can occur. There are reports of haemoptysis stopping after bilateral nephrectomy but the indications for this desperate manoeuvre are speculative. Good results from plasmaphoresis, with removal of antibody to glomerular basement membrane have recently been reported.

Diabetes

Proteinuria sometimes progressing to a nephrotic syndrome, chronic renal failure and urinary tract infection are the renal hazards of diabetes. It is not established that inadequate control of diabetes increases the incidence of these complications, but when they are present it seems prudent to pay careful attention to anti-diabetic therapy. In this context it should be realised that in patients with renal failure the degree of glycosuria may be a misleading guide to diabetic control. In advanced renal failure the insulin requirements may decrease.

The indications for restriction of salt, water and protein are similar to those in other renal diseases. When a nephrotic syndrome develops early in the course of diabetes a renal biopsy is indicated at least in children, in view of the report that in these circumstances, the biopsy may show only minimal abnormalities in the glomeruli and that steroids may then induce remission. Otherwise the usefulness of renal biopsy is limited, the correlation between histological abnormalities and prognosis in an individual case being poor. Many diuretics impair carbohydrate tolerance and for the diabetic patient with edema but without serious renal failure ethacrynic acid is the diuretic of choice as it does not have this side effect.

Urinary tract infection must be treated vigorously. Bladder catheterisation should be avoided whenever possible, particularly in diabetic coma, the management of which should be regulated by blood sugar determinations.

Hypophysectomy and adrenalectomy are not yet established in the management of diabetic nephropathy despite claims of improvement after these operations.

Gout

The treatment of acute attacks of both primary and secondary gout need not be modified by the presence of renal impairment. For long term treatment allopurinol (300–800 mg/day) is the drug of choice and avoids the risks of increased renal urate deposition and uric acid calculus formation carried by uricosuric drugs. The effective dosage of allopurinol does not appear to be affected by renal failure and can be regulated by its effect on plasma urate levels as in non-uraemic patients.

Allopurinol increases the urinary excretion of xanthine but there is to date, no evidence that this is harmful. It has been alleged that reactions to allopurinol occur more often in renal failure but their incidence remains acceptably low.

Myelomatosis

A high fluid intake is advised as dehydration may accelerate cast formation within the renal tubules leading to intrarenal obstruction. Claims that intravenous pyelography may precipitate acute renal failure have been disputed, but certainly fluid restriction should be avoided prior to this investigation.

Hypercalcaemia should be treated urgently with steroids, and hyperuricaemia with allopurinol.

The development of acute renal failure is usually fatal, but where the patient's condition is otherwise acceptable and a precipitating cause for the renal failure can be defined (e.g. dehydration or hypercalcaemia) it is reasonable to perform dialysis as recovery from the renal failure in such circumstances has been recorded.

Amyloidosis

There is no specific therapy. In 'secondary' amyloidosis the finding of renal involvement makes radical treatment of the underlying disease imperative where this is possible. The use of steroids, e.g. in rheumatoid arthritis, poses a special problem in view of the evidence that steroids may increase amyloid formation. This latter contention is not proven and it is probably reasonable to continue steroid therapy if this is warranted on other grounds.

When renal amyloidosis is found without predisposing disease it is important to search for evidence of myeloma. Even when the latter diagnosis cannot be made analysis of plasma and urine proteins may disclose a monoclonal immunoglobulin dysproteinaemia. Treatment with melphalan can remove the evidence of dysproteinaemia in such patients but it is not known whether the further formation of amyloid is reduced by this treatment.

RENAL CALCULI

A high fluid intake is advisable for all patients with renal calculi. As the calcium content of tap water may be considerable (e.g. 6–12 mg/100 ml) (1.5–3.0 mmol l^{-1}) this factor must be considered in patients with hypercalciuria, but it is generally believed that the benefits bestowed on stoneformers by urinary dilution outweigh this possible disadvantage.

Ureteric colic is treated with analgesics such as pethidine and the progress of the stone is monitored by straight abdominal films and excretion urography.

Specific preventative therapy depends on any demonstrable metabolic defect underlying stone formation.

Hypercalciuria

If hypercalciuria is due to hypercalcaemia the cause of the latter must be sought, paying particular attention to the diagnosis of hyperparathyroidism.

Hypercalciuria without hypercalcaemia may be part of a syndrome of renal tubular dysfunction needing treatment in its own right, e.g. renal tubular acidosis, when treatment with alkalis, sodium and potassium salts may be indicated.

Usually however hypercalciuria is an isolated finding in patients with renal calculi. Present day treatment is concentrated on dietary factors in this abnormality. It is important to check whether the patient has been taking any vitamin D containing preparation. Measures which lower urinary calcium excretion include; a low calcium diet, involving the use of softened water for cooking and drinking and often causing considerable domestic upheaval and agents which reduce dietary calcium absorption, e.g. cellulose phosphate (15 g/day) or sodium phytate (6 g/day).

Controlled observations on the long term effect of these measures on stone formation are lacking, although there are favourable short term reports particularly for the use of bendrofluazide.

Uric acid stones

These usually occur in a persistently acid urine and adequate alkali therapy (sodium bicarbonate 8–10 g/day) is often successful at preventing their recurrence. Allopurinol is indicated for patients with increased urinary urate excretion or hyperuricaemia. It may be of particular value in preventing the complications of hyperuricaemia occurring in patients with leukaemias and reticuloses when urate excretion may be very high, especially during treatment with cytotoxic drugs or radiotherapy.

Cystine stones

Maintenance of urinary alkalinity (e.g. with sodium bicarbonate 10 g/day or more) and avoidance of urinary concentration are often successful in preventing stone formation in patients with cystinuria. However, this treatment involves attaining a urine output of at least 3 litres/day with the necessary production of large volumes of dilute urine at night. D-penicillamine forms a soluble complex with cystine, is effective at preventing stone formation and may even achieve the dissolution of existing stones. However, this treatment is expensive and potentially hazardous. It is best reserved for those patients not responding to the more simple measures given above.

PERITONEAL DIALYSIS

Requirements

Although peritoneal dialysis can be carried out in the general ward, the space and staff required makes the procedure more appropriately done in an intensive care ward or area. Modern sterile disposable peritoneal catheters with metal stylet and giving sets are usefully combined with a sterile disposable plastic bag for collection of effluent. The whole system then remains closed except for the moment when fresh bags (or bottles) of the dialysis solution are put up. Two solutions are required, one approximately isotonic and the other hypertonic, so that the rate of fluid removal can be controlled. It is usual to warm the solution to body temperature. Since tap water is likely to contain organisms it is preferable to warm the bags without wetting them; warming pads or a small incubator may be used. A chart is needed on which to plot hourly temperature, pulse, respiration and blood pressure recordings. Records must also be kept of the volumes of fluid run in and run out and of any additions to this fluid. It is customary to add heparin (500 u/litre) and potassium (4 mEq/l) after correction of hyperkalaemia. It is also useful to record the time taken to run the fluid in and out since this is a measure of the efficiency of the system.

Method

The bladder is emptied and the anterior abdominal wall prepared as for surgery. Using full asepsis the catheter is inserted under local anaesthesia through a small scalpel incision at a point one third of the distance from the umbilicus to the symphysis pubis in the midline. Other sites over the lower abdomen may also be used. If the patient can either tense or blow forward the anterior abdominal wall it improves the confidence of the operator. If not, some will advise running in 2 litres of fluid through a needle before inserting the catheter. This takes time. As soon as the catheter is definitely inside the peritoneum the stylet is withdrawn and the catheter is then passed down into the pelvis as far as it will comfortably go, avoiding pushing too hard because this may kink the catheter. The catheter is supplied with marks so that the direction of its curve is known. If more than 5 cm protrudes as in a small patient it may be convenient to cut this off before fitting the giving set. Only occasionally with the modern catheter is a purse string suture needed to retain the catheter and prevent leakage. In some units a gauze dressing with adhesive strapping is applied, and redressed after antiseptic washing once a day. Others suggest open techniques with frequent application of antiseptic lotion or antibiotic creams.

Most adults will be comfortable with 2 litre exchanges of dialysis fluid, but if this causes discomfort 1 litre exchanges should be used. The rate of exchange must then be doubled since the clearance achieved is related to the volume of dialysis fluid used per hour. The first 3 exchanges should be carried out as fast as the system will permit so as to flush out fibrin from the catheter and minimise the chances of an early blockage. The drainage period should be limited to a maximum of 40 minutes (20 minutes for 1 litre exchange) since it is usual for the volume of fluid to run out, to be less than that run in during the early stages. The inexperienced are worried by this if they have not been warned to expect it, and dialysis becomes less and less efficient as each exchange becomes more and more prolonged. It should be pointed out that to build up a residual volume so that dialysis is continual rather than intermittent is an advantage. With later exchanges, and as hypertonic solution is used, a negative fluid balance is readily achieved. When it is established that the system is working well, it is convenient to organise an hourly or half-hourly routine for the exchanges. The time taken for the fluid to run in and out then dictates the 'dwell' time when the exchange is left in the peritoneum.

The amount of dialysis required depends on the degree of uraemia when dialysis is begun and on the rate of catabolism. It is usual to commence with a 36–48-hour period. The catabolic patient with ARF will need continuous dialysis;

stable patients with terminal renal failure have been managed for long periods of time on as little as 36–48 hours/week.

The dialysis effluent should be monitored for infection by daily cultures and microscopy for pus cells. Protein losses can exceed 100 g/day and plasma may be needed to restore blood volume if the blood pressure falls. Routine physiotherapy should be instituted because pulmonary complications are common.

3

THE LOCOMOTOR SYSTEM

J. A. MATHEWS

INTRODUCTION

Specific treatments are available for some rheumatic disorders. Rather more often the treatments used in acute and chronic disease of joints are not specific but are helpful as supportive treatment in a wide range of conditions. To avoid unnecessary repetition the non-specific methods will be described in more detail for the commonest inflammatory joint disease—rheumatoid arthritis, and for the commonest degenerative joint disease—osteoarthrosis. Where a disease has a specific method of treatment, it is usually used in conjunction with supportive measures.

INFLAMMATORY JOINT DISEASE

IDIOPATHIC

Rheumatoid arthritis

No single cause of rheumatoid arthritis has been found. The disease has a familial incidence, is commoner in women, may be precipitated by many factors, and after an initial inflammatory phase seems to be prolonged, by an autoimmune process. Rheumatoid disease is a systemic disorder but in most patients synovitis dominates the early clinical picture and produces the features of arthritis—hot, swollen, painful, stiff joints. In children the systemic features are more often prominent with fever and weight loss, but this happens less often in adults. The local inflammation may affect any synovial joint, bursa, or tendon sheath in the body, and if sufficiently severe or prolonged may produce secondary mechanical changes such as joint instability and subluxation, or tendon rupture. The synovitis may affect one joint (monarticular) or many joints (polyarticular), and the onset may be gradual or sudden. It is impossible to predict accurately the course of the disease, but the following features are generally thought to be associated with a good prognosis: sudden onset;

duration under one year; male sex; the absence of rheumatoid serum factor (Rose–Waaler and latex tests) or nodules. The diagnosis is suggested by the early appearance of radiological erosions, and confirmed by finding rheumatoid factor or nodules.

Treatment of rheumatoid arthritis may be directed at the inflammatory disease, whether systemic or local, or at the mechanical sequelae, or both when appropriate.

TREATMENT (EARLY RHEUMATOID ARTHRITIS)

It is not always possible to confirm the diagnosis at this stage as rheumatoid factor tests are often negative and nodules absent. Treatment must then remain symptomatic if possible. In view of the widespread but incorrect belief that the disease is always progressive, it is valuable to try to gain the confidence of the patient by explaining the true situation. In particular it should be stressed that the disease is crippling in only a minority, and that a great deal can be done to help at all stages.

Rest. If the patient is systemically ill recovery is hastened by starting treatment with a period of 2–3 weeks total bedrest. Whilst in bed the patient should have a good back support, a firm mattress, a bed cradle and a foot support. The temptation to make the patient comfortable with a pillow behind the knee should be resisted as this predisposes to flexion deformities of hips and knees. No special dietary, vitamin, or hormone supplements are of any value, but night sedatives should be given when necessary. Joint inflammation also settles more rapidly with splintage and even complete immobilisation for several weeks leads to surprisingly little residual stiffness. If inflamed joints are painful at rest, they should be splinted in the position of optimum function. Resting splints may be made of plaster of paris or moulded plastic, and are often needed for wrists and knees. Static muscle exercises should be given by a physiotherapist, and it may be an advantage to remove splints and move joints passively through their full range once or twice daily. Two spells each day lying prone also help to prevent flexion contractures of the hips and knees. As the activity of the disease subsides, the patient should be encouraged to undertake more activity, and be gradually mobilised.

Local steroid injections. If only a small number of joints or tendon sheaths or bursae is affected they may be aspirated and hydrocortisone acetate injected, 0.5–2 ml (12.5–50 mg) according to the size of the joint. Occasionally hydrocortisone acetate produces a "flare" in the joint, probably an example of crystal synovitis. This is sometimes avoided by using methylprednisolone acetate or triamcinolone hexacetonide, and these are claimed to have a longer action. Steroids must not be injected if there is a possibility of joint infection and should be avoided in unstable joints.

Salicylates. Soluble aspirin is conventionally the drug of first choice but sometimes causes indigestion or gastric ulceration and bleeding. A dose of 2 to 4 g daily is given in divided doses. An enteric coated preparation may avoid gastric side effects and benorylate has been shown to have approximately equal potency and cause less faecal blood loss.

Butazones. Phenylbutazone may be substituted for aspirin, or be added to it if extra effect is needed. As marrow suppression occasionally occurs, a preliminary blood count is essential to avoid confusion between blood dyscrasias caused by the disease and those due to treatment. Peptic and oral ulceration, fluid retention, and skin sensitivity, are other hazards. Phenylbutazone is usually taken orally, 100 mg t.d.s., but may be given as a suppository of 250 mg at night to relieve morning stiffness. Care must be taken not to exceed a regular total daily dose of 300 mg. Antacid and enteric-coated preparations are also available for patients in whom indigestion is produced.

Oxyphenbutazone is an alternative preparation with similar indications, side effects and doses. However the same side effect is not always produced by the two preparations in the same patient, and it may be worth changing to avoid a minor complication.

Indomethacin. This is an alternative to butazones, which probably causes less haematological side effects. However, peptic ulceration and cerebral side effects (headache or muzziness) can occur by whichever route is given. The usual oral starting dose is caps. indomethacin 25 mg t.d.s., and this may be increased to 50 mg t.d.s. A night time suppository of 100 mg is useful in combating morning stiffness, but care should be taken to avoid exceeding a total daily dose of 150 mg for long-term administration.

Fenamates. These drugs are useful alternatives which avoid both gastric and haematological side effects, but they sometimes cause severe diarrhea. Caps. mefenamic acid 250 mg t.d.s., or caps. flufenamic acid 100 mg t.d.s. are prescribed.

Paracetamol is a mild analgesic which may also be useful for mild rheumatoid arthritis—dose 1 g t.d.s.

Propionic acid derivatives. Drugs of this group have been introduced in recent years and seem to be relatively safe and convenient alternatives to the above drugs. Recommended doses tend to rise as confidence about safety increases. The group includes ibuprofen, naproxen ketoprofen and fenoprofen. Alclofenac is chemically related. Morphine and its derivatives and mixtures containing phenacetin are not safe for long-term administration.

Continuing disease activity

If the disease activity continues the diagnosis can usually be confirmed by the appearance of rheumatoid nodules or positive rheumatoid factor tests. When the diagnosis is certain, there is clinical or radiological evidence of disease progression (appearance of cortical bone erosions), the disease has failed to settle in one year, and the majority of symptoms are due to disease activity and not mechanical deformity, more specific antirheumatoid therapy is indicated.

Sodium aurothiomalate. The main toxic effects of gold salts are dermatitis, marrow suppression, and renal damage; therefore skin allergy, blood dyscrasias, and albuminuria are contraindications to their use. Treatment must be preceded by a blood count and each injection by an enquiry into skin symptoms (notably itching), and a urine test for albumin. Other marrow suppressant drugs (commonly phenylbutazone) must be stopped, and monthly blood counts performed. Myocrisin is given by intra-muscular injection, test doses of 10 and 20 mg on separate days, then 50 mg weekly until a full course of 500 mg has been achieved. If remission has occurred, it may be worth continuing with 50 mg monthly until 1 g has been given. Beneficial effects are not usually felt for 2 months.

Penicillamine. After many years of tentative use D-penicillamine has been shown to be helpful in active rheumatoid disease. In terms of the base it is preferable to start with a small dose of 125–250 mg daily increasing by monthly increments to a total daily dose of 750 mg. Unfortunately dangerous blood dyscrasias and proteinuria occur and require regular monitoring. Rashes and taste disturbance may also be troublesome. Nevertheless the efficacy of the drug is comparable to that of gold.

Antimalarials. These also act slowly, and the recognition of irreversible retinitis has led to decreased use. Rashes, bleaching of hair, corneal deposition, and exacerbation of psoriasis may occur. However, with expert ophthalmic supervision their use may occasionally be justified. Tabs. chloroquine phosphate 250 mg or hydroxychloroquine 200 mg are given once or twice daily for up to 1 year.

Steroids. These have a small but definite place in treatment. Extreme caution is needed in the use of steroids to suppress chronic diseases, as once started the drug can seldom be stopped. The aim should be to restrict the dose to that which can be tolerated long term. Prednisone or prednisolone are used, are of identical potency, and are indicated in several situations: 1. Severely active early disease uncontrolled by the simpler measures described, may be partially suppressed by up to 10 mg of prednisone daily. It is better policy to start with a small dose of steroid and gradually increase it to the minimum needed, than to start with a large daily dose and attempt to reduce it to an acceptable level. The disease cannot be 'stamped-out' by large doses of steroids, and if a high dose is used early it is seldom possible to reduce it to a satisfactorily low dose. 2. Crippling early morning stiffness may occur in the absence of obvious disease activity. This stiffness is sometimes dramatically relieved by giving 5 mg prednisone at night (but it is worth trying the phenylbutazone or indomethacin suppositories first). This steroid dose is seldom the cause of major side effects. 3. Between these two extremes is the patient with chronic and progressive disease in whom social or economic pressures make it worth 'buying' a small number of years of relative freedom, and running the risk of steroid side effects later. 4. A special case for larger doses of prednisone exists when there are potentially lethal systemic features to the disease, often involving arteritis. Nail-fold vasculitis *per se* does not demand steroid treatment.

Immunosuppressive drugs. Azathioprine and cyclophosphamide have been used in rheumatoid arthritis, and azathioprine has been shown to have a steroid-sparing effect. Azathioprine is used in a total daily dose of 2.5 mg/kg body-weight, and should be considered for those patients who are unable to tolerate the dose of steroids they need. Monthly blood counts are needed for control. Cyclophosphamide may be slightly more effective but the risk of marrow suppression, alopecia and azoospermia restrict consideration

of its use to only most aggressive forms of the disease.

TREATMENT (CHRONIC RHEUMATOID ARTHRITIS)

All too often the disease cannot be adequately suppressed and severe disability results. Fortunately a great deal can be done to match the patient and the environment to each other; both can be modified.

Modification of patient. Weak muscles. These can be strengthened by intensive physiotherapy concentrating on 'static' or isometric contraction of muscles to obtain maximum muscular effort with minimum joint stress. Faradic stimulation may help to initiate recovery of movement in severe chronic weakness.

Contractures. It is possible for minor but disabling contractures of joint capsules to be corrected by manual stretching. Heat is useful as a preliminary local analgesic and may be applied by wax baths to the hands and feet, or via short wave diathermy or radiant heat to larger joints. More stubborn contractures may need correction by serial plasters, and a manipulation under anaesthetic (often with local steroid injection) is sometimes necessary to hasten progress.

Supports. Stress may be diverted from unstable or painful joints. Polythene wrist splints, knee splints, walking aids, and surgical shoes are frequently of great help and lively splints can be used to overcome weakness.

Surgery. The choice of operation is difficult as the pattern of progressive joint involvement cannot be accurately predicted. Decisions must be taken with an orthopaedic surgeon. Early synovectomy delays damage to a diseased joint and is worth while if the disease is confined to a small number of joints. Recently ruptured tendons should be repaired. Late 'salvage' operations must be carefully chosen as an unsuccessful operation is demoralising. Synovectomy and debridement of a joint is a useful pain relieving procedure and where joint stability is not essential excision arthroplasty is possible, and is often successful for painful metatarsal heads or a painfully limited elbow. Medical synovectomy by irradiation has recently been reappraised particularly for the knee; yttrium-90 as a resin colloid can be injected into the joint and sometimes gives lasting relief of inflammation. Treatment is not without risk and burns, effusions and fever have occurred. If stability must be maintained a replacement arthroplasty is preferable, and increasingly successful operations on hips and knees are currently being performed. Silastic prostheses are helpful in some small joints. Guaranteed lasting freedom from pain and permanent stability is achieved by arthrodesis, but this can seldom be recommended in a polyarthritic disease whose progress is uncertain.

Modification of environment. Despite all treatment this disease sometimes produces severe disability. When this occurs, the help of the occupational therapist, medical social worker, disablement resettlement officer, domiciliary services, local authorities, and voluntary organisations may be needed. The patient's ability to travel can be modified by a wheelchair or motor propelled vehicle, the home adapted to the disability, and work modified or the patient re-trained. Many of these modifications are most effective when initiated early.

Complications. The numerous non-articular features of rheumatoid disease usually need treatment along expectant lines; steroids are frequently not a sinecure and should be reserved for complications that are life-threatening.

Amyloid disease carries a poor prognosis and is not helped by steroids. Local nerve pressure should be surgically relieved, as in the carpal-tunnel syndrome. Septic joints occur in rheumatoid patients, especially if on steroids, and must be thought of in a monarticular 'flare'. 'Anaemia of inflammation' is common, and seldom responds to oral or parenteral iron. Iron-deficiency anaemia may be due to salicylate induced gastrointestinal bleeding, and must be treated by stopping the offending drug and giving iron. The upper cervical spine is commonly affected by the disease with subsequent atlanto-axial subluxation. Mid-cervical changes may lead to a myelopathy. During preparation for surgery special care must be taken to avoid abnormal or violent neck movements. Occasionally the capsule of a swollen knee joint ruptures allowing synovial fluid to escape into the calf. The symptoms and signs mimic a deep vein thrombosis but arthrography can confirm the diagnosis so that treatment is directed to the knee and not the vein.

Psoriatic arthritis

Apart from the presence of skin lesions this condition differs from rheumatoid disease in several important ways. There is seldom severe systemic upset, although an elevated ESR, anaemia, and weight loss may accompany the synovitis. The synovitis is usually less proliferative and destructive than that in rheumatoid arthritis, but occasionally mutilating arthritis occurs. Clinically the arthritis is often asymmetrical, may affect the terminal interphalangeal joints of the fingers and toes, sometimes affects the sacro-iliac joints and spine to give an atypical spondylitis.

Psoriatic arthritis is not associated with rheumatoid nodules or serum factor, and with the rare exception of amyloid, it is not complicated by the many non-articular features of rheumatoid disease. The prognosis for both local joint destruction and systemic illness is therefore better.

TREATMENT

Rest. It is not often necessary to confine these patients to bed as there is seldom systemic illness. The affected joints may benefit from local splints and steroid injections.

Drugs. Those of use are the same as in early rheumatoid arthritis. Phenylbutazone in particular has a reputation for being most effective in psoriatic arthritis. Gold is not recommended for psoriatic arthritis since its effectiveness in this condition has not been demonstrated, and there may be more danger of severe skin reactions. Antimalarials should also be avoided as they too may provoke severe skin reactions. The indications for steroids are similar to those in rheumatoid arthritis but occur less often. Methotrexate has been claimed to be useful in severe combined skin and joint disease, but the danger of marrow suppression precludes its general use. Other cytotoxic drugs have also been tried.

Surgery. Indications and techniques are similar to those in rheumatoid arthritis.

Reiter's disease

The syndrome of urethritis, conjunctivitis, and arthritis, is precipitated either by the urethritis or by dysentery. The patient is nearly always male and may be ill with fever, high ESR, and anaemia. The urethritis may be accompanied by prostatitis and cystitis, and recurrent bouts of iritis occur. Keratodermia blenorrhagica sometimes affects the soles of the feet, and mucous membrane lesions may occur in the mouth and on the glans penis. Occasionally the cardiovascular system is affected with heart block, pericarditis or aortic incompetence.

The locomotor features may involve 'soft tissues'; both plantar fasciitis and Achilles tendinitis are common. The arthritis is often asymmetrical affecting the legs more than arms. The knees, metatarsophalangeal joints, and the interphalangeal joints of the hallux and other toes are frequently involved.

Most initial attacks settle in a few months, but recurrence is common, and after several attacks severe foot deformities often remain. Occasionally the sacro-iliac and spinal joints are affected mimicking ankylosing spondylitis.

TREATMENT

The systemic illness is often sufficiently severe to justify admission to hospital. The venereologist should be consulted, and usually a 7-day course of a broad spectrum antibiotic is ordered to treat the urethritis. Where there are eye complications the ophthalmic surgeon should be consulted; chloramphenicol eyedrops are usually recommended to prevent secondary conjunctival infection, and atropine or steroid eyedrops may help the iritis. Skin and mucosal lesions should be treated with simple hygienic measures. No specific treatment is available.

Joints are often very acutely painful and swollen, and are helped by rest, local steroid injections and splints. Supervised static exercises are again valuable for maintaining muscle strength. Special footwear is often necessary to support deformed feet.

Drugs. Tabs. phenylbutazone 100 mg t.d.s., or caps, indomethacin 25 mg t.d.s. are all probably more effective than salicylates. Sometimes the two preparations are needed in which case one should be given orally and the other by suppository. Systemic steroids may be needed if there is severe systemic disturbance which fails to settle with rest, but often their effect is disappointing.

Surgery. This may be helpful for the crippling foot deformities.

Prophylaxis. Contacts of the patient should be examined and treated as necessary. Exposure to repeated venereal infection may precipitate a relapse of the disease, and should be avoided.

Polymyalgia rheumatica

This syndrome of aching muscles in the elderly is not primarily a muscle disease but probably represents an inflammatory condition of central and proximal joints and bursae. There are many causes of the syndrome, among them myeloma, neoplasia, polymyositis and rheumatoid arthritis. Usually no underlying disease is found, and in these idiopathic cases there is a strong association with cranial giant cell arteritis, and occasionally with arteritis of major vessels elsewhere. Thus it is important to make an attempt to uncover any sinister cause of the syndrome before embarking on symptomatic suppressive treatment.

The idiopathic syndrome is commoner in women and may be diagnosed on the history of severe limb girdle stiffness in an elderly patient, the finding of limited central and proximal joint movement, and a high ESR. Unfortunately a very few patients with this syndrome have a normal ESR even in the presence of cranial arteritis; this slightly limits its value as a screening investigation. Electromyographic findings and muscle biopsies are normal.

TREATMENT

If symptoms are relatively mild, and the ESR only moderately raised (say up to 50 mm Westergren), phenylbutazone or indomethacin often relieve "muscular" symptoms. However, arteritis will not be adequately suppressed, and it has even been suggested that symptomatic improvement may lead to its being overlooked. As cranial arteritis has been found occasionally in patients with no local symptoms or signs and even with a normal ESR, a counsel of perfection includes routine temporal artery biopsy. Unfortunately the biopsy may not include a diseased segment of artery and a normal result neither excludes the diagnosis nor provides a complete reassurance.

When the stiffness is "crippling", or the ESR markedly raised (say above 50 mm) steroids are usually needed for control. Immediate steroid suppression is imperative when arteritis is suspected, as untreated involvement of cranial arteries may lead to blindness or strokes. The suppressive action of steroids makes it desirable to complete investigations before these drugs are started, and a temporal artery biopsy is helpful. Failure to take this biopsy makes it more difficult to advise about long term management. Tabs. prednisone 20–60 mg daily is started and the dose titrated slowly down to the minimum needed to relieve symptoms and maintain a normal ESR. A maintenance dose of prednisone 5–15 mg daily may be needed for 1½ or more years, the natural history of the "idiopathic" disease. The final steroid reduction is controlled by repeated ESR estimations and observation of symptoms and signs, the objectives being to keep the patient comfortable and the ESR below 20 mm.

An alternative school of opinion maintains that as no amount of investigation can absolutely exclude the possibility of cranial arteritis and its serious consequences, all patients with polymyalgia rheumatica should be treated with steroids. This opinion presupposes that the risk of treating a larger and miscellaneous group of disorders by steroid suppression is less that that of occasionally failing to detect and treat cranial arteritis, a hypothesis which has not been put to the test.

Ankylosing spondylitis

This is an inflammatory disease predominantly of the spine and usually affecting young men. A strong association with the HLA–27 leucocyte antigen has been demonstrated. The sacro-iliac joints are affected first, and the process classically ascends the spine. Occasionally the disease starts in a peripheral point, and atypical forms occur in association with Reiter's disease, psoriasis, and chronic intestinal disorders. Iritis is a common complication; aortitis and amyloid disease are rare. The cervical spine may become rigid and fragile, and may be fatally fractured.

Pathological changes similar to those in rheumatoid disease may be found in synovial joints but usually there is a greater tendency to new bone formation and ankylosis. Vascular fibrous tissue invades intervertebral discs and vertebral bodies leading to calcification and ossification.

The early clinical features are recurrent low backache often with marked morning stiffness, and positive sacro-iliac tests. The ESR is usually raised, and rheumatoid nodules and serum factor absent. X-rays may show erosion and sclerosis of the sacro-iliac joints early in the disease and ossification of intervertebral ligaments later.

TREATMENT

Preservation of mobility is the key to treatment. Comparatively short periods of enforced rest lead to marked stiffening. Normal active life should be encouraged, but violent sport or hobbies avoided. Breathing exercises are important, and there is a clinical impression that exercise regimes designed to counteract the kyphotic tendency help. Patients should use a firm mattress and should lie prone on a firm surface for 15 minutes twice daily.

Drugs. In mild cases the anti-rheumatics used initially for rheumatoid arthritis will reduce symptoms. Phenylbutazone 100 mg t.d.s., is very effective and has stood the test of time. If it is successful but cannot be tolerated, the antacid- or enteric-coated version may be used, or oxyphenbutazone substituted. Indomethacin 25 mg t.d.s. is an effective alternative. Systemic steroids are rarely justified and then only for uncontrolled disease activity, but their effects are disappointing. Intra-articular steroids are helpful for affected peripheral joints.

Radiotherapy. Deep X-ray therapy usually relieves the pain of spondylitis. As it does not influence the natural history, but increases the risk of leukaemia its use is reserved for special circumstances: 1. Patients unwilling or unable to take regular drugs under supervision. 2. Active disease uncontrolled by drugs. 3. A peripheral joint.

Surgery. Synovectomy and arthroplasty operations have similar indications to those in rheumatoid arthritis. A stiff hip is particularly disabling in a patient with a stiff back and invites arthroplasty. Where severe incapacitating kyphosis has developed, spinal osteotomy should be considered.

CRYSTAL SYNOVITIS

Gout

The arthritic features of gout are caused by the local deposition of urate crystals. This urate deposition results from persistently elevated blood uric acid levels, and these in turn are caused either by a genetically determined error of uric acid metabolism, or by an undue stress being placed upon normal uric acid metabolism or a combination of these circumstances. The additional stress may be due to high purine intake, abnormal turnover of nucleoprotein, or impaired renal urate handling. Frequently latent gout becomes overt when an undue stress is superimposed upon a covert metabolic error. Gout is commonest in adult males, occurs in postmenopausal females, and is rare before puberty.

Gouty arthritis should be suspected when arthritis of almost unrivalled acuteness occurs in the hallux metatarso-phalangeal joint, in the mid-tarsal joint, or less commonly in other peripheral joints. Gout rarely affects central joints and never in the first attack. Occasionally gout has a poly-articular onset and may resemble rheumatoid arthritis.

A suspected diagnosis of gout is sustained by finding repeatedly elevated blood uric acid levels. Caution in interpreting uric acid levels is necessary as they may be elevated by many drugs (notably thiazides and small doses of salicylates), and because normal values vary with the technique used by the laboratory. Confirmation of the diagnosis requires the identification of urate crystals in inflammatory joint fluid, synovial biopsy specimen, or the identification of a tophus. "Punched-out" areas in bone X-rays do not confirm the diagnosis as they may be confused with rheumatoid erosions.

TREATMENT

Acute attacks. The patient will spontaneously rest and protect the joint, and may find a cold compress or spray comforting. Adequate fluid intake is encouraged. Colchicine is traditional and effective treatment. 1 mg is given at the first notion of an attack, followed by 0.5 mg 2-hourly until pain is relieved or nausea or diarrhea supervene. Oral phenylbutazone is more effective. 200 mg should be given 6-hourly in the first day followed by 200 mg 8-hourly the second day, then 100 mg t.d.s. until the attack has settled. Intramuscular phenylbutazone 600 mg has no advantage in speed of action, but may be used in the presence of vomiting. Unfortunately if injected near a nerve it produces irrecoverable paralysis, so the placing of the injection must be made with great care. Oral indomethacin is a useful alternative and may be given 200 mg in the first day, reducing to 25 mg t.d.s. Intra-articular steroid injections are dramatically effective where feasible, but are often precluded by the technical difficulty of injecting an acutely painful, small joint. Intractable attacks may be relieved by ACTH gel 40 units or tabs. prednisone 25 mg daily, but relapses occur on withdrawal.

Interval treatment. Once started this type of treatment should be continued indefinitely, as the metabolic disorder is not reversible. Therefore the diagnosis must be beyond reasonable doubt. Uric acid lowering drugs are given if: 1. acute attacks are occurring frequently; 2. the blood uric acid is repeatedly 2 mg % (0.12 mmol/1) or more above the laboratory's upper limit of normal; or 3. clinical tophi or bone "cysts" are present. Uricosurics are the traditional first choice. Tabs. probenecid 0.5 g is started once daily after food, working up to 1.5 or 2 g daily. Should this dose be ineffective, or produce nausea, vomiting, or a rash, sulphinpyrazone should be substituted. Tabs, sulphinpyrazone 50 mg daily is given, gradually increasing to 50–100 mg t.d.s. If neither of these uricosuric drugs can be tolerated, or renal function is impaired or stones found, or gross uric acid overproduction and excretion is occurring, a xanthine oxidase inhibitor should be used. Tabs. allopurinol 100 mg daily should be started, and slowly increased to a therapeutic dose of 100–200 mg t.d.s Rashes may occur but other side effects are rare, and this drug is replacing uricosurics as the first choice. Any drug which lowers the blood uric acid should be started in small doses as acute attacks of gout are induced by changes of blood level. During the first month and covering any increase in dose of these drugs, colchicine 0.5 mg t.d.s., phenylbutazone 100 mg t.d.s. or indomethacin 25 mg t.d.s. should be given prophylactically. Similar prophylactic cover for operations is necessary. Restriction of intake of high purine foods produces a modest fall in uric acid levels but severe restrictions are seldom necessary. However reduction of obesity may well produce a worthwhile reduction in uric acid levels. Alcohol temporarily elevates the blood level and produces attacks of gout and intake should be moderated.

Surgery may be useful to remove mechanically disadvantageous or unsightly tophi. This is helpful in reducing the pool of uric acid to be cleared by the interval drugs.

Pseudogout

Crystals of calcium pyrophosphate may induce a synovitis resembling that of classical gout. Pseudogout tends to affect larger joints especially the knees, and seldom affect joints which are not the site of radiological chondrocalcinosis articularis. Chrondrocalcinosis is occasionally associated with a chronic polyarthritis. In contrast with classical gout, the big toe is scarcely ever affected, there is no diagnostic blood test, and tophi do not occur. Pseudogout is one of two types of arthropathy associated with haemochromatosis.

The diagnosis is suspected when chondrocalcinosis is found in a patient with arthritis, and is confirmed by the identification of calcium pyrophosphate crystals in synovial joint fluid. These can be distinguished by polarised light techniques from urate crystals. Generalised chondrocalcinosis itself may be associated with prolonged hypercalcaemia, alkaptonuria, and haemochromatosis as well as hyperoricaemia and these causes should be investigated.

TREATMENT

Acute attacks are a further example of crystal synovitis and may be treated similarly to gout— with phenylbutazone or indomethacin. However they are best treated by aspiration of the joint fluid and injection of steroid. Phenylbutazone, indomethacin and perhaps salicylates may help the chronic forms.

HAEMOPHILIC ARTHRITIS

Bleeding into joints occurs at some stage in most patients with factor VIII deficiency and causes acute arthritis of a severity matched only by crystal synovitis, infective arthritis, and rheumatic fever. The knee is the most commonly affected joint, followed by the ankle, elbow, shoulder and hip. Bleeds also occur into muscles and along tissue planes.

Following the haemarthrosis red cells are lysed within the joint, and the haemosiderin phagocytosed by synovial cells. Recurrent bleeds lead to capsular fibrosis, and in chronic arthropathy there may be contractures and enlargement of bone ends. Subcortical bleeds cause ischaemic lesions of bone ends and secondary degenerative changes follow. When there is a history of preceding trauma the bleed is often more severe.

Attacks may affect males of any age, and haemophilia should even be considered in adult males with painful joint swelling and haemorrhagic effusions. Constitutional disturbance is relatively mild, and rheumatoid factor tests negative.

TREATMENT

The acute arthritis needs immediate treatment to minimise the risk of permanent damage. Analgesics, ice packs, and splints relieve pain while the patient is sent to the nearest haemophilic centre. An intravenous infusion of antihaemophilic globulin (AHG) is given immediately. If there is obstruction to vessels or nerves near the joint, or if the joint is grossly distended, aspiration is strongly indicated and should be carried out as the infusion starts. Even with lesser degrees of joint distension aspiration hastens recovery and relief of pain but this advantage must be weighed against the pain of the procedure. The skin and joint capsule are infiltrated with local anaesthetic through a fine bore needle, and the aspiration made through a wide bore needle. When the pain and swelling start to settle, static exercises to the muscles controlling the joint must be started to prevent the rapid muscular wasting. Domestic self-treatment is becoming available and offers hope of additional relief.

Chronic arthritis often follows despite the best attempts at its prevention. When mild contractures occur, they may be corrected by gentle physiotherapeutic stretching, and the patient himself can often help with these manual procedures. If contractures are more severe, serial splints or manipulation under anaesthetic may be needed but the latter must be carried out under AHG cover. Occasionally pathological fractures occur through porotic bone near chronically affected joints, and it may be difficult to differentiate the associated haemorrhage from an intra-articular bleed. It is possible to modify the load on a joint and reduce the incidence of bleeding, for example by providing a weight relieving caliper for the knee.

Reconstructive surgery can help in isolated cases and synovectomy is under trial in an attempt to prevent recurrent bleeds. It is sometimes necessary for these patients to live in a sheltered environment particularly during school and training years.

BONE INFECTIONS

Osteomyelitis—acute onset

This painful condition is an acute emergency. The staphylococcus is the commonest cause, and the infection enters the metaphysis of a bone via the blood stream. Occasionally the streptococcus, pneumococcus, salmonella, or brucella may be responsible. The organism multiplies in the bone marrow causing fever, tachycardia, leukocytosis, and severe pain. There is local tenderness of bone and later redness and swelling. The pus may isolate areas of bone which form sequestra, and nearly always causes periosteal elevation. X-ray changes are late, a patchy porosis appearing at about 2 weeks, followed by periosteal new bone, and later still dense sequestra.

TREATMENT

When possible blood cultures and aspiration should precede antibiotics, but if these investigations are not rapidly available antibiotics must be started. The potential seriousness of the condition and the danger of delay indicate the need for a broader spectrum antibiotic than penicillin. Bacteriological advice should be sought and in the event of delay cloxacillin or fucidin should be started.

Chronic Sequelae. Incomplete resolution may lead to recurrent flares, sinuses, or sequestra. These should be treated with antibiotics or by excision.

Osteomyelitis—chronic onset

Tuberculosis is the commonest cause of chronic bone infection; vertebrae are most commonly affected but occasionally flat bones (rib or skull), or a finger (dactylitis) may be involved. Spread is to adjacent vertebrae and the symptoms merely a dull ache and vague ill-health. Osteoporosis follows, and two infected vertebrae with the enclosed disc may collapse causing an angular kyphos. Abscess formation sometimes causes local spinal cord damage with paraplegia, and pus may track to point at a distance. The diagnosis is suspected from the general condition, the chronic history, loss of spinal movement, and the presence of a cold abscess. It is confirmed by the radiological appearance, and biopsy is rarely needed for confirmation.

TREATMENT

This consists basically of antituberculous drugs, and rest in a spinal bed. Surgery may be needed to remove necrotic tissue, to stabilise the spine, or to decompress the spinal cord.

DEGENERATIVE JOINT DISEASE

Osteoarthrosis

Degenerative disease of joints causes pain, deformity and limitation of joint movement, often in older people.

The basic pathology involves hyaline cartilage, whose status quo is normally maintained by the balance between wear and repair. There may be an unknown genetic fault in cartilage make-up which makes it wear more quickly (Primary OA), or there may be undue stress on the joint following inflammatory disease, obesity, malalignment or incongruous joint surfaces (Secondary OA). The earliest pathological change is dulling and softening of the cartilage surface accompanied by reduction in the staining of mucopolysaccharides. Later a tangential flaking of the cartilage is followed by the formation of deep fissures. Fragments of cartilage break off and lie in the cavity. Small fragments migrate into the synovium and are then phagocytosed. The ensuing reaction leads to fibrosis and to contracture of the joint capsule. Hyperaemia of the bone end ensues and stimulates formation of cartilage at the joint margin; some of this becomes calcified and ossified. These changes lead to the radiological changes of reduction in joint space (especially at the weight bearing area), and osteophyte formation. Cartilage may be worn away completely leaving a dense bony surface, a process called eburnation, and occasionally fragments of cartilage break off and form loose bodies in the joint. Pain is thought to arise either from hyperaemic bone or from capsular stretching, and it seems to be the latter mechanism which accounts for pain occurring frequently in joints whose extremes of range are used.

One or more joints may be affected. Swelling of the joint often feels bony hard, and fluid and soft tissue swelling are less obvious. There is no diagnostic test for this condition, and there are no systemic features. The ESR is normal, and radiological changes including osteophyte formation often occur in symptomless joints. Therefore the diagnosis is clinical and rests upon finding symptoms and signs and later radiological changes in joints susceptible to osteoarthrosis. The pattern of joints affected varies with the cause. Primary OA often affects the terminal interphalangeal joints (Heberden's nodes), the carpo-metacarpal of the thumb, as well as weight bearing joints. Secondary OA affects the joints damaged by the predisposing cause, whether it be rheumatoid arthritis, gout, or an old fracture.

TREATMENT

This is influenced by the number, distribution and severity of the joints affected. As in other chronic painful diseases the patient's pain threshold must be assessed so that complex treatments are not ordered when gentle reassurance is required. Any underlying disorder should be treated, and whenever weight bearing joints are affected obesity reduced.

Pain relief. Heat may be applied with wax baths, infrared lamps, or short-wave diathermy, and unless accompanied by skilled physiotherapy is better provided by the patient using domestic methods. Hot water bottles, electric blankets, hot baths, and electric fires all provide temporary relief. The useful drugs are similar to those for early rheumatoid arthritis. Aspirin is often helpful, and codeine compound may add to its affect, but many patients prefer phenylbutazone or indomethacin. Sometimes acute "flares" occur, possibly due to joint haemorrhage or damage to cartilage following minor trauma. An intraarticular steroid injection is then effective. Sometimes a few days' bed rest relieves pain, and fortunately degenerative joints do not stiffen as quickly as inflammatory joints.

Improvement of range. Repetitive capsular strains are painful, and may be relieved by stretching the capsule. This stretching can be achieved gently by a physiotherapist using heat as an analgesic, or may be obtained more quickly by manipulation under anaesthetic.

Reduction of stress. Patients should be instructed not to "work off" their pain. Stress should be lessened by resting the affected joint when possible. In weight bearing joints this involves avoiding unnecessary standing, and the use of a walking stick.

Specific examples of treatment

Terminal interphalangeal joints. Wax baths, analgesics and exercises are useful. Steroids and surgery have no place.

Carpo-metacarpal of thumb. Recurrent pain is occasionally relieved by a suitable splint, and a local steroid injection may help. Excision arthroplasty or arthrodesis is needed when pain is severe.

Wrist. This usually follows rheumatoid arthritis or injury. A polythene splint or steroid injection may help, but arthrodesis is occasionally required.

Elbow. This frequently does not cause symptoms

as extremes of range are rarely required. Splints are helpful, and arthrodesis and arthroplasty occasionally useful. Stretching is rarely possible and attempts may be harmful. Tendon lesions are frequent near the elbow, and must be distinguished from joint disease. Tendon lesions respond to hydrocortisone acetate infiltration or local frictions.

Shoulder. This is rarely the site of primary OA, and pain is more often caused by a capsulitis which can be identified by its characteristic pattern of restriction of movement. Local steroids often relieve pain, and passive stretching may hasten recovery of range. Tendon lesions are common and again can be differentiated clinically from joint capsule constricture as they are associated with pain on resisted movement but a full passive range. After accurate localisation they are effectively treated by steroid injections or frictions.

Hip. Short-wave diathermy, passive capsule stretching and analgesics suffice for mild degrees. A walking stick is frequently helpful, and should have a rubber tip. Osteotomy is sometimes used to relax the joint capsule, but when severe, arthrodesis or arthroplasty may be needed. In cases where the acetabular cup is shallow it may be deepened by forming a shelf or by acetabular osteotomy.

Knee. If analgesics fail, a polythene splint may help. The quadriceps muscle wastes quickly and should have intensive static exercises. Arthrodesis, osteotomy, and arthroplasty all have a place. If the main disease is of the patello-femoral joint tibial advancement or patellectomy should be considered.

Hallux metatarso-phalangeal. A rockered sole often eases pain, but occasionally arthroplasty or arthrodesis is necessary. Silastic prostheses are useful here.

Disc prolapse and spondylosis

These degenerative or traumatic disorders of the spinal column may give bouts of pain and limitation of movement, usually affecting the low lumbar or low cervical regions.

Minor injuries to the posterior longitudinal ligament sometimes combined with degenerative changes in disc material allow posterolateral or posterior bulging of the intervertebral disc.

1. A small protrusion disturbs the symmetry of the articulations between vertebrae and leads to asymmetrical limitation of spinal movement. Impingement on the pain sensitive dura mater leads to pain of rather vague and apparently extra-segmental reference. With cervical protrusions pain is referred to the shoulder, inter-scapular region, or the head; from lumbar protrusions it is referred to the low back, sacro-iliac region or buttock. Dural irritation is usually accompanied by dural signs – limitation of femoral or sciatic stretch tests.

2. If the protrusion is larger nerve root pain may follow. Commonly this is C7 distribution from a cervical lesion, and L5 or S1 (sciatica) from a lumbar disc protrusion. Motor, reflex, or sensory deficits may occur.

3. A very large cervical protrusion may damage the spinal cord, causing spastic paraparesis, and in the lumbar region the cauda equina may be damaged leading to bladder symptoms. These features can occur in the absence of gross radiological changes, but diminution of intervertebral joint space and osteophyte formation are often seen. In the presence of a narrow spinal canal similar sequelae can be produced by smaller protrusions.

Apophyseal and neurocentral joints also undergo degenerative changes which may cause pain and limitation of movement. It is difficult to know how frequently these joints are the cause of symptoms, or how often radiological changes which are found reflect the disturbed anatomy at the disc joints. Occasionally a large osteophyte will cause a root palsy by obstructing a cervical intervertebral foramen.

These mechanical disorders of the spine are suggested by an episodic history, relief by rest, and the complete absence of systemic upset. A slowly progressive onset, unremitting pain, symmetrical limitation of movements, neurological signs, or involvement of more than one nerve root should raise the suspicion of a more serious pathology. Sacro-iliac tests are negative.

TREATMENT

Conservative. As pain from these lesions is often self-limiting, active intervention is seldom essential. Analgesics and rest are the foundations of treatment and should be matched to the severity of pain. Salicylates, compound codeine, dihydrocodeine, pethidine or morphine may be needed. Rest is most effectively achieved in bed, as only when recumbent is the bodyweight diverted from the discs. The cervical spine should be maintained in a neutral position by adjustment of pillows, and the lumbar spine supported by boards beneath the mattress to achieve a neutral and pain-free position. Lesser degrees of rest may be obtained whilst ambulant by supplying a semi-rigid collar, or a lumbo-sacral belt with steel supports, or a plaster of paris or polythene corset. When bed rest has allowed almost complete relief of pain, gradual mobilisation should be encouraged.

Accessory treatments. Manipulation may hasten reduction of either cervical or lumbar disc prolapse and is indicated in acute lesions causing limitation of movement and dural pain. Manipulation is contraindicated in the presence of severe pain, root pain, neurological deficit, disturbance of micturition, vascular disease, or when there is any doubt about the diagnosis. Cervical manipulations are performed with manual traction, and most manoeuvres involve rotation away from the side of maximum pain.

Traction seems to hasten relief of root pain, presumably by reducing the extent of disc protrusion. The main indication is root pain in the absence of neurological deficit, and traction may also be tried if manipulation has failed. Traction is best given daily. Cervical traction of 20 lbs. (9 kg) should be applied with the patient supine, but stronger and more effective traction may be given with the patient sitting, lumbar thoracic harness, and a force of up to 120 lbs (50 kg) applied through a harness pulling on the pelvis.

Epidural analgesia gives temporary relief from severe sciatica or lumbago. This is particularly useful for the few days of intense pain which accompany root interruption. 40–50 ml of 0.5% procaine in normal saline (with no preservative or adrenaline) is injected through the sacral hiatus, and usually produces several hours of analgesia; sometimes pain does not return completely. Corticosteroids can be added to the injection in an attempt to relieve local inflammation and there is evidence that recovery of symptoms is speeded. Most uni-radicular palsies recover in one year, but supportive measures (e.g. a toe-spring) may be needed meantime.

Prophylaxis. Indoctrination of the patient into habits which spare the lumbar spine stresses while flexed are helpful, and these habits can be reinforced by supplying a correctly fitted lumbo-sacral belt. It may be necessary for the patient to change his occupation to avoid harmful stresses. The place of exercise regimes is unclear but all too often they seem illogical.

Operative. Laminectomy and disc removal, or spinal fusion should be considered in conjunction with an orthopaedic or neuro-surgeon for several clinical situations. 1. Frequent incapacitating recurrences not prevented by simpler measures. 2. Insufficient relief by other methods. 3. Serious neurological features (long tract signs from cervical protrusions, progressive or multiple root involvement, or bladder symptoms in lumbar protrusions).

4

DERMATOLOGY

P. F. D. NAYLOR

INTRODUCTION

In this short account of dermatological treatment, attention will be given to general principles rather than detail. Local applications employed in treatment should be kept to a minimum and therefore only the commoner ones which are in use will be mentioned. Proprietary blends of active chemicals such as steroids and antibacterial agents are constantly changing and any list is likely to be out of date before it is published. The principles of treatment, however, and the active drugs available in dermatological practice change more slowly.

The first essential in treatment is accurate diagnosis. A large proportion of dermatological conditions are exogenously determined and appropriate modification of the environmental factors may play a major part in treatment. This is particularly so in eczema. It is not sufficient to diagnose eczema and then apply a potent combined steroid–antibacterial cream. Every effort must be made by careful history taking to determine the skin sites first involved and the pattern of spread. Only in this way is it possible to suspect and diagnose an allergic contact or a primary irritant eczema. Once such an eczema has become widespread the original pattern may be forgotten by the patient and no longer able to be discovered by the doctor. If the cause is not identified and removed in an exogenous eczema, then the condition is likely to persist indefinitely in spite of the most vigorous local treatment. It may be possible to suppress temporarily a primary irritant eczema with locally applied steroids, but it is the realisation by the patient of the environmental factors involved and their avoidance which will determine the long term success or failure of treatment. A further example of the importance of accurate diagnosis is in the treatment of intertrigo when infection with yeasts and fungi must be distinguished from seborrheic eczema or flexural psoriasis. Although it is difficult to exaggerate the importance of accurate diagnosis and its influence on effective treatment, for the sake of brevity, this will not be reiterated in each section.

ECZEMA

Exogenous eczema

When the causes of the eczema have been identified and, if possible, removed, the next most essential part of treatment is to obtain complete mental and physical rest for the patient. The patients who most persistently assert that rest is impossible are usually most in need of it and if the patient is leading a busy life the best way in which the necessary relaxation may be found is sometimes by admission to hospital. Quite frequently mild sedation is necessary and an antihistamine by mouth such as promethazine hydrochloride or chlorpheniramine seems to accomplish this and reduce the skin irritation.

In the acute stage the skin may be cleansed and cooled by sponging with physiological saline or a dilute solution of potassium permanganate. This may be followed by the local application of a calamine lotion containing 0.25% mild silver protein or a steroid lotion. If there is secondary infection a steroid lotion containing the appropriate antibiotic or one of the hydroxyquinoline derivatives such as clioquinol is often helpful. As the skin heals and dries then the lotions may be replaced by the same ingredients in a cream base. With further improvement an ointment base may be tolerated as a vehicle for the active ingredients. At this stage, tar is occasionally more effective than local steroids and may be used in gradually increasing concentrations. If scratching is playing a part in perpetuating the skin changes, then occlusive dressings with bandages impregnated with hydrocortisone or tar may be extremely useful. It is exceptional for the use of systemic steroids to be justifiable. If at any stage secondary infection is severe, then a systemic antibiotic may be necessary. The following should always be avoided in topical applications due to the risk of sensitisation: penicillin, sulphonamides, antihistamines and local anaesthetics.

Bathing, which must be prohibited during the initial stages, may be gradually introduced using emulsifying ointment BP in place of soap for cleansing purposes; an important practical point is to warn the patient that this will make the bath extremely slippery. When the eczema has settled, then patch testing may be undertaken if indicated in order to look for hypersensitivity to specific agents.

Before the patient returns home it is important that a full and careful explanation be given of the ways in which his life must be modified. Too many patients return home without realising that after an attack of primary irritant eczema it is necessary to protect their skin against irritants for an indefinite period, nor may patients with allergic contact eczema realise that the allergy is likely to persist for the rest of their lives.

After returning home the patient should, whenever possible, have a period of convalescence before a gradual return to full activity.

Atopic eczema

The course of this disorder is usually one of periodic exacerbations and remissions throughout childhood, fortunately with a tendency to improve, in the majority of patients as puberty approaches. The exacerbations may be related to climatic factors or periods of emotional stress but there may be no obvious precipitating factors. Diet has no effect on the disease. Treatment is directed at helping the child by sedation and local therapy and the parents by encouragement through the difficult periods. Sedation at night with antihistamines is helpful as these children are often extremely wakeful and seem to be able to endure long periods without sleep. If the family becomes demoralised by lack of sleep or the patient's skin is deteriorating, a period of in-patient treatment may be helpful. Local applications containing tar or hydrocortisone are the most useful. Some patients show a strong preference for either cream or ointment bases. The newer potent steroids should only rarely be used and never for more than a few weeks as they may easily cause dermal atrophy or systemic side effects. Recurrent boils sometimes complicate the situation and an antibacterial cream combined with hydrocortisone may be employed such as 1% hydrocortisone acetate in chlorhexidine cream BPC; occasionally ultraviolet light baths are helpful. The skin is often very dry and emulsifying ointment BP may be used for cleansing purposes. Systemic steroids may, on very rare occasions, be justified. Vaccination for the patient and the whole family must be avoided because of the danger of eczema vaccinatum.

Seborrheic eczema

This variety of constitutional eczema is sufficiently different from the varieties of eczema already discussed to warrant a separate description of the treatment. Mild dandruff may be treated by rubbing into the scalp at night salicylic acid and sulphur cream BPC either half or full strength. This should be left on overnight and removed in the morning with a medicated shampoo containing coal tar. The process may be repeated twice weekly. If there is a great deal of irritation and erythema a steroid lotion or cream may be used or, even better, a steroid in a non-greasy base specially formulated for the scalp. If there is infection and crusting a combined steroid–antibacterial cream may be used. Aqueous cream with sulphur and salicylic acid may also be used for eczematous patches over the sternum in the same way as for dandruff.

The generalised eruptive petaloid seborrheids which trouble these patients should be treated by bed rest and mild sedation with an antihistamine by mouth in the acute phase together with the local application of oily calamine lotion containing $\frac{1}{2}$ or 1% strong coal tar solution or 1% hydrocortisone lotion or cream.

The intertriginous eczema and fissuring in the groins, perineum, axillae and retro-auricular areas usually respond very well to a steroid-antibacterial cream, such as 1% hydrocortisone cream with 1% clioquinol. This is also very helpful for the frequently associated pruritus ani and aqueous cream BP should be used for cleansing purposes in place of soap when bathing and should also be used after defaecation.

Napkin rash

This is due to the irritant effect of wet alkaline napkins on the skin, together with infection by yeasts and bacteria. An important part of treatment is the correct laundering of napkins. After washing they should be carefully rinsed to remove all traces of soap or detergent and should then be soaked in an antiseptic such as benzalkonium chloride to kill urea splitting organisms which make them alkaline and extremely irritating to the skin. Frequent changing of the napkins is essential to keep the skin as dry as possible. Hydrocortisone lotion or cream containing clioquinol may be used in the acute stage and nystatin ointment should be used if there is considerable infection with *Candida albicans*. Zinc and castor oil ointment is a helpful protective local application when the rash is healing.

PSORIASIS

This is one of the commonest and most persistent eruptions. It is almost always possible to obtain a good measure of control but the time taken by different patients to do this varies a great deal. As relapse is unfortunately very common after reduction of intensive treatment then each patient must be encouraged to decide how much time to devote to his eruption; this will depend upon the severity of the psoriasis and how much it worries the individual patient. Treatment consists almost entirely of local applications and these vary with the type of psoriasis.

Guttate psoriasis

This widespread eruption of small psoriatic lesions, which may be precipitated by a streptococcal throat infection, usually tends to improve spontaneously. The speed of improvement sometimes seems to be increased by local applications such as oily cream containing 1–2% strong coal tar solution. An alternative is ultraviolet light baths but these should not be given in the early acute phase. Quite frequently the clearing is not complete and then local applications are required as described under chronic psoriasis.

Chronic psoriasis

If the psoriasis is of limited extent then treatment may be carried out by the patient at home. Local applications should be used after a bath when the scales should be removed by gentle scrubbing. After drying, the preparation should be applied accurately to the lesions and covered with a light dressing. A suitable local application contains tar and salicylic acid such as:— salicylic acid 2; strong coal tar solution 6; emulsifying ointment to 100. An ointment which patients find more acceptable is beclomethasone dipropionate ointment diluted 1:4 as follows:— 0.025% beclomethasone dipropionate ointment 25%, white soft paraffin to 100%. This may also be applied at night under polythene occlusion.

If, however, the eruption becomes acute or more widespread, a period of in-patient treatment will be needed. Beclomethasone dipropionate ointment diluted 1:4 may be used for acute widespread psoriasis. Dithranol is extremely effective but messy to use and should be reserved for the less acute eruptions. A trial area should be treated initially with 0.1% or 0.25% Dithranol Paste BPC and, if well tolerated, the treated area may be extended and the concentration of dithranol increased gradually up to 1%. The dithranol

by day can be alternated with the diluted beclomethasone dipropionate by night and this may produce rapid clearing of the lesions. The effect of tar and dithranol is enhanced by ultraviolet light but this should be used with caution as an acute exacerbation of the psoriasis may be produced by over-treatment. Tar baths may be helpful particularly when a patient with widespread psoriasis is being treated at home. 15–30 ml of strong coal tar solution should be added to a bath.

Flexural psoriasis

This may occur in the perineum, axillae and under the breasts. The most effective treatment is the local application of one of the strong steroids such as betamethasone valerate cream or ointment and these may be more effective when combined with clioquinol. If these are used for any length of time in the flexures, dermal atrophy and striae are unfortunately quite common. Fungi and yeasts may flourish in the flexural lesions and may need appropriate treatment.

Psoriasis of the scalp

This usually responds quite well to coal tar and salicylic acid ointment BNF. This should be massaged into the scalp at night, usually twice weekly is sufficient, and shampooed out in the morning with a medicated shampoo containing coal tar. If the patient finds this regime very troublesome then the newer potent steroids may be acceptable when formulated specially for the scalp. Occasionally, betamethasone valerate cream with 0.1% dithranol is very effective.

Local applications are ineffective for psoriasis of the nails.

Systemic treatment

Oral triamcinolone often produces a dramatic clearing of lesions. Control is only maintained, however, by increasing the dose with the risk of unpleasant side effects. Often when the dose is reduced this causes a severe rebound effect which may be pustular. This can be a very serious and even fatal complication.

When psoriasis is of such severity as to incapacitate a patient or to prevent him from working then it may be justifiable to administer the folic acid antagonist, methotrexate. This is a treatment which carries considerable risk and should only be done under circumstances where the necessary biochemical investigations may be routinely performed. It is rarely justifiable during the reproductive period of life. However, under special circumstances, it may produce well worth-while improvement.

Diet

At the moment there is no evidence that special diets have any specific part to play in the treatment of psoriasis. Obese patients with flexural psoriasis may benefit from a weight-reducing diet.

ACNE

Complete control of this troublesome and disfiguring condition is often difficult but it is usually possible to obtain sufficient improvement to make the rather time-consuming treatment worthwhile. In more severe cases treatment is important in that it will prevent or reduce scarring. Treatment will have to be continued until spontaneous remission of the disease occurs. These facts should be kindly but firmly explained to patients to avoid misunderstanding and disappointment.

Local treatment is aimed at the removal of blackheads and excess sebum and causing a mild desquamation. Blackheads should be removed carefully and completely by the patient with a proper expressor, a few being done each day; the help of a parent is valuable for difficult or inaccessible ones. Removal of sebum should be carried out, before going to bed, with a detergent solution such as cetrimide solution BPC. A detergent washing tablet is often helpful and may be applied with a shaving brush which is used to massage the skin at the same time. The cleansing agent should be removed by thoroughly rinsing the skin with water and after drying, one of the following local applications should be applied: calamine lotion with 4–8% precipitated sulphur for the face, back and chest; a cream containing 10% benzoyl peroxide for the face, resorcinol and sulphur paste BPC—full or half strength, for the chest and back. A wide range of other local applications is available but control is generally possible with simple measures if these are carried out carefully and regularly. The local applications should be left on overnight and then removed with the usual toilet soap in the morning. If this regimen produces too much erythema and a sore skin the sebum removal should be limited to alternate nights.

Cystic and pustular acne are particularly persistent and may cause severe scarring. They sometimes respond very well to tetracyclines by mouth starting at 250 mg four times a day for a week

and gradually reducing to 250 mg twice daily. The drug should be taken before meals and courses should last 6–8 weeks but may be repeated. Persistent cysts may respond well to freezing with carbon dioxide snow for 10–15 seconds; some may require surgical drainage or diathermy puncture.

Courses of ultraviolet light may be helpful for all types of acne but should be carried out under medical supervision. Occasionally, dietary factors are important but the patient is often well aware of these and avoids the offending things. Chocolate should be avoided and carbohydrate restricted. Hormone therapy and superficial X-ray therapy should not be used.

An endocrine cause for acne should be borne in mind and menstrual irregularities enquired about and hirsutes noted. Special investigations may be needed along these lines. It should be remembered that acne may be caused by environmental factors such as chlorinated aromatic hydrocarbons, sometimes used in the manufacture of electric cables, and also oils.

Acne rosacea

These patients should try and avoid the factors which they know produce flushing of the face, but this is often difficult. An excessive consumption of tea or alcohol should be discouraged. Tetracyclines by mouth in a dose of 250 mg once or twice daily before meals may be dramatic in their effect. Helpful local applications are 1% or 2% precipitated sulphur in aqueous cream applied with massage at night and hydrocortisone cream BPC in the morning. The potent steroid applications should not be used as these may make the condition worse and also produce telangiectasia.

SKIN INFECTIONS

The skin is susceptible to attack by a wide range of organisms both bacterial and fungal. In many of these conditions there exist constitutional factors which predispose the patient to such attacks. Only the common infections are here described.

Impetigo

This is the most superficial of the bacterial infections and is most often the result of staphylococcal infection but may be a combined staphylococcal and streptococcal infection. It is almost always susceptible to local anti-bacterial agents and only rarely are systemic antibiotics needed.

In impetigo of the scalp the possibility of pediculosis must be borne in mind.

A swab should be taken at the first attendance for bacterial culture and sensitivities to be performed. Treatment need not await the results but may be modified at the next attendance if the clinical response has been disappointing. All lesions should be gently cleaned three or four times daily with cetrimide solution BPC; if this is poorly tolerated then physiological saline may be used. This should be followed by the local application of an anti-bacterial agent; chlortetracycline ointment BPC is one of the most effective of these and sensitivity reactions are rare; its use, however, should be limited to out-patients because of the risk of bacterial resistance developing. Another very effective agent is a mixture of 0.25% neomycin and 0.25% gramicidin in an ointment base. It is usually possible to eliminate the infection in 1–2 weeks. Children should be kept away from school and each child should use his own towel in the home.

Recurrent boils and carbuncles

This is a frequently encountered problem and very often the underlying cause remains obscure. Eczema is a common background and diabetes must be excluded. The object of treatment is to reduce the staphylococcal population of the skin and eliminate the staphylococci carried in the nose and perineum. Cultures and sensitivities should be carried out from a boil and also from the nose and perineum; in family outbreaks the whole family should be investigated in this way and carriers of staphylococci should be treated. Chlorhexidine 0.1%—neomycin 0.5% cream should be applied to the nasal vestibuli twice daily for 2 weeks. Chlorhexidine cream BPC should be applied to the perineum twice daily and also to the skin round the boils. The use of an antiseptic soap helps to reduce the skin population of staphylococci. Systemic antibiotics may be needed if the boils are large and localising poorly and surgical drainage should be carried out when appropriate.

Chronic paronychia

The predisposing factors are wet work and a poor peripheral circulation in this chronic infection of the nail fold with bacteria and yeasts —usually *Staphylococcus albus* and *Candida albicans*.

The only effective remedy is to keep the appropriate fingers completely dry for a period of 3–6 months. This should be done by wearing cotton gloves for all housework to reduce the necessity for frequent hand washing. All wet work should be done in rubber gloves with cotton gloves underneath; the rubber gloves should not be worn for longer than 5 minutes at a time. Essential personal washing should be done with waterproof finger stalls on the appropriate fingers with an elastic band round the base of the finger. A great deal of encouragement to follow this regimen is needed by most patients. Local applications are only of secondary importance but magenta paint BPC or 3% clioquinol cream may be useful.

Fungal infections

The diagnosis of all suspected fungal infections should be confirmed by microscopical examination and, where facilities allow, should be identified by culture. It is important not to mistake a fungal infection for eczema as the local application of strong steroid preparations may make a fungal infection considerably worse.

Acute and severe tinea of the feet or groins is usually better treated with the patient resting in bed. If there is secondary bacterial infection and cellulitis then systemic antibiotics may be needed. Local treatment initially should be limited to sponging or soaking the affected area in physiological saline or aqueous 1:8000 potassium permanganate. This may be followed by the local application of calamine lotion with 0.25% mild silver protein or possibly hydrocortisone lotion with clioquinol. As the local inflammatory reaction settles then more potent anti-fungal agents may be applied as in chronic infections.

Chronic tinea of the feet may be treated as follows: local application of compound benzoic acid ointment BPC (Whitfield's ointment) at night and light cotton socks should be worn in bed. The feet should be washed in the morning and powdered with zinc undecenoate dusting-powder BPC. Open-stitch nylon socks should be worn during the day and sandals in preference to shoes. Chronic tinea of the groins may be treated with half strength compound benzoic acid ointment BPC or zinc undecenoate ointment BP. Pityriasis versicolor affecting the limbs and trunk may be treated by the local application of a 10% aqueous solution of sodium thiosulphate once or twice daily.

The anti-fungal antibiotic, griseofulvin, is effective against a wide range of fungi and is particularly useful in widespread fungal infections, in fungal infection of the nails and in ringworm of the scalp. It is fungistatic and works by being incorporated into the new keratin being formed and thereby preventing invasion by the fungus; it therefore takes time in which to work, and for example in ringworm of the scalp, treatment must continue until non-infected hair has grown out—a period of 6–8 weeks. The infected portions of the hairs should then be removed with clippers. Tinea of the nails may require griseofulvin therapy for 6–12 months or even longer. It is not effective against *Candida albicans*. The drug is given in a dose of 250 mg twice a day. In all superficial fungal infections relapses are common.

INFESTATIONS

Scabies
The ascaricide most usually employed is benzyl benzoate application BP which is the 25% emulsion. Equally satisfactory is gamma benzene hexachloride—usually the 1% cream. The latter preparation is rather less irritating to the skin and is as effective as benzyl benzoate.

The method of using either is the same. The application is creamed-on after a bath, to the whole body surface except the face and scalp. The process is repeated on the second day without bathing. On the third day the patient is instructed to bath, to dress in clean clothing and to change the bed linen. Clothing should be laundered, cleaned or left to hang for 2 weeks. The whole family must be treated in this way even if symptom free as itching may not occur for several weeks after infestation has occurred and its absence must not be taken to mean freedom from infestation. Irritation may persist for 2–3 weeks and does not necessarily imply failure of treatment. When treatment does fail it is usually due to faulty technique in applying the acaricide or failure to treat other members of the household.

Pediculosis
The drugs employed are either Dicophane (DDT) Carbaryl or gamma benzene hexachloride (gamma BHC). These are available in a range of preparations as powder, cream, lotion and shampoo.

SKIN TUMOURS

Virus warts
Before starting treatment the diagnosis must be verified by seeing the presence of a papillary structure within the lesion. To do this it may be necessary to pare away the superficial keratin with a sharp scalpel.

A large proportion of warts disappear without treatment within a year or so. For this reason treatment should not be too energetically pursued if it involves the production of scarring or upsetting a child. Simple remedies consist of paring the lesion daily and painting it accurately with the following:—formalin 5%, salicylic acid 12%, acetone 12%, collodion to 100%. The effect of this may be enhanced by prior maceration either with 40% salicylic acid plaster or zinc oxide self adhesive plaster. This treatment may be carried out by the patient. More resistant lesions may require treatment by freezing with carbon dioxide 'slush'—a mixture of solid carbon dioxide and acetone; this may be applied accurately to the wart with a fine brush for 3–4 minutes. Plantar warts may be frozen with carbon dioxide snow in a wooden holder applied with firm pressure until a white rim of frozen skin appears around the periphery of the applicator — this usually takes about 5 minutes but may be less. Liquid nitrogen, applied with an orange stick and cotton wool, may also be used for freezing warts but much shorter freezing times are needed than with carbon dioxide. Occasionally warts have to be curetted under local or general anaesthesia and the base treated with electrocautery or a silver nitrate stick. Even with great care the recurrence rate is over 10% and another disadvantage is the production of scarring. It is often difficult to be sure when there is a recurrence of warty tissue in a scarred area on the sole and this may lead to further curettage and scarring. If a large number of warts is present it is wise to treat only a few at a time, whatever method is employed, as treatment of warts in one area not infrequently leads to involution of them all.

Small genital warts should be treated by painting the lesions accurately with 25% podophyllin in alcohol or acetone followed by powdering with talc. The patient is instructed to bath and wash off the podophyllin after about 6 hours. Local reactions may be severe and for this reason if the warts are extensive a trial area only should be treated initially. If the treatment is well tolerated it may be repeated on alternate days. Larger lesions should be dealt with surgically under a general anaesthetic.

Seborrhoeic warts
These are conveniently treated by curettage under local anaesthesia. They may be very numerous and, since they never go malignant and the sole

reason for their removal is a cosmetic one, only the ones on exposed skin need be dealt with.

Basal cell carcinomata

It is always desirable to obtain the histology of these lesions as mistakes in diagnosis can occur even when the clinical picture does not seem in doubt. This may be done by biopsy before embarking on treatment or, if the lesion is small, excision biopsy may be carried out. Treatment is by excision, curettage or radiotherapy. The choice of treatment will depend upon the histological type of lesion, its site and size and to some extent on the local facilities available. Surgery is the treatment of choice for lesions which are histologically very invasive. Curettage is probably better avoided altogether unless the operator is experienced in this method of treatment. There should be adequate follow-up of patients.

Keratoses and squamous cell carcinomata

Although keratoses are common in the middle-aged and elderly on sun-exposed skin only a very small proportion progress to squamous cell carcinomata which are capable of metastasising. Such a transition is heralded by a period of rapid growth in the size of the keratosis. Keratoses may be dealt with by freezing with carbon dioxide snow or slush or by curettage. When multiple lesions are present, treatment by painting them daily for 10 days with a 1% solution of fluorouracil in propylene glycol is often successful. Where malignant change is suspected the lesion should be excised and examined histologically. The management and follow-up of patients with multiple keratoses is probably better left in the hands of people experienced in this field.

Cellular naevi and melanomata

A patient usually seeks advice about a mole either for cosmetic reasons or because the lesion has changed in some way. If treatment is asked for on cosmetic grounds the only method which should be employed is complete excision followed by histological examination of the lesion. The decision whether or not to do this is a question of balancing the patient's dislike of the mole against his dislike of the appearance of the scar which is likely to result. Factors to consider are the size and site of the mole and the skill of the operator and should be discussed frankly with the patient before a decision is taken. Moles may sometimes require removal when they are being rubbed by clothing.

Change in a mole may consist of an increase in size, a change in the amount or distribution of pigment, inflammation, ulceration and bleeding or even itching. Any such change in a mole should be followed by its complete excision as soon as possible and by histological examination. The extent of the operation required is often a difficult decision at the time of the primary excision. If the histological examination shows the lesion to be malignant and invading, further surgery may be necessary. The degree of malignancy and hence the extent of the surgery required should not be decided by quick smear techniques but should be based on the appearance of paraffin sections. Endolymphatic injection of radioactive substances following excision seems to be a promising method of increasing the survival rate; the incidence of complications is much less than following a block dissection of regional glands.

5

HYPOTHERMIA AND EXPOSURE

W. R. KEATINGE

GENERAL CONSIDERATIONS

Hypothermia is arbitrarily defined as a rectal or esophageal temperature below 35 °C. There is progressive mental slowing, confusion and unconsciousness as the body temperature falls from this level, but vital functions are seriously affected only when temperature falls below 28–30 °C. There is then a danger of sudden death from ventricular fibrillation. Below 18–25 °C the heart is incapable of maintaining an effective circulation even if it remains in normal rhythm. On rewarming the main hazard is that blood volume will have fallen progressively during hypothermia, so that vasodilatation produced by warming can lead to a failure of venous return to the heart and a serious fall in arterial blood pressure.

Prevention or reversal of these hazards is the main object of the management of accidental hypothermia, which causes most of the deaths of healthy people exposed to cold water or air, and the management of secondary hypothermia in which body cooling results from drugs or disease. Before considering the management of the various forms of hypothermia in more detail it is useful to have some general principles in mind.

Survival in accidental hypothermia depends most on the steps taken by the victim to retard body cooling, and on the immediate actions taken by his rescuers. These steps are often the reverse of what common sense dictates. Even when they are not, neither victims nor rescuers normally take the right actions unless they know clearly what to do in advance. It is therefore a major medical responsibility to advise potential victims, aquatic and open air clubs, and rescue organisations. What happens in hospital, both with accidental and secondary hypothermia, is of lesser importance but still influences the chances of survival considerably. The most important general principle at this stage is that it is easier to kill a viable patient by well intentioned but ill-considered treatment than it is to save a patient who would otherwise have died. When in doubt it is better at this stage to expect spontaneous recovery than to institute drastic treatment before full diagnostic information is available.

PREVENTION AND EMERGENCY TREATMENT

Immersion hypothermia

Because of the high thermal conductivity and specific heat of water, body temperature falls rapidly during immersion and most shipwreck victims die of hypothermia rather than drowning. Thin men can cool to dangerous levels within 30 min in water at 0 °C; they ultimately die of hypothermia in water as warm as 23 °C, and without protection even fat men die in water colder than 12 °C.

Before entering the water after a shipwreck survivors should be advised to put on thick clothing as well as the usual lifejacket, since even conventional non-waterproof clothing greatly retards body cooling in cold water. If the water is colder than 12 °C the clothing should include gloves and footwear, since cold vasodilatation otherwise greatly increases heat loss from the extremities, and since the extremities can otherwise freeze in sea water that is near its freezing point of −1.9 °C. Exercise increases the rate of which body temperature falls in cold water, and survivors should be advised to float still with their lifejacket or wreckage while they wait for rescue. They should not swim about if they can avoid it.

Confusion or unconsciousness after rescue suggests a dangerous degree of hypothermia. A heart rate below 45–50/min, which must be counted by palpation of the heart as peripheral arteries are constricted in hypothermia, will provide sufficient confirmation if no thermometer is available. People with this degree of cooling are liable to die from hypothermic arrest of the heart after rescue, because of continued loss of heat from the body core to the cold skin. The only effective way of preventing this, or of restoring cardiac action if hypothermic arrest does occur, is to put the patient into a bath of water at 40–44 °C. If no thermometer is available the water should be as hot as the rescuer's hand can stand. It is probably useful to leave the limbs out of the water, to minimise any risk of ischaemic damage from heating them before their circulation is restored. Even if the victim is apparently dead every effort should be made to locate a bath quickly; one patient has been revived after as long as 60 min of hypothermic cardiac arrest. Cerebral damage is probably inevitable if the delay is much longer than this. While cardiac arrest persists cardiac massage and mouth-to-mouth artificial respiration may help to preserve life if trained people are available to give them. They could be given at half the usual rate, in view of the reduced metabolism in hypothermia.

If the patient has a regular and improving heart beat and respiration after about 20 min in the hot bath he should be removed from it, dried, and lain flat under blankets to finish rewarming slowly. In cases of hypothermic cardiac arrest nothing is lost by continuing the bath for longer, and giving cardiac massage and artificial respiration until the patient either shows signs of life or is clearly dead. It is in any case important to remove the patient from the bath as soon as the risk of hypothermic cardiac arrest is over, in order to minimise the risk of sudden vasodilatation and a consequent dangerous fall in blood pressure.

Hypothermia in walkers and climbers

The obvious preventive advice, that people should not undertake walking or climbing expeditions that they lack the physical fitness or the expertise to complete, is more readily given than received. One important and more acceptable piece of practical advice is that once it becomes clear that shelter cannot be reached by dark it is better to stop and prepare a bivouac in good time than to continue and risk collapse from exhaustion without one.

Since cooling in air is relatively slow the victim is seldom undergoing rapid chilling of the body core, and so is seldom in danger of death from cardiac arrest, at the time of rescue. At the same time victims of cold air exposure have usually been hypothermic for longer than immersion cases, so that a hot bath carries a greater risk of producing a serious fall in arterial pressure. Unless hypothermic cardiac arrest or extreme slowing of the heart and respiration demand a hot bath, cold air exposure cases can simply be lain flat under blankets in a sheltered, and preferably warm, room and allowed to rewarm slowly.

People exposed to cold air have frostbite more often than immersion victims. If tissues are still frozen when the patient is seen they should be treated by plunging the affected part into hot water (40–44 °C). The limb should then be dried, exposed to air and protected from injury.

Hypothermia in infancy and old age

The high ratio of surface to mass in infants, particularly in premature infants, makes them liable to falls of body temperature in cool environments that present no problem to adults. No general susceptibility to hypothermia is produced by old age, but a few old people have defective metabolic responses to cold and readily become hypothermic in poorly heated houses. Infants show a similar but temporary special susceptibility to cold after a period of cold exposure, perhaps because of depletion of the brown fat that is known to be the source of many newborn animals' metabolic response to cold.

The most important measures in these conditions are preventive ones, to advise parents that too much fresh air in winter without adequate clothing can mean a dead baby, and to ensure that old people's houses have adequate heating. As regards treatment, the victims should be placed in a room or incubator at 32–34 °C, since their defective capacity for metabolic response to cold may make it impossible for them to restore normal temperature if they are simply wrapped in blankets. After recovery they continue to need special protection from cold; an infant will remain highly susceptible to hypothermia for at least a week or two, and an old person may remain so for much longer.

Hypothermia due to drugs or disease

Narcotic agents including alcohol, and hypoglycaemia, diabetic coma, myxedema or lesions of the hypothalamus can all induce hypothermia by impairing one or more of the mechanisms for maintaining body temperature. Since moderate hypothermia helps to preserve life in most of these conditions no active warming should be undertaken until an accurate diagnosis can be made, and preferably not until the patient is in hospital where the underlying condition can be effectively treated. The same is true to a lesser extent in hypothermia due to catastrophic illness such as massive cerebrovascular accidents or infection, although hypothermia is then often little more than a part of the process of dying. In all these cases it is generally best to do no more by way of emergency action than to lie the patient flat and wrap him in blankets to prevent further cooling until he is transported to hospital.

HOSPITAL TREATMENT

By the time that a patient reaches hospital or a room equipped for resuscitation body temperature has almost invariably stabilised or started to rise, so provided the patient is still alive the danger of subsequent death from progressive cooling of the heart and brain is over. Most victims of hypothermia who are not suffering from some other fatal condition recover from this point if left alone, and the most important points about management at this stage are negative ones. Ventricular fibrillation can be precipitated by unnecessary insertion of an airway or an esophageal temperature probe during hypothermia, because of the reflex bradycardia that irritation of the throat produces. If such procedures are unavoidable, prior injection of atropine (up to 1 mg intravenously) will reduce the risk; subcutaneous absorption is often very slow in hypothermia. Ventricular fibrillation can also be precipitated by vigorous cardiac massage and artificial ventilation, which causes a profound fall in pCO_2 in hypothermic patients.

If an airway is unavoidable it should be inserted with great care. Otherwise the patient should be lain flat and covered with blankets. ECG should be recorded, blood pressure measured by a sphygmomanometer, and body temperature followed by a rectal thermistor while the patient is unconscious and by a zero-gradient aural thermometer, which follows changes in cardiac temperature more closely, when consciousness returns. Facilities for positive pressure respiration, cardiac massage and electrical defibrillation should be kept close by but used only if ventricular fibrillation appears. Atrial fibrillation is common in hypothermia; it does not require treatment. Antifibrillatory drugs should not be given prophylactically to chilled patients, as many of these drugs have been shown actually to produce ventricular fibrillation or cardiac arrest in hypothermic animals. If repeated ventricular fibrillation demands an attempt to reduce ventricular irritability, cautious administration of 0.1–0.8 mg/kg of lignocaine hydrochloride intravenously in 1.5% solution is probably the safest course. Hydrocortisone or other steroids are often given in hypothermia. They are almost certainly harmless in single moderate dose, but there is no clear evidence that they are beneficial.

In patients with hypothermia secondary to disease the underlying condition must be diagnosed at this stage. This is often difficult to do so while body temperature remains low, but enough signs of the causal condition are usually present to allow a diagnosis provided it is kept in mind that hypothermia itself produces cardiac slowing and arrhythmias, clouded consciousness, high blood glucose and slow utilisation of any injected glucose. Any blood samples required to confirm a clinical diagnosis must be taken from an artery, or from a vein in an arm that has been in water at 40 °C for 10 min to retore blood flow. Casual peripheral venous samples taken from an ischaemic limb in hypothermia can be highly misleading.

After the diagnosis is made it may be necessary to accelerate rewarming if the patient is obese, as spontaneous rewarming in such people is often inconveniently slow. The most satisfactory way to do this is to immerse one arm in water at 40–44 °C. Such acceleration of rewarming is needed particularly for patients in diabetic coma, as they are resistant to insulin while body temperature remains low. If arterial pressure falls below 70 mmHg as body temperature rises it can usually be restored by raising the foot of the bed and discontinuing active rewarming. If hypotension persists, intravenous dextran solution can be given to expand the blood volume.

As the patient's body temperature rises it is advisable to measure blood pH, blood glucose and serum K, particularly if the patient fails to recover full consciousness and normal respiration when his deep temperature has reached 35 °C. Severe metabolic acidosis has been reported during rewarming following prolonged hypothermia. A blood pH below 7.2 calls for up to 200 mEq of sodium bicarbonate intravenously. A blood dextrose below 50 mg/100 ml calls for 20–50 ml of 50% dextrose intravenously and potassium may then be needed as well.

After body temperature has returned to normal any non-freezing cold injury of the limbs (e.g. 'immersion foot') will show itself as persistent hyperaemia and pain; if severe this will be followed by persistent distal anaesthesia and weakness and later by necrosis and contractures of muscle. Injury by frostbite will again show itself as hyperaemia, pain and anaesthesia, but in severe cases this will be followed by gangrene affecting mainly the skin. Both conditions are best treated after the initial rewarming simply by elevating the affected limbs to reduce edema, keeping them dry, and giving the patient analgesics to relieve pain. Intravenous heparin and dextran,

c

and hyperbaric oxygen, have all been used in frostbite but as they are not of proven value and carry some risk they are not advisable in routine treatment. Surgery has no place, at least until any dead skin has sloughed; it can do great harm at an earlier stage by damaging viable tissue. Months later sympathectomy can be useful in relieving the excessive sweating and sensitivity to heat and cold that are a frequent late result of severe immersion injury.

6

COMMON ENDOCRINOLOGICAL AND METABOLIC DISEASES

D. R. LONDON

NUTRITIONAL OBESITY

The immediate aim of treatment is to achieve weight reduction. However, it is equally important to re-educate the patient into more normal dietary habits. The first of these objectives is much more easily attained than the second.

Dieting

In order to produce weight loss in obesity it is necessary to reduce the calorie intake of the patient.

In mild obesity (10–20% above predicted weight) it is enough to prescribe a free diet except for a number of specified foodstuffs of high carbohydrate content.

Should the general advice contained in the free diet sheet prove inadequate then it may be necessary to spell out in more detail what the patient should be eating. Since it is impracticable for the home dieter to weigh every item another diet has been devised to give advice on amounts to be eaten.

If all other methods fail, the excessively obese patient (>30% of desirable weight) may be taken into hospital for total starvation. Although this has been carried out for periods up to 4 months it is more usual to totally withdraw food for only approximately 2 weeks. Prolonged treatment of this sort has caused death through heart failure and should not be prescribed for the elderly or for any patient who might have a cardiac abnormality; there is also a suggestion that even the young and previously healthy myocardium might be at risk. However, if total starvation is indicated, vitamin and potassium supplements should be given together with allopurinol. This last drug is used to prevent the symptomatic hyperuricaemia that might otherwise complicate the fast.

A liquid diet such as "Complan" or "Metercal" provides approximately 900 calories a day and may be the only way some patients can be persuaded to reduce their dietary intake.

Another way a "packaged diet" can be provided is by a variety of commercially available biscuits containing protein, vitamins and methyl cellulose. These are usually supplemented with milk and are particularly useful for inducing weight loss in those who are minimally obese and who do not wish to adhere to a complex dietary regime.

Dietary aids. Artificial sweeteners such as saccharin allow the dieter to enjoy a sweet taste from a non-carbohydrate, acaloric source.

Starch reduced bread allows the patient to have bread with a low carbohydrate content. When eating this, it is necessary to limit the amount ingested.

Appetite suppressants. Although the treatment of obesity depends on reducing the food intake of the patient it may on occasion be necessary to administer a substance that reduces the appetite. This aid to dieting should be prescribed reluctantly, as an important factor in the long term success of a dietary regime is that the patient should become tolerant of the hunger initially produced by reducing the intake. If hunger is removed by a drug then the patient cannot recognise and conquer it. This leads to difficulty in inducing a permanent change in eating habits. For this reason, and also for the sake of cost, it may be preferable to prescribe courses of an anorectic agent alternating each month with a placebo.

The indications for drug treatment are:

1. Patients who have great difficulty in keeping to a diet.

2. Depression, either preceding or following weight loss.

The drugs most useful in the suppression of appetite are:

Phenmetrazine: 50–75 mg day in divided doses or as slow release capsules.

Diethylpropion: 75–100 mg day in divided doses or as slow release tablets.

Phentermine: 15–30 mg daily.

Fenfluramine: 20 mg–40 mg twice daily.

Since phenmetrazine and phentermine produce restlessness and insomnia, they should be administered early in the day. Fenfluramine is said to have a sedative effect and is given at 10 a.m. and 4.00 p.m. Only fenfluramine should be given to patients with hypertension or heart disease or to a depressed patient within 2 weeks of stopping antidepressive therapy with monoamine oxidase inhibitors. Because of the risk of addiction and as there are more effective drugs, amphetamines should not be prescribed.

Another class of drugs that has been found to depress appetite are the biguanides, oral hypoglycaemic agents used in some cases of diabetes.

It has also been suggested that bulk, taken as methyl cellulose granules or biscuits, reduces appetite. However, the evidence obtained from controlled trials is that this approach to appetite reduction is ineffective.

Other methods for weight reduction that are either ineffective or dangerous include laxatives, thyroxine or tri-iodothyronine tablets and chorionic gonadotrophin injections. Jejuno-colic shunt operations have been carried out but are generally reckoned to have too many side effects. *Exercise.* Walking 3 miles a day utilises about 300 calories. This exercise, additional to that normally taken by the patient, will result in weight loss of 2–4 lbs a month. If the subject is young and fit, he will lose an equal amount of weight if he plays tennis or swims for 30 minutes a day or bicycles for 45 minutes a day.

Any patient, who is on a weight reducing programme, should be seen at least monthly, or preferably weekly, by their attending psysicians in order that they may be encouraged, sympathised with or cajoled into adhering to their diet. The closer the supervision of the patient, the more likely the success of the treatment.

ANOREXIA NERVOSA

The first aim of treatment requires that the patient's nutritional status is restored to normal. This normally necessitates admission to hospital in order that the intake of food can be closely supervised and the patient separated from her parents. The diet is gradually increased from 1500–5000 calories in the course of 2 weeks. At the start of treatment the patient is kept in bed and given 100–300 mg/day of chlorpromazine which can be increased by 150 mg/day to the limit of tolerance; this helps overcome the patient's fear of food. Pari passu with this, 1 hour after breakfast insulin is begun, first 10 u; the dose is then increased until mild hypoglycaemia results. As soon as this appears a large meal is given; in this way food is seen by the

patient to be beneficial. Once the patient is gaining weight psychotherapy can be given; indeed patients suffering from this condition, which has a high relapse rate, require the prolonged supervision of a skilled psychiatrist.

DIABETES MELLITUS

The management of each individual case is a continuing process of trial and error. It is therefore possible to provide only guide lines rather than detailed instructions.
Aims of therapy. Before detailing the types of treatment available for diabetes, it is necessary to state the objectives to be accomplished.

Reasoning from the known biochemical abnormalities in the disease would suggest that a practical index of successful treatment would be to restore the blood glucose level to normal. However, this accomplishment, even if it were universally possible, might result in considerably more disruption to the patient's life than if the blood glucose remained relatively uncontrolled. Although there is some evidence to show that with insulin-requiring diabetics the better the control the fewer the complications, it is not apparent whether this is because better control leads to fewer complications or because patients with a milder disease, who have a tendency to develop fewer complications, are more easy to control. Until this problem can be resolved the aim of treatment should be to maintain the patient in good health by:
1. Correcting diabetic symptoms.
2. Avoiding the complications of treatment, particularly hypoglycaemia.

The agents used in the treatment of diabetes mellitus are:
1. Diet.
2. Insulin.
3. Sulphonylureas.
4. Biguanides.
Diet. There are two reasons for dieting the diabetic:
1. Weight reduction.
2. Control of carbohydrate intake.

Dieting is valuable in the elderly obese patient in whom weight reduction is indicated.

In the young, besides as a means to weight loss where indicated, it is necessary to prescribe a diet in order to control the carbohydrate intake. The advantage of the patient eating a measured amount of carbohydrate is that the effect of other treatments, such as insulin or oral hypoglycaemic agents are less variable when the carbohydrate intake is held relatively constant. There is, moreover, evidence to suggest that patients who have an entirely unrestricted intake develop more complications than those whose diet is controlled. The patient may be given a list of portions of various foods containing a fixed amount, normally 10 g of carbohydrate. Using such a list as a guide it is relatively simple to have a daily intake approximating to the general amount advised by the physician.

The actual amount of carbohydrate to be recommended varies from patient to patient; those taking insulin tend to require more than those treated by other means. An adult of normal weight will need a daily intake of 120–250 g taken at such times that the dietary tendency to hyperglycaemia is countered by, and itself counters, the maximal hypoglycaemic action of the administered insulin. If insulin is not required then the carbohydrate load should be spread out over the day so that the patient is at no time excessively hyperglycaemic.

If the diabetic is obese, then the carbohydrate intake should be limited to 100 g or less. However, it must be remembered that severe carbohydrate restriction is itself a cause of ketonuria.

Although it has been suggested that animal fat might contribute to the atherosclerosis of the diabetic, not enough evidence has yet accumulated to justify the prescription of a diet low in animal fat and high in unsaturated fat as a useful therapeutic measure in the prevention of diabetic vascular disease.

Insulin. The indications for insulin therapy are:

1. Ketosis, when not due to starvation.
2. In childhood, adolescence and young adulthood.
3. Temporarily, to cover an illness or surgical operation in some patients taking oral hypoglycaemic agents.

The reasons for choosing a particular insulin are given below.

Insulin	Indications
Soluble	Ketosis. Coma when large amounts (> 80 u) per day are required. Where requirement is rapidly changing. (e.g. Childhood diabetes.)
Actrapid	As for soluble. Allergy or resistance to bovine insulin.
Isophane	Used in preference to protamine zinc as action begins earlier, lasts a shorter time — thus reducing risk of nocturnal hypoglycaemia — and is more consistent.

Sulphonylureas. These drugs are used extensively in the treatment of maturity onset diabetes and are effective in controlling the disease in a large proportion of this group of patients.

There are however a number of contraindications to the use of sulphonylureas:

1. Ketosis, not due to over restriction of carbohydrate.
2. Total pancreatectomy.

The obese diabetic who can be controlled by diet alone should, in the first instance, be encouraged to lose weight rather than be prescribed a sulphonylurea. If the patient, despite exhortation, remains obese or if weight loss does not control symptoms and blood glucose, then a biguanide or sulphonylurea can be given.

The drugs most frequently used are chlorpropamide, acetohexamide, tolbutamide and glibenclamide. Although side effects are rare, it has recently been authoritatively suggested, though by no means universally accepted, that the administration of tolbutamide, a sulphonylurea, is associated with an increased mortality due to cardiovascular causes.

If the diabetes is not controlled by a sulphonylurea and diet then either a biguanide can be added to the regime or the patient will require insulin.

Biguanides. Although the mechanism of action of this group of drugs remains unclear they may be used:

1. With sulphonylureas to achieve control in some maturity onset diabetics, thereby avoiding the need for insulin.
2. In some obese maturity onset diabetics the anorexia produced may reduce the food intake with consequent weight loss; this, in turn, leads to control of the blood glucose.

Unfortunately, however, there is a high incidence of side effects including lactic acidosis which may necessitate stopping the drug. In addition, these agents, like the sulphonylureas, have been incriminated for causing an excess cardiovascular mortality in diabetes.

Transfer from insulin to oral hypoglycaemic agents. If there is no history of ketosis and if the insulin requirement does not exceed 40 u/day, it may be possible to replace insulin with a sulphonylurea.

When chlorpropamide, a preparation that is slow in manifesting its maximal effect, is to be given, the insulin is withdrawn gradually over 5 days once the oral treatment has been begun. Throughout the period of changeover daily measurements of urine sugar and ketones must be made together, if possible, with daily blood glucose estimations. If there is any sign of developing ketosis insulin should be reinstituted.

Exercise. The diabetic should take a moderate amount of physical exercise. Any unusual increase in physical activity introduces instability into the therapeutic regimen with a requirement for either more carbohydrate in the diet (and sugar for emergencies) or less insulin.

Choosing the treatment. Possible schemes for deciding the optimum treatment for the individual diabetic are shown in Tables 1 and 2.

Control may be defined as a blood glucose normal or near normal throughout the 24 hours. Since it is usually impossible to obtain frequent blood specimens, preprandial venous blood glucoses <110 mg% (6 mmol l⁻¹) may be taken to indicate good control. A urine collected over this period should be glucose and ketone free.

The diabetes is not controlled if the preprandial blood glucose exceeds 150 mg% (8 mmol l⁻¹), if the urine consistently contains more than 0.5% glucose or if there is any ketonuria.

Between these two extremes lies a degree of chemical control that may be acceptable, given the patient's individual circumstances.

It is however essential that, apart from restoring the chemistry towards normal, the treatment removes the symptoms of the disease.

Urine testing and control of treatment. In the long term management of the disease it is desirable to have the patient test his own urine.

The urine should at all times be ketone free. Apart from an occasional trace (<0.5%) the urine should remain glucose free when the patient is dieted and/or receiving oral agents.

During stabilisation and at times of unsatisfactory control the urine should be tested immediately before all meals.

For day-to-day adjustments of dose the urine should be tested before the injection and when the insulin is exerting its maximal effect.

Insulin should be given initially as soluble insulin (SI) or Rapitard 20 u twice daily in the more severe cases or, in milder subjects as Isophane or Lente 20 u daily. Treatment may then be modified by blood sugar measurement and by following the urine glucose (Clinitest) providing the patient has a normal threshold.

Insulin resistance. If this occurs the patient should be changed to porcine insulin (Actrapid). If this is ineffective steroid therapy (prednisone 10 mg thrice daily) may reduce the insulin requirement. In a minority of patients large doses of SI are required (using insulin 320 u/ml).

Childhood diabetes. Diabetic children almost invariably require insulin. For psychological reasons an attempt should be made to control the disease with one injection a day of a long acting preparation, although, if the child presents with ketoacidosis, the initial stabilisation must be performed with frequent doses of SI. As soon as possible the child should be taught self-injection. The diet must be adequate in calories but

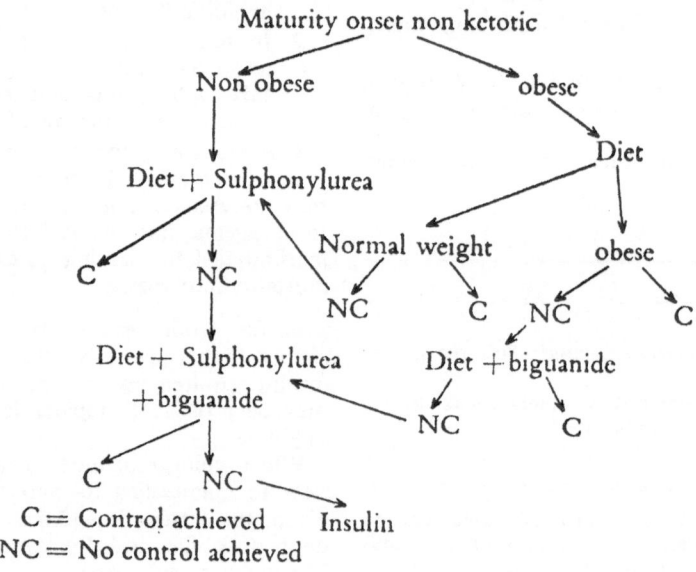

Table 1

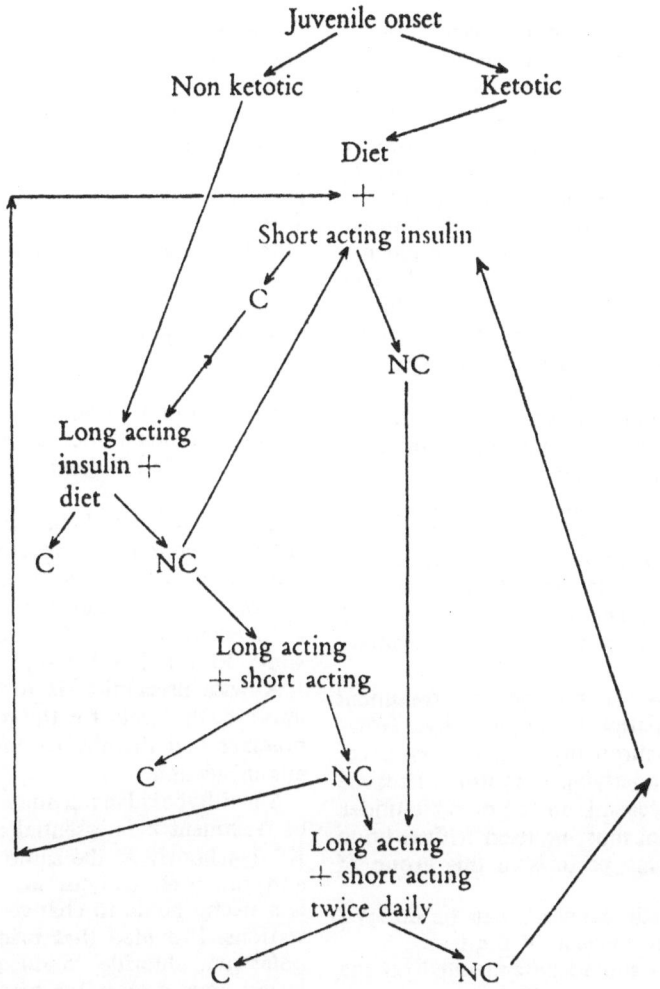

Juvenile onset

Non ketotic   Ketotic

Diet
+
Short acting insulin

C

NC

Long acting
insulin +
diet

C   NC

Long acting
+ short acting

C   NC

Long acting
+ short acting
twice daily

C   NC

C = Control achieved
NC = No control achieved

Table 2

moderately restricted in carbohydrate. Care is needed to balance the carbohydrate intake against the exercise/insulin requirements to avoid excessively frequent hypoglycaemic reactions.

Pregnant diabetics. Carbohydrate intake should be 150–250 g/day. From the second trimester onwards there is usually a rise in insulin requirements as indicated by blood glucose changes. Ketosis must be avoided for its effect on the fetus. From 32 weeks the patient should be admitted to hospital. The blood sugar should be monitored during labour to anticipate hypoglycaemia. The obstetric problems that arise are best managed by a specialist obstetrician.

Intercurrent illness. Even if the patient becomes anorectic, there will be a temporary rise in insulin requirement. The dose should be increased early in order to prevent ketoacidosis.

Surgery. Apart from the very mild case the surgical diabetic will require insulin. The occasional well-controlled maturity onset patient need only change his normal regime by omitting treatment on the day of operation.

It is wise to stabilise the patient on soluble insulin 2–3 days preoperatively. For an elective procedure under general anaesthesia, it is preferable to schedule the operation for the morning. If the urine is sugar free then 10–20 g of glucose should be given intravenously – oral glucose should not be given within 8 hours of surgery owing to the risks of vomiting and inhalation of the vomit. If ketosis is present the operation must be delayed until the condition is brought under control. During a long operation the patient should be watched for signs of hypoglycaemia – tachycardia and sweating. Also, the blood sugar should be estimated. If hypoglycaemia seems probable on clinical grounds, intravenous glucose should be given. Postoperatively a blood sugar should be taken to assess the need for insulin; if it is required then it should be accompanied by glucose given by a suitable route. Because of the heightened risks of infection, catheterisation should be avoided as a means of obtaining urine samples.

When the patient has passed through the immediate postoperative period the normal regimen of insulin administration can be resumed, accompanied by a normal carbohydrate load given in an appropriate manner.

For emergency surgery every case must be managed individually. The best guide to treatment comes from measurement of the blood glucose and bicarbonate. If the patient is ketotic, this becomes the therapeutic priority unless the emergency is so dire as to require immediate operation.

Complications. There is no specific treatment for diabetic nephropathy or angiopathy. However some cases of neuropathy benefit from careful control of the underlying condition. Because of the risk of hypoglycaemia in the diabetic under treatment, propranolol must be used with caution for the relief of angina pectoris in this group of patients.

The onset of diabetic gangrene can be delayed by careful attention to hygiene of the feet.

A vascular surgeon should be consulted on the management of circulatory insufficiency.

The rare specific diabetic cataract can be reversed if found early and the diabetes controlled. Control of blood glucose may induce refractive errors that disappear spontaneously after a few weeks. Some patients with diabetic retinopathy are benefited by pituitary destruction. However, the criteria for employing such a procedure are very strict and only a limited number of candidates are suitable.

Coma and pre-coma

Ketoacidosis. The seriousness of this condition demands that the patient should be treated in hospital. Initially a blood glucose estimation should be carried out and repeated every two hours until the physician is satisfied that the glucose is falling at an adequate rate.

Insulin is the basis of treatment. When the diagnosis has been made soluble insulin should be injected 5–10 u i.m. hourly until the blood glucose is less than 200 mg% (11 mmol l⁻¹). The patient can then usually return to a regime approximating to that obtaining before the onset of ketoacidosis. As the blood glucose level approaches the renal threshold, treatment can be based on urine testing. The risk of hypoglycaemia is in this way reduced—as a further precaution blood glucose measurements can be carried out.

Fluid and electrolytes. An intravenous infusion should be started when the first dose of insulin is given. Total fluids given should be approximately:

1 litre in first 1 hour
4 litres in first 12 hours
6 litres in first 24 hours

The fluid should be basically 0.9% sodium chloride, containing approximately 30 mEq of sodium bicarbonate in each of the first 3 litres. Alternatively the number of milli-equivalents of bicarbonate needed can be calculated from the sum: 10 mmol × [25 – plasma bicarb (mmol/l)].

A wise precaution is to insert a long catheter into a central vein for the measurement of venous pressure and thereby to control the rate of fluid administration.

Since hypokalaemia may develop in the course of treatment it is essential to monitor the plasma K⁺ 2–4 hourly at the same time as blood glucose and other electrolytes are measured. The ECG is a useful guide to changes in potassium concentrations. Provided that urine output is adequate, potassium chloride 25 mEq/hour is given in the intravenous drip 1–2 h after beginning treatment or immediately if the plasma concentration is low. The potassium deficit that will eventually require correction is approximately 200 mEq.

When treatment is begun the stomach contents should be aspirated through a tube and nothing given by mouth. After 24 hours of satisfactory treatment it is usually possible to begin feeding by mouth with carbohydrate drinks.

The treatment of diabetic ketoacidosis is not complete until the cause has been located and treated appropriately.

Hyperosmolar coma. This should be treated with moderate amounts of insulin – smaller than those required for ketoacidosis – and 0.45% sodium chloride i.v. Fluid requirements may be large, and the venous pressure should be monitored. Not all patients with this condition will require permanent insulin treatment.

Lactic acidosis. This is treated with intravenous sodium bicarbonate and, if possible, by removal of the cause of the lactate accumulation.

Hypoglycaemia. If possible the patient should immediately ingest carbohydrate-containing food or drink at the onset of symptoms.

When stupor or coma is present 10 g of glucose should be given i.v.; some patients, however, may require up to 100 g before the blood glucose is restored to normal. This should be done as quickly as possible to prevent permanent brain damage.

An alternative but less rapidly effective treatment, is to administer glucagon 0.5–1.0 mg i.m.

Soon after recovery the patient should be given a carbohydrate load by mouth to prevent relapse. The cause of the hypoglycaemia should be sought and the treatment regime modified if necessary.

In prolonged hypoglycaemia coma the patient should be tube fed and the blood glucose maintained at approximately 200 mg% (11 mmol l^{-1}). Cases of 'irreversible' coma should also receive intravenous hydrocortisone.

HYPOGLYCAEMIA

This should be treated according to the cause.

Insulin-induced hypoglycaemia in the diabetic has already been discussed (q.v.).

A pancreatic islet-cell tumour should be removed. When this course is impossible hypoglycaemia can be treated with diazoxide, glucocorticoids and glucagon. Streptozotocin has also been used in this situation.

Reactive hypoglycaemia may be difficult to treat. Measures that have been advocated include a low carbohydrate diet, frequent small feeds rather than a few large meals, and prohibition of tobacco.

Neonatal hypoglycaemia is treated with intravenous glucose using the blood glucose as a yardstick. Treatment is normally necessary for only the first week of life.

Idiopathic hypoglycaemia in childhood may be treated with corticosteroids, diazoxide or by long-acting zinc glucagon. In the acute attacks intravenous or oral glucose should be given.

Leucine sensitivity should be managed in the same way as idiopathic hypoglycaemia, since it is impracticable to prescribe a leucine-free diet.

THYROID

Hyperthyroidism

There are three ways of suppressing thyroid overactivity:
1. Antithyroid drugs
2. Radioactive iodine
3. Surgery

Drugs. The indications for this form of treatment are:
 (i) A small diffuse goitre
 (ii) Gross hyperthyroidism with cardiac involvement (see below)
 (iii) Pregnancy
 (iv) Childhood
 (v) The patient is being treated for the first time
 (vi) The preparation of a patient for radioactive iodine or surgery
The disadvantages are:
 (i) The goitrogenic effects. Thus, antithyroid drugs should not be used as the definitive treatment in patients with retrosternal prolongation of the goitre
 (ii) The recurrence of the hyperthyroidism in 40% of the patients when therapy is eventually stopped
 (iii) Side effects, of which the most important is agranulocytosis. These are unusual with the drugs currently in use

The drugs most frequently used are carbimazole or methimazole. Starting dose: 15 mg 3 times a day, maintenance dose: 5 mg once daily –5 mg 3 times a day.

Methylthiouracil or propylthyrouracil starting dose: 150–200 mg thrice daily. Maintenance dose 50 mg one to three times daily. In order to prevent the onset of iatrogenic hypothyroidism it is wise to maintain the starting dose no longer than 2 months and then to reduce the treatment at monthly intervals approximating to a schedule which, for carbimazole, is:

> 1st month 45 mg/day in divided doses
> 2nd month 30 mg/day in divided doses
> 3rd month 20 mg/day in divided doses
> 4th month 15 mg/day in divided doses

The therapy should be altered according to the patient's condition; if he shows signs of relapsing the dose should be increased, if hypothyroidism appears, the drug should be decreased. Treatment should be maintained for at least 6 months after the patient has become euthyroid. If hyperthyroidism recurs when treatment is stopped, either radioactive iodine or surgery should be employed.

It may be possible to prevent enlargement of the gland that occurs when anti-thyroid drugs are given by simultaneously administering triiodothronine or thyroxine.

Radioactive iodine (^{131}I). This is indicated when the thyrotoxic patient
 (i) is over 40 years old;
 (ii) has heart disease (see below);
 (iii) has intercurrent disease;
 (iv) is mentally ill.

It is contraindicated in:

(i) Patients under 40, because of the possible risk of inducing thyroid cancer or leukaemia.

(ii) Pregnancy.

(iii) Toxic nodular goitre in areas where goitre is endemic and there is thus a heightened risk of thyroid cancer.

The important complications of radioiodine therapy are:

(i) Hypothyroidism, which occurs at a rate of 10% per annum and remains a recurrent risk throughout the patient's life.

(ii) Thyroid storm, a rare event, but particularly serious in the cardiac patient. This occurs 1–2 weeks after therapy.

(iii) A transient tracheitis or thyroiditis.

Since radioiodine is very slow in exerting an effect, it is sometimes wise to make the patient euthyroid with drugs before giving the radioactive material.

Surgery. This should be performed:

1. When the patient has a large goitre
2. When the patient has a solitary nodule that might be cancerous
3. When drug treatment fails in a person under 40 years old
4. In retrosternal goitre
5. Pregnancy, during the second trimester, as an alternative to drugs

It is contraindicated in the old, the ill and the mentally unstable.

Preparation for surgery

(i) Render the patient euthyroid with antithyroid drugs

(ii) Admit to hospital. Stop drugs

(iii) Administer either potassium iodide 100 mg/day in milk or Lugol's iodine 1.0 ml/day for approximately 2 weeks. This manoeuvre decreases the increased vascularity of the gland produced by the antithyroid drug

Alternatively:

Administer propranolol (see below) for 2–3 weeks then (iii) as above.

Propranolol. There is evidence that this drug, used in a dose of 40 mg four times daily rapidly controls some of the clinical features of hyperthyroidism. In particular it induces a diminution of malaise, palpitations, sweating and nervousness, with a concomitant reduction in pulse rate and tremor. Particular caution should be exercised in the presence of cardiac failure. If the heart failure worsens the agent should be either stopped or given in a lower dose.

It has also been given instead of the antithyroid drugs to patients receiving ^{131}I or being prepared for surgery.

Ophthalmic manifestations. If the exophthalmos warrants treatment, simple measures such as padding the eye or the wearing of dark glasses may be tried.

Should the condition increase in severity tarsorrhaphy may be necessary to prevent corneal ulceration.

Orbital decompression is the ultimate in surgical treatment for malignant exophthalmos where sight is threatened.

There is no medical way of managing exophthalmos that is universally accepted. Some claim that triiodothyronine 125 μg/day given with the antithyroid therapy reduces the incidence and severity of exophthalmos.

There is a suggestion that the instillation of guanethidine eye drops (2 drops twice daily, of a 10% solution) may lessen exophthalmos. However, if this treatment is continued for 2 months or so, punctate keratitis may appear. Should this happen a 5% solution should be substituted; this allows the keratitis to heal but maintains the improvement in the exophthalmos.

Finally, some patients with malignant exophthalmos show an improvement with very large doses of corticosteroids – up to 150 mg/day of prednisone. Unfortunately, however, steroid dosage at this level inevitably leads to side effects, so the dose should be gradually reduced as soon as the eye signs allow.

Pretibial myxedema. This is best treated with occlusive dressings of topical corticosteroids.

Myxedema

In this condition the secretion of the thyroid gland can be replaced either with L-thyroxine (T_4) or liothyronine (T_3). There is no longer any place for desiccated thyroid in the drug cupboard.

T_4 0.1 mg is approximately equivalent to T_3 0.02 mg. Unless the patient is receiving immediate replacement therapy after total thyroidectomy it is usual to increase the treatment very slowly until maintenance levels are reached. This is because the myocardium may not recover at a rate fast enough to permit it to cope with the demands made on it during the period of recovery of the rest of the body. If the patient has angina pectoris it is better to use T_3 than T_4 as the shorter duration of action of the former enables the effects of overtreatment to be rapidly stopped. Alternatively the addition of propranolol by reducing the cardiac effects of the hormone, may allow continuation of the substitution therapy.

The usual course is to begin at a T_4 dose of 0.05–0.1 mg/day and then to increase the dose in weekly stages of 0.05 or 0.1 mg until a maintenance dose of 0.15–0.2 mg/day is reached. If an equivalent dose of T_3 is given it should be divided so that it is taken 2 or 3 times a day. In many cases it is possible to make the patient euthyroid. However, in those with severe underlying heart disease, it may be preferable to undertreat so that some degree of hypothyroidism remains.

Hashimoto's thyroiditis
This is treated with T_4. This will reduce the size of the gland and make the patient euthyroid.

ADRENAL

Cushing's syndrome
The choice of treatment for this condition is contingent on the underlying pathology.

If, as is most likely, the patient is suffering from adrenal hyperplasia due to an abnormality of the hypothalamico–pituitary–adrenal axis, the choice of therapy lies between destruction of the pituitary gland or total removal of the adrenal glands.

The pituitary gland may be destroyed by surgical removal, cryosurgery or local implantation of radioactive seeds.

This is currently the treatment of choice providing that:

(a) Adrenal hyperplasia due to pituitary hyperactivity has been diagnosed with certainty.

(b) The treatment is carried out at a specialist centre.

(c) The patient does not wish to remain fertile.

(d) The patient is no longer growing.

If any one of these criteria is not satisfied adrenalectomy is indicated. The drawbacks to this operation are:

(a) The technical difficulty.

(b) The occurrence of a pituitary tumour, that may not become manifest until after adrenalectomy, in approximately 10% of patients with Cushing's syndrome.

The main disadvantage of hypophysectomy is the ensuing panhypopituitarism in a proportion of those operated.

Following either operation the patient must be managed as for adrenalectomy (q.v.). However, the hypophysectomised patient does not usually require mineralocorticoid but will need substitution of thyroid (q.v.) and, possibly, also sex hormones. Diabetes insipidus following hypophysectomy is usually transient and may be controlled by DDAVP (desaminocys-D-arginine vasopressin) either 0.002 mg i.v. or i.m. twice daily or 0.01 mg intranasally twice daily.

Adrenal hyperplasia due to corticotrophin (ACTH) originating from a non-endocrine tumour may, if indicated, be treated by total adrenalectomy or removal of the source of ACTH if this is surgically feasible. In Cushing's syndrome due to adrenocortical adenoma or carcinoma the appropriate gland should be totally removed under steroid cover. The drug treatment of inoperable adrenal carcinoma with metyrapone, or aminoglutethimide is generally unsatisfactory although remissions with these agents have, on occasion, been reported.

Addison's disease
The treatment of this condition requires the administration of a glucocorticoid and a mineralocorticoid.

Apart from the situations detailed below, the following are normally given:

Glucocorticoid. Tabs. hydrocortisone 20 mg in the morning and 10 mg in the evening.

Mineralocorticoid. Tablets fluorocortisone 0.05–0.2 mg/day (usually 0.1 mg/day) in a single dose. If the patient cannot be relied upon, or if he should become ill and be unable to take his tablets, the risk of the rapid development of a severe Addisonian crisis can be reduced by the intramuscular administration of deoxycortone pivalate 25–50 mg once a month instead of the oral mineralocorticoid.

In hot climates, it may be necessary to administer sodium chloride tablets since, even in treated Addison's disease, it may not be possible to achieve maximal sodium conservation.

Intercurrent illness will require an increase in the dose of hydrocortisone to 100 mg/day. If there is doubt that the steroid is being absorbed it may be given parenterally as cortisone acetate. It is important to note that intramuscular cortisone acetate does not act until approximately 12 hours after injection.

Addisonian crisis requires the repeated i.v. injection of 200 mg hydrocortisone sodium succinate in an intravenous saline and, if the patient is hypoglycaemic, glucose infusion. Before treatment is begun, blood should be sampled for cortisol, glucose and electrolyte measurements. Treatment should be begun without waiting for the result.

Corticosteroid cover for surgery
1. *Adrenalectomy*: the following drugs should all be given.

(a) Cortisone acetate intramuscularly.

100 mg daily; day before operation, day of operation, days 1–3 post operatively.

75 mg daily, days 4–6.

50 mg daily, days 7–9.

Then hydrocortisone 30 mg permanently.

If the postoperative recovery is not uneventful, it may be temporarily necessary to continue the cortisone at the higher dosage.

As soon as the patient can be treated by mouth the same dose may be given in tablet form in divided doses 2–3 times a day.

(b) Hydrocortisone sodium succinate.

Day of operation: 100 mg intramuscularly with premedication, or 100 mg intravenously at the time of induction of the anaesthetic. Ampoules of the preparation should be available in the operating theatre; this will avoid unnecessary delay in the administration of the hormone should it be required urgently. Further doses of 50–100 mg i.v. may be given if there is a fall in systolic blood pressure to below 90 mmHg; it should be noted that post-operative hypotension however is more often due to haemorrhage than to steroid deficiency.

(c) Mineralocorticoid.

This should be instituted as soon as the cortisone therapy has been reduced to 50 mg daily. (For details vide management of Addison's disease).

2. *Patients already receiving steroid therapy.* The regime is the same as for adrenalectomy, except that if the patient is taking more than 75 mg a day of cortisone or its equivalent (15 mg of prednisone) they will require to continue this in addition to the amounts recommended for adrenalectomy.

Patients coming to operation within 6 months of receiving steroid therapy should be managed according to the schedule set out for adrenalectomy except that they can finally be weaned from the steroid at the end of the convalescent phase.

GONADS

Male

Eunuchoidism due to primary testicular insufficiency is treated with an androgen. Of the preparations available those most frequently employed are:

Fluoxymesterone tablets 5–15 mg daily.

Testosterone enanthate in oil 250–500 mg every 2–4 weeks.

Delayed puberty or selective gonadotrophin deficiency may be treated by Human Chorionic Gonadotrophin (HCG) injections 1500 i.u. 3 times a week.

Some patients with infertility due to defective spermatogenesis may benefit from gonadotrophin prepared from menopausal urine (HMG).

Female

Gonadal dysgenesis is treated with ethinyl estradiol 50–100 μg/day. Alternatively cyclic progestogen and estrogen using one of the oral contraceptive preparations may be administered.

The infertility produced by the polycystic ovary syndrome may respond to ovarian wedge resection, corticosteroids, clomiphene or gonadotrophins. The last two approaches should only be undertaken in centres where intensive endocrine monitoring can be performed. The hirsutism found in the polycystic ovary syndrome may occasionally benefit from treatment with oral contraceptives or corticosteroids in low dose (10 mg or less of prednisone daily).

The beneficial effects of such therapy may take 3–6 months to appear.

PITUITARY

Acromegaly.

The indications for treating this condition are
1. Visual field defects
2. Insulin resistant diabetes mellitus
3. Hypertension
4. Intractable headache
5. Other evidence of progressive disease

If the visual pathways are affected, the treatment is surgical, otherwise there is the additional choice of radiotherapy administered either externally or by the implantation of radioactive seeds (^{90}Yt or ^{198}Au) into the gland. A promising new treatment is bromocriptine for lowering growth hormone levels.

Hypopituitarism

The cause of this should be found, and if possible, remedied. If there is secondary hypofunction of the adrenals, thyroid and gonads, it is important that the adrenal deficiency is treated first, as the prior administration of thyroid hormone may precipitate an Addisonian crisis. The target gland deficiencies should be treated as for myxedema and Addison's disease, except that mineralocorticoid substitution is usually unnecessary.

The gonadal deficiency can be managed with continuous androgen therapy in the male. In the female, cyclical estrogens are given for 3 weeks in every month. Infertility can sometimes be overcome by the injection of human gonadotrophin preparations administered under specialist supervision.

It is possible to treat pituitary dwarfism in children with human growth hormone; this requires close clinical and metabolic control, as the supply of this hormone preparation is severely limited.

HYPERPROLACTINAEMIA

In some hypogonad males or females with or without galactorrhea, elevated serum prolactin levels are found. These may be treated according to the cause, such as drug withdrawal or pituitary surgery where appropriate. Prolactin levels may also be lowered by the administration of bromocriptine.

Diabetes insipidus

This may be controlled by desmopressin injections or nose drops, lysine vasopressin nose drops, chlorothiazide or chlorpropamide tablets. It is possible to overdose with the antidiuretic hormone preparation thereby inducing water intoxication. Diabetes insipidus is usually transient following hypophysectomy and does not require treatment for longer than a week or two.

METABOLIC BONE DISEASE

Rickets and osteomalacia

This requires calciferol and, in the initial stages of treatment, calcium supplements. If tetany occurs, it may be necessary to give intravenous calcium.

If the cause of the rickets is dietary, the deficiency should be rectified either by public health measures or by permanent supplementation with small amounts (400 u/day) or vitamin D. If the rickets is secondary to other diseases, then these should be treated; when this is impossible the vitamin D therapy will have to be continued and the treatment monitored with plasma calcium, phosphorus and alkaline phosphatase estimations. Some patients may require very large doses (50 000–500 000 u/day) to restore the calcium and bone to normal.

HYPERCALCAEMIA

The prime aim of therapy is to remove the cause of the condition. However if the serum calcium is so high as to be life threatening, or if the underlying disease is untreatable, symptomatic measures should be used. These include the oral or intravenous administration of phosphate and, in some instances, corticosteroids by mouth.

PAGET'S DISEASE

Calcitonin has been used with success in the management of this condition, as has mithramycin.

7

SEXUALLY TRANSMITTED INFECTIONS

J. L. FLUKER

GENERAL REMARKS

It is essential to obtain the patient's maximum co-operation and as far as possible to prevent default, as many patients when symptoms have disappeared feel that further treatment is unnecessary. A full explanation of the reasons for treatment should always be given according to the patient's intelligence. It is wise also to treat the patients' families as well and to consider the whole as a unit. For every infected patient there must always be another and far better results will be obtained if both partners can be treated, if not together in confidence, at least under the same roof. For example it is no good telling a husband that he is cured and may resume a normal sexual life if it is not noticed that on the preceding day, his wife had had a positive culture returned for gonorrhea. Reinfection and further trouble would only follow. Indirectly this also helps to inculcate a sense of responsibility into patients towards others, the lack of which may be so important a factor in the spread of this type of infection.

SYPHILIS

There is an enormous amount of literature about the treatment of syphilis and numerous different treatment schedules have been used. Those described here have the merit of simplicity and of being generally applicable. The important principle of treatment is that there should be a continually maintained low concentration of penicillin in the blood stream for a minimum period of 8 days. In order to preserve an adequate margin of safety somewhat longer periods of treatment are recommended. The best form of penicillin to use is procaine penicillin G by itself or suspended in aluminium monostearate to delay absorption. A daily injection of 600 000 or 900 000 units of either preparation will provide adequate blood levels. In cases of sero-negative primary syphilis when *Treponema pallidum* has been recovered from the sores but the blood tests are all nega-

tive, a course of ten such injections is adequate, but in late primary syphilis with positive blood tests and in all cases of secondary syphilis and early latency within the first 2 years of infection, 15 such injections should be given. When daily attendance is not possible or is unlikely to be secured a single dose of 2.4 megaunits of benzathine penicillin should give an effective blood level for about 2 weeks. This type of injection is rather painful and may cause the patient to default.

Follow up is required for 2 years. Blood tests should be done 2 weeks after the end of treatment and thereafter monthly for 3 months and then 3-monthly until 2 years have passed. During the second year the cerebrospinal fluid should be examined. In just under 0.5% of cases it will be abnormal. In such an event re-treatment will be required as otherwise the patient may develop neurosyphilis. In sero-positive cases it may take up to 6 months before all the blood tests have reverted to negative, but such slow reversion is not an indication for further treatment.

Infectious relapse occurs in under 2% of sero-negative primary cases and in just over 4% of all other cases of early syphilis. It is usually preceded by serological relapse which can be detected during follow up, before the occurrence of actual lesions which are often fleeting and superficial but are likely to be infectious. If such relapse occurs the disease will continue into the latent phase. All the available evidence suggests that after 2 years the disease is in fact permanently cured and the patients may be discharged. Exceptions are so few that any further follow up with consequent anxieties for the patient, is not justified. In fact, the great majority of relapses occur during the first year.

The Jarisch-Herxheimer Reaction

This is a focal and generalized exacerbation of symptoms which follows treatment with almost any reagent except perhaps bismuth or mercury. It is believed to be due to the liberation of endotoxins consequent upon the death of large numbers of treponemes but this explanation is purely theoretical. The reaction varies from a transient feeling of malaise to a severe exacerbation of all the symptoms coupled with generalized aching in the limbs, headache and high pyrexia occasionally with rigors. It is essential to warn patients that this may occur—which it does in over 50% of cases. It does no harm at this stage of the disease.

Alcohol should be discouraged while treatment is actually being given, solely because it is believed to lower the efficacy of antibiotic therapy in general. Most text books suggest that sexual intercourse should be banned for 2 years but it is doubtful if many authorities insist upon this now. If a couple living together are both infected provided that observation is maintained there seems no valid reason why intercourse should not be permitted with each other after treatment of both has been finished. When one of the pair is uninfected at least 3 months observation of both should elapse and ideally the uninfected partner should know all the facts. In this way, any infection of the latter will become evident and treatment be given. Intercourse with others should be avoided for at least 1 month, preferably for 3–6 months. Where these conditions are not fulfilled somewhat more frequent blood testing may reveal an incipient relapse before any damage has been done. If patients are warned that any relapse would render them once again infectious to others and that a reversal of seronegativity would give early warning of this, they are more likely to complete surveillance. Indirectly this gives an opportunity without a hint of moralizing, of inculcating a sense of responsibility towards others in those in whom it is lacking.

When patients are allergic to penicillin the treatment of choice is with tetracycline or erythromycin 500 mg four times a day for 15 days. The follow up should be for at least 2 years. This treatment is less satisfactory partly because there is no guarantee that the patients will always remember to take the tablets. There are no indications today for the use of arsenicals nor is there evidence that the addition of bismuth to penicillin produces superior results.

In latent and late syphilis the general principles of treatment are similar. At least 15 injections of penicillin should be given and in the more severe forms of tertiary syphilis, as many as 20 or 30 in the first course. Opinions differ as to whether further maintenance courses of treatment are required. Many maintain that one long course is adequate. Some physicians, however, prefer to add maintenance courses of penicillin, usually consisting of 10 injections each, although larger doses of 1.2 or 2.4 megaunits may be given at weekly intervals for 6–8 weeks. At the very most four such courses should be given and if it is intended to give more than one course the patients should be informed at the beginning as otherwise the apparently haphazard administration of further courses may be very demoralizing. It is probable that patients with very early cardiovascular or neurological lesions, for example patients with an accidentally detected aortic diastolic murmur, early tabes or general paresis, may benefit from further courses as it is obviously important to prevent any spread of the syphilitic process but there is no evidence that patients with cardiac failure or in the late stages of neurosyphilis really benefit from unduly prolonged treatment.

The Jarisch-Herxheimer reaction may occur in both cardiovascular and neurological cases. It is rare in the former and may consist of attacks of anginal pain or exceptionally, an actual coronory thrombosis. In neurological cases, particularly in general paresis, convulsions may occur and rare instances of death have been reported. Sometimes there is marked exacerbation of the clinical picture. There is some evidence that the severity of these reactions may be reduced by the prior administration of steroids for example prednisone 20–30 mg daily for 3 days with commencement of penicillin on the third day. Prior administration of bismuth for 3 weeks was common practice but in cases of general paresis is inadvisable as the sooner treatment is begun the better the results.

The fallacy that 10 injections is all that is required to cure any stage of syphilis is now discredited. Three examples will suffice, of how such treatment led to disaster. A patient of 36 with general paresis was given 10 injections of penicillin and no follow up. Six months later a fatal exacerbation occurred. Another patient with early tabes was given 10 injections. An X-ray examination of the aorta at that time disclosed no abnormality—4 years later he had an aortic aneurysm. Another patient with latent syphilis had pneumonia and was given the equivalent of 10 injections. Four years later he had marked tabes dorsalis. His wife also had syphilis of the aorta. This underlines the importance of examining all possible contacts of syphilis patients at any stage of the disease immediately the diagnosis has been confirmed.

Apart from their use for the prevention of Jarisch-Herxheimer reactions in late cases of syphilis, steroids are generally contraindicated except in interstitial keratitis where they are valuable locally; in some cases of Charcot joints and those of VIIIth (auditory) nerve deafness. In gummatous processes too rapid treatment with penicillin is believed sometimes to result in excessive scar formation with the so-called therapeutic paradox and it is likely that an initial course of bismuth for 3 weeks 0.2 g twice weekly intramuscularly, coupled with oral potassium iodide 1 g three times a day for 2 weeks may prevent this.

Maternal syphilis

The infection reaches the fetus across the placenta. Treatment with penicillin will prevent this and a course of 10 injections is all that is required to ensure a normal child. Follow up of the child should be at 1 month and at 6 months. Cord bloods are unreliable owing to the mixture of maternal reagin or treponemal antibodies. Passive transfer of such antibodies may take place in the infant and positive results at 1 month, provided that the child is fit, should be disregarded and the tests repeated. At 6 months they should all be negative. However, the presence of IgM antibodies in the fetal blood as detected by the Fluorescent Antibody Test is normally diagnostic of congenital infection and an indication for treatment.

Some authorities assert that it is only necessary to treat the first pregnancy but Moore (1949) found that after treatment had been withheld in 390 pregnancies, three syphilitic infants were born. The writer had a case of a patient who, 22 years after her initial infection and after 8 normal pregnancies in every one of which she had received anti-syphilitic treatment, produced a child with active congenital syphilis, (Fluker 1962). It would therefore seem wise to treat all such pregnancies, except possibly those in women who have had only sero-negative primary syphilis, and have been discharged as cured. Active congenital syphilis at birth is very rare in the United Kingdom but when it does occur the infant may be acutely ill and the sooner penicillin treatment is given the better. The suggested dosage is 150 000 units daily over a period of from 10–15 days. The mortality rate may be quite high and there is some evidence that the Jarisch-Herxheimer reaction may be contributory so that the administration of steroids should be considered, at any rate for the first 2 or 3 days.

Gonorrhea

In uncomplicated gonorrhea, so far as penicillin is concerned, one injection to provide an adequate blood level for 24 hours is all that is required. In the early days of penicillin treatment 300 000 units of procaine penicillin G was adequate but owing to the fact that numerous strains of gonococci have acquired varying degrees of insensitivity it is usual to begin with considerably larger dosages ranging from 1.2 to 5.0 megaunits. If treatment is effective by the third day in the male the discharge should have ceased and the urine should be clear without haze and with few or no shreds. Further tests should be done at the end of 1 week, 2 weeks and 4 weeks, at which stage prostatic massage should be carried out. The prostatic bead should not contain any pus, still less, of course, gonococci. Blood tests for syphilis should be done at the beginning and at the end and in certain cases if there is any risk of previous exposure to syphilis, or in districts where the latter disease is prevalent, further blood tests should be done at the end of 3 and even 6 months. In practice this is not often possible because very few patients will attend for that length of time. Homosexual patients and others pursuing a free and easy sex life should be encouraged to have regular check-ups at 3- to 6-monthly intervals.

In women, urethral and cervical smears and cultures should be performed on the third day, at the end of a week, 2 weeks and 4 weeks but with special emphasis on the time immediately following the first period after treatment. Similar considerations as in the male apply with regard to blood tests. Sexual intercourse should be avoided for at least a month and alcohol, which, because it is excreted in the urine, tends to aggravate this type of infection, for the first few days.

In 1971, the British Clinical Co-operative Group in a survey of 194 clinics in the United Kingdom, found that in the treatment of males, 83 (43%) administered a routine dosage of 1.2 megaunits of procaine penicillin or less, and 27 (14%) one of 2.4 megaunits. However, amounts well in excess of this are used and the determining factor in the size of dosage should be the relative sensitivity or otherwise in that locality of the strains of gonococcus. The proportion of insensitive strains differs widely in different regions and sometimes in the same place over a period of time. If as suggested by Evans (1966) an *in vitro* minimum inhibitory concentration of 0.3 units/ml denotes full sensitivity of a given strain of gonococcus, then a dosage of 1.2 megaunits of penicillin is likely to achieve almost a full cure rate in infections with such strains. Rates varying from 13.2% of strains showing a minimum inhibitory concentration as high as

0.125 to 1.0 units/ml in London (Medical Research Council 1961), to 44.3% in Australia in 104 strains ranging from 0.1 to 3.5 units ml (Smith and Levey 1967), and again in London, 35% (Gray, Phillips and Nicol 1966 and 1969) have been reported.

As it is only necessary to have an adequate blood concentration for 24 hours to cure uncomplicated gonorrhea, this means that an increased dosage is required to increase the blood levels if relatively insensitive strains of organism are involved. Mere prolongation of treatment on a small dosage or splitting one large dose into two or more over a 24-hour period is ineffective. Probenecid which by blocking renal excretion of penicillin results in significantly increased serum levels, has been increasingly used of late. Hilton (1959) treated 64 patients who had received procaine penicillin 1.2 megaunits with probenecid 0.5 g 6-hourly for four doses without any treatment failure. Serum penicillin levels at 21 and 30 hours after penicillin ranged between 0.15 and 48 units/ml.

Gray, Phillips and Nicol (1970) using probenecid 1 g orally followed by an injection of benzyl penicillin 5 megaunits with lignocaine in 8 ml—given to 200 patients, found one failure among 185 returning for follow-up, a cure rate of 99.5%. Olzen and Lomholt (1969) having similarly treated 832 cases of uncomplicated gonorrhea, obtained a success rate of 99%.

Fluker and Hewitt (1969) treated with ampicillin 2 g orally followed at once by an injection of 3.6 megaunits of procaine penicillin, 60 cases of *treatment failure* following penicillin dosages ranging from 0.9 to 3.6 megaunits of procaine penicillin with cure of 54 of the 57 followed (94.5%). Onyeabo (1970) adding probenecid 2 g to the foregoing (PPPP) cured 306 (98.7%) out of 310 cases all in women and previously untreated.

It is thus clear that for rational and effective treatment with penicillin, the sensitivity of the local strains of gonococcus must be known and that where there is a substantial proportion of relatively insensitive strains, massive dosage is required. Without this data, comparisons of different treatment schedules in the various centres is quite meaningless. The close co-operation of microbiologists is vital.

Patients who are allergic to penicillin or have lesions as yet undiagnosed that might be syphilitic must not be given penicillin nor in the latter instance, tetracyclines, erythromycin, chloramphenicol and cephaloridine for fear of masking that infection. Generally co-trimoxazole (trimethoprim 80 mg with sulphamethoxazole 400 mg per tablet) administered morning and evening for 7 days or three tablets similarly for 4–5 days in most series reported, has given cure rates in excess of 90%. Lastly, an injection of kanamycin 2 g gives a cure rate of over 95% as reported by Wilkinson, Race and Curtis (1967), Hooton and Nicol (1967) and Fluker and Hewitt (1970). However, both its expense and more particularly its potential toxicity on the cochlea preclude its routine use. Other antibiotics such as tetracyclines, including doxycycline, erythromycin, spiramycin and streptomycin are in general considerably less effective but an injection of Spectinomycin 2 g is highly so.

In the case of complications in either sex but particularly in salpingitis, treatment should be continued for at least 7–10 days or longer if necessary. Tetracyclines which are bacteriostatic rather than bactericidal may not be the wisest choice of antibiotic in these cases. In the case of bartholinitis, if an abscess forms it must be drained preferably by aspiration and any resulting cyst marsupialized subsequently. In cases of salpingitis, bed rest is desirable and any abscess formation must be treated surgically. Sterility may follow owing to bilateral blockage of the fimbriae.

Rectal gonorrhea in male homosexuals is a prominent feature in certain clinics of large cities but in many other centres is still uncommon. The results of penicillin treatment are less good. The following results are based on work done at the West London Hospital. Onyeabo (1971) using PPPP in 192 cases had 18 failures in 180 followed—a cumulative failure rate of 11.2%. Waugh (1971) using co-trimoxazole (as Bactrim) giving two drapsules twice daily for 7 days had a cumulative failure rate of 12.6%—eight failures in 66 cases followed from an initial total of 72 and in a later series 12 failures in 105 cases followed (11.4%). It is interesting that in Waugh's second series no less than seven patients developed early syphilis, a penile chancre after 15 days, anal chancres after 5, 27, 56 and 91 days, sero-positive primary syphilis at 90 days (chancre not located) and secondary syphilis at 48 days. In Onyeabo's series there was only one case of syphilis. In homosexual cases at least, surveillance should therefore last for not less than 3 months. Fluker and Hewitt (1970) treated 100 cases with procaine penicillin 1.8 megaunits and 100 with kanamycin 2 g both by injection. The numbers followed were 96 and 90 respectively with failures in 26 and 14 respectively, the cumulative failure rates being 28.3% and 17.1%. This illustrates the necessity for high penicillin dosage. The importance of cultures both in the diagnosis and surveillance of treated rectal cases cannot be overemphasized. Finally there is no longer any place for the routine use of streptomycin to which antibiotic the resistance of numerous strains of gonococcus is absolute.

Gonococcal ophthalmia neonatorum which in the United Kingdom is a notifiable condition, is also potentially a very dangerous one in which the eyes may be destroyed completely within 48 hours. Parenteral injection of penicillin is required but local treatment is the more important with douching of the eyes and the instillation of penicillin eye drops at the rate of 1 per minute into each eye until the discharge has ceased. The manoeuvre may be repeated if the discharge subsequently recurs.

Non-gonococcal urethritis

Those cases of urethritis secondary to some general medical or surgical conditions will depend upon treatment of that particular condition and do not concern us here. This leaves three types of urethritis. Firstly the non-specific urethritis of unknown aetiology. Secondly, urethritis due to trichomonas and thirdly that due to *Candida albicans*. The first type is by far the most common. The least unsatisfactory treatment is with tetracycline, either oxytetracycline or tetracycline usually given as 250 mg four times a day for 7–21 days. The cure rate is probably about 80%. Patients should be seen at the end of one, two or three and 5 or 6 weeks. The discharge disappears and the urine clears much more slowly than in gonorrhea, but by the end of a week or 10 days there should be no symptoms. Unfortunately, relapse is very common during the first few weeks though it rarely happens thereafter, and no patient should be guaranteed cure in a shorter period. About 80–85% of patients are in fact cured but the remainder will need further treatment. A second line of defence is a single injection of streptomycin associated with a sulphonamide for 7 days. All the evidence suggests that this combination is three times as effective as either alone but the cure rate which used to be claimed as approaching 80% does not now seem to be much more than 60–65%. Thirdly, if both the other methods fail, a course of urethral irrigations for from 10–14 days using either 1:10 000 oxycyanide of mercury or 1:10 000 potassium permanganate may effect a cure.

In certain relapsing cases that initially respond to tetracycline, it may be worth restarting the tetracycline at full dosage for 21 days, followed by half dosage, this is to say 250 mg twice a day, for a further 10 or 14 days, and a pro-

longed period of 3–6 weeks or more on 250 mg daily. This seems to prevent relapse in a limited number of cases. Other antibiotics are usually much less effective and the least effective of all is penicillin. Those patients whose infection persists or recurs after 3 weeks or so should invariably have the prostate examined and this in any case should be done at the end of 5 or 6 weeks before the patient is discharged. If the trouble persists for more than 8 weeks investigations to exclude stricture including an urethrogram, urethroscopy and bouginage will be advisable. In very difficult cases a full urinary tract investigation will be required. Operation is often the best method of treatment as careless instrumentation of the lower genito-urinary tract may cause serious renal infection.

THE TREATMENT OF PROSTATITIS

This is extremely unsatisfactory but the best method seems to be a prolonged course of tetracycline accompanied by weekly or even bi-weekly prostatic massage for about 6 or 8 weeks. Some cases seem to respond after a holiday. Alcohol and sexual activity should be eschewed as long as there is any evidence of active urethral infection.

Reiter's Disease

Reiter's disease which consists of urethritis, arthritis and eye manifestations sometimes associated with skin and buccal eruptions presents a difficult problem. The urethritis must be treated on the lines already indicated. Bed rest is advisable and where acute arthritis is present, immobilization is required often using a pillow in the early stages. Later on a bi-valved plaster may be helpful. Nevertheless complete immobilization is inadvisable as this over a period may lead to a stiff joint. If the joint is very distended with fluid, especially the knee, aspiration with steroid replacement may be helpful. Delayed resolution over a period exceeding a month is another indication for this treatment. Phenylbutazone in a total dosage of 400 mg daily seems to have a slightly specific effect and to be better than other analgesics but the occurrence of blood dyscrasias must be remembered. Steroid therapy is disappointing but in acute cases that persist for more than a month may be tried in a dosage equivalent to not less than 40 mg of prednisone daily. If the eye is involved, irrigation will be required with bland drops for a simple conjunctivitis, but if anterior uveitis is found, mydriatics and steroid therapy are indicated and an ophthalmologist's advice should be sought. It should be remembered that Reiter's disease is not gonococcal arthritis. This latter is an arthritis in which gonococci will be found in the joint fluid. It is part of a septicaemic condition.

Trichomoniasis

Trichomoniasis in both male and female is best treated with metronidazole 200 mg 3 times a day for a week. Results are excellent and at least 85% of patients are cured. In the event of failure the dosage may be doubled. Equally good results are obtained with metronidazole 2 g (400 mg × 5) in a single dose, (Woodcock, 1972). In the female, failure is often due to reinfection from the male consort and although a few males show evidence of urethritis from this cause, the majority who are infected are symptomless carriers. If both partners are treated, sexual intercourse should be avoided until treatment is complete. In the event of complete failure, nitrimidazine is often effective; othewise acetarsol pessaries, two morning and evening, may be employed in the female.

Although no evidence has been adduced that metronidazole or nitrimidazine causes fetal damage during the first trimester of pregnancy, nevertheless it is usual to withhold them during that time. Nifuratel 200 mg three times a day by mouth may be tried together with pessaries. However, the results obtained from this preparation at least in Great Britain are less satisfactory, (Fowler and Hussain, 1968).

Candidiasis

Candidiasis in both sexes is very troublesome. The most satisfactory treatment in the female is either with nystatin pessaries one morning and evening or two at night for at least 2 weeks—there is some evidence that reinfection may occur from the rectum. If this is confirmed by the isolation of *Candida albicans* from the stools or from rectal swabs, or where such investigations are impracticable, when it is suspected, oral nystatin, one tablet four times a day for a week, is a useful adjuvant. Amphotericin B pessaries, one at night for 14 days, may also be effective. Sometimes it may be necessary to continue treatment for at least 2 months and to use any or all of these remedies in quick succession. In the male, urethral irrigations may be required as nystatin which is not absorbed from the alimentary tract is ineffective.

When there is local inflammation due to *Candida albicans* either vulvitis in the female or balanoposthitis in the male, then nystatin cream is helpful. This latter infection in the male is not uncommon. In those rare cases when the male develops a hypersensitivity of the skin to an infection in the female partner, this may be suppressed by local steroid treatment but obviously elimination of the trouble in the female genital tract is the only permanent solution.

FEMALE CONTACTS OF MALE PATIENTS WITH NON-SPECIFIC GENITAL INFECTION

Females should always be examined and if any lesion is found it should be treated on its merits. If only a cervicitis is found or nothing else, the particular treatment which has cured the male partner—usually a tetracycline—is the only logical step to take, and may prevent reinfection of the male. Very often when recurrence occurs in the male it is due to an overlooked focus of infection—for example, prostatitis or developing stricture.

Chancroid

Chancroid or soft sore is not very common in the United Kingdom except in certain port clinics. The important thing is to remember that the condition may coexist with syphilis and that syphilis cannot be excluded without 3 months observation following treatment, with repetition of blood tests to exclude it. Sulphonamides are usually effective in a course of 5 days or alternatively a daily injection of streptomycin, either alone or with sulphonamides for 5 days is curative. Tetracyclines are also effective but these are better avoided on account of the possible masking of syphilis. If a bubo forms it will have to be drained and aspiration is the best treatment. Phagoedena, once so destructive, is never seen today, at least in the United Kingdom. It used to result in partial or complete gangrene of the penis.

Lymphogranuloma venereum

This again is seen only in the major ports of the United Kingdom, but is common in many subtropical areas. Once the diagnosis has been established, treatment is required for a minimum of from 10 to 14 days. Sulphonamides may be used, full dosage for a week dropping to half dosage for the second week. Tetracyclines are also useful, 500 mg four times a day from 10 to 14 days, or more recently triacetyloleandomycin in a similar dosage and in a recent series 11 out of 14 cases were permanently cured (Fluker, 1963). If a bubo forms then aspiration will be required. Rectal stricture is sometimes seen in females and dilation of this may be required, together of course, with the appropriate chemotherapy or antibiotic treatment. If one of the above remedies fails, then another should be tried and it will be extremely unlikely to meet a case resistant to all three.

Granuloma inguinalae

The writer has no experience of this condition whatever, which is extremely rare in the United Kingdom. Antimony, once used, no longer has a place in treatment. Streptomycin intramuscularly is effective. A total of 20 g is adequate in most cases, given over a period of 5 days. If a smaller but somewhat safer dosage is used, this is effective but slower. Tetracyclines are also suitable—a dosage of 500 mg for 10 to 20 days being curative and probably safer than streptomycin but syphilis must be excluded before their use.

Yaws

Yaws does not occur in the United Kingdom in its natural form but latent cases are sometimes seen, in whom the diagnosis from syphilis is often extremely difficult. Normally this condition requires less penicillin than syphilis, but if treatment schedules similar to those of syphilis are given, cure of either condition can be guaranteed and this amount of treatment is an additional safeguard in the event of an error of differential diagnosis between the two conditions.

Condylomatosis or genital warts

The term 'venereal warts' is undesirable, genital is the correct epithet. These lesions are very common and are frequently transmitted by sexual intercourse. Consequently peri-anal lesions are common in male homosexuals. Treatment in both sexes in early cases is with the resin podophyllin which should be applied to the warts usually as a 25% solution in spirit. This solution should *never* be given to patients to apply themselves as most serious reactions may thus occur. Care should be taken to prevent the solution from burning the surrounding skin, and it should always be washed off after 6 hours. The warts turn white and usually after three or four re-applications will separate. Lesions on mucous membranes sometimes do better from the application of trichloracetic acid. If, however, the warts are particularly hard or very deep seated, local applications are ineffective and diathermy is required—usually under a local anaesthetic. Intra-vaginal or cervical warts in the female are better dealt with under general anaesthesia. Peri-anal

or intra-rectal warts usually respond poorly to local applications and become exceedingly sore and tender. Much the best treatment is with repeated diathermy, preferably under a local anaesthetic. These lesions have a tendency to recur and although surgery under a general anaesthetic with admission to hospital may temporarily get rid of them, the limited follow up possible in the ordinary surgical outpatients is insufficient to prevent generalized recurrence, whereas, if they are dealt with a few at a time under local anaesthesia, the end results are often much superior. All predisposing causes such as trichomoniasis or candidiasis in the female should of course be removed. Above all, gonorrhea and syphilis must be excluded, particularly their proctological manifestations in patients with perianal warts.

Balanoposthitis in the male

There are several causes of this but general principles of treatment include improved hygiene with retraction of the prepuce during micturition and consequent prevention of urinary contamination of the lesions which invariably aggravates them. The invariable testing of the urine for sugar with diagnosis and treatment of any accompanying glycosuria is an integral part of the correct management of every case. Balanoposthitis is often an important symptom of diabetes mellitus. In mild cases a local application of copper sulphate, 1 in 500 is very useful. In those cases where there are deep slits or fissures a dye such as 1% gentian violet is the best application and where there is much secondary infection as in acute erosive balanoposthitis a sulphonamide is helpful. If there is phimosis and a purulent sub-preputial discharge, sub-preputial irrigations with normal saline once or twice daily are indicated, together with a sulphonamide. On no account should any anti-syphilitic antibiotic be given as in these latter cases there may be an underlying primary sore and if such treatment were started the sore might have disappeared by the time that retraction of the prepuce becomes possible without the condition being cured and with accurate diagnosis now invalidated completely. Whenever there is a possibility of this having happened, a diagnosis of syphilis should be assumed and full treatment and follow-up given.

The widely held belief that cases of sexually transmitted infections should be isolated in special wards or forced to discontinue their work unless physically ill, is sheer nonsense. Obviously, surgical gloves should be worn by those performing darkground tests. That is all that is necessary.

The follow-up of contacts is essential especially in families and this must not exclude latent or late syphilis. Failure to do this may result in tragic developments in the neglected spouse and middle aged or elderly people in such a situation need not always be told the underlying cause of their troubles.

Patients should normally be asked to bring their known contacts and in teaching them how to do this, it may be possible to instil some sense of responsibility towards others, lack of which is often one of the basic causes of their troubles. A skilled welfare officer may be invaluable in helping patients, especially young girls and homosexual males to cope with their problems.

In conclusion, it should be realised that the treatment of this group of patients does not simply consist in the exhibition of antibiotics but that the highest skill and art of medical practice may be needed to develop and exploit to the patients' full advantage the remarkable power over the individual which this very intimate and special doctor–patient relationship often gives to the physician.

8

THE NERVOUS SYSTEM

R. W. ROSS RUSSELL

BACTERIAL MENINGITIS

Specific therapy is available for most types of bacterial meningitis and the isolation of the causative organism from the CSF or blood must be the first objective. Early treatment is imperative and should be given as soon as specimens for culture have been obtained. Treatment given before taking specimens is probably the reason why in many reports about a quarter of the specimens yield no organism; treatment could not therefore be soundly based and this must be an important factor in the continuing mortality in this disease.

In selecting the appropriate antibiotics for treatment before culture results are available it is important to remember that the causative bacteria vary at different ages. In general the commonest causes are *N. meningitidis*, *H. influenzae* and *Str. pneumoniae*. *H. influenzae* is the commonest cause in infants and young children but rare in older children and adults. *N. meningitidis* is also frequent in children and the commonest cause in young adults, *Pneumococci* are found most often in old age and as a secondary infection. In neonates the spectrum of infecting organisms is quite different; coliforms are common as are haemolytic streptococci of Lancefield Group B; *N. meningitidis* and *H. influenzae* are rare. When secondary meningitis supervenes after chronic ear infection, sinusitis, trauma or lumbar puncture, the infecting organisms can be any of a large number of organisms including *Staphy. aureus*.

The principles of treatment of meningitis are early diagnosis, early intensive chemotherapy and the early detection and treatment of complications. Early diagnosis depends on CSF examination and the diagnosis can frequently be made from immediate staining of the spun deposit; CSF should not be chilled or refrigerated. The CSF is often turbid but a clear fluid does not exclude significant pleocytosis or meningitis. Visible haziness is produced when the cell count exceeds 500/mm³. In pyogenic meningitis polymorphs are usually present in large numbers,

hundreds or thousands/mm³ and protein is in the range 100–500 mg%. The sugar content is less than 50 mg% (3 mmol/1) and in the established cases less than 25 mg% (1.5 mmol/1).

Specific therapy

At the initial lumbar puncture if the fluid is turbid 5000–10 000 units soluble penicillin may be given intrathecally.

N. meningitidis. Sulphadiazine: adult dose 1–1.5 g 6-hourly for 4 days and penicillin 1 mega unit 6-hourly for 7 days. For children 100 mg/kg. Lumbar puncture will be required to check progress after about 48 hours, but in the uncomplicated case it is usually unnecessary to repeat it thereafter. Ampicillin oral, i.m. or i.v., 1–4 g/day may be used as an alternative to penicillin. Carriers should receive sulphadiazine as above.

Str. pneumoniae. Either:
(a) penicillin 1 mega unit i.v. 2-hourly until improvement occurs then penicillin 1–2 mega units i.m. every four hours for ten days; or
(b) penicillin 10–15 000 units intrathecally each day until 24 hours after the CSF is sterile, and penicillin i.m. 1 mega unit four times daily for 10 days. This infection is often associated with otitis media, sinusitis, skull fracture or congenital defects. These may need surgical treatment. Lumbar punctures will be required, whichever treatment is used, to check the responses and to detect relapses, which are relatively common. Treatment should in any event be continued for 10 days or until all signs have settled for at least one week. Response to treatment is usually slow and cerebral abscess occurs more frequently than in other forms of meningitis.

H. influenzae. Chloramphenicol—1–2 g i.v. 6-hourly for 24 hours followed by 1 g i.m. 6-hourly for 5–7 days with sulphadiazine as above.

Urgent undiagnosed case. Chloramphenicol 1–2 g 6-hourly by intravenous injection.

Streptococci, staphylococci and other organisms. The treatment of meningitis due to other organisms will depend upon sensitivity tests; cooperation with the bacteriologist is essential. It may be necessary to employ cephaloridine, cloxacillin, gentamicin or carbenicillin in certain cases, particularly those following head injury or neurosurgery. A variety of unusual organisms may occasionally cause meningitis in patients with disordered immunity. Specific therapy may be available (e.g. ampicillin for *Listeria*, amphotericin B for *Cryptococcus*).

Other treatment. If vomiting and dehydration are severe, especially in infants, parenteral fluids may be required. Hypotension, coma or an extensive purpuric rash are indications for intravenous hydrocortisone 100 mg 3-hourly, supplemented by oral treatment. Young children and all patients with a history of epileptic seizures should be given phenobarbitone.

Tuberculous meningitis

In all cases of meningitis with a lymphocytic cellular reaction the CSF should be examined and cultured for acid-fast bacilli. The cell count is variable (usually 25–500/mm³) and CSF sugar is usually in the range 20–40 mg% (1–2 mmol/l). Culture of tubercle bacilli takes several weeks and treatment cannot await the results of sensitivity tests. Bacilli may show a primary resistance to standard drugs or resistance may be acquired during treatment (secondary resistance).

Combined therapy with streptomycin, isoniazid and rifampicin is mandatory as initial treatment. Streptomycin (1 g/day) i.m. is sufficient and intrathecal therapy is no longer necessary for uncomplicated cases. Treatment should continue for 2 months. INAH is given orally in doses of 15 mg/kg/day in adults and 20 mg/kg/day in children who tolerate it well. Nine months treatment is recommended. Rifampicin is given by mouth (450–900 mg/day as a single dose) and continued for 9 months. For resistant strains and severe infections pyrazinamide (3 g daily) is available.

Viral meningitis

In the United Kingdom the enterovirus group (Coxsackie, Echo) are now the commonest pathogenic virus causing meningitis in the summer months. During the remainder of the year mumps predominates. No specific therapy is available or necessary.

Herpes simplex may be responsible for a severe meningoencephalitis with a high mortality. The diagnosis is established by identifying the virus from brain biopsy. Intravenous idoxuridine first introduced as specific therapy has now been superseded by cytosine arabinoside 2 mg/kg

i.v./day. Cerebral edema is a prominent feature and dexamethasone 4–12 mg/day is also recommended.

EPILEPSY

General management. In patients with idiopathic epilepsy the brain is structurally normal but epilepsy may also be a symptom of brain damage. Both groups of patients need suppression of epileptic activity and in the latter group removal of the primary cause may be possible. In idiopathic epilepsy, seizures usually begin in childhood or adolescence, occasionally in adult life. Seizures may be provoked by fever, or intercurrent illness. As the child matures there is a tendency for epileptic seizures to become less frequent and only about one third of childhood epileptics continue to have seizures in adult life.

Many epileptic patients become aware of factors which provoke attacks such as drowsiness, lack of sleep, fever, visual flicker, nervous tension, premenstrual fluid retention and alcohol. Others recognise abnormalities of mood, headache, or involuntary myoclonic jerking as a prelude to an attack.

Seizures vary greatly in type and frequency and in the ease with which they may be controlled. A recent advance in the management of epilepsy is the monitoring of serum levels of anticonvulsants although the precise significance of these levels is still open to doubt. Estimation of serum levels is useful in the management of patients with toxic symptoms, in patients who may not be taking drugs or in patients taking a combination of drugs which may be interacting. Drugs are often combined but the use of more than two drugs at a time is confusing and unnecessary.

First choice drugs for major seizures. Phenobarbitone is the initial drug of choice for many types of epilepsy. The dose is 30–150 mg/day in divided doses according to age, being adjusted to give a plasma level of 15 μg/ml (60 μmol l⁻¹). Toxic manifestations usually occur at the level of about 25 μg/ml (100 μmol l⁻¹) consisting of drowsiness, ataxia, confusion and dysarthria. It usually takes about 2 weeks to achieve stable blood level when the patient is beginning treatment. Phenobarbitone is broken down slowly and probably need be taken only once per day.

Hyperactive children with seizures respond poorly to phenobarbitone and the behaviour disorder may be made worse. Patients taking anticoagulants require extra care in monitoring the dose. Occasional patients develop a megaloblastic anaemia which responds to folic acid. *Phenytoin.* Phenytoin is a most useful drug for many types of focal and generalised epilepsy. It is given by mouth and absorbed very rapidly. By intramuscular injection its effects are slight and unpredictable. About 10 days are usually necessary to reach a stable plasma level. The drug should be given once per day rather than in divided doses. Phenytoin is metabolised mainly in the liver and the rate of metabolism is markedly influenced by other drugs notably by phenobarbitone (which increases the rate of phenytoin breakdown) and by sulthiame (which leads to increase in serum levels by inhibiting breakdown of phenytoin). The effective plasma levels are in the range of 10–20 μg (40–80 μmol l^{-1}). Phenytoin (and probably phenobarbitone) if taken for long periods have important side effects on vitamin D metabolism and tend to cause osteomalacia. Alkaline phosphatase is frequently raised in patients on long term phenytoin, and serum calcium and bone X–rays may also be abnormal. Other toxic effects of phenytoin are gum hypertrophy, cerebellar ataxia and dysarthria. The cerebellum may be permanently damaged by chronic overdose. Unusual side effects include skin rashes and lymphadenopathy. Megaloblastic anaemia due to folate deficiency is common and serum levels of folate should be checked periodically.

Primidone. Primidone is largely metabolised in the liver to phenobarbitone. There is some doubt whether its anticonvulsant activity is due only to phenobarbitone or whether it exerts an independent anticonvulsant action. The drug is a useful substitute for phenobarbitone especially in cases of temporal lobe epilepsy. It is often given in combination with phenytoin but should not be given with phenobarbitone because of the risk of toxicity. The dose varies from 250 to 1000 mg/day by mouth and is adjusted to give a plasma phenobarbitone within the range of 10–20 μg/ml (40–80 μmol l^{-1}). Its major side effects are drowsiness, vertigo, nausea and vomiting; these are most commonly seen at the initiation of treatment. The drug is normally used as a substitute for phenobarbitone in patients whose seizures cannot be controlled with a combination of phenobarbitone and phenytoin.

SPECIAL TYPES OF EPILEPSY

Temporal lobe epilepsy: in this type of epilepsy there are partial lapses of consciousness and periods of automatism. Attacks may occur in children as a sequel of birth trauma or cerebral anoxia; in adults they usually result from an intrinsic cerebral tumour. It is the most difficult variety of epilepsy to control and patients may also present a behaviour disturbance between attacks. A combination of phenobarbitone and phenytoin should be tried, but is often disappointing. Primidone and phenytoin is the most satisfactory drug regime in many patients. If this is unsuccessful phenytoin may be combined with a benzodiazepam, such as Clonazepam, 4–6 mg/day, or with diazepam. The latter drug is particularly useful in those patients with marked behaviour disturbance between attacks. Carbamazepine is also well worth a trial in this variety of epilepsy. The dose is 400–800 mg/day by mouth and the effective serum level 60–80 μg/ml (250–360 μmol l^{-1}). It can be used in combination with other drugs. There is some risk of serious haematological side effects especially in elderly patients who may also notice drowsiness, dysarthria and ataxia.

Petit mal. In this common variety of childhood epilepsy the drug of choice is ethosuximide given initially in a dose of 500 mg/day, increasing slowly to 1.5 g or until control is achieved. The usual plasma level is 40–80 μg/ml (300–600 μmol l^{-1}). If major seizures are also present phenobarbitone or phenytoin are required in addition. If ethosuximide fails to control the attacks troxidone may be used (900 mg/day). In this case repeated white cell counts are desirable. Clonazepam (see below) and acetazolamide (250–375 mg/day) are also sometimes effective.

Second line drugs. The following drugs may be found useful in patients with grand mal or temporal lobe epilepsy whose seizures respond poorly to the standard regime:

Sulthiame, dose 200–600 mg/day. This probably acts mainly by increasing plasma levels of phenytoin and it is always given in combination. It may produce hyperventilation as a side effect. Clonazepam is a recently introduced benzodiazepine with more pronounced oral anticonvulsant activity than diazepam. The dose is 2–8 mg/day in divided doses and the therapeutic plasma level 25–75 μg/ml (100–250 mmol l^{-1}). It is compatible with other anticonvulsants and can also be administered intravenously. The major side effect is drowsiness.

Sodium valproate is thought to inhibit breakdown of gamma amino butyric acid. The dose is 80–160 mg/day in divided doses. It may produce drowsiness if given in combination with phenobarbitone; it potentiates the effect of phenytoin. Other side effects are nausea and vomiting due to gastric irritation. The therapeutic plasma level is in the range 50–100 μg/ml (300–600 μmol l^{-1}). It is incompatible with monoamine oxidase inhibitors.

SURGICAL TREATMENT OF EPILEPSY

Surgical excision of a localised cortical epileptogenic focus in the temporal lobe may be considered when seizures are poorly controlled by medication and when repeated EEG examinations show a persistent epileptic focus in a localised and accessible part of the temporal lobe, preferably in the non-dominant hemisphere.

STATUS EPILEPTICUS

Failure to recover consciousness between seizures adds considerably to the dangers of epilepsy and immediate hospital treatment is required. The condition most commonly results from a structural lesion especially involving the frontal lobes. It may also complicate infections such as meningitis or cerebral abscess and is most frequently seen in patients who have suddenly withdrawn anticonvulsant therapy. Emergency treatment is directed at maintaining a clear airway, at stopping the seizures and preventing hyperpyrexia and cerebral edema. The best initial drug therapy is intravenous diazepam 10 mg repeated every 15 minutes up to 400 mg. There is some risk of respiratory depression. Alternative treatment is intravenous infusion of paraldehyde 5 ml in 500 ml saline by slow intravenous drip. This well tried remedy is often effective but carries some risk of pulmonary edema. In resistant cases intravenous phenytoin, or intravenous chlormethiazole (continuous i.v. infusion, 700 mg/hour) may be tried or the patients may be anaesthetised for a short time using intravenous barbiturate anaesthetic such as thiopentone and maintaining adequate oxygenation.

Petit mal stasis is an uncommon condition most often seen in children and responds best to intravenous diazepam. Myoclonic jerks are often seen in combination with epilepsy and if infrequent require no treatment. They respond best to the benzodiazepam group of drugs such as nitrazepam 7.5 mg/day.

NARCOLEPSY AND CATAPLEXY

Uncontrollable attacks of sleep during the day (narcolepsy) may be associated with involuntary generalised muscle weakness provoked by emotional stress (cataplexy). Other features are attacks of sleep paralysis and hypnagogic hallucinations. The syndrome is not associated with epilepsy. Amphetamine (5 mg twice daily) is the most satisfactory remedy for narcolepsy. There is a danger of addiction but many patients remain well controlled on a small dose for long periods. This is the only indication for the use

of amphetamine. Cataplexy responds best to clomipramine 30–150 mg/day.

MIGRAINE

General management. It is helpful to explain to the patient with migraine that the pain originates in over-active blood vessels and that liability to attacks will continue throughout life, although becoming less pronounced after middle age. Many patients discover provoking factors such as nervous tension, physical exertion, ingestion of alcohol or certain foods such as cheese or chocolate and learn to avoid them. Oral contraceptive drugs may produce migraine for the first time or may provoke attacks in a migrainous subject. Migraine usually disappears during pregnancy. Migraine is essentially a paroxysmal condition and seldom causes continuous or daily headaches. When such headaches occur in a migrainous subject there is usually a superimposed anxiety or depressive reaction requiring separate treatment. Migraine sufferers are suggestible and a placebo effect is common with any new remedy.

Treatment of the attack. Mild attacks respond to simple oral analgesics such as soluble aspirin or codeine phosphate 3 mg. Attacks of moderate severity may often be terminated by an ergotamine preparation, ergotamine tartrate 2–4 mg sublingually or by a compound tablet of ergotamine 1 mg, caffeine 100 mg taken by mouth. The effect of caffeine is to increase the absorption of ergotamine. If severe nausea is present, a combination of ergotamine with an antihistamine is indicated (ergotamine 2 mg, caffeine 100 mg, cyclizine 50 mg). In severe attacks a subcutaneous injection of ergotamine tartrate 1 mg or a suppository containing ergotamine may be effective. An ergotamine medihaler (0.36 mg/dose) is available but carries a considerable risk of overdosage. The major contraindication to ergotamine is cardiac ischaemia or peripheral vascular disease.

Prevention of attacks. Frequent attacks of migraine or migrainous neuralgia may often be prevented by regular administration of a small dose of ergotamine combined with a sedative. A suitable preparation is ergotamine 0.3 mg, belladonna alkaloids 0.1 mg, phenobarbitone 30 mg. When headaches wake the patient from sleep the drugs should be taken on retiring. Long term daily treatment with ergotamine requires careful supervision but small quantities are taken daily without ill effect by large numbers of patients.

Methysergide, a serotonin antagonist, has been introduced as a preventative drug in patients suffering frequent disabling attacks. The drug is often effective but carries a considerable risk of side effects. These occur in about 20% of patients and consist of arterial occlusion, retroperitoneal or retropleural fibrosis, vertigo, vomiting. Sudden withdrawal of the drug may provoke severe migraine. The dose is 1–2 mg/day to a maximum of 6 mg and the drug is sometimes used in combination with ergotamine. Methysergide should not be taken continuously for longer than three months.

Clonidine is used as a preventative treatment for migraine in a dose of 0.025–0.075 mg/day; its effect is unpredictable, but a few patients appear to benefit. The following drugs may also be tried in resistant cases of migraine:

Cyproheptadine 12 mg/day, prochlorperazine 15 mg/day, propranolol 40–120 mg/day, amitriptyline or other tricyclic antidepressants 75 mg/day, indomethacin 75 mg/day, pizotifen three tablets daily (2175 μg).

Migrainous neuralgia

Attacks of migrainous neuralgia often occur in groups separated by long intervals of freedom. The most effective treatment is preventative, using a compound ergotamine preparation as for migraine. Most attacks are nocturnal and the drug is effective taken in the evening by mouth or by suppository. About every week or so the drug is stopped to ascertain whether treatment is still necessary. Methysergide may also be prescribed for resistant cases (dose 2–4 mg taken at night). Clonidine is also worth a trial.

Herpetic neuralgia

Root pain and hyperaesthesia commonly occur at the time of the skin eruption in herpes zoster. There is some evidence that corticotrophin 40 units/day for 5 days not only eases these symptoms but may lessen the incidence of post-herpetic neuralgia. Topical idoxuridine (40% in dimethyl sulphoxide) applied to the lesions may have a similar effect.

Severe constant spontaneous pain and cutaneous hyperaesthesia are features of the intractable condition of post-herpetic neuralgia. Non-narcotic analgesics such as aspirin, paracetamol (1000 mg/day), dextropropoxyphene (250 mg/day), mefenamic acid (1000 mg/day) may give relief. The narcotic analgesics are best avoided, because of the risk of addiction. Local peripheral nerve block with procaine or phenol is sometimes helpful for a limited period. Cutaneous vibratory treatment which has a temporary anaesthetising effect on nerve endings may alleviate hyperaesthesia.

Patients with post-herpetic neuralgia are often obsessional and depressed, and may be helped more by anti-depressive than by analgesic treatment. Phenelzine 30–45 mg/day with chlordiazepoxide 20 mg/day (and with the appropriate dietary restrictions) is recommended. Herpes zoster may be symptomatic of an underlying neoplastic or lymphomatous lesion.

Trigeminal neuralgia

In this condition which occurs almost always in the elderly, attacks of severe lancinating pain occur in one or more divisions of the trigeminal nerve on one side; pain is provoked by touching the skin, eating and by cold. Attacks are episodic and long periods of freedom occur. In repeated attacks the pain remains unilateral but may spread to affect other divisions of the nerve. General measures include the avoidance of precipitating factors and the treatment of depression. Mild attacks may be helped by simple analgesics but in most cases the specific remedy, carbamazepine, is still required. This is given orally 200 mg/day in divided doses, increasing if necessary slowly to 1000 mg/day, or until toxic effects occur (ataxia, drowsiness, nausea, skin rashes). Rapid suppression of severe pain occurs although a mild sensation may continue. This dose is maintained at the minimum level which will suppress symptoms; it is unwise to continue treatment for longer than 6 months because of the danger of granulopenia. The drug does not prevent future relapses.

If no relief occurs, surgical treatment may be necessary. This consists of alcoholic injection of the trigeminal ganglion or division of its sensory root. This produces a permanent cure, but the patient should be warned of the loss of facial sensation which ensues.

CEREBRAL VASCULAR DISEASE
Indications for treatment

The arterial disorder underlying most common types of vascular disease is atheroma, a process causing fibrous and fatty change in the intima of large and medium sized arteries. These changes may be aggravated by hypertension, which in addition causes thickening and hyalinosis of small arteries and arterioles. Deposition of platelets on roughened arterial surfaces initiates thrombosis and the resultant mixed thrombus may occlude the vessel or become organised and incorporated into an atheromatous lesion.

By the time symptoms of cerebral ischaemia develop, atheromatous degeneration is usually widespread and probably irreversible by medical treatment, although it might possibly have been prevented by treatment early in life. In occlusive vascular disease treatment may be directed at prevention of fibrin formation and of hypertension. Fibrinolytic therapy is not used at present in the cerebral circulation due to the risk of allergic reactions and of haemorrhage, and drugs acting on platelet aggregation are still being evaluated.

Transient cerebral ischaemia

This common symptom has a number of causes including recurrent embolism from heart or arterial wall, systemic hypotension or diminished cardiac output, diversion of blood to extracerebral tissues, or hypertensive vascular spasm. Either anaemia or polycythaemia may also predispose to its occurrence. Since attacks are rarely observed, it is often impossible to be certain of the aetiology. Assessment of treatment is also difficult, since attacks often cease spontaneously. Approximately 30–50 percent of patients develop a completed 'stroke' within 5 years. Prognosis is better in the vertebrobasilar than in the carotid territory.

Arteriography is necessary for the investigation of ischaemic attacks within the carotid territory, unless there is severe hypertension, widespread vascular disease or advanced age.

If a localised accessible carotid stenosis is found, endarterectomy abolishes attacks in the great majority of patients. Visualisation of the other carotid artery or of all the other extracranial arteries is advisable before operation. Arteriography is not routinely undertaken for vertebrobasilar ischaemia unless there is clinical evidence of common carotid, innominate or subclavian occlusion.

Anticoagulant treatment with coumarin drugs (dose controlled by regular prothrombin estimations) effectively abolishes or reduces transient attacks although the incidence of completed or fatal stroke is not materially altered. Anticoagulant treatment for a period of 12 months is recommended for all patients with transient ischaemia who are unsuitable for surgery and who have no medical contraindications (peptic ulcer, liver disease). Many common drugs (e.g. aspirin) may change the required dose of anticoagulants.

Patients having transient ischaemic attacks from bland embolism in association with chronic rheumatic carditis require continuous anticoagulant treatment indefinitely unless the cardiac lesion is surgically corrected, when this treatment may sometimes be discontinued.

Attacks associated with transient hypertension or hypotension should be treated by appropriate regulation of blood pressure. Iatrogenic postural hypotension is commonly due to sedative or psychotropic drugs. Successful treatment of anaemia, dysproteinaemia or cardiac failure may also result in the cessation of attacks of cerebral ischaemia.

Major stroke

Stroke in evolution. In a few patients the neurological deficit produced by ischaemia may evolve slowly over hours or days. The cause is usually an extension of arterial thrombosis, often in the cartoid artery, or the development of cerebral edema. Rapid and early anticoagulant treatment should be given; heparin 10 000 units 6-hourly intravenously followed by warfarin or subcutaneous heparin (5000 units twice daily) continued for one month as this has been shown to improve prognosis. If brain swelling or raised intracranial pressure is suspected, dexamethasone 2–4 mg intramuscularly may be given in the acute stage. A stroke in evolution may be difficult to distinguish from subdural or intracerebral haematoma or from cerebral tumour, all of which may require surgical treatment. Arteriography and CSF examination may be necessary to exclude other non-vascular lesions but the results of surgery on the carotid artery during the acute phase are poor.

Completed stroke. In most patients, the onset of cerebral infarction is rapid and the condition has stabilised before admission to hospital. Nothing can be done at present to restore ischaemic cerebral damage or the patency of occluded intracerebral arteries. Treatment is aimed at prevention of complications, by ensuring adequate air-way, oxygen therapy (if cyanosis is present) prophylactic antibiotics and physiotherapy for chest infection. Vasodilators, such as 5% CO_2 inhalation, increase blood flow to normal brain but probably not to infarcted areas. There is no evidence that they are beneficial. If consciousness is depressed attention to hyperpyrexia, water and electrolyte balance, nutrition, and the care of the skin and bladder are necessary. Dexamethasone 4–12 mg/day is given to reduce cerebral edema during the acute stage. Anticoagulants are of no value in preventing further strokes except in cases of embolism from the left atrium, when treatment should be started immediately after the stroke and continued indefinitely. Anticoagulants may however, decrease the incidence of venous thromboembolism in bedridden patients during the acute phase. In all patients surviving a completed stroke, early ambulation and physiotherapy are encouraged.

Hypertensive vascular disease

Patients with chronic hypertension tend to suffer multiple minor strokes, often mistaken for transient ischaemic attacks. Unlike the latter, the effect is cumulative and the end result is a state of dementia, pseudobulbar palsy, with bilateral pyramidal and extrapyramidal signs. Early treatment of severe hypertension is recommended in the hope of arresting the underlying arteriolar degeneration. Improved prognosis for recurrent stroke has now been shown. Severe episodes of hypotension should be avoided since cerebral ischaemia may be aggravated but in general the dangers of treating high blood pressure in the presence of cerebral vascular disease appear to have been overestimated. Although vasodilator drugs such as cyclandelate may cause short term increase in cerebral blood flow, they are of doubtful value in the treatment of chronic cerebrovascular disease.

Subarachnoid haemorrhage

Subarachnoid haemorrhage usually arises from rupture of an aneurysm near the circle of Willis. Less common causes are leakage of a cerebral arteriovenous malformation, subarachnoid extension of intracerebral haemorrhage, rupture of a small hypertensive artery, paroxysmal hypertension (which may be drug induced) or head trauma. In some cases no cause can be found. In aneurysm cases, there is a large initial mortality (approximately 40%) due to cerebral compression and edema. Such patients die within 6–48 hours and no treatment is available beyond routine care of coma. Conscious patients and those whose condition is stable or improving after 48 hours require full arteriographic investigation to identify a bleeding aneurysm. A number of surgical techniques are available, such as ligation of the carotid or parent intracerebral artery, trapping, clipping or wrapping the aneurysm and evacuation of intercerebral haematoma. All procedures carry some risk and this must be weighed against the dangers of re-bleeding. The incidence of death from a second haemorrhage is considerable during the first 2 weeks, thereafter diminishes rapidly and is relatively small after 6 weeks. In general, in patients seen within 2 weeks and having aneurysm of the distal carotid or posterior communicating artery, treatment is by carotid ligation or by direct surgical treatment of the aneurysm. Middle cerebral and anterior communicating aneurysms are treated by direct surgery. In patients surviving for 6 weeks after bleeding and in patients with no demonstrable aneurysm, conservative treatment is indicated. This entails at least one month of strict bed rest with hypotensive therapy if chronic hypertension is present.

Subdural haemorrhage

The chronic evolution of a subdural haematoma is thought to result from venous bleeding following minor head trauma and is commonest in elderly patients. Treatment is by surgical evacuation with removal of the surrounding membrane.

Intracerebral haemorrhage

Spontaneous intracerebral haemorrhage occurs almost only in hypertensive patients and arises from rupture of small intracerebral arteries in the basal ganglia, cerebellum, pons or hemisphere white matter. Bleeding is less rapid than in subarachnoid haemorrhage. Some haemorrhages remain small and localised but the majority extend into the subarachnoid space.
Immediate treatment. In hemisphere or pontine bleeding, death in 6–48 hours is frequent. There is no indication for early surgical treatment; supportive care of comatose patients is instituted. In patients who show no further deterioration after 72 hours arteriography may be undertaken to find the size and situation of the haematoma. If no spontaneous improvement occurs or if signs of raised intracranial pressure develop, surgical evacuation of the haematoma may be indicated if in an accessible situation (e.g. subcortical white matter). In suspected cerebellar haemorrhage, radiological investigation is recommended, since early surgical evacuation improves prognosis.

Cranial arteritis

In this variety of vascular disease the external rather than the internal carotid branches are affected. The disorder is painful but usually recovers completely; involvement of the arteries to the optic nerve or retina (arising from the ophthalmic artery) may, however, lead to permanent visual impairment. It is always desirable to confirm the diagnosis by biopsy of a temporal artery but treatment should be given immediately since in some patients visual complications may be prevented. Prednisone is started at high dose, 60 mg/day, and the dose is reduced at weekly intervals by 10 mg. Relief of headache and muscle pain is rapid. The maintenance dose should be the smallest dose which adequately controls symptoms and keeps the sedimentation rate within normal limits. It may be necessary to continue treatment for many months and sometimes for years. Proximal muscle weakness may be caused both by giant cell arteritis (polymyalgia rheumatica) and by corticosteroid treatment.

PARKINSON'S DISEASE—DRUG TREATMENT

Medical treatment in Parkinson's disease aims to suppress the symptoms of tremor, rigidity and akinesia but does not arrest the disease. Drugs are available to raise the cerebral content of dopamine and to reduce cholinergic activity. For an early case benzhexol, orphenadrin and benztropine have central anticholinergic and antihistaminic actions but few peripheral atropine-like side effects; there is little to choose between them. Benzhexol is a suitable initial treatment in a dose of 4–8 mg/day. Eight-hourly treatment is necessary. The dose may be increased slowly until an optimal effect is reached or until side effects become troublesome (dry mouth, urinary retention, constipation, vertigo, confusion). The maximum tolerable dose is 20–40 mg/day. There is usually substantial relief of rigidity although tremor and akinesia are less affected. Excessive salivation is well controlled. Tolerance varies and if side effects are troublesome then benzhexol may be replaced wholly or partly by one of the other alternatives. There is little point in prescribing more than two drugs at a time. Anticholinergic drugs should be given with caution in the presence of glaucoma or prostatic enlargement and sudden withdrawal of drugs should be avoided since it may provoke a parkinsonian crisis.

L-dopa is now established as the most effective treatment for parkinsonism at all stages of the disease. Approximately one-third of patients show marked improvement, one-third some improvement; the remaining third cannot tolerate the drug because of side effects. Akinesia, dysphonia, dysphagia and oculogyric crises which respond poorly to anticholinergic drugs may be greatly helped. The effect on tremor is less predictable but considerable improvement can be expected if the drug is tolerated. Patients with symptoms of dementia are seldom helped and often made worse.

Nausea and vomiting are frequent side effects and may respond to treatment with metoclopramide 10 mg 8-hourly, cyclizine 50 mg 8-hourly, or anticholinergic drugs. Other side effects include involuntary movement of the lips and tongue, choreathetosis, postural hypotension, cardiac dysrhythmias and insomnia. Some patients notice periodic short term exacerbation of parkinsonian symptoms (on–off phenomenon) sometimes related to variations in serum levels of L-dopa.

L-dopa is administered in a dose of 250 mg t.i.d. increasing slowly to a maximum of 4–5 g/day. The drug should always be given after food, and a very frequent dosage schedule, two- or three-hourly, may be necessary.

L-dopa is increasingly frequently prescribed in combination with a peripheral decarboxylase inhibitor. This reduces the incidence of peripheral side effects, notably nausea and vomiting. The most widely used preparation of this type is Sinemet containing 250 mg L-dopa per tablet, with carbidopa 25 mg. This has an action equivalent to 1 g L-dopa.

Amantadine (100–200 mg/day) originally introduced as an anti-viral agent has been found by chance to improve parkinsonism; although a less powerful drug than L-dopa its actions are similar and the two may be used together. Side effects are similar to those of L-dopa. The drug is suitable for mild cases, elderly patients or those intolerant to L-dopa.

Bromocriptine, a derivative of the ergot alkaloids, has a direct stimulating effect on central dopaminergic receptors. It has a long period of action. Side effects (similar to those of L-dopa) can usually be avoided by starting with a very small dose. Preliminary reports of its use in parkinsonism are encouraging.

Parkinsonian tremor is aggravated by nervous tension; the beta adrenergic blocking agent propranolol (80–120 mg/day) has a beneficial effect in a few patients though the majority are little helped.

Surgical treatment. Stereotactic lesions in the thalamus may abolish or lessen parkinsonian tremor in the contralateral limbs without loss of voluntary power and is a valuable treatment for patients with disabling unilateral tremor which does not respond to L-dopa. Substantial improvement is usually obtained though the tremor tends to re-appear again in a mild form after some months and the underlying disease appears to progress. Elderly patients or those with bilateral disease, dysphagia, dysphonia, dementia or severe disturbance of equilibrium respond poorly to operation.

Operative morbidity and mortality is increased in hypertensive patients.

General measures. Every effort should be made to keep the patient mobile and at work although writing, talking and tasks involving manual dexterity become increasingly difficult. Physiotherapy can be most useful in treating patients with disturbance of equilibrium and gait and in those with flexion dystonia. Elderly patients should be in hospital when beginning L-dopa treatment. Although many patients with Parkinson's disease become moderately or severely incapacitated within 5 years of onset the disorder may remain static and well controlled for many years. Patients often become depressed and require reassurance that neither mental deterioration nor rapid progressive invalidism need ensue. Additional drug treatment for depression may be required; it should be noted that mono-amine oxidase inhibitor drugs are incompatible with L-dopa.

Other varieties of parkinsonism. Akinesia and rigidity are commonly seen in patients treated with phenothiazine drugs for psychiatric disorders. If the condition is acute intravenous benztropine gives dramatic relief. Less severely affected patients usually respond to oral anticholinergic drugs. Postencephalitic parkinsonism may respond well to L-dopa in small doses but intolerance is frequent. Arteriosclerotic parkinsonism frequently shows pyramidal as well as extrapyramidal features and dementia is common. The response to L-dopa is disappointing and mental symptoms may be aggravated. Progressive supranuclear ophthalmoplegia (Steele–Richardson syndrome) is not helped by L-dopa.

Other involuntary movements. Benign essential tremor (familial tremor) may respond to alcohol but there is a considerable hazard of addiction. Propranolol (Inderal 40–160 mg/day) gives worthwhile relief to some patients. Sydenham's chorea is a self-limiting condition and if mild is adequately controlled with phenobarbitone. If movements are more violent haloperidol 1 mg/day or tetrabenazine 75 mg/day may be used. Tetrabenazine is the drug of choice to control the involuntary movements of Huntington's chorea although there is a considerable risk of depression. The same drug can be used in the treatment of hemiballismus, and is worth a trial in patients with blepharospasm, torsion dystonia and writer's cramp, although the results are unpredictable.

POLYNEURITIS

Symmetrical lesions of motor and sensory peripheral nerve fibres, the maximum damage falling on the longest fibres, comprise a common syndrome of multiple aetiology. In general terms the prognosis is favourable if the underlying cause can be remedied, since in many cases axons survive, the blocking of conduction being due to segmental demyelination. Remaining fibres may slowly regenerate and peripheral sprouting may re-inervate denervated muscles.

The metabolic peripheral neuropathies of diabetes, polyarteritis nodosa or rheumatoid disease, uraemia or porphyria may improve with control of the underlying disease.

Toxic peripheral neuropathy caused by drugs usually responds to prompt withdrawal of the drug, but the neural damage may be permanent (as in thalidomide neuropathy). Drugs interfering with metabolic pathways may require supplementary treatment (e.g. pyridoxin in isoniazid neuropathy). Neuropathy from heavy metal poisoning may require specific treatment with penicillamine.

In deficiency states neuropathy can in theory be due to lack of a specific B vitamin (thiamine, nicotinamide, pantothenic acid) alone or in combination with alcoholism. In practice, multiple deficiency is always present and large doses of a multiple vitamin preparation are recommended, with parenteral therapy in acute cases. In genetically determined neuropathy (peroneal muscular atrophy, hereditary sensory neuropathy, Dejerine–Sottas neuropathy) the course is usually slowly progressive and unresponsive to treatment. A possible exception is Refsum's disease where the accumulation of an abnormal metabolite (phytanic acid) may perhaps be improved by dietary means.

Acute infective polyneuritis

Acute infective polyneuritis is a self-limiting, rapidly progressive, predominantly motor neuropathy which may complicate a number of infectious fevers, immune reactions, or may occur in isolation. A major advance in treatment has been the management of respiratory complication by mechanically assisted ventilation and by preventing the inhalation of pooled pharyngeal secretions. Establishment of an adequate airway is the first requirement in severely paralysed patients. Involvement of the respiratory or pharyngeal nerves may necessitate tube feeding, tracheostomy and assisted respiration and regular chest physiotherapy and bronchial aspiration for adequate ventilation and to prevent pulmonary collapse and infection. A vital capacity of less than one litre, the recurrence of restlessness or cyanosis due to hypercapnia or hypoxia are indications for tracheostomy. Pooled pharyngeal secretions are aspirated regularly and a cuffed tracheostomy tube is a further safeguard against inhalation.

There is some evidence that steroids (prednisone 60 mg/day) or corticotrophin (ACTH 40 units/day) may improve the prognosis. A short 2-week course of treatment is recommended. Although the majority even of severe cases recover, and assisted respiration should be continued for months if necessary, a few patients show irreversible denervation. The disease may also follow a chronic relapsing course and some cases relapse when corticosteroids are withdrawn.

General measures in severe polyneuritis

1. Paralysis and sensory loss necessitate careful positioning and frequent turning to prevent pressure sores.

2. Urinary retention may require an in-dwelling catheter and continuous drainage, combined with a high fluid intake and sulphonamide treatment to minimise urinary infection and stone formation.

3. Loss of weight and muscle wasting is often severe; a high-caloric and protein diet is required during recovery.

4. Limb pain in early stages is often severe and may require pethidine (50 mg i.m.). It should be used with caution because of the dangers of respiratory depression.

5. Electrolyte disturbances, especially potassium deficiency, may complicate steroid therapy.

6. Daily passive exercises and light splinting may be needed to prevent contractures, especially of the tendo-achilles.

7. Hallucinations and affective disturbances may be due to paralysis and sensory deprivation, to drugs and to the environment of the intensive care unit.

8. Autonomic disturbances such as hypotension, cardiac arrhythmias, absent sweating and baroceptor reflexes occur frequently. Orthostatic hypotension and syncope are preventable by appropriate positioning of the patient and by leg bandages.

VITAMIN B₁₂ DEFICIENCY

The neurological damage produced by deficient vitamin B_{12} affects peripheral nerves, spinal cord, optic nerves and cerebral hemispheres. Cases presenting with neurological involvement frequently have no anaemia although the bone marrow is megaloblastic. Treatment is begun urgently as soon as the diagnosis is established since spinal cord damage may progress rapidly, and is often irreversible. A daily injection of 1000 μg hydroxocobalamin is given for 2 weeks. The same dose is then given twice weekly and continued until no further improvement occurs. The dose is then gradually reduced. For maintenance therapy, a single injection of 1000 μg every 3–4 weeks is adequate.

There is usually an immediate improvement in general well-being and mental symptoms. Distal sensory loss, paraesthesia and optic nerve symptoms improve more slowly. Symptoms in-dicative of cord damage such as sphincter disturbance may show little change. Occasional patients show sensitivity to hydroxocobalamin and cyanocobalamin may be substituted. A high-protein diet with supplements of other vitamins is advisable. In cases of optic neuropathy, tobacco and excess of alcohol are contraindicated.

MULTIPLE SCLEROSIS AND PARAPLEGIA

Only supportive and palliative treatment is available for multiple sclerosis but the acute episodes of focal demyelination, e.g. retrobulbar neuritis, and partial spinal cord lesions, show a strong tendency to full symptomatic recovery. No treatment may be necessary if the patient already shows evidence of improvement, but if the condition is deteriorating or showing no spontaneous resolution, within a few days, corticotrophin in high dose (80 units/day for 1 week; 40 units/day for 1 week) or dexamethasone 8 mg/day may accelerate recovery although prognosis and future relapses are probably unaffected. Cases with cerebellar or vestibular disorder respond poorly to treatment. There is no evidence that long-term corticotrophin treatment is of value.

Treatment of chronic multiple sclerosis. Paraplegia with ataxia and variable sensory loss is a common end result of many types of pathology in the spinal cord. Treatment aims at reducing spasticity and flexor spasms, preventing contractures, pressure sores and urinary complications.

Spasticity. This results from heightened reflex activity of spinal fusimotor neurones following removal of the inhibitory influences of pyramidal and extra-pyramidal pathways. Drugs having a depressant effect on synaptic activity at cord or brain stem level such as diazepam 5–20 mg/day, meprobamate 800–1600 mg/day, and tigloidine hydrobromide 1000–2000 mg/day may be used. Baclofen 40–60 mg/day or dantrolene 50–400 mg/day are the most recent and effective drugs for spasticity. In general, the effects decrease on continued treatment. Drowsiness and ataxia are troublesome side effects. Best results are obtained with diazepam and by temporarily substituting another drug when this loses its initial effectiveness.

In cases retaining moderate voluntary power but disabled by spasticity reduction of reflex activity by ice packs applied to the muscles or by chemical damage to sensory and motor roots of the cauda equina may improve motility. Cases with unilateral spasticity are most suitable. 1 ml of phenol 5% in glycerine is injected intrathecally in the appropriate region with careful positioning of the patient. Some cutaneous sensory loss may result but is seldom severe. Sphincter disturbance may be aggravated if lower sacral segments are damaged. Injections of small quantities of phenol around peripheral nerves or into the motor point of spastic muscles avoid this danger and may be equally effective.

Contractures are best prevented by frequent passive movements, by measures to combat spasticity and by suitable positioning in bed; avoiding flexion at the hip and knee and extension at the ankle; established contractures may require surgical treatment. Active muscle exercises are of great value at all stages; standing and walking between bars encourages the development of tone in anti-gravity muscles, and discourages a tendency to flexion. Patients may also develop useful movement by employing muscles above the level of the lesion. Established contractures may be treated by tenotomy or tendon transplant.

Avoidance of urinary infection largely determines the length of survival of the paraplegic patient. Aseptic catheterisation, (e.g. by 'no-touch' technique) in the early stages is essential. Spastic or mechanical outflow obstruction renders the infection of residual urine almost inevitable, and may be relieved by surgical treatment in suitable cases. Urgency and precipitancy of micturition may be helped by benzodiazepam or by surgical distension of the bladder.

MUSCLE DISEASES

Myasthenia gravis

The intermittent course of the disorder makes the assessment of treatment difficult. The aim is to give sufficient anticholinesterase drugs to enable the patient to lead a normal life, though it is seldom possible to restore full muscle power. Excessive dose of anticholinesterase may itself cause muscle weakness and muscles in different parts of the body may show varying degrees of responsiveness. Relapses are often caused by intercurrent infection. Hyperthyroidism is frequently associated with myasthenia gravis and requires separate treatment. A myasthenic syndrome usually responding poorly to anticholinesterase may occur with oat-cell carcinoma of the bronchus.

The most widely used drug is neostigmine bromide 15 mg by mouth 2 to 12 times daily. The period of action is up to 4 hours and if necessary the longer acting pyridostigmine 60–120 mg, one to four times daily may be added. Abdominal colic if troublesome may be relieved by oral atropine 0.6 mg. In some cases a potentiating effect is found by adding ephedrine 15 mg to each dose of neostigmine.

Assisted positive pressure respiration may be necessary in severe myasthenia, especially if a chest infection develops. If muscle weakness is due to over-treatment, a period of assisted respiration may restore responsiveness. Weakness in the limbs responds best to anticholinesterase drugs and the effect on ocular, facial and bulbar weakness is less satisfactory. If disability remains severe on full doses of anticholinesterase drugs after some months, or if increasing muscle weakness especially in respiratory or swallowing muscles becomes evident, a thymectomy should be considered. Response to the operation is best in young females with a short history of myasthenia. Purely ocular myasthenia may be little affected, and patients with malignant thymic tumours respond poorly to all forms of treatment.

A valuable recent addition to the therapy of myasthenia is the alternate day corticosteroid regime. Prednisone 100 mg/day is given on alternate days while anticholinergic drugs are progressively reduced. Initially weakness may increase and the treatment should be carried out in hospital. Steroids are continued at high dose for months; side effects are unusual.

Myositis

Suppression of the inflammatory process, relief of muscle pain and tenderness, and improvement of muscle power is usually possible with corticosteroids. Treatment should begin at a large dose 40–60 mg/day, reducing over a few weeks to the smallest maintenance dose which gives relief of symptoms. Treatment may have to be continued for many months and side effects (peptic ulceration, vertebral collapse) are frequent. Skin lesions are little affected. A remission may occur, especially in children.

Muscle cramps, myotonia

An effective treatment for most types of nocturnal muscle cramp, irrespective of the cause, and for all types of myotonia, is quinine bisulphate 300–600 mg at night or t.i.d.

It may be given combined with benzodiazepam 5–10 mg/day.

9

BLOOD DISORDERS

G. I. C. INGRAM, P. KINGSTON, B. H. McGIBBON,
G. L. SCOTT and G. WETHERLEY-MEIN

INTRODUCTION

In this section no attempt has been made to consider all possible régimes of treatment for all recognised blood disorders. The principles of treatment of common or important conditions have been discussed and lines of treatment, based on these principles, have been suggested.

IRON DEFICIENCY

The background to treatment

Iron deficiency, though common, is easily mismanaged and treatment is perhaps most effectively based on an understanding of iron balance.

In the normal adult the body iron is distributed between the red cells (2500 mg), the respiratory enzymes of somatic cells (600 mg) and the available iron store (800 mg). The normal daily loss (1.5 mg in men and 2.5 mg in menstruating women) is easily balanced by absorption from a normal diet which, in the United Kingdom, for example contains approximately 15 mg of iron.

The iron deficient patient certainly cannot absorb more than 10 mg of iron from such a diet and, since 20 ml of blood contains about 10 mg of iron, an average loss of more than 20 ml per day will establish negative iron balance with progressive store depletion and subsequent anaemia. Somatic cellular iron depletion with epithelial changes may be associated with the anaemia but, in a few patients, may precede it.

In iron deficiency absorption is enhanced and, although many variables alter the proportion of orally administered iron which is absorbed, the dose is, in the present context, the most important. With, for example, oral ferrous sulphate the compromise between maximal absorption and minimal intolerance is achieved with approximately 200 mg given three times daily. This will induce a net absorption of about 50–60 mg of elemental iron. Although these figures are only very approximate it can be calculated that absorption of this order will not only meet the demands of maximal possible erythropoiesis but will also balance iron depletion caused by any rate of blood loss which could be accepted as chronic rather than acute.

Against this background certain principles of treatment can be suggested.

Principles of treatment

Diagnosis. Except in situations where facilities for precise diagnosis are not available empirical administration of iron to anaemic patients should be avoided. In the absence of iron deficiency it is ineffective and in certain conditions, such as thalassaemia and sideroblastic anaemia, it may be harmful. It is perhaps even more important to emphasise that iron deficiency is inevitably the by-product of some primary disorder, such as chronic blood loss or malabsorption, and that recognition and treatment of the primary condition is often of more importance to the patient than treatment of the iron deficiency itself.

Management. In the anaemic iron-deficient patient effectively administered iron will be preferentially used for haemoglobin synthesis, the haemoglobin level will revert to normal and there may, therefore, be complete symptomatic improvement while the iron stores are still depleted. At this stage, in the absence of clear explanation and firm encouragement, there is a natural tendency for the patient to discontinue iron. In the patient in whom the cause of the iron deficiency has been removed this is of little importance since a state of positive iron balance will exist and the store and somatic cellular iron will be gradually repleted and maintained by normal absorption from a normal diet. In the patient who must continue in negative iron balance – for example the young woman with dysfunctional menorrhagia – discontinuation of therapy as the haemoglobin level returns to normal, with reversion to negative iron balance. is the commonest cause of recurrent iron deficiency. Such patients *must* be maintained on a continued iron supplement.

Since symptoms are probably not a valid index of marginal iron deficiency the effectiveness of maintenance should be checked by measurement of haemoglobin level and, if somatic iron deficiency without anaemia is suspected, by determination of serum iron and binding capacity after withdrawal of therapy for one week.

Failure to respond to adequate therapy in true deficiency is most commonly due to failure to take the iron but an associated infection or deficiency of B_{12} or folate should be excluded.

Choice of preparation

A very large number of effective iron preparations are available and only the principles of their use will be discussed.

1. Provided the dose is adequate the rate of response to any effective iron preparation is determined by the erythropoietic capacity of the marrow and not by the route of administration. Providing the patient does not suffer from a malabsorption syndrome, and even the majority of patients with this condition can absorb ferrous iron, oral therapy will produce as rapid a rise in haemoglobin as parenteral therapy.

2. There is little to support the view that sophisticated oral preparations reduce intolerance or that in practice additives, such as ascorbic acid, significantly increase absorption.

3. Combined preparations of iron and other haematinics have no place in therapy, except possibly in pregnancy where a combination of iron and folic acid is not illogical and may be convenient.

4. The vast majority of iron deficient patients can be effectively and inexpensively treated with oral ferrous sulphate (200 mg t.d.s.). Parenteral therapy, using iron dextran or iron sorbitol complexes intermittently or as total dose infusion (iron dextran), is relatively expensive, not without risk and should be reserved for patients who either cannot absorb oral iron, cannot be relied upon to take it or have genuine intolerance for oral preparations.

MEGALOBLASTIC ANAEMIA

The background to treatment

Megaloblastic anaemias are almost invariably due to deficiency of vitamin B_{12} or folic acid or both.

Proper management requires an accurate diagnosis of the B_{12} and/or folic acid deficiency and an understanding of how these deficiencies can arise.

Causes of vitamin B_{12} or folic acid deficiency. Vitamin B_{12} is absorbed from the terminal ileum in the presence of intrinsic factor which is secreted by the gastric mucosa. Deficiency of this vitamin is almost always the result of impaired absorption; only rarely is it due to inadequate dietary intake. Defective absorption can arise because of:

1. Lack of intrinsic factor, as in pernicious anaemia or after gastrectomy.
2. Reduced absorptive capacity of ileal mucosa due to resection or mucosal disease (as in 'malabsorption syndromes').
3. Competition for vitamin B_{12} by intestinal parasites, or bacteria (as in 'blind loop' syndromes).

Folic acid is absorbed from the duodenum and jejunum. Inadequate dietary intake is probably not uncommon, especially with prolonged cooking of foods, and may contribute to deficiency due to:

1. Increased demand for folic acid when cellular turnover is rapid, as in physiological states (e.g. pregnancy) or pathological conditions (e.g. chronic haemolysis or malignancies).
2. Malabsorption syndromes (as above).
3. Administration of drugs (e.g. anticonvulsants or folic acid antagonists).

Diagnosis. Diagnosis depends first on examination of the bone-marrow to demonstrate that erythropoiesis is unequivocally megaloblastic, and secondly on establishing the type and cause of the vitamin deficiency. The diagnosis may be suggested by the clinical features but confirmation is required by special investigations, e.g. assay of serum B_{12} and red cell and serum folate, tests of vitamin B_{12} absorption, etc.

Management of patients with severe megaloblastic anaemia (Hb < 5 g%) requires particular care.

1. Routine blood transfusion is contra-indicated because of the very real risk of lethal circulatory overload but if response to B_{12}/folic acid is likely to be inhibited by the presence of a complicating factor such as infection, then *exchange* transfusion should be considered.
2. After specimens have been obtained for B_{12} and folate assay, initial treatment of the severely anaemic patient should be with *both* haematinics,
3. Attention has been drawn to the danger of hypokalaemia during response to treatment in patients with severe megaloblastic anaemia and suggests the need to monitor the serum potassium

levels and administer potassium supplements when indicated.

General principles of management

1. The cause of a deficiency should be eliminated if possible.
2. The deficiency should be corrected by administering the appropriate vitamin or vitamins.

(a) *Vitamin B_{12}*, preferably in the form of hydroxocobalamin, is given by intramuscular injection. To replenish body stores and to obtain an optimal response 1000 μg may be given on alternate days for four doses. Thereafter 500 to 1000 μg should be injected weekly until the haemoglobin concentration becomes normal. Maintenance doses (e.g. 1000 μg every 2 months) must be continued *for life* when the cause of the deficiency is irreversible, as in pernicious anaemia. There is no good evidence that neurological damage is more rapidly reversed by giving more vitamin B_{12} than is required to maintain full haematological remission.

(b) *Folic acid* is usually given orally (daily dose of 5–15 mg) but may be given intramuscularly to patients who are vomiting or for initiating treatment in malabsorptive states. Prophylactic administration in pregnancy is desirable, especially during the last trimester. The optimal dose in pregnancy is debatable but probably should not be less than the minimal daily requirement of 300 μg. Higher doses may be necessary in the presence of iron deficiency, intercurrent infections or multiple pregnancy.

Folic acid may usefully be combined with iron for prophylactic treatment in pregnancy but indiscriminate use of multivitamin preparations containing folic acid is to be deplored since this may delay the diagnosis of vitamin B_{12} deficiency until irreversible neurological damage has occurred.

THE REFRACTORY ANAEMIAS

This is a heterogeneous group of conditions which have in common an anaemia which, in the vast majority of patients, fails to respond to any specific therapy. The haemoglobin must therefore be maintained, often for long periods, by blood transfusion. A central part of effective treatment is the proper management of these repeated transfusions. The importance of non-traumatic infusion, preservation of veins, the selection and preparation of blood and the management of iron overload should be studied carefully.

The treatment of the anaemia of infection,

chronic disease and renal failure is considered later and only some specific points in the management of thalassaemia, sideroblastic anaemia and aplastic anaemias will be considered here.

Thalassaemia

Patients with thalassaemia 'minor' rarely need more than a correct diagnosis and the avoidance of transfusion and iron therapy.

While there are a few children with thalassaemia 'major' who can maintain haemoglobin levels between 6 and 7 g% with infrequent transfusions the majority require regular transfusion from the age of 6 months. For well being and normal growth the haemoglobin should be kept above 8 g% but the more transfusion is required to achieve this, the more rapidly will tissue iron overload develop. However, it has not been shown that thalassaemic patients treated in this way have a shorter life span than those on a low transfusion régime. Chelating agents should be used, but are disappointing. Splenectomy, which may produce a slight but valuable reduction in the transfusion requirement should be considered particularly when some association of considerable splenomegaly, inadequate response to transfusions and neutropenia or thrombocytopenia indicate a hypersplenic state. Folic acid deficiency is common and prophylactic folic acid (300 μg daily) should be given.

THE SIDEROBLASTIC ANAEMIAS

This is a heterogeneous and rare group of anaemias and, while in many patients repeated transfusion becomes the only effective treatment, a proportion of patients respond to specific therapy. In the primary group some, generally younger, patients will make complete and sustained response to continuous small doses of pyridoxine (1–50 mg daily). In others, larger doses of pyridoxine (e.g. 100–600 mg daily) may, sometimes after many months, usefully modify transfusion requirements. Even in the absence of folate deficiency folic acid (5–10 mg daily) should also be given and in all patients adequate trials of pyridoxine, folic acid, crude liver extract, ascorbic acid and niacin—singly or in combinations, should precede the acceptance of transfusion as the only effective treatment.

Among the secondary sideroblastic anaemias those due to drugs, such as isoniazid, cycloserine, pyrizinamide, phenacetin and paracetamol should respond to withdrawal of the drug or treatment with pyridoxine.

Acellular marrow failure (aplastic anaemia)

For obvious reasons a drug or environmental aetiology should be sought and excluded. Remission is rare and occurs either spontaneously, as in some children at puberty, or in a small proportion of patients treated with anabolic steroids. Of these oxymetholone seems at present the most useful, having produced good responses in some cases. Doses used have been between 2 and 6 mg/kg daily for two months or more. Therapy is continued at a lower dose if there is remission to lessen the problem of side effects (virilisation, fluid retention and cholestatic jaundice). Marrow transplantation has proved a successful form of treatment in a few instances, but the selection of suitable patients and donors, as well as the subsequent management, poses many problems.

In this group in particular the management of transfusion, infection and thrombocytopenia is important.

Pure red cell aplasia

Prednisone may be useful and the dose should be 40–60 mg daily in adults and approximately 2 mg/kg/day in children. The dose should be cut down rapidly after 3 or 4 weeks, although smaller maintenance doses may be needed if there is a response.

THE ANAEMIA OF INFECTION AND CHRONIC DISEASE

A considerable proportion of patients with prolonged, severe chronic infection or with chronic non-infective processes such as rheumatoid arthritis develop an anaemia. In most cases the anaemia is of production failure type with occasionally a mild haemolytic component. There is often an associated abnormality of iron metabolism, resembling but easily distinguished from that of iron deficiency, which may prompt iron therapy. Such therapy is ineffective since the abnormalities of iron metabolism are almost certainly secondary to a general disturbance of protein metabolism of which failure of haemoglobin synthesis is a part. In fact these anaemias are refractory to all specific therapy and even when there is a co-incidental cause of anaemia, such as true iron or folate deficiency, response to specific therapy will, in the presence of continued infection or chronic disease, be considerably or completely inhibited.

The treatment of this type of anaemia is the treatment of the primary disease and resolution of the chronic disease or infection is usually followed by a spontaneous rise in haemogloblin.

In certain situations, for example as a preparation for surgery or when anaemia is severe, transfusion may be necessary. In general, however, if a patient can, unaided, maintain a haemoglobin level around 9 g%, attempts should not be made to maintain a transient normal haemoglobin level by repeated transfusion as this adds risk without conferring significant benefit.

HAEMOLYTIC ANAEMIA

Haemolytic anaemia may be due to intrinsic defects of the red cell, usually congenital, or to extrinsic causes, usually acquired. Most patients with chronic haemolytic anaemias establish an equilibrium whereby a satisfactory haemoglobin level is maintained by increased erythropoietic activity. Decompensation may occur if the marrow activity is suppressed by infection and, therefore, all infections in patients with haemolytic anaemia should be treated vigorously. Folate depletion is likely to occur, especially if demands are increased, as by pregnancy, and although routine folate supplements are not indicated careful observation is needed to anticipate potential deficiencies. Iron is rarely required in haemolytic states, as increased erythropoietic activity stimulates iron absorption, and it should never be given without laboratory proof of iron deficiency because of the danger of iron overload. Blood transfusion should be avoided in chronic haemolytic anaemia unless decompensation occurs, because it disturbs the established equilibrium and may contribute to haemosiderosis.

INTRINSIC RED CELL DEFECTS

Congenital (excluding the haemoglobinopathies)

Of the many known congenital defects of the red cell, only two are commonly of importance clinically, hereditary spherocytosis and glucose-6-phosphate dehydrogenase (G6PD) deficiency.

Hereditary spherocytosis

Most patients maintain acceptable haemoglobin levels in the absence of infection or pregnancy, but in occasional patients the condition may be either so severe that haemolysis is present at birth or so mild that it is discovered as an incidental finding in middle age. A frequent complication is biliary obstruction and cholangitis due to pigment stones. The only effective treatment is splenectomy which, although not curing the red cell defect, prevents their premature destruction. Elective splenectomy should be recommended in all patients but especially in those who are anaemic or who have had an aplastic crisis or who have pigment stones. The results are usually excellent, although the operation should, if possible, be deferred until after the age of 8 years as there is evidence of an increased incidence of septicaemia in younger splenectomised children.

Glucose-6-phosphate dehydrogenase (G6PD) deficiency

This disorder affects principally Negroes and the Mediterranean races but most subjects have no haemolysis unless treated with oxidant drugs; a list of the most important drugs is given in Table 1. Before a potentially G6PD deficient patient is given a high-risk drug, screening tests should, ideally, be performed on his red cells to exclude this defect. If haemolysis occurs, it is usually self-limiting as only the older cell population is susceptible. No treatment is available apart from withdrawal of the drug and blood transfusion if indicated.

Table 1. Drugs in current use which have caused haemolysis in G6PD deficient subjects

Antimalarials. Primaquine, chloroquine
Sulphonamides and Sulphones. Sulphadiazine, sulphadimidine, sulphamethoxypyridazine, salicylazosulphapyridine, dapsone
Antibiotics, etc. Chloramphenicol, nitrofurantoin
Antipyretics. Phenacetin, codeine
Antituberculous drugs. Para-aminosalicylic acid (PAS)
Synthetic analogues. Synkavit (menadiol sodium diphosphate) (especially in newborn infants)

ACQUIRED
Paroxysmal nocturnal haemoglobinuria (PNH)

This rare disorder is the only known example of an acquired intrinsic red cell defect. At the present time, there is no specific treatment other than blood transfusion. Patients are often sensitive to transfused plasma which may accelerate haemolysis and in such cases red cells washed in saline should be used. Iron is rarely needed in patients receiving regular transfusions, and it should never be given without demonstration of iron deficiency as there is evidence that it exacerbates haemolysis. Splenectomy is of no value and the place of steroids has not been established, but if marrow aplasia is a feature the use of

androgens is reasonable (see review by Dacie, 1967b).

Acquired haemolytic anaemia due to extrinsic causes

Haemolysis may be a complicating feature of many diseases, but as a rule, no specific treatment is indicated apart from treatment of the primary condition or blood transfusion. Only the treatment of the autoimmune and microangiopathic haemolytic anaemias will be discussed in detail here.

Autoimmune haemolytic anaemia (AIHA)

The AIHA's may be divided into "warm" and "cold" antibody types depending on the nature of the antibody. As the treatment is different in each case serological studies are essential. Either type may be primary and idiopathic or secondary to infectious disease, lymphoma, chronic lymphatic leukaemia, collagen disease, carcinoma or drugs. A thorough search for a primary cause should be made as the anaemia often responds to treatment of this condition.

"Warm" antibody type. The first line of treatment is corticosteroids. Prednisone, or equivalent, should be given in doses of up to 60 mg daily, depending on the severity of haemolysis. This dose should be reduced as rapidly as possible to a level which adequately controls the haemolysis. Most patients respond, although the antiglobulin test may remain positive. Some patients seem to benefit from the use of ACTH, although they fail to show improvement with synthetic steroids.

Blood transfusion should be avoided if possible as the donor cells are usually rapidly destroyed but blood should not be withheld if anaemia is endangering life. Serological investigations may reveal that the antibody has specificity, usually within the rhesus system, in which case it may be possible to select appropriate blood for transfusion.

If steroids fail to control the haemolysis, or if side effects limit their use, splenectomy should be considered. If significant splenic sequestration can be demonstrated by the use of ^{51}Cr labelled red cells, splenectomy should certainly be recommended, but in severe cases it should be performed even in the absence of this evidence as many patients benefit to some extent.

If the above measures fail to control the disease, immunosuppressive drugs should be tried. The data available at present on the use of these drugs in AIHA are inconclusive, but some patients with warm antibodies have undoubtedly improved. Most experience has been gained with azathioprine given in a dose of between 100–200 mg daily. The present evidence suggests that these drugs should be used only after more conventional therapy has failed.

"Cold" antibody type. AIHA of this type may complicate infections or may occur as a chronic disease in elderly people. The former are usually transitory and do not require treatment. Similarly, most patients with the chronic cold haemagglutinin disease need no treatment beyond protection from the cold. Corticosteroids are usually of little value and splenectomy is not recommended. Blood transfusion should be restricted as far as possible because donor cells are usually destroyed more readily than the patient's own cells. More success has been claimed for the use of immunosuppressive drugs in this condition, and these drugs are probably the treatment of choice. Chlorambucil is the most widely used drug, the dose being from 2 to 4 mg/day.

Microangiopathic haemolytic anaemias

These anaemias are found in such conditions as the haemolytic–uraemic syndrome in children, malignant hypertension, eclampsia, thrombotic thrombocytopenic purpura, abruptio placentae and disseminated carcinoma. Haemolysis is the result of red cell fragmentation which is probably secondary to intravascular coagulation occurring in the small blood vessels. Treatment initially should be directed to the primary cause. The effective control of blood pressure and renal failure is particularly important. Anaemia should be corrected by blood transfusion. Corticosteroids are of doubtful use, and may be contraindicated in intravascular coagulation. Recent evidence suggests that in severe cases the outlook is improved by heparin therapy which blocks further intravascular coagulation. Sufficient heparin must be given to produce a significant lengthening of the whole blood clotting time and the dose may need to be of the order of 10 000–20 000 units daily.

SICKLE-CELL DISEASE, HAEMOGLOBIN C DISEASE AND HAEMOGLOBIN E DISEASE

SICKLE-CELL SYNDROMES

The term 'sickle-cell syndromes' or 'sickle-cell states' covers a number of genetically distinct conditions, which have in common the presence of sickle haemoglobin within the red blood cell. It is customary to divide these syndromes or states into two categories, the common and virtu-

ally symptomless sickle-cell trait carrier, and the remaining conditions grouped together as 'sickle-cell disease'.

Sickle-cell disease

There are three common types of sickle-cell disease: sickle-cell anaemia, sickle-cell thalassaemia and sickle-cell haemoglobin C disease. Characteristically, the clinical course of sickle-cell anaemia is the most severe, whereas the patients with sickle-cell thalassaemia vary widely in their clinical disability, some of them being symptomless.

The clinical course of a patient with sickle-cell disease is marked by a variable number of intermittent crises which disturb the 'steady state' condition of the patient. Once established the crisis may prove refractory to treatment and, because of this, the clinician should aim to maintain the steady state and prevent the onset of crises by the provision of medical support and the institution of accepted public health practices.

The management of patients with sickle-cell haemoglobin C disease in some ways causes the most worry. For a great deal of the time they may well be symptomless, but they can suddenly react to stress such as pregnancy, infection or anaesthesia with an unexpected and fatal infarctive crisis.

Sickle-cell trait

The sickle-cell trait carrier is perfectly fit unless subjected to unphysiological hypoxia, e.g. anaesthetic accident or high altitude unpressurized flying. Whether violent exertion can precipitate a crisis at moderate altitudes is not certain. The amount of sickle-cell haemoglobin present in the blood of the sickle-cell trait carrier varies from 25–45%. One would expect that the carrier with the higher percentage of sickle-cell haemoglobin is more likely to react unfavourably to an hypoxic stress.

MANAGEMENT OF PATIENTS WITH SICKLE-CELL DISEASE, DURING THE STEADY STATE

The haemoglobin level of patients with sickle-cell disease is highly variable. Some patients with sickle-cell thalassaemia and sickle-cell haemoglobin C disease may have haemoglobin levels within the normal range whereas, at the other end of the scale, patients with sickle-cell anaemia may be very little incommoded despite steady state haemoglobin levels which may be anywhere between 5 and 10 g%.

1. *Transfusion.* A patient with sickle-cell anaemia has an oxygen dissociation curve shifted to the

right, i.e. their haemoglobin is less avid for oxygen and will release more oxygen to the tissues. This functionally advantageous right shift in the oxygen dissociation curve accounts for the remarkable activity displayed by sickle-cell anaemia patients with haemoglobin levels as low as 5 g%. Needless transfusion may be harmful, for the resulting increase in blood viscosity may precipitate an infarctive crisis.

2. *Nutrition*. Good nutrition must be maintained.

3. *Infection* must be prevented by: a. public health measures that improve community and individual hygiene. b. Immunisation against infectious diseases. c. Malarial prophylaxis and the treatment of intestinal parasites (if appropriate). d. The use of long term prophylactic antibiotic therapy is debatable but prompt and vigorous treatment of early infections (especially respiratory) is essential and requires readily available good medical supervision.

4. *Folic acid* is desirable as a continuous supplement but must be considered essential in pregnancy. Iron is contraindicated unless iron deficiency has been proved and it is considered beneficial to elevate the patient's haemoglobin level.

5. *Excessive cold* should be avoided. If excessive heat, with sweating, is inevitable, dehydration should be prevented.

6. *Bicarbonate therapy*. If, despite the above measures, infarctive crises still occur, the effect of long term prophylactic treatment with oral sodium bicarbonate (in sufficient dose to keep the urine alkaline to litmus) should be assessed.

7. *Ophthalmic care*. Ophthalmic examination, permitting early treatment of retinal lesions, may well prevent the occasional case of sickle-cell disease ending with blindness.

8. *General*. It is wise to avoid situations that might precipitate crisis. For example, whilst the patient should be encouraged to undertake as full a life as is possible, it may well be sensible to forbid any competitive athletics. There is a risk, albeit in all probability a small risk, that patients with sickle-cell disease may develop an infarctive crisis, especially splenic, during air flight in pressurized planes, which travel at an altitude equivalent to 5–8000 ft. If alternative means of transport are convenient, they should be advised.

MANAGEMENT OF CRISES

INFARCTIVE CRISIS

The commonest form of crisis in patients with sickle-cell disease is the infarctive crisis. This is caused by sickled red cells obstructing blood flow, which leads to tissue anoxia and ultimately tissue death. Apart from the spleen, infarctive crises in bones, chest and abdomen are particularly common. Other sites are legion—the patient may present with diagnoses as divergent as meningitis and priapism.

The major factors liable to provoke infarctive crises are: (1) Low blood oxygen tension, (2) Vascular stasis, promoted by circulatory collapse, cooling, shock and prolonged applications of tourniquets. Increase in blood viscosity, caused for example by dehydration, can also provoke an infarctive crisis. (3) The part played by low blood pH in precipitating an infarctive crisis is not certain. Theoretically, there are grounds for believing that acidosis may be harmful.

The slowing of the local circulation caused by the blockage due to the sickled cells itself causes further hypoxia, acidosis and stasis. A vicious circle is thus set up, encouraging further sickling to occur at that site. No treatment is likely to unblock a vessel obstructed by sickled cells; one can only hope to prevent vascular obstruction spreading to other sites.

General treatment

1. Keep the patient at an equable temperature. Sweating causes dehydration and cold may precipitate a sickling crisis.

2. Search for and vigorously treat underlying infections.

3. Maintain hydration by oral and, if necessary, intravenous fluid.

4. Analgesics will be required, but it is important to remember that the patient may also be G6PD deficient and react with a haemolytic crisis. Addictive drugs should be avoided if alternatives would give adequate relief.

Specific treatment

Although the regimes described below have all been advocated, no adequate assessments by controlled trials have been undertaken.

Anticoagulant treatment. Bone pain may be caused by marrow infarction and may herald a pulmonary embolus. Heparin has been advocated in the presence of bone pain (especially post partum) both as a prophylactic measure against pulmonary infarction, and also in its treatment. Intravenous magnesium sulphate, which has an anticoagulant and vasodilatory action, has also been recommended (1–2 ml of 50% $MgSO_4$ is injected slowly every 4 hours, the dose being reduced in children).

Alkalinisation. Sufficient oral sodium bicarbonate to maintain the urine alkaline to litmus has been recommended both prophylactically and in the treatment of infarctive crisis.

Urea therapy. The clinical use of urea in the infarctive crisis was a logical advance from the *in vitro* observation that high concentrations of urea can break the bonds that form between sickle haemoglobin molecules during the sickling process. Unfortunately, such high levels are not obtainable *in vivo*, and the benefits of urea therapy are problematical. Vigorous urea therapy may well result in harmful dehydration.

Cyanate therapy. An erythrocyte will sickle when the sickle haemoglobin molecules reach a certain level of oxygen desaturation. If due to acidosis the oxygen dissociation curve of a patient with sickle-cell disease is moved yet further to the right (the Bohr effect) the sickle haemoglobin becomes even less avid for oxygen and, therefore, there will be a greater quantity of reduced sickle haemoglobin within a red cell at a given pO_2 level. The functional advantage (increasing yet further the unloading of oxygen) that acidosis gives to a patient with sickle-cell disease must be balanced against this increased liability of the blood to sickle at a given pO_2 level. The aim of alkali therapy is, by preventing acidosis, to maintain the oxygen dissociation curve in the position found in the steady state, i.e. when the patient has the functional advantage of a moderate shift of the oxygen dissociation curve to the right without attendant sickling crisis. By using a drug such as cyanate, haemoglobin can be made more avid for oxygen and the curve shifts to the left. This is the rationale for the use of cyanate in sickle-cell disease but, unfortunately, the use of such an anti-sickling agent is not without disadvantages. Not only is cyanate a toxic drug (it combines with the NH_3^+ terminal of all polypeptide chains, including red cell enzymes) but also the cyanated haemoglobin that it produces is an inefficient unloader of oxygen. The patient will respond to this situation in the same way as a patient with an abnormal haemoglobin that is too avid for oxygen, by increasing the quantity of circulating haemoglobin. In sickle-cell disease where blood flow is critical, such a development may prove undesirable.

Exchange transfusions. There may be a place for exchange transfusion in treating the patient whose clinical condition is deteriorating despite vigorous orthodox treatment. An exchange transfusion is also advisable in the preoperative preparation of patients with sickle haemoglobin for surgery (such as cardiac surgery) likely to involve hypoxic periods. In these situations a regime should be calculated to ensure that 50% or over, of the patients red cells are replaced by normal donor red cells. This can be achieved either by a true exchange, blood being withdrawn at the time of the transfusion, or, in anaemic patients, by one or preferably two careful infusions of packed red cells, care being taken not to overload the circulation.

Should a patient with sickle-cell disease require a blood transfusion, fresh blood should be used. Stored blood is of low pH and, because of the low 2, 3-diphosphoglycerate content, is for some hours remarkably avid for oxygen.

APLASTIC CRISIS

The aplastic crisis, caused by marrow depression, is detectable by a fall in the 'steady state' haemoglobin level accompanied by a reduction of the reticulocyte count. The aplastic crisis is commonly associated with infections, especially of a viral type. Because of the decreased red cell survival, even a short lived depression of marrow activity can, in sickle-cell anaemia, cause a sudden catastrophic fall in haemoglobin level and transfusion is then needed to maintain life. A marrow output failure of megaloblastic type may also result from a deficiency of folic acid, and it has already been mentioned in the management of the steady state, that prophylactic administration of folic acid is desirable in all patients with sickle cell disease and is imperative during pregnancy.

SEQUESTRATION CRISIS

This form of crisis, although described in adults, particularly affects infants and young children. There is sudden massive pooling of red cells, especially in the spleen and immediate transfusion is needed to maintain life.

HAEMOLYTIC CRISIS

The red cell life span varies according to the variety of sickle-cell disease and is particularly shortened in sickle-cell anaemia. The red cell life span may, perhaps as a result of infection, be further reduced (the haemolytic crisis) below the 'normal' steady state figure previously found for that particular patient. Such a patient with a haemolytic crisis has a high reticulocyte count and can therefore, be distinguished from a patient with an aplastic crisis, the latter complication probably being far more common.

It has already been mentioned that ethnic groups liable to carry the sickle-cell gene may also be deficient in glucose-6-phosphate dehydrogenase. Untoward haemolytic reactions may occur in such patients on receiving many commonly used drugs (e.g. sulphonamides).

Characteristically, after the age of 5 years, the patient with sickle-cell anaemia has an impalpable spleen because of previous multiple splenic infarcts. Rarely this does not occur; there may be splenomegaly, especially in the more benign case, and the patient may then suffer from hypersplenism. This is recognised by the excessivly low haemoglobin level (tranfusion may be needed to support life), associated with thrombocytopenia and leucopenia. Under these unusual circumstances splenectomy may be beneficial although, in malarial areas, the spleen may shrink in response to anti-malarial therapy. An enlarged spleen, whilst it is the exception rather than the rule in sickle-cell anaemia, is commonly found in both sickle-cell thalassaemia and sickle-cell haemoglobin C disease.

SPECIAL PROBLEMS IN SICKLE-CELL DISEASE

THE MANAGEMENT OF LEG ULCERS

The patient with sickle-cell anaemia who resides in the New World or in Britain has probably up to a 50% chance of developing a chronic leg ulcer. It is unusual for these to be found prior to puberty and, in Africa, leg ulcers appear to be relatively uncommon. Sickle-cell ulcers, as well as being unsightly, may easily render the patient unemployable. Conservative treatment (Eusol washes have proved to be of value) supervised by an interested medical attendant facilitates healing by ensuring that the ulcer is kept clean. Both adequate instruction and materials should be given so that out-patient treatment can be continued at home. In cold climates it appears reasonable to avoid undue chilling of the extremities. The results of grafting are often disappointing. If in the exceptional case the only final resort is skin grafting, there may well be a case for encouraging healing by a simultaneous transfusion program aimed at reducing the proportion of the patient's red cells to below 50% of the total.

THE MANAGEMENT OF PREGNANCY

Despite every care some risk, though probably a small one, is associated with pregnancy, especially during the last trimester and in the post partum period. Careful supervision should aim at the early detection and treatment of complications, which may arise with alarming suddenness. The principles of management of the patient are basically no different from those previously discussed, the administration of folic acid in particular having done much to reduce the previous high mortality figures. The aim of the obstetrician is to avoid a long, exhausting and ultimately infected delivery. If a caesarian section is carried out, the anaesthetist must be prepared to work with a haemoglobin level lower than that acceptable in a patient without sickle-cell disease. If pregnancy precipitates an uncontrollable run of complications, exchange transfusions repeated at intervals until after the post partum period should be considered.

SURGERY

General anaesthesia

Because general anaesthesia for a patient with sickle-cell disease is a hazardous, and at times a fatal, undertaking unnecessary operations should be avoided. In particular, the diagnosis and treatment of abdominal pain in patients with sickle-cell disease is a difficult problem. If the pain is caused by an infarctive crisis surgical interference is almost certainly contraindicated. If surgery is essential local anaesthetic procedures, if unassociated with hypotension, are preferable.

Pre-operative management

If feasible, operation should be carried out only when the patient is in the 'steady state'. If this is not possible, infections should be treated and folic acid given. In the event of a major operation prophylactic antibiotic therapy to prevent post-operative pulmonary infection is desirable. The presence of a low pre-operative haemoglobin level, especially if it is known to be a 'steady state' level does not necessarily demand a pre-operative transfusion. It is unlikely for example that a patient with a haemoglobin level above 7 g% will need pre-operative blood. The exact haemoglobin level that would require pre-operative transfusion must depend upon the individual circumstances, e.g. whether this is a steady state haemoglobin level, the nature of the operation, the risk of haemorrhage and the availability of blood. It is at levels between 5 and 7 g% that the decision whether to transfuse or not becomes difficult. If major thoracic surgery is required, it would be wise to consider an exchange transfusion regime prior to the operative procedure. Excessive premedication may result in dehydration and some degree of respiratory depression before the start of the operation.

Operative management

The temperature of the operating theatre should be such that neither sweating nor excessive cooling of the patient occurs. Tissue blood flow should be maintained by avoiding cardiac depression and excessive vasodilatation or vasoconstriction. If use of a tourniquet is essential it should be applied after exsanguination of the extremity and even then for the shortest possible time. Unless it is minimal, blood loss should be replaced by fresh blood and hydration maintained by suitable intravenous fluids. 5% dextrose, which encourages red cell swelling may play a part in retarding the sickling process. If pre-operative alkalinisation was not possible, 50 mEq of sodium bicarbonate may be administered intravenously over a 90 minute period. Adequate (30–50%) oxygen must be given and drugs causing either respiratory or cardiovascular depression avoided.

Post-operative management

Perhaps surprisingly, this appears to be the most dangerous period. Supervision of oxygen therapy must be maintained until full recovery from anaesthesia occurs. If practicable, oxygen for a further 24 hours is desirable. Early mobilisation should be encouraged and hydration maintained. The onset of severe bone pain may herald marrow infarction and a pulmonary embolus. Anticoagulant therapy should be considered in these circumstances if the patient's post-operative condition permits. If they occur, infections should be vigorously treated.

MANAGEMENT OF THE SICKLE-CELL TRAIT

Sickle-cell trait carriers are fit and are capable of leading normal lives. During anaesthesia, simple precautions, ensuring adequate oxygenation from induction to full post-operative recovery, are essential. Dehydration, lengthy application of tourniquets and circulatory stasis should be avoided. Even if these precautions are successfully taken, patients with the sickle-cell trait may be at some risk during major thoracic surgery associated with hypoxia, and the advisability of a pre-operative exchange transfusion should be considered under these very unusual circumstances.

MANAGEMENT OF PATIENTS WITH HAEMOGLOBIN C DISEASE AND HAEMOGLOBIN E DISEASE

The *carriers* of haemoglobin C and E are symptomless and require no management. The abnormal homozygotes who suffer from Haemoglobin C disease and Haemoglobin E disease have a chronic haemolytic anaemia of mild or moderate severity which, as a result of infection, may be worsened by a superimposed aplastic or haemolytic crisis. They do not suffer infarctive or sequestration crises. Uncomplicated Haemoglobin C thalassaemia is relatively mild whereas Haemoglobin E thalassaemia (common in South East Asia) may result in severe clinical disability.

Such patients require good nutrition, folic acid supplements being advisable and essential in pregnancy. Infections should be prevented along the lines outlined in the management of sickle-cell disease. If haemolytic or aplastic crises occur, transfusions should be given if indicated. As splenomegaly is usual in all these disease states, the possibility of superimposed hypersplenism should always be considered when assessing the patient's clinical and haematological state.

THE LEUKAEMIAS

The ultimate aim of the treatment of the leukaemias is based on the concept that these disorders may be curable if the self-renewing population of abnormal leukaemic cells can be completely eliminated from the body. While this goal is not yet generally attainable, the recent exploitation of specific nutritional and antigenic differences between normal and leukaemic cells has increased the hope that it may eventually be reached. At present, however, treatment depends mainly upon the use of cytotoxic drugs to suppress or control, the leukaemic process (chemotherapy) together with meticulous supportive care. The usefulness of subsequent immunotherapy has yet to be fully assessed.

In *acute leukaemias,* the aim of chemotherapy is, first, to produce the greatest possible reduction of the leukaemic cell mass so that a complete clinical and haematological *remission* is obtained, and second, to *maintain* this remission for as long as possible. In *chronic leukaemias,* especially the chronic myeloid form, chemotherapy at present aims at restraining the abnormal cellular proliferation. In all myeloproliferative disorders, uric acid turnover may be high, and increased by treatment. This may need to be controlled with allopurinol, in a dose of 200–400 mg daily.

Acute leukaemias

As far as response to treatment is concerned, acute leukaemias are usually divided into two cytological categories, 'lymphoblastic' and 'myeloid' forms. The latter group, which includes the myeloblastic, monocytic, myelomonocytic and promyelocytic varieties, remit much less frequently than the 'lymphoblastic' type. Since over 90% of acute leukaemias in children appear to be 'lymphoblastic', whereas this form is rare in adults, it is convenient to consider treatment of children and of adults separately.

Treatment in children

1. *Current conventional regimes* for treating acute lymphoblastic leukaemia in children are based upon the observations that: (a) Some drugs, e.g. prednisone and vincristine, are more effective for *inducing* a remission, whereas others, e.g. 6-mercaptopurine and methotrexate are better used for *maintaining remissions*. (b) Remissions are more frequently induced if drugs are used in combination although, for maintaining remissions, it is less clear whether drugs are best used simultaneously, sequentially or cyclically.

Thus to induce a remission, the combination of prednisone (e.g. 40 mg/m²/day by mouth) and vincristine (from 0.5 to 2 mg once a week by intravenous injection) is effective in about 90% of cases. The addition of rubidomycin makes this virtually 100%.

For maintaining remission it is now clear that some form of continued therapy for 2–3 years is necessary. Various regimes are used and, since experience and controlled trials are continually leading to modifications, it would be misleading to recommend a definitive system of treatment in the present context. The following example is, therefore, only illustrative of the general pattern of current conventional treatment.

1. Once clinical and haematological remission has been induced the patient is 're-induced' at 4 week intervals with an injection of vincristine associated, as in the primary induction course, with high prednisone dosage for one week.

2. Between these re-induction courses interval maintenance is aimed at by daily oral 6-mercaptopurine (e.g. 75 mg/m²/day and oral or parenteral methotrexate (e.g. 15 mg/m²/once weekly).

3. Prophylactic treatment of leukaemic meningeal involvement to meet the increasing incidence of this complication in otherwise successfully managed children, is initiated soon after induction of the initial remission. It involves cranial irradiation and intrathecal methotrexate and the present results of this regime indicate that it should be part of the conventional approach to treatment.

2. *More aggressive regimes* are being designed to obliterate the total leukaemic cell population after the induction of initial remission, particularly in children with high initial leucocyte counts. These regimes, which usually involve high dose administration of various chemotherapeutic drugs, serially or in combination, require the backing of specialised services for the prevention and management of infection, thrombocytopenia and other by-products of extreme marrow depression. The need for exploration of this aggressive and hazardous approach is undisputed, but at present, there is no clear evidence that it confers advantages which make it superior to properly managed 'conventional' therapy of the type described.

Treatment in adults. Acute 'lymphoblastic' leukaemia in adults is treated on the same basis as the disease in children but remissions are less frequently obtained. Acute myeloid leukaemias have proved, until recently, particularly resistant to chemotherapy. Cytosine arabinoside and rubidomycin are the agents of choice for induction at present (remission rate of 40–50%) but their use should probably be reserved for centres able to cope with the profound myelosuppression they can cause. Death from haemorrhage or infection is a particular hazard during the first few weeks of treatment in acute myeloid leukaemias. Similar principles of cyto-reduction maintenance therapy obtain as in the treatment of acute lymphoblastic leukaemia. It is possible that immunotherapy may prove of benefit in the management of acute myeloid leukaemias.

Referring patients. Patients with leukaemia should be referred if possible to a hospital which has appropriate facilities and experience for proper management of treatment, including radiotherapy. However, the evidence at present available suggests that the marginal advantages in survival which derive from treatment in *highly* specialised units may not necessarily outweigh the disadvantages arising from disruption of family life or removal of a child far from the home environment.

Chronic myeloid leukaemia

Patients with chronic myeloid leukaemia can be kept in good health for long periods if the abnormal proliferation of granulocytes is carefully controlled. Busulphan is the chemotherapeutic agent of choice. It is started orally at a daily dose of 0.065 mg/kg body weight and continued until the leucocyte count has fallen to 15 000–20 000 mm³. The drug should then be stopped (because the count generally continues falling for a few weeks) but resumed as required, on a long term, continuous or intermittent basis to maintain the leucocyte count within normal limits.

In 60–70% of cases, the disease progresses to a terminal 'blastic' phase for which there is no effective definitive treatment but which may respond briefly to the regimes described for the treatment of acute myeloid leukaemia. In other patients, intractable bone marrow failure, possibly the result of prolonged or excessive chemotherapy, develops and death usually results from anaemia, infection or uncontrollable haemorrhage. In a few patients there is transition to a myelofibrotic state and the treatment of this is discussed later. In some patients prolonged busulphan therapy may produce skin pigmentation or, occasionally, pulmonary fibrotic changes—the so-called 'busulphan lung'.

While splenectomy in the *late* hypersplenic state carries a considerable morbidity, *early* elective splenectomy is at present under controlled trial. Its long term benefit is as yet not established.

Chronic lymphatic leukaemia

In this condition a gradual accumulation of abnormal lymphocytes in blood, bone marrow and lymphoid tissue may be associated with neutropenia and defective synthesis of immunoglobulins. Patients are therefore particularly vulnerable to infection and when this occurs vigorous treatment with antibiotics and, in severe infections, with γ-globulin, is at least as important as chemotherapy.

The role of chemotherapy is best determined in the individual patient by assessing, by observation, the activity of the process in that patient. The process may remain static for long periods in some patients, particularly the elderly, and if they remain well treatment is then probably unnecessary. In most cases, however, the presence or development of active disease demands control, and intermittent high dose courses or long term, low dose regimes of chemotherapy may be required. In patients with very active disease manifested by progressive anaemia, persistently rising leucocyte count and rapidly enlarging lymph nodes and spleen there is an indication for aggressive combined therapy using, for example, oral chlorambucil (0.15 mg/kg body weight/day), prednisone (40 mg/day) and intravenous vinblastine (5–10 mg once weekly). The duration of such regimes is determined by the clinical re-

sponse and their marrow depressant effect. In the majority of patients, in whom treatment is necessary but the disease less active, Chlorambucil alone is probably the drug of choice although other alkylating agents, especially cyclophosphamide, may occasionally be more effective. Chlorambucil is given by mouth, the recommended initial daily dose being 0.15 mg/kg body weight, reducing to lower maintenance levels.

Chlorambucil should not be used in the presence of significant depression of the bone marrow. In such cases treatment should be started with prednisone (e.g. 40 mg daily by mouth) and continued until adequate haemopoietic function is restored. The steroid may then be tailed off as treatment is begun with chlorambucil. Prednisone is also of value for treating the acquired autoimmune haemolytic anaemias which can occur. Long courses of corticosteroids should, however, be avoided because of the risk of infection, although if there is slow response to adequate chemotherapy, a short course combined with chemotherapy may induce a more rapid resolution.

Some patients develop troublesome local enlargements of lymph nodes but have no indication for systemic chemotherapy. In such cases external irradiation of the affected glands may give considerable relief.

General symptomatic and supportive therapy in the leukaemias

Supportive measures to control morbidity are important and particularly so when normal bone marrow function is impaired. Anaemic patients may require blood transfusion and acute haemorrhage due to thrombocytopenia may be controlled by transfusion of platelets.

The presence of an unresponsive autoimmune haemolytic anaemia or a hypersplenic syndrome may be an indication for splenectomy and in chronic lymphatic leukaemia, in contrast to the acute and chronic myeloid leukaemias, excellent results may be obtained in very carefully selected patients. Infections must be promptly and energetically treated with appropriate antibiotics used in effective doses. Finally, the importance of continuing personal support of the patient and relatives cannot be emphasised too strongly.

POLYCYTHAEMIA, THROMBOCYTHAEMIA AND MYELOFIBROSIS

Primary proliferative polycythaemia (primary polycythaemia, polycythaemia vera), thrombocythaemia and myelofibrosis are, clinically at least, closely related conditions and although a proportion of patients presenting with one of these conditions will at some time undergo transition to another they are, in the present context, best considered separately. Although the treatment of the other forms of polycythaemia—renal, anoxic, and relative—is usually the treatment of the primary condition, some specific aspects of their therapy need discussion here.

Renal polycythaemia

In general no patient with polycythaemia should be treated until a renal cause has been excluded. If a relevant renal lesion is established surgical removal, after reduction of the venous haematocrit by venesection, is the treatment of choice and will be followed by a fall in the plasma erythropoietin and reversion of the red cell mass to normal. Venesection is a poor substitute but, if surgery is contraindicated, may relieve polycythaemic symptoms.

Anoxic polycythaemia

This condition, though generally regarded as a logical compensatory response to anoxia, may be more disadvantageous than beneficial. This is particularly so in the elderly, in whom a combination of arterial disease and high haematocrit (>55%) may result in major vascular occlusion due to increased blood viscosity. Careful venesection to a venous haematocrit of 50–55% reduces this risk and is not usually associated with any increase in anoxic symptoms. This regime is particularly useful in the polycythaemia of chronic infective pulmonary disease where high plasma fibrinogen levels may produce considerable additional increase in viscosity.

Relative polycythaemia

The apparent polycythaemia associated with burns and severe dehydration demands restoration of normal plasma volume. In the Gaisbock 'stress' polycythaemia syndromes differential diagnosis from the true polycythaemias by demonstration of a normal red cell mass will establish that modification of the red cell mass is unnecessary. Venesection may, surprisingly, produce symptomatic relief.

Primary proliferative polycythaemia (polycythaemia vera)

In this condition, which is generally accepted as an autonomous proliferation of red cell precursors, there is a wide spectrum of clinical and haematological behaviour in terms of rate of increase of red cell mass, associated leucocyte and platelet proliferation, splenomegaly, symptoms,

course and complications. It is therefore advisable, before deciding on any particular line of treatment, to make an assessment of each individual patient in these terms. The treatment can then be designed to meet the needs of the patient. On this basis patients can be rather arbitrarily divided into three main groups although, in practice, there is often considerable overlap and there may be, with time, transitions from one to the other.

In the first group a marginal increase in venous haematocrit (<55%) and red cell mass (<200 ml above expected normal) may be found incidentally without polycythaemic symptoms, splenomegaly, granulocytosis or thrombocythaemia. Aggressive treatment of such patients is not necessary since observation over time may show that they maintain an unchanged steady state for many years. This group, sometimes classified as 'benign polycythaemia', can be spared the possible risks of chemotherapy or ^{32}P unless they show transition to the second or third group. There is, however, increasing evidence that even in this marginal group there is an increased risk of vascular occlusive lesions particularly if there is associated hypertension or vascular disease and venesection to a venous haematocrit of 45–48% is advisable.

In the second group subjective symptoms may or may not have been observed by the patient but there is an unequivocal elevation of red cell mass (>200 ml above normal) and venous haematocrit (>55%) and there is often palpable splenomegaly, granulocytosis and thrombocythaemia. In this group it is absolutely essential to reduce the red cell mass even in the absence of symptoms in order to eliminate the considerable risk of thrombotic episodes. In this group symptoms, if present, and the risk of thrombotic complications are related to the increased viscosity produced by the enlarged red cell mass. This may be reduced by venesection alone, by irradiation with ^{32}P, by chemotherapy or by some combination of these forms of treatment. There is general agreement that immediate symptomatic relief and removal of the risk of thrombotic lesions is initially best achieved by venesection. The venous haematocrit should be reduced to between 45 and 50% as rapidly as possible and venesections of 500 ml two to three times a week will normally achieve this in two to three weeks. Disagreement as to how it should be maintained at this level centres around the use of radioactive phosphorus and the arguments for and against this are considered later.

In the third group symptoms are not only those of increased blood viscosity but may be also related to associated proliferation of granulocytes and platelets or to the development of gross splenomegaly. In this group the initial treatment of choice is again venesection but although the usually moderate granulocytosis (<20–30 000/mm³) itself requires no treatment there is an indication for control of the granulocyte proliferation if there is associated gout, high blood urate or itching. Similarly, even in the absence of thrombocythaemic symptoms, high platelet counts (>500 000/mm³) must be reduced, particularly if the platelets are of abnormal morphology or function, for these patients are at risk of severe spontaneous or post-traumatic bleeding or of micro-vascular occlusive lesions.

The relative roles of venesection, ³²P and chemotherapy in the maintenance of the venous haematocrit at an acceptable level and in the control of granulocyte and platelet proliferation need some consideration. Irradiation, using ³²P is certainly simple and usually effective in controlling red cell, granulocyte and platelet proliferation but it is now widely accepted that it produces an increased incidence of acute leukaemic transformation in polycythaemics. In practice, therefore, there is a strong argument for maintaining those patients in the first two groups, with symptoms and complications predominantly due to viscosity, by venesection alone. Once the venous haematocrit has been returned to normal by adequate initial venesection the majority of these patients will only require subsequent single venesections of 500 ml every 3 to 4 months. It is important to recognise that, although this form of treatment has an attractive simplicity, it demands more careful and more frequent observation by the doctor and more co-operation from the patient than the usually longer acting ³²P therapy. Inadequate supervision with lack of control of a slowly rising venous haematocrit can result in avoidable thrombotic episodes and may explain the increased morbidity and mortality which uncontrolled observations have suggested may occur in venesected as opposed to ³²P treated patients. Venesection of course, carries no radiation hazards but its long term effect is partly, but not entirely, dependent on the induction of iron deficiency and in some, but surprisingly few patients this may produce its own signs and symptoms. Asymptomatic iron deficiency, demonstrable by low serum iron and high serum iron binding capacity, requires no treatment in these patients. The rare occurrence of symptomatic glossitis, angular stomatitis, etc., is an indication for considering an alternative therapy to venesection. Iron should be administered cautiously otherwise there will be rapid reversion to the polycythaemic state.

Chemotherapy or ³²P is necessary first, if it becomes essential to reduce the platelet or granulocyte proliferation, secondly in the rare cases where venesection is either impracticable or ineffective in controlling the red cell mass and, finally in the uncommon non-myelofibrotic patients with gross symptomatic splenomegaly. While there is no evidence that chemotherapy is less likely to induce acute leukaemic transformation than ³²P the established leukaemogenic effect of ³²P suggests that there should be adequate trial of some chemotherapeutic agent before the use of ³²P is considered. Busulphan is probably the drug of choice for inhibition of erythropoiesis and granulopoiesis and for the management of an associated thrombocythaemia. In the average adult oral busulphan 2–6 mg/day, with dose and duration of therapy controlled by response and monitoring of leucocyte and platelet counts is safe and often effective. In patients without thrombocythaemia busulphan may produce an unacceptable thrombocytopenia before there is control of cellular proliferation or reduction in splenomegaly. There is some unconfirmed evidence that under those circumstances chlorambucil, 2–4 mg/day, may be more effective in reducing spleen size and that cyclophosphamide, 50–150 mg/day, may produce less thrombocytopenia.

Prejudice against the use of ³²P is not universal and many experienced workers regard it as the treatment of choice. Nevertheless, for the reasons already given, it is suggested that the majority of patients can be effectively treated by venesection alone or by a combination of venesection and chemotherapy. In a small number there is a clear cut indication for ³²P therapy. These are patients who do not make an adequate response to the venesection/chemotherapy regimes or in whom, for various reasons, the careful supervision it requires is impracticable. These indications are enhanced in patients in the sixth and seventh decades in whom death from unrelated causes is likely to precede transition to acute leukaemia. Methods for calculating the optimal dose of ³²P are established and in the average adult this approximates to a single initial intravenous dose of 5 mCi, usually after reduction of the haematocrit by venesection. The effect is slow but prolonged, most patients only requiring repeat therapy, determined by rate of relapse, at intervals of 9–18 months.

Acute gout occurs in about 30% of patients with primary polycythaemia and obviously requires immediate treatment with, for example, phenylbutazone (200 mg q.d.s.). About 70% of patients have raised blood urate levels and particularly when such patients are being treated with chemotherapy or ^{32}P oral allopurinol (*ca.* 400 mg daily) should be given prophylactically to avoid not only the precipitation of acute gout but also to obviate the risk of renal complications.

Itching, particularly after a warm bath, occurs as the presenting symptom in about 8% of patients and may be the most distressing complaint. There is some evidence which suggests that liberation of histamine from granulocytes, particularly basophils may be a factor. It is therefore reasonable, in such patients, to treat with antihistamines, (perhaps the most effective being oral cyproheptadine hydrochloride, 100 mg t.d.s. or 200 mg at night if drowsiness precludes daytime therapy) and to reduce the granulocyte mass by chemotherapy but, it is usually difficult in severe cases to achieve more than partial relief.

Thrombocythaemia

The mechanisms by which the high abnormal platelet counts found in this condition produce haemorrhage or microvascular occlusive lesions are complex and not clearly understood. Empirical chemotherapy with reduction of the platelet count to the normal range is, however, extremely effective. Busulphan is the drug of choice and the régime is identical with that used in the treatment of chronic myeloid leukaemia. Although the initial rate of response is often slow continuous maintenance therapy is usually unnecessary since the platelet count once reduced, may remain at a normal level for many months without treatment. The slowly rising platelet count of relapse precedes the recurrence of symptoms and is easily controlled by a short course of busulphan.

In occasional patients who present with a severe bleeding syndrome, transfusion may be necessary but a short course of corticosteroids (prednisone 20 mg t.d.s. for 7–10 days) may be surprisingly effective.

Myelofibrosis

This is one of the few myeloproliferative disorders in which diagnosis is not necessarily an indication for treatment. The natural progression of the disease, commonly presenting in the 5th and 6th decades, is slow. The elderly patient with a modest anaemia and considerable splenomegaly will often remain in a steady state, well and working for a number of years if spared the complications of enthusiastic therapy. At some stage an unacceptable degree of anaemia, unmanage-

able by tranfusion and often associated with gross splenomegaly will make treatment necessary. In the vast majority of patients irradiation, chemotherapy and corticosteroids are ineffective and may produce marrow depression before modifying spleen size. There is a strong case for splenectomy at this stage since the anaemia, transfusion requirements and thrombocytopenia may be considerably modified by elimination of the nonspecific hypersplenic component. This operation should not be undertaken as a prophylactic measure in the well, steady state myelofibrotic, should not be postponed until the operative risk is unacceptable and should not be rejected on the invalid grounds that the spleen in myelofibrosis is a useful site of haemopoiesis.

HODGKINS DISEASE

It is now realistic to talk of cure for patients with early Hodgkins disease (Stages I and II) i.e. only one group of lymph nodes involved, or more than one group provided they are confined to one main anatomical region. Since treatment and prognosis are largely determined by the distribution of disease on presentation, accurate staging is essential, for which lymphography and in some patients laparotomy may be needed in addition to the usual clinical tests. Prognosis is indirectly related to histology for, although all histological types seem equally radio-sensitive the more malignant types usually present at a later stage (III or IV).

With the possibility of cure the interests of the patient. who may require both radiotherapy and chemotherapy during the course of the disease, are best served by a close co-operation between radiotherapist and chemotherapist, preferably working in a combined clinic and effectively interchanging information with the family doctor.

Indications for radiotherapy and chemotherapy

Stages I and II should be treated with radical radiotherapy and cure should be the objective. In Stage III radical radiotherapy should be considered but, in both Stage III and Stage IV systemic symptoms are common and these require treatment by chemotherapy. Focal lesions are still best treated with local radiotherapy and, particularly with mediastinal lesions, the relative timing of radiotherapy and chemotherapy is important. In acute cord compression initial neurosurgery may be essential while chemotherapy or radiotherapy may be equally effective in patients with slower onset.

Choice of chemotherapeutic agents

There is now good published evidence that the remission rate is increased by the use of intensive chemotherapy using several drugs. Evidence is also accumulating that survival is prolonged and that the life so obtained is of good quality.

Thus it would appear at present that combination therapy of this type is definitely indicated. However, such therapy may not always be practicable and the use of single drugs is worthy of note as an inferior, but occasionally the only possible form of treatment.

The choice of drug will largely depend on the systemic symptoms. If these are mild one of the oral alkylating agents, such as chlorambucil or cyclophosphamide, is indicated. If they are severe or lesions are extensive intravenous therapy, with vinblastine for example, is likely to be more rapidly effective. The most rapid responses, for urgent relief of pressure symptoms, may be produced by intravenous mustine hydrochloride. Both mustine and cyclophosphamide may be given intrapleurally or intraperitoneally in the management of pleural and peritoneal lesions.

Dosage, duration and control of chemotherapy

Quadruple chemotherapy

Careful monitoring of the Hb, WBC and platelets is necessary with any form of chemotherapy, but is particularly important when using multiple drug treatment, although the use of prednisone in the regime does allow bolder use of the other drugs than could be considered otherwise. Published regimes are generally variants of the following:

Week 1: Mustine hydrochloride 6 mg/m² × 1 i.v.
Vincristine 1.4 mg/m² × 1 i.v.

or

Vinblastine 5–10 mg × 1 i.v.
Procarbazine 100 mg/m² orally daily
Prednisone 40 mg/m² orally daily

Week 2: Same as week one providing peripheral count is satisfactory.

Week 3: No drugs except prednisone which should be cut down to zero over 3 or 4 days.

Vinblastine is generally considered preferable as it is more effective generally in Hodgkins disease than vincristine and the incidence of neurotoxicity with the latter often forces discontinuation. Careful modification of dosage is needed when the peripheral count is low due to bone marrow involvement with disease or to previous radio-therapy or chemotherapy. It is rarely useful to increase prednisone dosage over 60 mg daily.

Careful premedication (see later) is essential both for the patient's well being and to ensure that continued treatment is acceptable to him.

Single drugs

If for some reason it is decided to use only a single drug, then it is considered preferable to use it in the maximum tolerated dose for short periods, with interval periods for marrow recovery.

The alkylating agents. With the short course, high dose regime the oral dose of *chlorambucil* is 0.2–0.4 mg/kg daily for 10–14 days. *Cyclophosphamide* may be given orally (100–200 mg/daily), or intravenously in a dose of 100–400 mg/daily for 5 days. It produces less thrombocytopenia than chlorambucil or mustine but chemical cystitis occurs in 3% of cases and alopecia in 20% when the total dose exceeds 3–4 g. *Mustine* (0.4 mg/kg in one total dose or in three daily divided doses) must be given intravenously over a period of 1–2 minutes, into a fast running saline or 5% dextrose infusion since paravenous leaks produce tissue necrosis. Premedication with chlorpromazine (50 mg) and phenobarbitone (100 mg) will usually diminish or prevent the nausea and vomiting which may follow this therapy. If this regime fails to prevent vomiting, then cyclizine, prochlorperazine, perphenazine or higher doses of chlorpromazine, should be tried.

Vinblastine. 0.1 mg/kg i.v. weekly, increasing the dose by 0.05 mg/kg to a maximum of 15 mg per injection until leukopenia (less than 4000 × 10⁹/l) occurs. After this a dose is given just below the leukopenic dose weekly or every 2 weeks. After remission the lowest dose necessary to maintain remissions should be used. Side effects are negligible at this dosage but watch must be kept for neurotoxicity; tissue damage occurs with paravenous injection.

Procarbazine. 50 mg increasing to 150–300 mg orally daily. Gradual increase usually avoids the otherwise common complaint of nausea. If necessary the same dose can be given intravenously. After 2–3 weeks on this dose a lower maintenance dose can be used or the drug can be used intermittently at higher dose. This drug is a methyl hydrazine derivative and may cause haemolysis with prolonged use. In addition the action of phenothiazines may be potentiated and hot flushes may occur when alcohol is taken.

Vincristine. 2 mg/m² at weekly intervals for 2–3 weeks. A single dose must not exceed 3.5 mg.

This drug may be useful if bone marrow depression limits treatment, but it should mainly be used in combination with other drugs. Neurotoxicity is related to total dose but constipation and paraesthesia with areflexia are not uncommon. Constipation can be avoided by using a mixture containing dioctyl sodium sulphosuccinate and methyl cellulose.

Prednisone. The indications for this drug are first, an autoimmune haemolytic anaemia (rare in Hodgkin's disease). Secondly, in conjunction with cytotoxic drugs as part of 'multiple drug therapy' and thirdly, when bone marrow depression is marked and continued chemotherapy or radiotherapy are necessary in the face of advancing disease. The useful dose rarely exceeds 60 mg daily and the usual disadvantages of long continued administration apply.

Supportive treatment

Infections. Patients with Hodgkin's disease are subject to unusual and repeated infections (e.g. torula meningitis). Meticulous investigation in the appropriate clinical context is part of management. Oral or more extensive moniliasis is a frequent complication and should be prevented if possible by giving nystatin or amphotericin B to suck if oral antibiotics are prescribed.

Symptomatic. Systemic symptoms of itching, fever and sweats should regress quickly if the disease is responding to treatment. Diazepam or phenergan with, if necessary, heavy sedation at night, are useful for itching. Blood or platelet transfusions (p. 107) may be needed at some stage if severe marrow depression occurs. Antiemetics may be needed during radiotherapy or intensive chemotherapy. Appropriate and sufficient analgesic drugs must be used when indicated.

The other malignant lymphomas

These present too wide a clinical and histological spectrum to be dealt with in detail here but it is important to recognise that some non-Hodgkin's lymphomas, particularly of diffuse or nodular lymphocytic type may, like some cases of lymphocytic leukaemia, run an unpredictably benign course without therapy. The majority will however require treatment.

The significance of staging, prognosis and indications for a particular form of treatment are less certain than in Hodgkin's disease. Generally speaking, localised disease is treated by radical radiotherapy—in some cases following surgical removal of the 'tumour' (e.g. primary lymphoma of tonsil or bowel). Even in generalised disease radiotherapy is the treatment of choice for local symptoms of pain, pressure on vital organs and to decrease large tumour masses.

Alkylating agents, prednisone, vinblastine and vincristine are the most useful drugs singly or preferably in combination. Autoimmune haemolytic anaemia is not uncommon and prednisone is particularly indicated in this complication (ref. p. 91. Haemolytic anaemias). Other cytotoxic drugs may be effective but less so than in Hodgkin's disease. Repeated bacterial infections may be a problem because of abnormalities in immunoglobulin synthesis.

MYELOMA AND MACROGLOBULINAEMIA

Myelomatosis

This disease is due to an abnormal proliferation of plasma cells which causes both local and generalised symptoms, and treatment must be aimed at reducing the plasma cell mass. Few of the symptoms are caused directly by the myeloma protein, but its level is related to the mass of tumour and does enable the response to treatment to be assessed.

Recent evidence suggests that two cytotoxic drugs, cyclophosphamide and melphalan are equally effective, and that their use results in improvement in both the length and quality of survival. Treatment may be continuous or intermittent and some marrow suppression should be produced if maximum therapeutic effect is to be achieved. With continuous therapy an initial course of 80–100 mg melphalan should be given over a period of 20–25 days, the total dose being controlled by twice weekly leucocyte and platelet counts. Treatment is stopped for 10 days and restarted on recovery of the platelet count to at least 100 000/mm^3 and the white count to at least 2000 mm^3. A maintenance dose of between 1 and 4 mg melphalan daily is given. Intermittent courses lasting 7–10 days with a break of a similar time between each course may be needed to maintain acceptable counts, but treatment should not be stopped entirely. Cyclophosphamide is used in a similar way, the initial dose being 100–150 mg daily, followed by 50–100 mg daily. However it is now thought that melphalan may be more effective when administered intermittently in high dosage (10 mg daily for 7 days). Prednisolone 40 mg daily may be administered concurrently. The optimal period between courses is six weeks. Both the dose of melphalan and the duration of the course should be reduced in the presence of impaired bone marrow function or uraemia. If severe thrombocytopenia or leucopenia occurs, either from bone marrow replacement or from cytotoxic therapy, corticosteroids, e.g. prednisone 20 mg daily, should be given. Anaemia should be corrected by blood transfusion. The best results are associated with a slow reduction in the myeloma protein level. A rapid fall in serum or urinary protein is a poor prognostic sign as these patients usually relapse quickly. If relapse occurs a change of treatment is unlikely to be successful.

Radiotherapy has no influence on the long-term prognosis, but is of great value in the treatment of local bone lesions which are causing pain or disability. Relief of pain from bone lesions is often striking, although healing of fractures seldom occurs.

Hypercalcaemia is a serious and frequent complication, often unrelated to the extent of bone involvement, and can cause coma and renal failure. The first essential is to ensure that the patient is fully hydrated, using intravenous fluids if necessary. Melphalan may produce a dramatic fall in serum calcium levels, but most patients respond to steroids in high dose, e.g. prednisone 40 mg daily.

The other serious complication and bad prognostic sign is renal failure which may be due to hypercalcaemia, Bence–Jones proteinuria, myeloma kidney, or amyloid. Hydration and correction of hypercalcaemia are imperative. Uraemia is not a contraindication to the use of cytotoxic agents but a smaller dose should be given and the blood count must be watched carefully.

Exceptionally high levels of myeloma globulin, usually in excess of 10 g/100 ml serum, may produce hyperviscosity symptoms, and plasmapheresis may be indicated (see below). Similar symptoms may occur if the myeloma protein is a cryoglobulin, and in this case exposure to cold must be avoided.

Macroglobulinaemia

The clinical picture of macroglobulinaemia differs from myeloma in that hyperviscosity and bleeding symptoms predominate and bone lesions are infrequent. These symptoms are directly related to the increased levels of macroglobulin and the primary aim of treatment must be to reduce the level of this protein. Two methods of treatment are available, cytotoxic drugs and plasmapheresis.

Cytotoxic drugs have been less successful in the treatment of macroglobulinaemia. Chlorambucil is the most widely used drug and as for myeloma, treatment should be continuous as long as the

blood count permits. The usual dose is 4–10 mg daily initially, and 2–4 mg daily thereafter for maintenance. Cyclophosphamide 50–100 mg daily is an acceptable alternative.

Plasmapheresis is a useful method of treatment of acute symptoms due to increased viscosity. In patients with chronic symptoms, intermittent plasmapheresis may be combined with chemotherapy but it is impossible to achieve a lasting reduction in macroglobulin levels by this method alone. The indications for plasmapheresis should be clinical and not biochemical as individual patient and protein variation affects the relationship between macroglobulin level and viscosity symptoms. Intensive plasmapheresis is distressing to the patient and can result in loss of normal plasma proteins, including clotting factors, immunoglobulins, and platelets. A reasonable method is to remove between 500 and 600 ml of plasma daily for about 10 days or until symptoms are relieved. This is best achieved by removing a unit of blood from the patient, centrifuging it, separating cells and plasma, and then returning the red cells to the patient. This process is then repeated until sufficient plasma has been removed. The retransfusion of the patient's own red cells eliminates the risk of transmitting serum hepatitis or of mismatching. Not more than one unit of blood should be removed from the patient without some form of replacement. If special plastic units are used throughout, the whole process can be completed in a closed system, so reducing the risk of contamination.

Steroids are relatively ineffective in the treatment of macroglobulinemia, although they should be given if bleeding is a prominent feature. Penicillamine has been used to try and depolymerise the macroglobulin molecules and so reduce viscosity. It is an expensive form of treatment which is not justified by the results obtained.

BLEEDING DISORDERS

I. MANAGEMENT OF THE LIFE-LONG BLEEDING DISORDERS

Haemostatic failure in the life-long bleeding disorders is nearly always due to a congenital defect of a single clotting factor. Bleeding episodes are treated by the intravenous infusion of the appropriate blood product to supply a quantity of the normal factor. For any but the most routine situations it must be possible to control treatment by monitoring the coagulation activity in the patient's blood.

Haemophilia (Factor VIII defect)

Therapeutic materials. If fresh normal *plasma* is administered the patient's factor VIII activity may be raised from zero to *ca.* 0.2 iu/ml (i.e. to *ca.* 20% of average normal) but to avoid circulatory overload higher doses must be given as concentrates. Concentrates of human factor VIII, e.g. 'cryoprecipitate' or lyophilized concentrates, are available through blood transfusion services and commercially. Concentrates from bovine and porcine blood may also be obtained commercially in Britain.

Management of bleeding episodes. The characteristic bleeding into joints and muscles and spreading haematomata deserve urgent anti-haemophilic treatment if pain is severe enough to require analgesia or to interfere significantly with function. Human Factor VIII from one of the above sources should be given in sufficient quantity to maintain the patient's plasma activity above *ca.* 0.10 iu/ml for a few hours. Adequate immediate analgesia must also be provided, but the ultimate relief of pain depends on the control of bleeding. Further doses of Factor VIII at *ca.* 6–12-hour intervals should be given until it is apparent that the pain is not returning and function is improving, but a single treatment applied within a few hours of onset, on an out-patient basis, will often suffice. There is good evidence that the provision of an emergency treatment service for haemarthrosis materially reduces the long-term incidence of crippling.

A tight effusion of the knee with pain at rest may be aspirated to relieve the pain, after generous anti-haemophilic cover, and with the utmost gentleness. Aspiration of smaller effusions should only be attempted when it is thought that blood will be easily withdrawn; evidence suggests that return of movement is more rapid, but not more complete, than after anti-haemophilic cover alone; subsequent attacks may be less frequent.

In haematuria the blood loss is usually less than would appear and the mere presence of blood in the urine can be ignored for a week or two. Factor VIII should, however, be given to raise the plasma activity to 0.30–0.40 iu/ml if the passage of clots is causing ureteric colic, if the urine is infected or if the patient is becoming anaemic. Repeated attacks should be investigated, but cystoscopy requires anti-haemophilic cover. In epistaxis, anti-haemophilic infusion should be combined with local treatment, e.g. limited electro-cautery of a bleeding point, or covering a diffusely bleeding area with a small piece of absorbable dressing. Ordinary packing may provoke further bleeding when it is removed. Intra-abdominal bleeding (e.g. the 'psoas syndrome') or bleeding into the central nervous system require more vigorous anti-haemophilic treatment and should be managed in hospital, and preferably in a haemophilia centre.

If the patient does not respond to anti-haemophilic treatment for a particular incident, the Factor VIII activity in the patient's plasma after infusion should be monitored and the dose suitably adjusted. If the activity obtained is disproportionately low his plasma should be tested for inactivation of Factor VIII. If this is demonstrated, Factor VIII must either be withheld entirely, in the hope that the antibody will die away, or given in massive doses temporarily to saturate circulating antibody and leave some residual therapeutic activity, after which a further rise in antibody titre may unfortunately be expected in a few days. The value of immunosuppressive drugs is not yet clear. The use of factor-IX concentrates is being investigated.

Management of post-traumatic bleeding. Following major trauma, the minimum haemostatic activity of Factor VIII is about 0.30 iu/ml, which must be maintained by divided or continuous infusion until the wound is reasonably consolidated. There is evidence from dental extraction and orthopaedic operations that the duration of anti-haemophilic cover may be reduced if the patient's fibrinolytic mechanism is concomitantly blocked by the administration of epsilonaminocaproic acid, 20 g/day or tranexamic acid, 4 g/day (adult doses). The management of elective surgery in haemophiliacs is best carried out in a haemophilia centre.

General management. Haemophiliacs should be registered at a haemophilia centre, where their treatment will be arranged and where many of them can be taught to administer their own intravenous infusions when treatment materials can be provided for them to keep at home and at work. Prompt self-treatment of bleeding episodes will accelerate resolution and also reduce the haemophiliac's dependence on professional help. The centre can also provide advice for school teachers and employers concerned with individual patients, and help patients to obtain maximum benefit from social services. The general aim should be to enable the haemophiliac to live as normally as possible, to attend ordinary schools and to seek ordinary employment within his capabilities.

Other clotting factor defects

Christmas disease (Factor IX defect) is managed on the same lines as haemophilia. Factor IX may be given as whole fresh plasma, or as a concentrate containing prothrombin and Factors IX and X, with or without Factor VII, which is becoming available from various centres. *Von Willebrand's disease* may be treated by whole fresh plasma which shortens the bleeding time for a few hours and allows the patient to synthesize Factor VIII normally for a day or two. This may initially be supplemented by Factor VIII concentrate if an immediate increase in Factor VIII is required. The bleeding in *congenital afibrinogenaemia* responds well to infusions of purified fibrinogen. Congenital deficiencies of other clotting factors may be treated by infusions of whole plasma or of the concentrate of prothrombin and factors VII, IX and X, as appropriate, along the same lines as haemophilia.

II. MANAGEMENT OF BLEEDING IN DISORDERS KNOWN TO BE ASSOCIATED WITH PARTICULAR CLOTTING DEFECTS

In liver disease, deficient clotting factors may be replaced before traumatic assaults, including liver biopsy, on the lines suggested above, under "Other clotting factor defects". Overdose with oral anticoagulants may be treated with vitamin K_1 (e.g. 2 mg) or, more rapidly, by replacement of the relevant factors on the lines suggested above. Haemorrhagic disease of the newborn and prematurity may be treated on the same lines with concentrates or whole plasma.

III. MANAGEMENT OF THE DEFIBRINATION SYNDROME

Principles of management

The defibrination syndrome is usually the result of continuous intravascular coagulation with secondary activation of fibrinolysis, although sometimes fibrinolysis may predominate. Management may be on three lines: first, to resolve the underlying disorder; second, to support the haemostatic reserve by intravenous infusion of those components which have been seriously depleted; and third, to block defibrination in the blood.

Indications for treatment

The need for treatment depends on the expected duration of the provocative underlying condition, the likelihood and danger of bleeding in the given situation (wounds, etc.) and the degree of depletion of the haemostatic reserve. In a rapidly resolving situation, such as the later stages of labour, no haematological treatment may be re-

quired because defibrination may be expected to remit spontaneously when the uterus contracts after delivery. If the patient is bleeding abnormally, where there is special risk of bleeding, or if bleeding would be serious if it occurred, the haemostatic reserve should be maintained above the critical level. Fibrinogen can be given as a concentrate in a dose of about 6 g; Factor VIII and fibrinogen can be given together as cryoprecipitate, as in the treatment of haemophilia, if available; other factors are best given as whole fresh plasma; platelets may also be given as platelet-rich plasma or platelet concentrates, although it is probably more important to replace the clotting factors first. The fate of infused materials should be monitored because the rate at which they disappear from the circulation will indicate the activity of the defibrination process. Replacement alone should not be continued for more than about 24 hours since the continuous deposition of fibrin may lead to serious microembolisation. Intravascular coagulation may be blocked by heparin or sometimes over the longer term with oral anticoagulants. At the beginning of anticoagulant treatment it may be wise also to restore haemostatic components which are seriously depleted, to prevent bleeding from anticoagulation; when the intravascular consumption of haemostatic factors is blocked by the anticoagulant the patient's own synthesis may be expected to restore normal levels in about 24 hours. Antifibrinolytic drugs should only be given if intravascular clotting can be excluded or blocked, or else the embolic component of the syndrome may be seriously aggravated.

THROMBOCYTOPENIA

Thrombocytopenia is a common cause of a generalised tendency to bleed spontaneously from small vessels, especially in the skin and mucous membranes (purpura). In the majority of cases, some more or less easily recognised cause is responsible for the reduction in the platelet count (secondary thrombocytopenia) but in a few patients no cause can be demonstrated by the usual methods of investigation (idiopathic thrombocytopenic purpura or ITP). Management of thrombocytopenia therefore requires not only an understanding of the methods of treatment, which are discussed below, but also an appreciation of the principles underlying differential diagnosis between the numerous causes of purpura.

Management of ITP

Treatment of ITP is based largely upon the administration of corticosteroids (usually prednisone and splenectomy together with local haemostatic measures and supportive therapy, particularly transfusion of blood or of platelets. The use of these measures depends upon the age of the patient and the severity and duration of the symptoms.

Treatment in children. Most cases of ITP in children run an acute, self-limiting course and the aim of treatment is to tide the patient over the acute phase in the hope that a spontaneous remission will occur. In mild cases no active treatment may be necessary but in more severe cases prednisone may be required in high doses (e.g. 2 mg/kg body weight/day), together with transfusion, to control bleeding. Because of the risk of side effects, prednisone should not be continued at high dosage for more than a few weeks by which time either a remission will have occurred or there will usually have been sufficient improvement to justify gradual withdrawal of the steroid. In a few cases, haemorrhagic manifestations may remain sufficiently severe to require continuing treatment with prednisone at the lowest effective dose (to control symptoms, not to achieve a normal platelet count), and if troublesome thrombocytopenia and bleeding persist for more than about 6 months, splenectomy may have to be considered.

Treatment in adults. ITP in adults, after an often acute onset, commonly follows a chronic course with recurrent remissions and relapses and long lasting spontaneous remissions are rare. Patients with a similarly severe degree of thrombocytopenia are not equally troubled by spontaneous bleeding. If bleeding is a problem, an attempt should be made to obtain a remission by using steroids as described above. If, after an adequate trial of prednisone, patients have failed to remit, or need a high maintenance dose to control bleeding, splenectomy is indicated. A sustained remission follows splenectomy in about two thirds of patients but in the remainder the operation has either no effect or a temporary response is followed by a relapse.

In such cases a further course of steroids may produce a remission or a small maintenance dose of prednisone may control symptoms. Immunosuppressive agents, e.g. azathioprine, have alternatively been used, since in such circumstances it is possible that an abnormal immunological mechanism is operating. Remissions have occasionally been so obtained but this approach requires further evaluation. More commonly in the absence of remission when long term therapy is required to control symptoms, the use of azathioprine may be helpful by enabling the dose of prednisone to be decreased to a more acceptable level. At splenectomy it is important that the surgeon should search for and remove accessory spleens and when a relapse follows an initial response to splenectomy, the possibility that some functional splenic tissue (e.g. a splenunculus) may remain should always be investigated. Exploratory laparotomy and removal should be considered. The treatment of ITP during pregnancy requires special consideration which is beyond the scope of the present discussion.

Management of secondary thrombocytopenias

Treatment should be aimed at alleviating or eliminating the underlying cause (such as drug ingestion). Steroids and transfusion of blood and platelets may be required to control severe bleeding but splenectomy is generally not indicated.

BLOOD TRANSFUSION AND THE USE OF BLOOD PRODUCTS

The administration of blood or blood products carries appreciable risks and should never be undertaken without weighing carefully the possible benefits against the potential hazards.

INDICATIONS FOR THE SPECIFIC USE OF BLOOD AND BLOOD PRODUCTS

Acute blood loss

This is the main indication for the use of whole stored blood. The decision to transfuse can usually be based on clinical judgement and observation of systolic pressure but in complex situations measurement of central venous pressure may be necessary. Since the immediate requirement is the correction of hypovolaemia rather than anaemia initial infusion of a blood substitute is as effective as, and considerably less dangerous than, inadequately cross matched blood. A dextran with a molecular weight of about 70 000 is the most satisfactory preparation. It is contraindicated in patients who have a bleeding diathesis. Freeze dried plasma is not recommended for, although it is an efficient blood volume expander, it contains unphysiological amounts of electrolytes and isoagglutinins and there is also a risk of serum hepatitis. Plasma protein fraction, a liquid preparation containing mainly albumin, is more physiological and is hepatitis free.

Whole fresh blood is only indicated when it is necessary to transfuse both red cells and factors lost on storage, such as platelets and Factors V and VIII. This may occur when a primary bleeding disorder causes considerable blood loss or when haemostatic defects follow massive transfusion. With massive transfusion (rapid infusion of more than 2 litres of stored blood) there are additional problems, for hypocalcaemia, hyperkalaemia and hypothermia may lead to cardiac arrest. Hypocalcaemia can be prevented by administration of 10 ml of 10% calcium gluconate per 500 ml of blood given. Hypothermia, perhaps the most important factor, can be prevented by warming of blood immediately before transfusion but it is essential that special equipment is used to warm the blood.

Chronic anaemia

When anaemia can be corrected by specific therapy (iron, B_{12}, folate) transfusion should be avoided and is unnecessary even in the severely anaemic patient. All patients with severe anaemia are especially liable to circulatory overload and when transfusion is essential, as in marrow failure, packed red cells should be given at not more than 70 ml per hour. A rapidly acting diuretic, such as frusemide (20 mg i.v.) should also be given. If the facilities are available exchange transfusion provides a safe method for increasing the PCV without causing circulatory overload.

Thrombocytopenia

Platelet transfusions may produce temporary but useful arrest of spontaneous or post-traumatic thrombocytopenic bleeding. In the absence of bleeding they have no prophylactic value except as immediate cover for surgery in thrombocytopenic patients. Platelets from at least 6 units of blood are required to produce a therapeutic effect in adults. They may be given as platelet rich plasma (volume 1250 ml) or, less effectively, as a platelet concentrate (volume *ca.* 150 ml) and the preparation should be used within 6 hours of collection for maximum benefit. Recent work suggests that platelet concentrates prepared and stored at 20 °C retain their effectiveness for up to 48 hours.

Hypoproteinaemia

Substantially salt free, freeze dried albumin preparations are available but should only be used for the treatment of specific episodes since long term maintenance of protein equilibrium by albumin infusion is impracticable.

Hypogammaglobulinaemia

Pooled adult human γ-globulin provides a source of antibodies against the common infective diseases. It is used in prophylaxis against certain infectious diseases and in the treatment of hypogammaglobulinaemia.

There is evidence that in congenital hypogammaglobulinaemia the incidence of infections is reduced if the γ-globulin level is kept above 250 mg/100 ml. The preparations available contain almost pure IgG and are unsuitable therefore for the treatment of IgA or IgM deficiency. The indication for γ-globulin therapy is that the serum IgG level should be below 200 mg/100 ml. The recommended dosage is an initial loading dose of 0.05 g/kg daily for 5 days followed by 0.025 g/kg weekly. The injections are given intramuscularly and are painful. Intravenous administration may lead to severe allergic reactions and should be avoided. γ-Globulin will not replace defective cellular immunity.

Hypogammaglobulinaemia may complicate other diseases, particularly chronic lymphatic leukaemia and myelomatosis but is not necessarily associated with increased infection. If recurrent infections do occur in these diseases γ-globulin replacement therapy should be tried using the dosage schedule already laid down. If the patient can tolerate the injections it is worth persisting as some patients are benefited considerably.

There is also a place for γ-globulin in the treatment of acute infections in hypogammaglobulinaemic patients who are not receiving regular replacement therapy. A short intensive course, as for the loading dose, should be given together with appropriate antibiotic cover. Severe infections in infants during the period of transient hypogammaglobulinaemia, which accompanies the decline of maternal antibodies, are another indication for γ-globulin therapy.

THE SELECTION OF BLOOD FOR TRANSFUSION

Whenever possible blood of the same ABO and rhesus group should be used. Group O cells may, in an emergency, be given to recipients of other ABO groups but large quantities of group O plasma should not be transfused because of the danger of a haemolytic reaction due to the destruction of the recipients red cells by isoagglutinins in the transfused plasma. The same restriction applies to the use of group A or B blood for group AB recipients.

Rhesus positive blood may be given to rhesus

negative recipients who have never previously been exposed to the rhesus antigen by transfusion or pregnancy but, as sensitisation may result, it should be given in exceptional circumstances only and never to the pre-menopausal woman. It must be emphasised that whenever blood of a different ABO or rhesus group is used it must be fully cross matched. If, in an emergency, the clinical situation is judged to be so desperate that cells must be given and transfusion cannot be deferred until properly cross matched blood is available then blood of the same ABO and rhesus group of the patient should be given rather than Group O rhesus negative blood.

THE MANAGEMENT OF SOME COMPLICATIONS OF TRANSFUSION

The prevention of circulatory overload and the management of massive transfusion have already been considered.

Haemolytic transfusion reactions

If a haemolytic reaction is suspected the transfusion should be stopped immediately and the units of blood and the giving set should be sent to the laboratory immediately together with two specimens of blood, one clotted and one heparinised, taken from a vein well away from the infusion site. There is no specific treatment but the patient's blood pressure must be maintained by the use of vasopressor agents and intravenous hydrocortisone. Maintenance of blood volume is of cardinal importance and a suitable volume expander should be given until more blood can be cross matched. Careful observation of fluid balance should be made and all urine passed should be sent to the laboratory. If renal failure does supervene appropriate treatment should be instituted.

If bleeding develops the possibility of an induced defibrination or fibrinolytic syndrome should be considered.

Febrile reactions

These are frequent in multiply-transfused patient and can often be prevented by the use of an antihistamine, e.g. chlorpheniramine, 10 mg i.m., or promethazine hydrochloride, 25 mg i.m., at the start of a transfusion.

Iron overload

Transfusion of twenty 500-ml units of whole blood gives an increase in body iron load of 4000–5000 mg. Patients who must be maintained by repeated transfusion for long periods may therefore develop transfusional siderosis. In such patients the removal of body iron by chelation should be attempted. Infusion of 4 g of desferrioxamine in 200 ml saline at each transfusion will only produce a urinary iron excretion of around 30 mg in the iron loaded patient. Increased dose does not give significantly increased excretion and more frequent intravenous or intramuscular chelation usually proves impracticable or intolerable. At present, therefore, chelation is inadequate but worthwhile.

Thrombophlebitis

The care of veins, particularly in repeated or prolonged infusions, is of paramount importance. The most effective single precaution that can be taken is to ensure that, in high risk situations such as haemophilia and the refractory anaemias, infusions are only set up by the most experienced operator available. Other points are:
1. In small or frightened children light general anaesthesia will often save trauma to vein, child and operator.
2. Dextrose solutions are irritant and should not be administered through the same giving set as blood or sludging and thrombophlebitis will occur.
3. A small cannula, preferably of plastic type, is less traumatic than a needle and should be used, particularly for prolonged infusions.

10

THE CARDIOVASCULAR SYSTEM

W. I. CRANSTON

CARDIAC FAILURE

Cardiac failure may be predominantly left sided, predominantly right sided, or a mixture of the two. Strictly speaking, cardiac failure is present when the ventricular function curve is flattened, i.e. when a given increment of filling pressure gives an abnormally small increment of stroke volume. An elevated venous pressure may also be present when the ventricular function curve is normal, but cardiac output is high. This is found in anaemia, thyrotoxicosis, beri-beri, acute nephritis and cor pulmonale.

It is impossible to decide clinically whether the ventricular function curve is abnormal in these conditions; in general, peripheral vasodilation suggests a more or less normal function curve, and vasoconstriction suggests an impaired one.

Left ventricular failure

This occurs when the function curve of the left side of the heart is significantly flatter than that on the right. Thus, to maintain the same stroke output from each ventricle, a very much higher filling pressure is necessary in the left atrium and ventricle. This high pressure requires an equal, or greater pressure rise in the pulmonary veins and capillaries. Consequently, there is an increased transudation of fluid within the lungs. Lymphatic flow will increase, and will to some extent counteract this effect, but the net result is the development of pulmonary edema. There is a decrease in lung compliance, and usually a marked interference with normal ventilation–perfusion relationships, resulting in arterial hypoxia, which may be of severe degree. Severe dyspnea and orthopnea are observed, and some relief is usually obtained if the patient sits up. This is probably because of some pooling of blood in the legs, resulting in a reduced right sided filling pressure and stroke output. Left sided filling pressure and stroke output also fall, until the stroke outputs from the two sides are balanced. Because the left sided function curve is flatter than that of the right, the fall in left

sided filling pressure is much greater than the fall in right sided filling pressure, and in this way relief is obtained.

Left ventricular failure may be due to a sudden impairment of left ventricular function, as following a myocardial infarct. Function is more gradually impaired in patients with hypertension, left sided valvular lesions, or ischaemic heart disease. There is some evidence to indicate that attacks of angina may be associated with transient impairment of left ventricular function. Not uncommonly, episodes of left ventricular failure may be induced, in patients with compromised ventricular function, by the onset of rapid arrhythmias or by over-transfusion.

Management

Many attacks of left ventricular failure are spontaneously self-limiting, especially in patients with insidious progression of left ventricular impairment.

If the patient is seen in an acute attack, morphine should be administered (15 mg i.m. or 10 mg slowly i.v.). Intravenous frusemide (20–40 mg) is of value in preventing subsequent attacks, but the duration of individual attacks of failure is usually so short that a diuretic action has little influence upon the attack in progress.

Oxygen is of value if it can be given, but the distressed and very dyspneic patient will often not tolerate its administration until the effects of posture or morphine have become apparent. These measures will control the attack of left ventricular failure in most patients, except some of those with extensive myocardial infarcts who may require treatment with digitalis. The desperately ill patient, and the patient who has been over-transfused, may require venesection, of 500–1000 ml of blood, or even more, in the latter case.

Management thereafter depends upon the cause of the attack. Hypertension should be treated. Patients with valvular lesions will require treatment with digitalis and diuretics and investigation to determine the appropriateness of surgery.

Congestive cardiac failure

Right sided cardiac failure or congestive cardiac failure may be due to an increased work load on the right ventricle, to impairment of the capacity of ventricular muscle to cope with a normal load, or to a combination of the two. Congestive failure may follow impairment of left sided function, without a preceding history of left ventricular failure.

An increased right ventricular work load may be due to valvular abnormalities or to an increased pulmonary vascular resistance, possibly with a high cardiac output, as in cor pulmonale. Impaired functional capacity of the ventricular muscle may be due to ischaemia, or to any kind of cardiomyopathy; congestive cardiac failure may follow any sustained tachycardia, though this is usually associated with impaired cardiac muscle function.

Congestive cardiac failure usually presents with breathlessness, edema, raised central venous pressure, and hepatic enlargement. Management can be considered in two parts:

(a) The general management of patients with cardiac failure.

(b) Treatment directed toward influencing the cause of cardiac failure.

The general management of congestive cardiac failure

The initial aim of treatment is to rest the myocardium; this means resting the patient. Patients with severe cardiac failure should be at rest in bed. They should be propped up, with the legs either horizontal or hanging down. If the legs are horizontal, it is usually easier to remove edema from the legs, but in severe cardiac failure, especially if left ventricular failure is present, it may be necessary, for the patient's comfort, to have the legs dependent. In this position there is theoretically a greater risk of development of deep vein thrombosis, so it is probably better avoided unless it is dictated by the patient's comfort. Many of these patients have lost their appetites and the diet should be light, and so far as possible, tailored to the patient's appetite rather than to any arbitrary scheme. Added salt should be avoided, but strict salt restriction is usually an unnecessary penance to impose upon the patient, at least until other treatments have failed. A commode is preferable to a bed-pan, because its use involves the expenditure of less energy.

The obese patient with cardiac failure will require weight reduction, but this is something which takes time and is a second order aim of treatment.

The mainstays of drug treatment are digitalis preparations and diuretics. Digoxin is given unless;

(a) there is evidence of recent digitalis treatment or,

(b) there is evidence of hypokalaemia.

Some patients in chronic cardiac failure are depleted of potassium, particularly if diuretics have been given; though serum potassium is a poor guide to total body potassium, a low serum level indicates a need for caution in the use of digitalis.

For a rapid effect, adult patients may be given an initial dose of 1.0–1.5 mg digoxin, followed by 0.25 mg 6-hourly until an adequate response is obtained or evidence of toxicity appears. Toxicity may be manifest by gastrointestinal disturbances, particularly nausea, or by the development of ectopic beats or other arrhythmia. Maintenance doses of digoxin usually lie between 0.25 mg once daily and 0.25 mg twice daily. Digoxin may be given intravenously, as a slow injection of 0.5–1.0 mg, if the patient has not previously received this drug; this method of administration may be particularly valuable in patients with left ventricular failure. Other digitalis preparations may sometimes succeed in patients who develop toxic effects with digoxin; daily maintenance doses of digitoxin usually lie between 0.05–0.2 mg, and of lanatoside C between 0.25 and 0.75 mg.

If possible, the patient should be weighed each day, since body weight usually provides a better index of response to treatment than fluid balance charts. The response to treatment is assessed, by falling body weight and disappearance of edema, reduction in central venous pressure and diuresis. In patients with atrial fibrillation, an additional guide is provided by the heart rate (not the pulse rate); it is usual to aim at a heart rate of 65–80/min at rest, in this condition. The development of toxic effects or a heart rate below 55/min is an indication for reducing the dose. It is commonly necessary to titrate the dose of the drug almost to the limit of tolerance, in order to obtain an adequate effect. After recovery from an episode of congestive cardiac failure, it may be necessary for the patient to continue to take a maintenance dose of digitalis, the size of which must be determined for the individual patient by trial and error. If the primary cause of the cardiac failure is remediable, the patient may not require such maintenance treatment.

Many different diuretics are available, and it is better for the practitioner to familiarise himself with one drug, and to use this as the drug of first choice, moving to other agents only if a definite indication exists. A rapid diuresis can be induced by intravenous frusemide (20–40 mg), or by intramuscular injection of 2 ml of mercuramide; the former will usually produce a more rapid, but shorter lasting diuresis than the latter. If there is less urgency, any of the benzthiazide diuretics, may be used, with due attention to potassium supplements. In general, it is better to employ potassium chloride preparations than those which do not contain chloride. Enteric coated potassium chloride tablets should not be used, because they may give rise to small bowel inflammation and perforation. Slow release tablets (Slow–K) or water soluble preparations (Sando–K) greatly reduce this hazard. Once the patients's dry weight has been attained, continuous treatment with diuretics may be necessary. At this stage, there is no advantage in using one of the more rapidly acting diuretics. Some have advocated the use of diuretics and potassium supplements on alternate days, but there is no convincing evidence that this kind of regime results in fewer side effects than continuous treatment with both agents. There is some conflict of evidence about the value of potassium supplements in maintenance treatment with diuretics; though some studies have indicated that these supplements are rapidly excreted, and do not affect the patient's exchangeable potassium, most physicians will continue to use them in patients with cardiac failure.

When a stable situation has been reached, it is necessary to consider the patient's future activities in relation to his capacities, and, as in all chronic diseases, it may be necessary to alter his mode of life.

Intractable congestive failure

Few heart diseases are completely curable, and thus, as patients become older, heart failure tends to become more and more difficult to treat. If the above measures have failed, complete rest is imperative. It is often possible to reduce edema in patients who are resistant to full digitalisation and the use of single diuretics, by a combination of diuretics. The object is to try to increase glomerular filtration rate at a time when the renal tubules are being influenced at a number of different levels. Several combinations are possible, but one which is usually effective is:

at time 0   Triamterene 100 mg orally
0 + 30 min   Mercuramide 2 ml i.m. (it is better to inject this into the upper limb, which is usually less edematous than the lower)

0 + 60 min   Frusemide 80–120 mg i.v.
0 + 90 min   Aminophylline 250 mg (slowly) i.v.

Combinations of this type may succeed in mobilising fluid after less drastic measures have failed. If these combinations are used frequently, and particularly if dietary sodium intake is severely restricted, there is a risk of decreasing glomerular filtration and the production of azotaemia. If a diuresis cannot be established, reduction of dietary sodium below 10 mEq daily may be required. With marked reduction of sodium intake, there is usually a further increase in aldosterone secretion, and a tendency for increasing urinary potassium loss, particularly if benzthiazide diuretics are being given. The dangers of potassium depletion are exaggerated by the digitalis which such patients should be receiving, and adequate potassium supplements must be maintained. In the late states of intractable cardiac failure, hyponatraemia is commonly found, and is of grave prognostic significance. These patients have an excess of total body sodium but an even greater excess of total body water, for reasons that are as yet uncertain. The addition of hypertonic saline is harmful, and the only measure that may help, is the restriction of fluid intake to less than 800 ml/day.

Nausea and vomiting are not uncommon in untreated cardiac failure, and are also common side-effects of digitalis preparations and of some potassium preparations. These symptoms can sometimes be difficult to assess and to treat. If no digitalis effect is evident upon the ECG, and in the absence of any arrhythmias which might be due to digitalis, it is reasonable to continue the drug, unless nausea is clearly related to the consumption of the tablets. In this case the dose may need to be reduced, or alternatively a different preparation of digitalis may be substituted. Plasma digoxin concentration is measurable by radioimmunoassay. Therapeutic ranges are between 1 and 3 mg/ml (1.3–2.6 nmol l^{-1}) in blood samples taken immediately preceding an oral dose of the drug. This can be of value in situations where one is uncertain whether certain symptoms are due to lack of, or excess of, digoxin. Patients at particular risk of digoxin intoxication are the elderly, and those with low glomerular filtration rates.

Treatment of the underlying cause of cardiac failure

(a) *Valvular and structural lesions.* The development of cardiac failure in patients with valvular lesions may be an indication for surgical treatment of the underlying abnormality; this decision will require cardiological investigation. Cardiac failure may be precipitated by subacute bacterial endocarditis in such patients.

(b) *Hypertension.* If a patient with hypertension shows signs of cardiac failure, this is an indication for treatment of the hypertension.

(c) *Pulmonary heart disease.* Cor pulmonale, usually secondary to obstructive airways disease, is a common cause of elevated venous pressure and edema. As previously indicated, this is not necessarily evidence of impaired right ventricular function, and the cardiac output is often high; the skin is often warm. Episodes of apparent cardiac failure are commonly precipitated by acute respiratory infections, sometimes manifest only by a change of sputum from mucoid to purulent. The most important aspect of management is to treat these infections energetically with antibiotics, appropriate oxygen therapy and physiotherapy. The use of digitalis and diuretics in this condition is controversial. There is a theoretical argument that the reduction of venous pressure by diuresis, might be followed by a fall of cardiac output and hence an increase in tissue hypoxia. There is, however, no convincing evidence that harm is produced by the use of digitalis and diuretics, and most physicians employ these agents in this condition. Patients with chronic respiratory disease, usually have high plasma bicarbonate concentrations, and sometimes carbonic anhydrase inhibitors (acetazolamide 500 mg daily, dichlorphenamide 50 mg daily) will induce a diuresis in patients who are relatively refractory to other agents.

Heart failure secondary to pulmonary emboli is also common, and may present in two ways. Firstly, there is acute failure due to recurrent massive (and usually multiple) pulmonary emboli, and secondly the insidious onset of predominantly right-sided cardiac failure in patients with no history to suggest thrombophlebitis. Diagnosis can be particularly difficult in the second group, and hangs upon the exclusion of significant airway obstruction in patients with pulmonary hypertension, but without other cause for cardiac failure. Treatment is as for cardiac failure generally, together with the use of anticoagulants. Oral contraceptives should be withdrawn from female patients if they are being used.

(d) *Beri-beri.* This condition is uncommon, but its importance lies in the fact that it can be cured. Warm extremities, a bounding pulse, tender leg muscles and a dietary history of deficiency suggest the diagnosis. Treatment is by the oral or intra-muscular administration of 50 mg thiamine, followed by dietary supervision.

(e) *Myocardial ischaemia.* Cardiac failure may arise insidiously, in patients with myocardial ischaemia. In this situation, it should be treated as indicated above. If propranolol has been used to control anginal pain, it will have to be withdrawn when cardiac failure develops, as it will further impair the function of the failing ventricle.

Cardiac failure may also arise acutely, following myocardial infarction. The common association of ventricular arrhythmias may make treatment difficult in these circumstances. If numerous ventricular extrasystoles are present, they may be controlled by intravenous lignocaine in a dose of 75–100 mg, followed by a continuous infusion at a rate of 1–2 mg/min. If the extrasystoles are controlled in this way, digoxin should not be withheld, and diuretics should be given, though the heart rate and rhythm should be frequently observed and the serum potassium regularly checked. In really severe heart muscle failure, with peripheral vascoconstriction, low blood pressure and oliguria, intravenous isoprenaline may be used as a continuous infusion at a rate of 0.1–2 μg/min. This procedure requires continuous monitoring, and facilities for defibrillation. The object is to control the infusion rate in such a way as to increase myocardial function without inducing serious arrhythmias, and the balance may be difficult to sustain. Concomitant administration of lignocaine may prevent or control ventricular arrhythmias, but it must be stressed that this kind of procedure should only be carried out where facilities for intensive care are available.

(f) *Arrhythmias.* Sustained high heart rates may cause many of the signs of cardiac failure, particularly in hearts already diseased. Treatment of the arrhythmia will often control the cardiac failure. If atrial fibrillation cannot be converted to sinus rhythm in patients with rheumatic heart disease, long term anticoagulant treatment should be instituted, as there is evidence that this decreases the risk of embolisation.

(g) *Anaemia.* Patients with severe anaemia frequently have raised jugular venous pressures, commonly with a high cardiac output. This state, like that in thyrotoxicosis, does not necessarily indicate impairment of cardiac muscle function and the signs usually regress when the underlying cause is treated.

(h) *Thyrotoxicosis.* Patients with thyrotoxicosis have a high cardiac output, and not infrequently a modest elevation of venous pressure, which does not indicate cardiac failure. True cardiac failure may arise, however, usually due to rapid atrial fibrillation in older patients. This should be treated by conventional methods, (though it may sometimes be difficult to control the heart rate with digitalis), while the thyrotoxicosis is controlled, usually with carbimazole or an equivalent preparation. Propranolol will suppress many of the manifestations of thyrotoxicosis, but it is unwise to use this in patients with cardiac failure. Once the patient is euthyroid, the atrial fibrillation should be corrected with cardioversion if it has not resolved spontaneously.

MYOCARDIAL ISCHAEMIA

The progressive narrowing of the coronary arteries by atheroma, common in many societies, results in two varieties of symptom complexes— angina pectoris and myocardial infarction. These descriptions of symptoms correlate only to a rough extent with pathological changes; most patients with angina pectoris have occlusion of at least one coronary artery, and many have areas of myocardial necrosis. The management of these conditions may be considered under two headings the treatment of the symptom complex, and the prevention or retardation of the under- lying advancing process of atheroma.

Management of the symptom complex

(a) *Angina pectoris.* Attacks of pain are brought on when the supply of blood to the myocardium is insufficient to meet its needs. Thus rational treatment requires an increase of blood supply, a decrease of requirements, or both. An increase in the effective availability of oxygen can be achieved by the treatment of severe anaemia, if this exists, but there are no other non-surgical methods of increasing effective blood flow in patients with coronary artery disease. Surgical treatment may include by-pass grafts of occluded arterial segments, or replacement of a diseased aortic valve, but these are specialised procedures and will not be further considered here.

The most important aspects of treatment con- cern the reduction of myocardial work. Myo- cardial oxygen consumption is roughly propor- tional to the work done by the heart; a simplified, but reasonably effective index of this work is given by the product of systolic blood pressure and heart rate. Thus either hypertension or tachy- cardia merits treatment. During or just before the attack, the sublingual administration of gly- ceryl trinitrate (0.5 mg) reduces the left ven- tricular work load by a peripheral vasodilator action. It transiently reduces arterial pressure, and, by dilating veins, causes a decrease in atrial

filling pressure and thus cardiac output. It there- fore reduces myocardial blood flow requirements in two ways, and it is the only drug, with the exception of amyl nitrite, which can be used during the acute anginal attack. Its use may be limited by faintness, headache, flushing, or a feeling of fullness in the head. Frequency of dosage is limited only by side effects of this kind.

Prevention of attacks of angina can be achieved in several ways. Reduction of weight will indirectly reduce the myocardial work load, and this should always be undertaken in patients who are obese. The long-acting nitrates have little or no demonstrable superiority to inert tablets, and there is little point in using them. Pro- pranolol does have a demonstrable effect, and in many patients it will increase exercise tolerance considerably. It reduces the myocardial work load by slowing the heart rate, reducing cardiac output and decreasing the velocity of ejection of blood with each ventricular contraction. It also has a modest effect in reducing arterial blood pressure. It should be used with great caution in patients at risk of heart failure, as it decreases the effectiveness of ventricular contraction. An initial dose of 10 mg thrice daily may be used. but frequently the patient requires larger doses of up to 240 mg thrice daily. A history of asthma should always be sought before using propran- olol, as this agent may exacerbate or induce attacks in susceptible patients. Newer β-blocking drugs such as acebutalol, alprenolol or timolol have less tendency to do this. Practolol should not be used because it has been shown to cause eye lesions, which may progress to corneal per- foration and blindness. It is not yet certain that the newer β-blockers will not cause chronic toxic effects like those of practolol. Diabetics on insulin may require careful observation if given pro- pranolol, as it may render hypoglycaemic attacks more severe.

In general, the patient with angina must live within his exercise tolerance, and this may re- quire modification of his employment and his home circumstances. This is an exercise in com- promise.

(b) *Myocardial infarction.* The acute problems of myocardial infarction are discussed in the next chapter and will not be further mentioned here.

Influencing the course of coronary artery disease

Many attempts have been made and are being made, to influence the progression of occlusive arterial disease in all parts of the circulation, but particularly in the coronary arteries. It is difficult to do this in a rational way, because the pathogenesis of arterial disease is not clearly understood. It is clear that there is a relationship between various serum lipids and arterial disease, and a probably independent relationship between arterial pressure and arterial disease. The striking variation in the prevalence and incidence of occlusive vascular disease in different populations and the indications that this difference is almost certainly in part due to environmental factors, encourages the view that it ought to be possible to influence the progress of this condition. Several approaches have been tried, based upon empirical findings. Almost all of these approaches require long-term dietary or drug manipulation, and the major problem that arises, as with all chronic diseases, is the difficulty of getting asymptomatic persons to accept modification of their way of life for a nebulous future benefit. The small effect of the known risk of bronchial carcinoma on cigarette consumption is an example of this sociological, rather than medical, problem. There is no reason to doubt that similar problems will arise with other prophylactic regimes.

(a) *Smoking.* There is good evidence that abstention from cigarettes will reduce the risk of myocardial infarction.

(b) *Anticoagulants.* Numerous trials of anticoagulants have been carried out, both in the acute phase following myocardial infarction, and in the prevention of subsequent infarcts. Most of these studies have some defects of design or control, and it is extremely difficult to carry out ideal clinical trials.

It is probably reasonable to employ anticoagulants to prevent pulmonary emboli after an acute myocardial infarction, if the patient is likely to remain in bed for more than two weeks. The evidence that long term anticoagulant treatment influences prognosis in patients who have had myocardial infarcts is conflicting, but it is probably safe to say that if the use of these drugs confers any benefit, it is a very small one, and it is very doubtful whether their long-term use is justified. There is also some rather conflicting evidence that the sudden cessation of long-term anticoagulants may be followed by a transiently increased risk of vascular occlusive episodes.

(c) *Influencing serum lipid patterns.* Two general approaches have been used:

(i) Altering the diet, either by reducing lipid intake, or by giving unsaturated fatty acids.

(ii) Altering the lipid pattern by drugs, such as clofibrate or cholestyramine.

There is good evidence that the pattern of serum lipids may be modified by these means,

but evidence that mortality is affected is less convincing. Trials on the use of polyunsaturated fatty acids have, on the whole, been disappointing. In some studies a decrease of mortality due to coronary heart disease has been largely or completely cancelled by an increase in deaths from other causes, so that the overall death rate has not been significantly improved.

The situation with clofibrate is only slightly less confused. A fairly definite advantage was shown in a primary prevention trial, carried out on persons largely free of evidence of previous coronary artery disease. Once again, however, this protection only appeared to relate to total episodes of coronary artery disease; death rate, which was small, was not significantly affected. It is perhaps more realistic to consider the effects of secondary prevention trials, on patients who have survived one episode of coronary artery disease; such patients, having already experienced tangible evidence of a dangerous condition will probably be more likely to adhere to a treatment regime. Here again, the evidence leaves something to be desired. Two controlled trials of this kind have been reported. Though it appeared that continuous treatment with clofibrate might be of some value, in patients who had angina before or after myocardial infarcts, the difference in total mortality was again quite small, and certain differences between the control and treated groups make interpretation difficult.

Thus, at present, it cannot be stated that measures which alter lipid patterns will significantly influence mortality, and the evidence available does not justify widespread measures of this kind. It is, however, wise to attempt to reduce lipid levels in patients with inherited hyperlipidaemias. It can, of course, be argued that these methods might be very effective if started early enough in life, but there is no evidence at all on this score.

(d) *Influencing fibrinolysis.* There is some evidence of impairment of fibrinolysis in patients with myocardial infarction, and evidence that this abnormality may be corrected by the administration of phenformin (50 mg daily) and ethylestrenol (4 mg daily). This regime also reduces platelet adhesiveness. As with all the other preventive regimes there is no conclusive evidence that this treatment influences survival, and it is not free of side-effects. If there is any evidence of renal failure, phenformin should not be employed because of the risk of lactic acidosis.

(e) *Surgery.* In recent years, there has been increasing use of surgical bypass of affected major coronary vessels by saphenous vein grafts. This procedure, though logical, has not been shown to influence long-term prognosis. The one situation in which it is reasonable to consider such treatment is in patients with severe angina uncontrolled by medical treatment.

SUBACUTE BACTERIAL ENDOCARDITIS

Prevention

Patients known to have rheumatic valvular disease should be given prophylactic antibiotics *immediately* before, and for 48 hours after dental surgery or minor surgical procedures. Ideally, the gingival margin should be swabbed within three days of the proposed treatment; if penicillin-resistant organisms are found, the appropriate antibiotic should be given. Otherwise benzyl penicillin in a dose of 2 megaunits daily should be employed.

Treatment

If the organism is known, its antibiotic sensitivity should be established, and the appropriate antibiotic given in adequate dose for 6 weeks. It is of considerable importance to establish, after treatment has been instituted, that the patient's own serum is bactericidal to his own organism, obtained before treatment.

It is becoming much more common to fail to isolate a micro-organism from patients who clinically have subacute bacterial endocarditis. The possibility of Q fever should always be considered, and if type I antibodies are detected the patients should be treated with tetracycline and/or lincomycin. In other patients with negative blood cultures, the choice of antibiotic can be difficult. It is usual to start with penicillin and streptomycin, the former given in large doses of 10–100 megaunits daily, depending upon the response, the dose of the latter depending upon the patient's age and blood levels. These large doses will usually have to be given intravenously, with an indwelling catheter. This demands great care, and aseptic introduction, in view of the risk of inducing septicaemia with contaminating organisms. The catheter should be changed every few days. The response to treatment is judged clinically, and by observation of temperature and sedimentation rate. Failure to achieve a response in about 14 days is an indication for stopping treatment for a few days, reculturing the blood, and if an organism is not found, treating with a different antibiotic.

Valvular damage can progress very rapidly during bacterial endocarditis, and intractable cardiac failure may be a problem. Some successes have been achieved by valve replacement during the course of bacterial endocarditis, though the mortality is high. If a patent ductus arteriosus is present, it should be closed, and with other lesions, surgery may prove helpful in desperate situations.

PERICARDITIS

Pericarditis arising from myocardial infarction, acute rheumatism, renal failure, or collagen vascular disease requires management of the underlying lesion. Pericarditis arising several weeks after cardiac surgery or myocardial infarction may be improved with steroids. Anticoagulants, if being used, should be withdrawn because of the risk of pericardial bleeding and consequent tamponade. Purulent pericarditis will usually be preceded by septicaemia, but may require pericardial aspiration for diagnosis.

Tuberculous pericarditis may be diagnosed on the findings in the pericardial fluid, though this is often unhelpful, and it is sometimes difficult to distinguish this condition from non-specific pericarditis, which is probably due to viral infection in many cases. If tuberculous pericarditis is confirmed a course of streptomycin, PAS and isoniazid should be given. The patient should be watched for the development of signs of constrictive pericarditis, which will require pericardiectomy.

In non-specific pericarditis, there is not uncommonly evidence of effusions elsewhere; the course is rather variable. In some patients, the condition resolves quite rapidly, leaving no sequelae. Only symptomatic treatment is required. In others, the condition may persist, with fever, pain, and in a number of cases, progression to constrictive pericarditis. Symptomatic relief is obtained using steroids, but considerable difficulty may arise if the possibility of tuberculosis cannot be ruled out. Either of two courses of action can then be adopted; to give steroids and antituberculous treatment, or to establish the diagnosis by open pericardial biopsy; the latter approach provides an opportunity for early pericardiectomy, if the pericardium is already fibrosed.

HYPERTENSION

Indications for treatment

The management of a patient whose arterial pressure is raised depends upon a number of factors, almost all of which are related to the patient, though a few are technical. The first is the level of the blood pressure. The measurement itself is liable to some technical errors, particularly in patients with fat arms. It is likely that a good deal of this kind of error may be eliminated by the use of sphygmomanometer cuffs containing a bag of sufficient length to encircle the arm completely, and it is to be hoped that manufacturers will be able routinely to supply such cuffs on all sphygmomanometers.

There is now very good evidence that blood pressure levels in any population are a continuous variable. There is also good evidence that the prognosis of patients is inversely related to the level of their pressure. This means that there is little point in attempting to provide a numerical definition of hypertension. What is important is an operational definition – the level of blood pressure at which the doctor is going to take some action. This level, of course, depends upon evidence that the treatment will be beneficial to the patient, and evidence on this point is still incomplete. There is, however, adequate evidence that treatment of patients with severe or malignant hypertension improves their outlook very considerably.

Absolute indications for rapid blood pressure control include:

(a) Malignant hypertension, with papilledema or 'cotton wool' exudates, is an indication for emergency treatment, since untreated malignant hypertension is very rapidly fatal.

(b) Left ventricular failure with pulmonary edema, if due to hypertension.

(c) Hypertensive encephalopathy, with impairment of consciousness and possibly fits; this will usually present with the retinopathy of malignant hypertension but occasionally this is absent. It is sometimes difficult to distinguish this condition from subarachnoid haemorrhage.

General indications for treatment

There is fairly conclusive evidence that asymptomatic middle-aged patients with diastolic blood pressures in excess of 120 mmHg, will have a better prognosis for life if their arterial pressure is reduced. This does not necessarily mean, however, that every patient whose diastolic pressure is above this level should be treated, and common sense must be employed. The decision that a patient with hypertension requires treatment, implies either long-term administration of drugs, or fairly extensive, uncomfortable, and sometimes hazardous investigation of an underlying cause. Thus, for example, there can be little argument for treatment of an asymptomatic, female aged

over 70, with a pressure of 180/120 mmHg. Treatment is not contraindicated by any of the following:

(a) Angina pectoris, or a myocardial infarct more than two months before.

(b) Cerebrovascular disease (unless the patient has such intellectual impairment that treatment might be difficult).

(c) Cardiac failure. } These conditions are positive indications for treatment.
(d) Renal failure.

In asymptomatic patients with diastolic blood pressure levels below 120 mmHg there is some evidence to suggest benefit from treatment, though this evidence is not beyond question. The presence of cardiac failure, however, in patients with mild hypertension is an indication for treatment. Except in emergencies, a number of blood pressure measurements should be taken before a decision is reached.

General aspects of treatment

As far as possible, the patient's activities should not be restricted. Weight reduction should be instituted in overweight patients, but in the absence of renal failure no other dietary restrictions are needed. Since patients with hypertension have a greater risk of developing myocardial infarcts than the population at large, and since there is evidence that a reduced incidence of myocardial infarcts follows the cessation of smoking, it is sensible to encourage this course.

If treatment with drugs is going to be undertaken, it will almost always have to be life-long, and continued supervision will be necessary. Certain patients will be able to manage their own drug regimes, on the basis of blood pressure measurements at home, but this does not eliminate the need for supervision.

Treatment of secondary hypertension

Hypertension may be due to a number of underlying causes. In general, extensive investigations should not be carried out, unless the physician considers that treatment is indicated, whether or not an underlying cause is found. Treatment should consist of elimination of the preliminary cause if possible, in the following ways:

Coarctation – surgical.

Phaeochromocytoma – surgical, preceded by premedication with phenoxybenzamine and propranolol.

Cushing's syndrome – surgical.

Aldosteronoma – surgical.

Renal disease. If involving both kidneys – as

for essential hypertension. If unilateral, the damaged kidney is non-functional, and the other intact – nephrectomy. If the damaged kidney is functional, the decision is a difficult one, and if the patient's blood pressure is readily controlled by drugs, it is often best to leave the damaged kidney alone. Urinary infection should be treated. Oral contraceptives can cause hypertension and may have to be withdrawn. Occasionally hypertension is a consequence of sodium retention due to drugs such as carbenoxolone, or even to excessive ingestion of liquorice.

Treatment of essential hypertension and secondary hypertension in which the primary cause is not eradicable

The object is to reduce the level of arterial pressure to as normal a level as possible, without side-effects which distress the patient. A diastolic pressure below 100 mmHg is usually the aim.

Adrenalectomy is not now performed; sympathectomy may very occasionally be of help in a patient who is unable or unwilling to continue treatment with drugs. The drugs used fall into two general categories: those which do not require meticulous attention to dosage, and those that do. The former can be used as the sole treatment for patients with mild or moderate hypertension, or in combination with the latter type in more severe hypertension. No single drug provides the ideal treatment, and individual patients' responses may make it necessary to change from one drug to another.

(a) *Non-emergency treatment of hypertension.* Patients with diastolic pressures below 120 mmHg can often be treated with fixed dose drugs alone, and, if there is no urgency, it is worth trying this approach, since it is relatively unlikely to give rise to side effects.

Thiazide diuretics are usually the best agents with which to begin treatment, unless the patient has gout or diabetes. There are many drugs of this type, and none has any particular advantage. Adequate doses are:

Chlorothiazide	250 mg twice daily or 500 mg once daily
Hydrochlorothiazide	25 mg twice daily or 50 mg once daily
Hydroflumethiazide	25 mg twice daily or 50 mg once daily
Bendrofluazide	5 mg twice daily or 10 mg once daily
Cyclopenthiazide	0.25 mg twice daily or 0.5 mg once daily
Polythiazide	1–2 mg once daily
Chlorthalidone (not strictly a thiazide)	50–100 mg daily

Frusemide and ethacrynic acid are shorter acting diuretics, which do reduce arterial pressure, but they have no demonstrated advantage over the thiazides, and are more expensive than the others.

Apart from the risk of precipitating gout and diabetes the main hazard is potassium depletion, and potassium supplements should generally be given: the dose depends on the patient's response, but 13 mEq of potassium chloride 2 or 3 times daily, as slow-release (*not* enteric-coated) or effervescent tablets are usually adequate. If hypokalaemia is a serious problem (and this is mainly the case when digitalis is used), triamterene 50 mg daily, spironalactone 50 mg daily, or amiloride 10 mg daily may be added but is seldom required. The normal diet usually contains up to 60 mEq of potassium daily; if a patient stops eating for any reason, he will lose this additional supply of potassium, and depletion may become more likely. The elderly, in particular, tend to have a low dietary potassium intake.

The diuretics will usually give a reduction of arterial pressure in about a week, and if this is of adequate extent, no other treatment is needed.

Should further reduction of arterial pressure be required, a blocking agent is a reasonable next choice; for most patients propranolol is satisfactory. It may be given alone or together with a diuretic. Propranolol has the advantage that it does not cause postural or exercise hypotension, and does not interfere with ejaculation. The dose requires titration, and will usually lie between 30 mg and 640 mg daily, though there are reports of successful treatment with doses as high as 4 g daily. Care must be exercised in patients at risk of cardiac failure, and the drug should not be given to patients with a history of airways obstruction. Acebutalol is a selective β-blocking agent which can be employed in these circumstances: it is not yet certain that this drug is free of serious long term side effects. It is given in a dose of 400–1000 mg daily.

Alternatively, a rauwolfia alkaloid can be employed, such as reserpine in a dose of 0.1 mg three times daily. This takes several weeks to produce a stable effect, and may cause depression.

Clonidine has more recently been introduced, and is of value in certain patients. Its action is probably central, and it does cause drowsiness in some patients. It does not cause postural hypotension. The dose requires regulation, and may range from 300 μg to 2000 μg daily. Sudden withdrawal may cause severe hypertensive rebound.

With more severe hypertension, or if the above

measures give inadequate control, one must employ one of the drugs, whose dose requires careful regulation (Table 1); with the exception of hydrallazine all these drugs interfere with sympathetic transmission and in consequence cause a greater fall in blood pressure in the standing position, with usually a further fall on exercise, often accompanied by dizziness or faintness. Pargyline is not a very satisfactory agent, as it is a monoamine oxidase inhibitor, and as such, may cause considerable side effects when certain foods or other drugs are taken. Hydrallazine is used quite extensively in the United States, but little elsewhere, because of its side effects and the danger, at high doses, of inducing a state like systemic lupus erythematosus. So far as the others are concerned, there is little difference in effectiveness or incidence of side effects, though methyl dopa causes slightly less postural hypotension than the others. (Prichard *et al.*, 1968). Dosage may need to be reduced in warm weather or infections. The drugs may be used in association with diuretics. If diuretics are given after a stable dose of sympathetic blocking agent has been attained, this dose will need to be roughly halved, or hypotension may follow.

Table 1

Drug	Dose range per day	Approximate duration of action (h)	Frequency of dose modifications
Bethanidine	15–400 mg	8–12	Every 2–3 days
Methyl dopa	750–4000 mg	18–24	Every 3–5 days
Guanethidine	10–300 mg	36–48	Every 5–7 days
Debrisoquine	10–300 mg	8–12	Every 2–3 days
Hydrallazine	25–400 mg	8–12	Every 2–3 days
Pargyline	25–200 mg	Slow onset	Every 1–2 weeks

It is better to become familiar with the use of one of these drugs, and to change only if the patient is inadequately controlled on the first one. The general plan is to start with a small dose, and increase this at intervals shown in Table 1 until adequate control is achieved, or until side effects limit further increase. Hypotension in the morning is quite common with most of these drugs. This can sometimes be alleviated, if one of the shorter acting drugs is used, by reducing the morning dose, if symptoms appear after it is taken, or the evening dose, if symptoms occur before the morning dose is taken. In patients with renal failure the dose increments should be made at greater intervals, as these drugs are excreted in the urine, and cumulative effects are more likely in the presence of renal failure.

Prazocin is a directly acting vasodilator with hypotensive activities, and can be used alone, or in combination with the above drugs. It should be started at a low dose of 1 mg twice daily, increasing to a maximum of 6 mg twice daily. Unexplained loss of consciousness has been reported frequently in patients starting treatment with a high dose. Minoxidine is an even more recent introduction; it may well be a very effective drug, but there is, as yet, inadequate experience of its properties.

Ganglion-blocking agents, such as pempidine or mecamylamine are now seldom used.

Certain patients, frequently those with renal disease, may present great difficulty in the control of blood pressure. A common situation is that in which the patient is receiving a sympathetic blocking agent and has a very high blood pressure while recumbent, with incapacitating hypotension when he stands up. The addition of diuretics seldom eases this situation; sometimes changing to a different sympathetic agent may help. If this fails, it is reasonable to maintain the sympathetic blocking drug at the maximum level that is tolerable, and then adding either propranolol or clonidine in increasing dosage. Oral diazoxide, in doses of up to 1500 mg daily, has been used in this situation, but carries the risk of the development of diabetes.

(b) *Acute blood pressure reduction*. Several methods are available:

(1) Intravenous diazoxide 200–300 mg injected rapidly

(2) Intramuscular guanethidine 20 mg

(3) Intramuscular pentolinium 1–3 mg

(4) Hexamethonium tartrate i.v. 2.5 mg followed by increments of 2.5–5 mg at 2–3-minute intervals, dose determined by B.P. readings.

Once initial control is achieved, treatment is as in the previous section.

Antihypertensive treatment and surgery

Thiazides alone do not require modification of the dose, but careful control of potassium levels is important. If possible, rauwolfia alkaloids should be discontinued 2–3 weeks before operation. Clonidine or prazosin should be discontinued 2–3 days pre-operatively.

Sympathetic blocking agents should be discontinued 1–4 days before operation, if good control has been maintained for some time; guanethidine should be withdrawn 7–10 days before. In the case of emergency operations the main hazard is that of marked hypotension from slight blood loss, and volume expansion may be needed. These patients will be very sensitive to infused noradrenaline.

E

Hypertension and pregnancy

Patients with pre-existing hypertension may become pregnant; in these patients, the risk to the fetus is greater than in normal pregnancies, mainly because of placental insufficiency, and early induction of labour is often necessary. Apart from this, arterial pressure should be kept under strict control, by the methods previously described. No evidence has been produced to indicate that any of the drugs listed has teratogenic properties.

Women whose blood pressures were previously normal may become hypertensive during toxaemia of pregnancy. Here, control of blood pressure, together with sodium restriction, will reduce the maternal risk; there is little convincing evidence that diuretics significantly improve the prognosis of the fetus, though they may decrease the amount of time that the patient has to remain in bed.

Diet

Diet may have to be modified in obese patients, in order to lose weight. In this connection there is evidence that fenfluramine does not interfere with the hypotensive action of any of the drugs mentioned in this section. Protein restriction may also have to be introduced in the presence of renal failure. Very occasionally, in extremely difficult cases, rigid sodium restriction may be necessary. With these exceptions, there is no indication for any dietary measures in the management of patients with hypertension.

Interactions

The treatment of hypertension must usually be continued for life, and it is therefore important that patients be warned of possible dangerous combinations. Tricyclic antidepressants will inhibit the action of guanethidine, bethanidine, debrisoquine and clonidine. The depressed hypertensive patient is often difficult to treat, particularly if his hypertension is severe. Apart from the interaction just mentioned, methyldopa, reserpine, or clonidine may make the depression worse. In such patients, thiazides, or propranolol are particularly useful, though occasionally propranolol may cause psychotic symptoms. Pargyline may improve both conditions. Monoamine oxidase inhibitors may be given together with sympathetic blocking agents, provided that the hypotensive drug is started first. If the monoamine oxidase inhibitor is taken first, there is a theoretical risk of some increase in blood pressure when the sympathetic blocker is started. Lithium salts are not contraindicated.

Any sympathomimetic drug may cause an increased rise of blood pressure in hypertensive patients. This applies to ephedrine, the amphetamines, and a large number of proprietary cold cures which contain sympathomimetics.

There is some evidence that methyldopa may to some extent inhibit the anti-parkinsonian action of L-dopa.

PERIPHERAL VASCULAR DISEASE

Dissecting aneurysm

There is growing though inconclusive evidence that surviving patients in whom a diagnosis of aortic dissection has been made, fare better if treated conservatively for 2–3 weeks before surgical intervention is attempted. This course is only practicable if essential arteries are spared. During this period the patient is kept strictly at rest. Hypertension, if present, should be treated and there is a theoretical argument for the use of intramuscular reserpine, 2.5 mg daily, in order to reduce the ejection rate of blood from the left ventricle. The nature of the surgical intervention depends upon the distribution and extent of the dissection.

Aortic aneurysm

The definitive and only effective treatment for aortic aneurysms is surgical. The prognosis of untreated aortic aneurysm is poor, so that surgical treatment should always be considered, unless the patient's general condition or vascular disease elsewhere precludes it.

Obstructive arterial disease

This is common, and generally affects the aorta, and its lower branches. The commonest clinical problems arise in the lower limbs. As with myocardial ischaemia, there are two main problems; influencing the course of the atheroma, and management of the symptoms produced by arterial obstruction. The first problem has not been solved. The methods employed and the evidence of benefit from these approaches, are similar to the situation in myocardial ischaemia, and will not be reiterated.

General measures include weight reduction, treatment of anaemia and the avoidance of vasoconstrictor agents such as ergot alkaloids.

The progressive occlusion of lower limb arteries causes intermittent claudication, followed by distal necrosis. The obstruction is usually in large arteries, except in diabetes, where small vessels may also be obstructed. The ideal treatment is to restore the patency of the obstructed arteries, and with obstructive lesions above the level of the knee, this is often possible by surgical means. The site of the obstructive lesion must be defined by clinical and arteriographic investigation, provided that the patient does not have serious vascular disease elsewhere.

If surgical treatment is not to be carried out, the patient will have to live within his exercise tolerance. Weight reduction may improve his walking distance. Peripheral vasodilator drugs are of no value in the management of intermittent claudication, because the limitation of flow is due to a structural narrowing of large vessels, which is not affected by vasodilators.

In these patients, the care of the feet must be exceptionally conscientious. Small superficial lesions of the skin may become severely infected, and may lead to loss of tissue. This is a particularly serious problem in diabetic patients, because of their increased susceptibility to infection and because peripheral neuropathy may cause sensory loss, so that minor trauma, as from an ill-fitting shoe, goes unnoticed.

As the disease progresses, the likelihood of tissue loss increases, and rest pain, with impending gangrene may be present. This may require powerful analgesics. The involved limb should be kept cool to reduce tissue metabolic demands, while the rest of the patient is warmed in an attempt to reduce sympathetic tone. Sympathectomy has little part to play in the treatment of intermittent claudication, but may be of use in some patients with rest pain, but without actual gangrene. Peripheral vasodilator drugs are not generally very useful, but may be given a trial. Once gangrene is apparent, small peripheral areas may, if uninfected, be allowed to separate spontaneously, while reflex heating is continued. Gangrene of any area larger than a toe is an indication for proximal amputation and rehabilitation.

11

CARDIO-RESPIRATORY EMERGENCIES

R. D. BRADLEY

Clarity of thought is indispensable, and becomes more so as the urgency of the situation increases. The patients under consideration will usually present with arterial hypotension and/or dyspnea. Diagnosis before treatment is of the essence in the management of such patients, and unless in imminent danger of death, it is vital to obtain a history and to examine the patient thoroughly. Premature treatment undertaken blindly is only likely to conceal the diagnosis for ever.

There is an inherent difficulty in keeping to this logical path of action, posed by the fact that as patients come close to death, from whatever cause, they tend to look the same and to lose those distinguishing features by which they may be separated one from another. In a small proportion of cases, it is necessary to restore the patient in order to make an accurate assessment, but rational treatment is impossible without a diagnosis. The resolution of this dilemma can only be achieved by making a first order diagnosis, applying appropriate restorative measures, and then, with the patient partially restored, seeking the final diagnosis and definitive treatment.

The proposition that haemorrhage and heart failure should be treated in the same way is clearly ridiculous, yet both may produce a state in which the salient features are hypotension and low cardiac output. To pronounce that all patients with major derangements of the circulation are in a "state of shock", and to look for some common mode of therapy for this state, is profitless. Even when it is possible to make an accurate physiological assessment of patients suffering from acute circulatory disorders of the same aetiology, it emerges that the disease patterns differ, and the treatment requires to be tailored to the needs of each. Thus, in patients suffering from septicaemia, the emphasis may be upon hypovolaemia, myocardial failure, or the breakdown of the normal pattern of perfusion in the peripheral circulation.

INITIAL MANAGEMENT

The possible courses of action are shown in Figure 1. The first action must always be to ensure that the patient has a clear airway. Subsequent management will be dictated by the state of the patient.

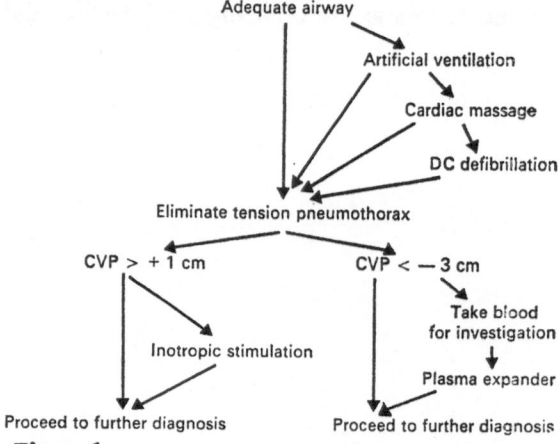

Figure 1

If the patient's ventilation is grossly inadequate, he should be artificially ventilated with whatever apparatus is available (Brook airway, 'Ambu' bag or endotracheal tube and anaesthetic bag), preferably with oxygen. If unconscious and pulseless, the circulation should be supported with external cardiac massage. If the patient remains in a state of cardiac arrest, the degree of metabolic acidosis should be determined and corrected (0.1 mEq sodium bicarbonate/kg body weight/mEq base deficit—where the base deficit is measured in mEq/1); arbitrary correction with 100 mEq sodium bicarbonate if the arrest has been brief, or 200 mEq for longer periods, is a suggested approximation if measurement is impossible. An ECG should be recorded. Ventricular fibrillation should be dealt with by DC defibrillation, starting with 100 joules. If the ventricular fibrillation persists or returns, intravenous lignocaine 1 mg/kg body weight followed by defibrillation will increase the probability of a stable rhythm. Asystole or fine ventricular fibrillation may be converted to coarse ventricular fibrillation, or some more favourable rhythm, by the intravenous use of 5–10 ml of adrenaline diluted 1/10 000 (100 μg/ml); 5–10 ml of 2% calcium chloride will increase myocardial tone, and therefore increase the effectiveness of cardiac massage in a grossly atonic heart.

Normally it is possible to proceed directly from ensuring that the patient has an adequate airway, to eliminating the possibility of a tension pneumothorax. There are two reasons for doing so at this early stage—the logical one, that the condition does not belong in either of the main groupings in the system of diagnosis to be described, and the practical one, that this is a treatable condition in which the patient's state is likely to deteriorate rapidly. In the absence of other pulmonary pathology, the physical signs are unmistakable—absent or grossly diminished breath sounds and resonance to percussion on one side of the chest, and mediastinal shift toward the opposite side.

CENTRAL VENOUS PRESSURE

Reference to Figures 1 and 2 will show the cardinal position of the central venous pressure (CVP) in terms of diagnosis. Should the venous pressure be assessed incorrectly, the diagnosis must inevitably be wrong. Every possible manoeuvre must be used to establish whether the level is raised or lowered, and if there remains any uncertainty, it must be measured with a catheter in some part of the venous system within the chest. The catheter can be advanced to this point from a basilic vein in the arm, or from the subclavian, femoral or internal jugular vein. As will be seen later, a centrally placed venous line is of enormous value for many of the measures which may subsequently become necessary.

Pressures in the venous system must be measured relative to some fixed point. The sternal angle is the most convenient reference point in clinical practice, and it is to this point that the figures quoted are related.

The possible range of normal mean venous pressures is of the order +3 cmH$_2$O to −5 cmH$_2$O. If the venous pressure is to be used as

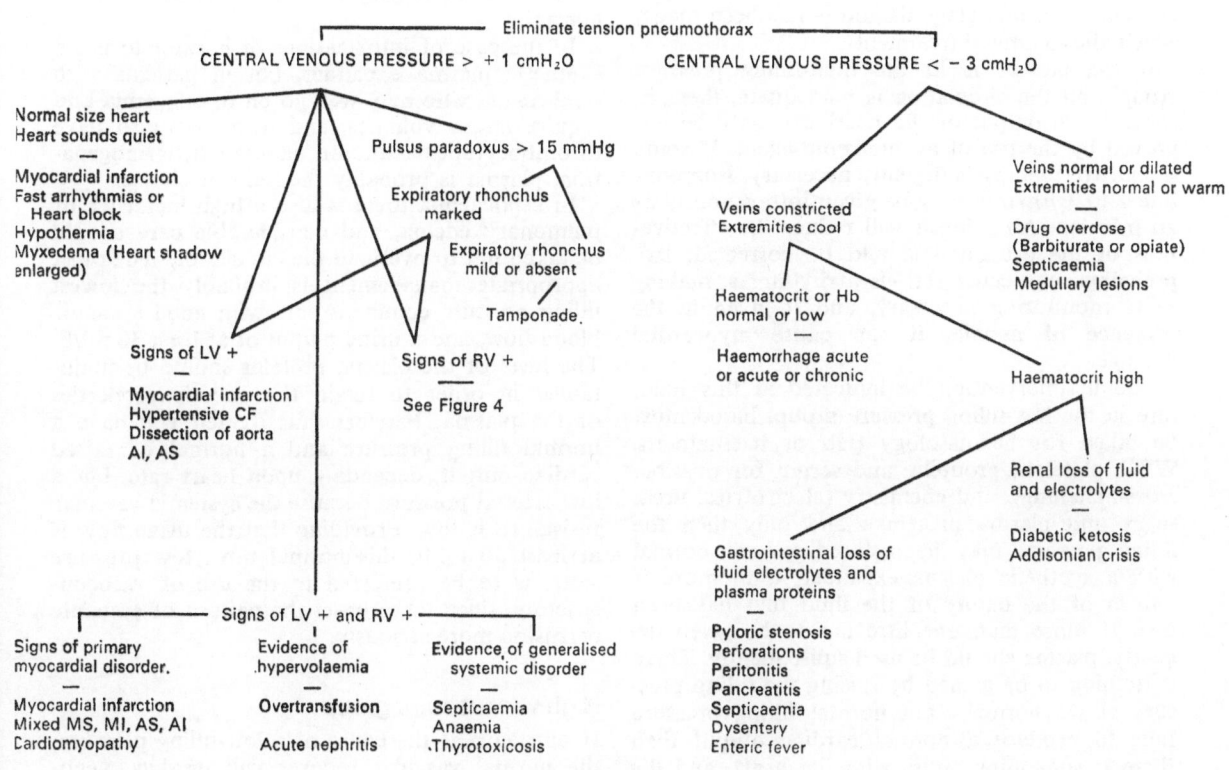

Figure 2

an arbiter in patients presenting with acute cardio-respiratory disorders, the centre of the watershed can be more closely confined. All those with pressures greater than +1 cmH_2O are placed in the high-filling pressure group, and those lower than −3 cmH_2O in the low-filling pressure group.

There will be a small number with mixed disease, and should a patient present with profound circulatory disturbance, whose filling pressure lies between the limits suggested above, it is well to consider the possibility of dual pathology.

Once the height of the venous pressure is known, a decision has to be made in the light of the patient's condition, for if this is deteriorating seriously, there is now information upon which to base logical supportive therapy without risk of concealing the diagnosis. There is a second consideration which may suggest such action— the patient may be in such a poor state that the physical signs upon which the diagnosis depends, will not be apparent until something has been done to improve his condition. Thus abdominal physical signs may be absent in a patient with a perforated peptic ulcer, until the circulation has been at least partially restored. The principle of diagnosis before treatment is not in fact being broken, for a first stage diagnosis has been made, which allows limited treatment.

If the patient is in the high-filling pressure group, and the circulation is inadequate, then, in general, the output of the heart can only be improved by the use of an inotropic agent. If some supportive therapy is urgently necessary, isoprenaline 1 to 2 μg/min may be given intravenously as an infusion. An acidosis will reduce the effectiveness of the drug and should be corrected. Isoprenaline may cause serious arrhythmias, making ECG monitoring necessary, and if given in the presence of anoxia, it can cause myocardial damage.

Should intervention be indicated at this juncture in the low-filling pressure group, blood must be taken for haematology (Hb or haematocrit, WBC, platelets, grouping and serum for possible cross-matching), and chemistry (electrolytes, urea, sugar and plasma proteins), and only then the filling pressure may be restored toward normal with a synthetic plasma expander, until more is known of the nature of the fluid that has been lost. If more than one litre has to be given urgently, plasma should be used subsequently. There is nothing to be gained by raising the filling pressure above normal. If a normal filling pressure fails to produce a normal cardiac output then there is something amiss with the heart, and the further administration of fluid may well do harm.

LOW VENOUS PRESSURE GROUP (−3 CMH_2O OR LOWER)

The further logical separation of patients with disorders in this group is not usually a matter of great difficulty.

Low venous tone group

If the cause of the fall in venous pressure is a drop in venous tone, as may occur in cases of barbiturate and opiate intoxication, certain medullary lesions and in some patients with septicaemias, then the limb veins will appear to be of normal calibre, or even dilated, the limbs will be of normal temperature, or warmer than normal (unless the patient has become hypothermic) and the skin usually dry.

These patients characteristically retain good flows, with arterial pressures as low as 50–60 mm Hg, provided that they remain lying flat, and will produce urine at normal rates when the arterial pressure is above 60 mmHg. If the cardiac output remains low despite an adequate filling pressure, an inotropic agent should be used.

The general circulatory treatment, as opposed to specific treatment aimed at the cause, should be directed to raising the filling pressure toward normal.

In the case of intoxications, it is safer to use a synthetic plasma expander, but in patients with septicaemia who may well go on to oligaemia and require larger volumes, and who may also have thrombocytopenia and/or undergo defibrinogenation, plasma is probably the fluid of choice.

In septicaemia there is also a high incidence of pulmonary edema, and considerable care should be taken not to overload the circulation. The most appropriate management is probably the lowest filling pressure commensurate with good systemic blood flow, and a urine output of at least 30 ml/h. The level of the plasma proteins should be maintained in order to retain the oncotic properties of the plasma. Patients thus treated will have a normal filling pressure and a normal or raised cardiac output, depending upon heart rate, but a low arterial pressure because the systemic vascular resistance is low. Providing that the urine flow is at least 30 ml/h, this normal flow, low pressure state, is to be preferred to the use of vasoconstrictors, since these upset the pattern of systemic perfusion more seriously.

High venous tone group

If oligaemia is the cause of a low-filling pressure, the normal vascular reflexes will produce venoconstriction and cold extremities, and the skin may or may not be sweaty. If the haematocrit or haemoglobin is normal, the probable cause is acute haemorrhage; if the haematocrit is low, acute or chronic haemorrhage. Should the haematocrit be high, renal or gastrointestinal losses of fluid, electrolytes and plasma proteins should be sought.

Common causes of gastrointestinal loss of this nature are pyloric stenosis, gastrointestinal perforations, peritonitis, pancreatitis, dysentery, enteric fever, and septicaemia. The loss may be into the lumen of the gut, or the peritoneal cavity, or both.

Renal losses on this scale occur in diabetic ketosis and Addisonian crisis.

The diagnostic scheme just described will, of course, break down, should a chronically severely anaemic patient in becoming oligaemic by loss of salt and water, raise his low haematocrit to normal. Although the diagnosis of acute haemorrhage will be incorrect, the conclusion that the oligaemia should be treated with whole blood remains true.

Ideally, oligaemia should be treated by replacement of whatever fluid has been lost. This has to be modified in practice by considerations such as the local availability of blood and blood products, their safety, and the limit set upon the use of synthetic plasma expanders by their effect upon the normal haemostatic systems, and the kidneys.

It might be thought also that the volume of the replacement should equal the volume which has been lost, and although this is probably ultimately true, it is not a particularly helpful concept. The volume which has been lost is not generally known, and although the remaining circulating volume can be estimated with isotopic techniques, replacement based upon measurements of volume in this way may cause the death of the patient. The reason for this apparent anomaly is the variability in the capacity of the vascular bed. There are few more powerfully constrictive influences upon the systemic venous capacity vessels than oligaemia.

The relation of venous tone and venous blood volume to central venous pressure can be shown diagrammatically. In Figure 3(a), the central venous pressure is plotted on the ordinate, and the change of volume of blood in the systemic venous capacity vessels on the abscissa.

A normal man would lie at or about the origin, with a volume of 3.5 litres in the systemic venous capacity vessels, a venous pressure of approximately 0 cm water, and a normal venous tone. The line AB represents the way in which the venous pressure would rise and fall as blood is either added to or removed from the system, if the venous tone is kept constant. This line might

be called an isophleb, a line of constant venous tone. There is a series of these isophlebs, each one representing the relationship between venous pressure and venous volume at a different level of venous tone. Figure 3(b) shows a number of such lines.

During haemorrhage, volume is lost from the venous bed but initially the drop in venous pressure is very small as the veins tighten down upon the shrinking volume.

The progress of events may be followed in Figure 3(c). As haemorrhage proceeds, the patient moves down the line OABCD. First the patient's foot veins will constrict, then the arm veins, and ultimately the venules in the skin of the face, giving the patient a characteristic pallor. With further haemorrhage, the venous pressure will fall quite sharply, and with it the cardiac output and systemic arterial pressure.

In ideal circumstances during transfusion the opposite path is retraced, and as the venous pressure approaches normal, the patient's venous system is observed to dilate; the re-appearance of the foot veins signalling a return to normality. Events may not follow such a simple course. There are a number of factors which may cause the venous system to remain tightly constricted, in spite of volume replacement. The most important appear to be anoxia, hypothermia, pain, and myocardial damage which may occur during the period of coronary malperfusion associated with a low cardiac output.

Figure 3(d) illustrates how it may come about that the venous pressure may rise to dangerous levels (E), before the volume of blood which was lost from the system has been replaced. This may be lethal if the heart is abnormal.

If the cause of the high venous tone is dealt with, or resolves spontaneously because of the increase in cardiac output associated with restoration of the filling pressure, the patient will return to normal along the hysteresis loop DEO. It is possible to avoid the danger involved in raising the filling pressure in this way, by observing the venous pressure and state of the peripheral veins, and not by measuring the blood volume. If, as the venous pressure rises toward normal, the peripheral veins do not dilate, a cause for the sustained high venous tone must be sought and corrected. It will then be possible to charge the systemic venous system to its normal capacity, the end point being signalled by dilation of the foot veins.

(The model of the venous system which has been presented, in which the filling pressure of the right heart is the product of venous tone and volume of blood contained in the venous reser-

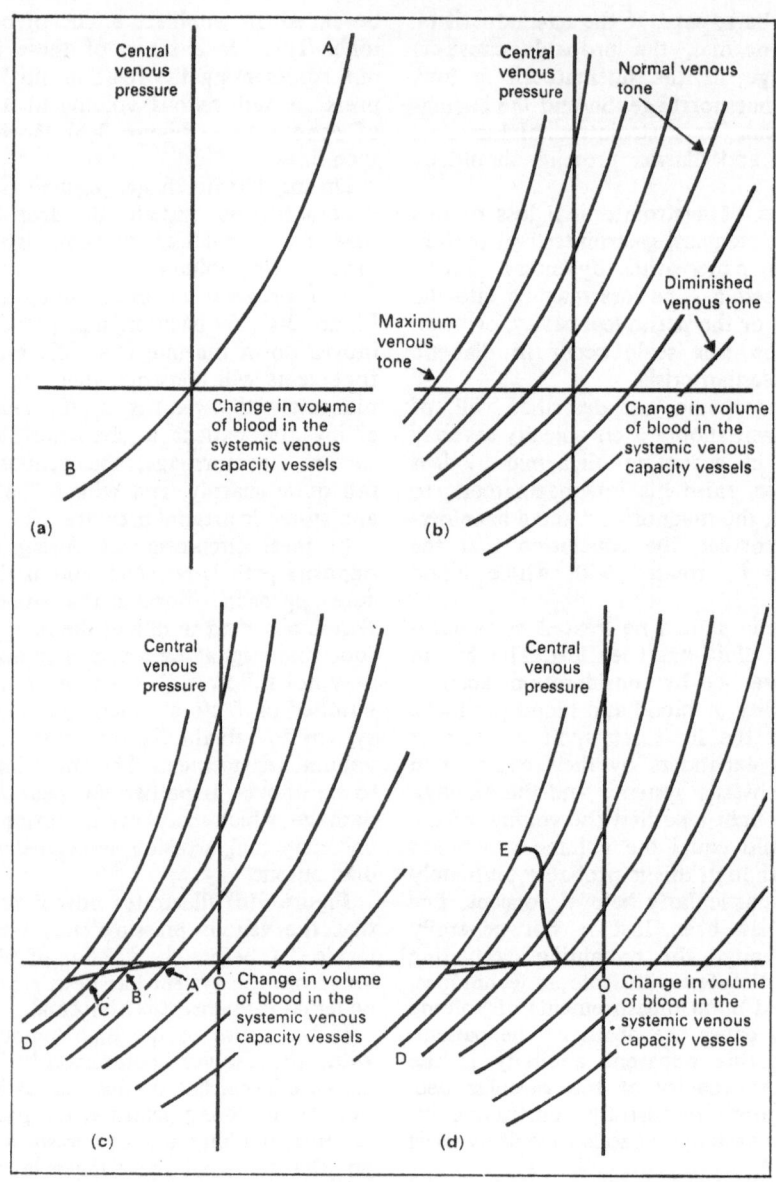

Figure 3

voir, is an over-simplification derived only from static considerations. The addition of dynamic considerations such as the 'sucking' effect of the right ventricle, modify the system but do not alter the conclusions.)

HIGH VENOUS PRESSURE GROUP (+1 cmH₂O OR ABOVE)

It is beyond the scope of this account to enter into the detailed diagnosis of all the conditions grouped under this heading in Figure 2. Some general principles are outlined in the figure; it will be seen that the breakdown into smaller groups of possibilities depends upon the assessment of the relative activity and size of the two sides of the heart. This assessment depends upon the clinical ECG and X-ray findings. Because of the difficulties of making an accurate estimate of each side of the heart, diagnosis is very much less simple here than in the low filling pressure group.

High venous pressure—normal heart size

The combination of an impalpable, or nearly impalpable right and left ventricle of normal size, a raised venous pressure and notably quiet heart sounds in a patient presenting acutely with hypotension or dyspnea, is most commonly due to myocardial infarction. Fast arrhythmias, heart block, hypothermia and severe myxedema can also produce these physical signs, but none of these conditions presents any diagnostic difficulty, apart from the possibility that they may be complicated by myocardial infarction.

Difficulty does arise when the signs of ventricular overactivity, which would place the patient in a different diagnostic group, are absent because of extreme reduction in cardiac output.

High venous pressure with right ventricular overactivity

The signs of right ventricular overactivity which characterise this group are a palpable right ventricular and pulmonary arterial heave, audible third and fourth sounds over the right ventricle, widened splitting of the second sound, and an intensification of the second element of the second sound. Not all may be present, and some, such as a third sound signifying dilation of the ventricle, are of greater significance than others, for example, a fourth sound which only implies atrial overactivity and may be heard in any condition in which there is an increase in sympathetic activity, even though the atrial pressure may be abnormally low.

Figure 4 illustrates the criteria for further subdivision within this group on clinical grounds.

If the skin veins are constricted and the extremities cold, the probable causes are myocardial infarction, acute mitral incompetence, mitral stenosis or a major pulmonary embolus. In all of these except the last the left atrial pressure is high, whereas in major pulmonary embolism uncomplicated by previous heart disease, the left atrial pressure is low. It is unfortunate, therefore, that there is no reliable physical sign related to this pressure which can be used as an arbiter, although a straight chest X-ray showing upper lobe diversion with prominent upper lobe veins, or a visible left atrium, is good evidence of a raised left atrial pressure.

Myocardial infarction of sufficient extent to produce signs of right ventricular overactivity will always be associated with ECG changes. It is only when these changes are compatible also with acute pulmonary embolism that diagnostic difficulty arises and special investigations may be required.

Acute mitral incompetence is almost always associated with a loud apical pansystolic murmur, and sometimes a thrill. The cause may be papillary muscle dysfunction or a ruptured cusp—the former associated with infarction, and the latter usually with bacterial endocarditis. Chronic mitral incompetence is, of course, associated with a dilated left ventricle. Previously undiagnosed mitral stenosis may present as an emergency, especially in pregnancy, but it is recognised by the characteristic mitral diastolic murmur, if present, or from a typical mitral configuration of the heart on chest X-ray.

If the skin veins are dilated and the extremities warm, then the likely diagnoses are pneumonia, a moderate pulmonary embolus or, if in addition the arterial carbon dioxide tension is raised, airway obstruction which may be acute or chronic.

Chronic airway obstruction and acute asthma presenting as cardio-respiratory emergencies usually declare themselves from the briefest of histories. Glottic or tracheal obstruction will usually be discovered if its existence is considered.

High venous pressure with left ventricular overactivity

The signs of left ventricular disturbance suggestive of this group of disorders, are a left ventricular heave, apical third and fourth sounds, reversed splitting of the second sound, and the presence of pulsus alternans. Again, the fourth sound is of less account than any of the other signs as it may be heard in any state associated with sympathetic overactivity. Relatively small degrees of pulsus alternans may be detected with a sphy-

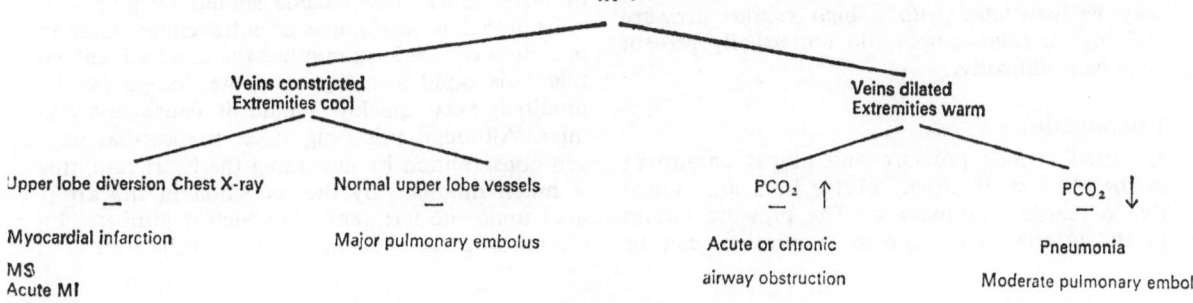

Figure 4

gmomanometer; this is often precipitated by an ectopic beat, and, unless the heart rate is of the order of 200/min, is a reliable sign of left ventricular dysfunction.

When acute left ventricular failure occurs against a background of systemic hypertension, it is often associated with a further rise in the arterial pressure. Myocardial infarction in this setting of enlargement of the left ventricle, may present diagnostic difficulty, unless the ECG changes are unequivocal, or there are enzyme changes, because the enlargement may well be due to previous infarction. Dissection of the aorta is usually suggested by the severity and sudden onset of substernal pain radiating to the back or legs, but asynchrony or absence of pulses and broadening of the mediastinum should be sought. Both aortic stenosis and aortic incompetence may present as emergencies, and are indicated by the appropriate murmurs and changes in pulse pressure.

High venous pressure with left and right ventricular overactivity

Patients in this category may be subdivided into those with primary myocardial or valvular disorders, those with hypervolaemia, and those with some general systemic disorder which occasions an abnormally high cardiac output.

Hypervolaemia and high output states are commonly accompanied by biventricular overactivity to palpation, and audible fourth sounds at the apex and left sternal edge. Primary myocardial disorder is suggested by third sounds heard over the ventricles, and by pulsus alternans.

Those with primary myocardial disorder or valvular disease include patients with myocardial infarction, cardiomyopathies, and varying combinations of mitral and aortic stenosis and incompetence.

Hypervolaemia will be diagnosed, provided that the conditions which may give rise to this are considered—that is, overtransfusion, acute nephritis, and drug induced water–salt retention. Generalised systemic disorders, such as severe anaemias, thyrotoxicosis, and septicaemia, which may be associated with a high venous pressure and high cardiac output, do not usually present diagnostic difficulty.

Tamponade

A raised venous pressure and pulsus paradoxus in the absence of airway obstruction, are indicative of cardiac tamponade. The pressure swings in the arterial pulse due to respiration, can be measured with a sphygmomanometer. The pressure at which the pulse is just palpable at the end of each expiration is recorded, and the pressure in the cuff lowered until the pulse can just be felt continuously throughout the respiratory cycle. The second pressure recorded at this point is then subtracted from the first. In normal subjects this pressure swing is less than 5 mmHg, but will rise to 15–30 mmHg in tamponade, and may be as high as 45 mmHg in severe asthma where it reflects the intrathoracic pressure swing.

If the heart shadow on chest X-ray is large, and there is a systolic descent in the venous pressure, the tamponade is due to a pericardial effusion. If the heart shadow is normal, or only slightly enlarged, and the descent in the venous pressure is post-systolic, or both post-systolic and systolic, the tamponade is due to pericardial constriction.

GENERAL PRINCIPLES OF ACUTE MANAGEMENT OF HIGH FILLING PRESSURE DISORDERS

The acute life-threatening problems which occur in this group of disorders are low cardiac output, pulmonary edema, arrhythmias, cardiac tamponade, pulmonary embolism, and airway obstruction.

Low cardiac output

In those situations within the high-filling pressure group of disorders in which the cardiac output is seriously impaired, the stroke output of the heart is low, and in contrast to the normal heart does not change significantly with alterations in filling pressure. Transfusion will not, therefore, improve the cardiac output, and since it may precipitate pulmonary edema, must be avoided.

Useful increases in cardiac output are only likely to be be obtained with inotropic agents such as digitalis and isoprenaline. The agent of choice will depend upon the heart rate and rhythm; if the rate is fast, or if there is flutter or atrial fibrillation, digitalis should be used. In the presence of a slow rate, or if there is any evidence of heart block, isoprenaline should be given.

Isoprenaline sulphate as an intravenous infusion in a dose of 0.5–5 μg/min has the great advantage that it is rapid in action, and the dosage can be modified very quickly should it cause arrhythmias. Although this drug raises myocardial oxygen consumption by increasing the heart rate, this is much modified by the reduction in the afterload upon the left ventricle which it produces by diminishing the systemic vascular resistance.

Acetyl strophanthidin has certain advantages over digoxin in acute situations, its effects appearing and passing off very much more rapidly. Digitalisation may be achieved with four intravenous doses of 0.1 mg given at 20-minute intervals.

Pulmonary edema

Pulmonary edema appears whenever the left atrial pressure or pulmonary venous pressure is raised above a critical value of approximately 24 mmHg. This critical value drops to the region of 12 mmHg if the concentration of the plasma proteins is halved. Pulmonary edema will also occur if the basement membrane of the pulmonary capillaries loses its normal properties, as it does locally in areas of pneumonia or pulmonary infarction, and in the generalised pulmonary capillary damage which may be sustained in septicaemia. Administration of high concentrations of oxygen in the inspired air will tend to correct the fall in arterial oxygen tension produced by pulmonary edema, but will not contribute to the dispersal of the edema.

If the edema has been generated by a high left atrial pressure, relief must be obtained by reducing this; the rate of disappearance of the fluid will increase according to the degree of reduction. In the case of left ventricular failure, the relation of the two sides of the heart is such that a small fall in right atrial pressure of 2 or 3 mmHg, such as may be obtained rapidly with intravenous morphia, will produce a fall in left atrial pressure as large as 10 or 15 mmHg.

If the heart is normal and the high left atrial pressure is due to overtransfusion, suitably large falls in left atrial pressure can only be obtained by dropping the right atrial pressure from 15 or 20 mmHg to the region of 5 mmHg. Pulmonary edema due to hypervolaemia cannot, therefore, be treated with morphia, but fast acting diuretics such as frusemide or ethacrynic acid should be administered intravenously, or if the patient is anuric or likely to die before the diuretics can operate, venesection must be undertaken. It will usually be necessary to remove about 1500 ml of blood to reduce the atrial pressures to reasonable levels, and, provided the blood is taken into suitable containers, the patient's own packed cells can be retransfused, when the circulating volume has been further reduced with diuretics.

Attention is seldom paid to the level of the plasma proteins in the treatment of pulmonary edema, but this is of particular importance in the context of septicaemia, in which the plasma proteins may be lost into the peritoneum and the gut, and there may be coexistent myocardial failure. When pulmonary edema occurs in septicaemia due to breakdown of the pulmonary capillary membrane, there is some evidence that massive doses of steroids may help, but this complication is often fatal. Intermittent positive pressure ventilation delivered through an endotracheal tube is a most valuable supportive measure in any patient with very severe acute pulmonary edema, from whatever cause. It may be necessary to curarise such patients, as they have a very considerable ventilatory drive and should not be allowed to breathe against the respirator as this will tend to make the edema worse.

Arrhythmias

This brief account of the treatment of acute arrhythmias refers essentially to those occurring in association with acute myocardial infarction, but is applicable in a wider range of heart disease.

In dealing with any arrhythmia, it is essential to correct arterial hypoxaemia, to measure and correct hypo- or hyper-kalaemia, and to consider digitalis intoxication as a cause. There is some evidence also that an acidaemia should be corrected.

Supraventricular and junctional arrhythmias. Sinus bradycardia and nodal bradycardia only require to be treated if the slow rate is producing ectopic beats or an inadequate cardiac output, indicated clinically by poor peripheral perfusion, urine flows of less than 30 ml/h, and drowsiness, or in the worst cases loss of consciousness

Intravenous atropine 0.5–1.0 mg is probably the least dangerous method of increasing the rate. An intravenous infusion of isoprenaline 0.5–5 μg/min will usually produce an adequate response, but if this fails pacing may be required.

Sinus tachycardia in excess of 110 beats/min is associated with a poor prognosis if the cardiac output is low, and digitalisation should be considered.

Atrial ectopic beats may presage other supraventricular arrhythmias, but do not require treatment.

Paroxysmal atrial tachycardia, flutter, and atrial fibrillation in the presence of myocardial infarcttion imply either left ventricular failure or direct involvement of the atria or sinus node in the ischaemic process. In either case, digoxin is the treatment of choice, rather than DC shock, as all these arrhythmias tend to be recurrent. A synchronised DC shock may be used if there is no response to digitalisation, and this should be done under lignocaine cover within the first 24 or 36 hours of digitalisation, before the possibility of intoxication arises. The use of β-adrenergic blockers may also be considered, but DC shock must never be used in the presence of these agents. Paroxysmal atrial tachycardia with block and nodal tachycardia may be treated in the same way provided that there is no possibility that they are manifestations of digitalis toxicity. If this possibility exists, the digitalis must be stopped, and adequate potassium supplements given. Support with a temporary transvenous pacemaker may be needed, if lignocaine and β-blockers are used to suppress ventricular dysrrhythmias arising as a result of digitalis intoxication.

Ventricular arrhythmias. Ventricular ectopic beats should be treated if they occur at a greater frequency than five per minute, if they occur within the T wave of the preceding beat, if they are multifocal in origin, or if they occur in runs of two or more. Ventricular tachycardia requires treatment as a matter of moderate urgency, and ventricular fibrillation as a matter of extreme urgency.

Ventricular ectopic beats and ventricular tachycardia should be treated initially with intravenous lignocaine 1 mg/kg body weight as a bolus followed by an infusion of 1–2 mg/min. In the case of ventricular tachycardia this should be followed by a DC shock. Ventricular fibrillation has already been dealt with in the section headed 'Initial Management'.

If lignocaine fails to control ventricular ectopic beats, or the return of ventricular tachycardia, or fibrillation, there are a number of other agents which should be tried. The least depressing in terms of ventricular function is phenytoin 125 mg intravenously over 5 minutes which may be repeated up to a total of 500 mg in 2 hours. Total dose should not exceed 1 g/24 h.

Procaine amide may be given intravenously in a dose of up to 50 mg/min for up to 1 hour, or from 2–6 g orally per 24 hours. Quinidine bisulphate 100 mg intravenously over 5 minutes followed by an infusion at 1–2 mg/min, although possibly the most depressing in its action on myocardial function, is also the most effective in the control of ventricular arhythmias, and may also be given by mouth in a dose of 1.5–3 g/24 h. Propranolol, bretylium tosylate and antihistamines have all been used, but appear to be less effective.

By virtue of being myocardial depressants all these drugs are relatively contraindicated in the presence of a low cardiac output, or atrioventricular conduction defects, or evidence of latent block such as bundle branch block, loss of septal Q waves, or widening of the QRS complex. If ventricular arrhythmias occur with severe conduction disturbances, pacemaking should be instituted first.

Heart block. Second degree and complete heart block associated with clinical evidence of poor cardiac output, Stokes-Adams attacks, or ventricular arrhythmias require treatment.

A few cases may respond to intravenous atropine 0.5–1 mg. The majority will respond to an isoprenaline infusion 0.5–5 μg/min; if this fails or provokes ventricular arrhythmias, transvenous cardiac pacing is indicated.

Cardiac tamponade

Where this is sufficient to cause dyspnea, and arterial paradox with a fall in arterial pressure such that the systolic pressure is varying between 90 and 60 mmHg, or lower with respiration, the pericardial sac should be aspirated immediately. It is convenient to introduce a soft catheter over a Seldinger guide wire. The catheter can subsequently be left to drain attached to an underwater seal. If the tamponade is not rapidly relieved surgical intervention is required.

12

DISEASES OF THE LUNG

K. B. SAUNDERS AND S. J. G. SEMPLE

The greater part of this chapter is devoted to the commonest therapeutic problems in lung disease, namely infection, airways obstruction, and respiratory failure, with particular reference to diseases characterised by airways obstruction (chronic bronchitis, asthma, emphysema). Some other forms of lung diseases are more briefly considered. The treatment of pulmonary tuberculosis is described in Chapter 13.

ACUTE PULMONARY INFECTION

Infection may involve the airways (acute bronchitis) or the pulmonary parenchyma (pneumonia) or both. Pneumonia may be a primary lesion caused by a specific organism ('the specific pneumonias'), namely *Str. pneumoniae, Staph. pyogenes,* or *Klebsiella pneumoniae.* More commonly, the pneumonia may follow an upper respiratory tract infection, or an acute bronchitis (aspiration pneumonia or bronchopneumonia). Such infection is particularly common in elderly or debilitated patients confined to bed, and in the post-operative state.

Acute viral infections of the respiratory tract

It is not possible to treat the virus infection directly, but the secondary bacterial infection which often follows may be treated as outlined below.

Mortality statistics show a rise in deaths from all causes during influenza epidemics, particularly from hypertension, rheumatic heart disease, chronic nephritis and diabetes. Immunisation against influenza is therefore recommended in the following conditions:

    (a) chronic lung disease (chronic bronchitis, emphysema, asthma, bronchiectasis, pulmonary tuberculosis and fibrosis)

    (b) chronic heart disease

    (c) chronic renal disease

    (d) diabetes

Acute bronchitis

There are only three therapeutic measures which are important in the treatment of uncomplicated acute bronchitis; these are the administration of antibiotics, the suppression of cough, and relief of pain.

Antibiotics should always be used in those specially at risk from bronchitis and also in those patients bringing up copious quantities of purulent sputum. It is difficult to give any clear cut indications for or against the use of antibiotics apart from these. In general the authors feel that antibiotics should be given to all patients with bronchitis who are coughing up purulent sputum on the grounds that the administration of antibiotics may reduce morbidity, shorten the period off work, and prevent permanent damage to the airways. Routine sputum culture is unnecessary, but should be reserved for those cases where there is no response to conventional treatment, or where pneumonia is suspected. Tetracycline (500 mg four times a day), ampicillin (500 mg four times a day), or co-trimoxazole (two tablets twice a day), for 3–5 days is all that is required to treat the majority of patients. Amoxycillin is a more recent derivative of ampicillin. It has a similar spectrum of antibacterial activity, and is better absorbed from the gastrointestinal tract. Claims that it attains a better bactericidal concentration in sputum have not been unequivocally established. It is given in a dose of 250 mg thrice daily.

Cough suppressants should never be given to patients in respiratory failure due to an exacerbation of chronic airways obstruction, for the survival of the patient may depend on the effectiveness of the cough. Moreover, most cough suppressants depress respiration. They should in theory not be given to patients with productive cough, especially during the day, for the airways are cleared of pus predominantly by coughing. However, suppression of cough and relief of pain will be necessary for some such patients at night to enable them to sleep, and are particularly indicated for those with a painful dry cough. The most useful suppressant for routine use is codeine phosphate which can be given in tablet form in a dose of 10–60 mg, or as linctus codeine (BNF), 4–8 ml. The main side effect is constipation. When cough is particularly persistent and troublesome then morphine or diamorphine may be used but probably only in the elderly or incurable patient because of the danger of addiction.

Water will only reach the respiratory passages if droplets of water of the right size and in sufficient quantities are inhaled. If the droplets are too large they will quickly settle out and not reach the lower airways; if they are too few in number they will quickly evaporate. In theory it is possible that the deposition of water in the airways might make the sputum easier to expectorate. There is no evidence that this is true nor can one be sure with the techniques used that the nebulisers or steam tents produce water droplets of the right size and in sufficient quantity in the inspired air to be of value. The recently developed 'plate' humidifiers may prove more efficient. They are not yet sufficiently developed for general use, but may be suitable for intensive care units (see Status asthmaticus). We do not therefore feel that the provision of an aerosol or steam tent is of value in the treatment of acute bronchitis, apart from bringing symptomatic relief in patients whose mouth and pharynx have become dry and uncomfortable due to persistent mouth breathing.

Pneumonia

The pneumonias are often classified on anatomical grounds as localised (lobar or segmental pneumonia) or generalised (bronchopneumonia). This classification has no therapeutic value, for the treatment depends on the infecting organism.

Occasionally, the clinical picture may point to a particular organism (the specific pneumonias). The recommended initial treatment is then as follows (all parenterally):—

Pneumonia	Organism	Recommended initial treatment
Pneumo-coccal	Str. pneumoniae	Penicillin G, 1 megaunit 6 hourly
Staphylo-coccal	Staph. aureus	Cloxacillin 500 mg 6 hourly and sodium fusidate 500 mg 8 hourly
Fried-lander's	Klebsiella pneumoniae	Cephaloridine 500 mg 6 hourly and gentamicin 60–80 mg 8 hourly

In practice it is rare to be able to identify the infecting organism on clinical criteria. Usually identification rests on the results of sputum and blood culture, and until these results are available an empirical approach must be taken (see below). Initial treatment will then be modified by subsequent tests of bacterial sensitivity, especially important in staphylococcal infection. If the isolated organism is insensitive to the antibiotic initially given, and there has been no clinical response, the bacteriologist will advise on the best antibiotics or continuation of antibiotics to be given.

GENERAL PRINCIPLES OF TREATMENT OF PNEUMONIA

(1) *Prophylaxis.* Elderly patients, smokers, patients with chronic cough and sputum with or without airways obstruction, and patients who are to have abdominal surgery, are particularly likely to get post-operative pneumonia. The incidence of the complication will be decreased by stopping smoking at least a week before surgery and by routine pre-operative and post-operative physiotherapy. Physiotherapy will also help to prevent hypostatic pneumonia in the elderly or debilitated who are confined to bed.
(2) *Antibiotic therapy.* In general, if the patient is less than 50, has no associated chronic respiratory disease, and has become infected outside hospital, the initial drug should be penicillin, for the causative organism will very frequently be a pneumococcus or a penicillin-sensitive staphylococcus. If the patient is over 50, has associated respiratory disease such as airways obstruction or bronchiectasis, or has become infected while in hospital, broad spectrum therapy is required. If the illness is not serious (low-grade fever, little systemic upset, minor X-ray changes), tetracycline, ampicillin, or co-trimoxazole is the initial drug of choice. Recently, strains of *Str. pneumoniae* resistant to tetracycline have been isolated, but this is at present a rare occurrence. Many surgeons prefer to treat post-operative pneumonia by physiotherapy alone in the first instance, reserving antibiotic therapy for cases where the fever does not resolve in 3 or 4 days. If the illness is severe, a more potent bactericidal combination should be used, and culture of the blood as well as the sputum is mandatory, for the patient may be too weak to clear secretions by coughing, and the blood may be the only source from which the pathogen may be grown. Penicillin and streptomycin have been frequently used in the past, but a hospital staphylococcus is often resistant to both drugs. Ampicillin 1 g

q.d.s. and cloxacillin 500 mg q.d.s. is an effective and relatively non-toxic combination, but will not control infection due to klebsiella, or *Pseudomonas pyocyanea.* A cephalosporin plus gentamicin is the best combination for these two uncommon organisms. The ototoxicity of gentamicin is a disadvantage if renal function is impaired, when dosage should be controlled by measuring blood levels.

In general ampicillin and cloxacillin are probably the best initial combination for the seriously ill patient.

(3) *General measures.* A productive cough should not in general be suppressed, nor should a cough suppressant ever be given to a patient with respiratory failure (see acute bronchitis). Unproductive cough may be treated with codeine or pholcodine linctus BPC, 4–8 ml. Pleuritic pain may be treated with local heat and simple analgesics (aspirin, paracetamol), but more powerful analgesics such as pethidine and morphine are also respiratory (and cough) depressants. It is safest never to use them. Confusion and delirium may occur in young patients with severe pneumonia, but in elderly patients even with apparently mild infection. If this is associated with carbon dioxide retention and hypoxia, the problem is that of respiratory failure, discussed below, and oxygen therapy should be given, but with great caution. Pneumonia rarely causes carbon dioxide retention unless there is associated chronic respiratory disease. If respiratory failure is not present, chlorpromazine 50 mg is the best sedative.

Arrythmias should be treated if they are causing circulatory embarrassment. The commonest is atrial fibrillation, when digitalis may be needed to control ventricular rate.

Finally, the clinical picture may be that of overwhelming septicaemia, with tachycardia, low blood pressure, oliguria, mental confusion and poor response to initial treatment. Such patients should be transferred to an intensive care unit if possible: if the central venous pressure is low, systolic blood pressure and peripheral perfusion may be restored by expanding the circulating blood volume with blood or plasma. Massive doses of antibiotics are needed, and large doses of steroids are usually given.

THE TREATMENT OF DISEASES CHARACTERISED BY AIRWAYS OBSTRUCTION

These diseases are:

(1) *Chronic bronchitis.* Definition: a disease characterised by chronic cough and sputum (in the absence of any other cause for these symptoms such as bronchiectasis, tuberculosis, or chronic heart failure).

(2) *Asthma.* Definition: a disease characterised by attacks of airways obstruction which are reversible, i.e. between attacks the lungs are clinically normal. Sophisticated tests of lung mechanics may show abnormalities between attacks even when simple spirometric tests give normal results.

(3) *Emphysema.* Definition: a disease characterised by abnormal accumulation of air beyond the terminal bronchiole, with destruction of pulmonary parenchyma, including alveolar walls.

These definitions can hardly be regarded as satisfactory; the first is made purely on symptoms; the second on clinical and functional characteristics; and the third is a pathological diagnosis for which the best evidence in life is the chest X-ray. Nevertheless they will suffice for the discussion of therapy which follows.

Causes of airways obstruction

An increased resistance to the flow of gas through the airways may have several causes:

(a) the airways may be blocked by edema fluid, mucus, or pus

(b) the airways may be obstructed by inflamed edematous bronchial mucosa

(c) the airways may collapse during expiration, especially if the bronchial walls are weakened and supporting parenchyma destroyed by disease

(d) the bronchial muscle may be inappropriately contracted

The functional diagnosis

The effect of isoprenaline in a classical acute asthmatic attack is obvious and requires no objective confirmation. However in patients with chronic airways obstruction, before embarking on a course of treatment which may last years, using expensive drugs which may have unpleasant side effects, it is necessary to make sure first that increased airways resistance is present, and, second, that it is responsive to the particular bronchodilator employed. Airways obstruction of clinical significance will be detected by the simple spirometric measurement of forced expiratory volume in one second (FEV_1) and forced vital capacity (FVC). If the ration FEV_1/FVC is less than 60%, there is airways obstruction. These measurements can be made as easily in general practice as in hospital practice. They can be repeated after giving a bronchodilator, when an increase in FEV_1 will give objective confirmation that the airways obstruction will be relieved by the drug. More sophisticated measurements of lung function are rarely required.

ASTHMA

It is customary to classify asthma as extrinsic or intrinsic.

EXTRINSIC ASTHMA

This is characterised by onset of the disease in childhood and by a family history of atopy (asthma, hay fever, eczema). The lungs are usually clinically normal between attacks. An asthmatic attack may be precipitated by exposure to some substance to which the patient is sensitive (e.g. cat fur, horse hair, or house dust containing mites), by an upper respiratory infection; by exposure to cold air; or by some psychological upset.

The general principles of the treatment of asthma are to prevent attacks when possible and to abort them quickly when they occur.

Psychological factors

Although there is no doubt that some patients with asthma are neurotic, there is no clear evidence that neurosis is more common in this than in any other disease. Sometimes an attack will be triggered by an emotional upset such as a barely avoided traffic accident, or an outburst of anger. The treatment is then that of the asthmatic attack, which will always include the psycho-therapeutic effect of a firm, confident, sympathetic approach. The question is whether the number of attacks can be decreased by long-term treatment of the psychological factors. Again the psycho-therapeutic effect of firm, sympathetic handling is the primary aim. One may hope, over a period of months or years, to bring the patient nearer to understanding the factors which underly the attacks, and to help him to avoid those situations which exacerbate the disease. However an attempt to do this abruptly will carry, to the patient, the implication that his condition is 'all in the mind'; this is invariably a serious, and sometimes irretrievable mistake. Some patients, particularly during periods of stress at home or at work, are helped by a mild sedative such as chlordiazepoxide 5-10 mg t.d.s. or diazepam 2-5 mg t.d.s. Sedation is never indicated during an acute attack. The patient is then anxious and agitated because he cannot breathe and because he fears he may die, a suspicion which occasionally proves correct.

Relief of the airways obstruction will then relieve the anxiety.

Allergic factors

It may be possible to show, by skin or inhalation testing, that the patient is sensitive to a certain substance. These are usually inhaled dusts (e.g. horse dander, house dust) or ingested proteins (e.g. shellfish). There are two possible approaches: first, to remove the offending substance from the environment as far as possible; second, to try to desensitise the patient. Unfortunately, neither approach has proved spectacularly profitable to the majority of asthmatic patients. Many atopic subjects will prove to be sensitive to a number of allergens; moreover, skin testing on different occasions may give different results. If in the clinical history there is a strong suggestion that one particular allergen is responsible for provoking the asthmatic attacks, and this is confirmed by testing, that allergen should obviously be avoided. This may be easy if, for example, it is an ingested substance such as shellfish, but impossible if it is an omnipresent hazard such as house dust. Measures such as replacing feather pillows, mattresses and stuffed furniture by foam materials may be beneficial, but may also involve a family in considerable expense. Again, if the clinical picture and the sensitivity tests strongly point to one particular allergen, an attempt may be made to desensitise the patient by a course of injections. Such a course may be time consuming, painful and expensive; occasional anaphylactic deaths have been recorded. Clinical benefit is far from guaranteed. In the case of pollen sensitivity however, a preseasonal desensitisation course has been shown to benefit most patients in a controlled clinical trial. In our opinion, this situation is the only one where such treatment has a proven likelihood of success. Desensitisation may turn out to be of benefit in patients with a house-mite allergy, but this is not yet sufficiently proven to be advised routinely.

Disodium cromoglycate

This drug offers the first direct attack on the immunological reaction responsible for asthma. It has been shown by inhalation tests to inhibit both the clinical reaction due to reaginic antibodies (Type I) and that associated with serum precipitins (Type III). Most clinical trials have shown a statistically significant benefit to patients with extrinsic asthma. This has been most obvious in children and young adults, and the benefit has been measured in terms of symptoms, reduced steroid and bronchodilator dosage, and lung function tests. The drug has to be given by inhalation in powder form, and since the powder itself may cause bronchospasm in some subjects, isoprenaline sulphate may be included. This cannot be regarded as a satisfactory method of administration and it is hoped that a more convenient preparation will be developed. The drug is initially given 6-hourly, or 3-hourly in severe cases. However, the optimum dosage for maintenance therapy has yet to be determined by proper clinical trial; we suggest one inhalation three times a day.

This drug has not yet been completely assessed; and the effectiveness of long-term therapy is not yet known. Nevertheless it is certainly worth a trial in cases of extrinsic asthma, particularly in children and young adults.

Treatment of Infection

Attacks of asthma may be precipitated by upper respiratory infections or acute bronchitis. If there is fever, cough or purulent sputum a wide spectrum antibiotic (tetracycline, ampicillin or cotrimoxazole) should be prescribed.

Bronchodilator therapy

In an acute asthmatic attack, a sympathomimetic drug should be given by inhalation. We prefer the newer drugs, orciprenaline, salbutamol or terbutaline which have minimal cardiovascular side-effects. These drugs also have a more prolonged effect than isoprenaline alone. The dosage recommended by the manufacturers should never be exceeded. If thee is no improvement within 2 hours, medical advice should be urgently sought, further treatment being discussed in the section on Status asthmaticus.

In some cases of severe asthma, the lungs may not return to normal between attacks: some degree of bronchospasm may be present almost continuously. Oral bronchodilator therapy is then appropriate. Again we prefer orciprenaline or salbutamol to ephedrine, which may cause difficulty of micturition and insomnia especially in the elderly, but theophylline derivatives such as choline theophyllinate are also satisfactory. There is little evidence that combinations of bronchodilators and barbiturates are more effective than a bronchodilator alone..

Corticosteroid therapy

Rarely, extrinsic asthma may be so intractable that continuous corticosteroid therapy is needed.

The danger of side-effects should then be weighed against the severity of the patient's respiratory disability. It may be possible to alleviate symptoms sufficiently by giving prednisone 5 mg q.d.s. on only three consecutive days in each week; corticosteroid side-effects are unlikely with this regime. However, regular therapy with prednisone 5–15 mg/day may be required; a dose greater than 10 mg/day will probably cause side-effects.

Beclomethasone dipropionate or betamethasone valerate may be given as inhalations in a dose of 100–200 μg four times daily without causing adrenal suppression or corticosteroid side effects. In some patients, inhaled steroids may be substituted for oral prednisone, which should be tailed off gradually. In others, the combination of inhaled with oral steroid therapy may allow the previous dose of oral prednisone to be reduced to more acceptable levels (i.e. less than 10 mg/day).

INTRINSIC ASTHMA

This is characterised by onset in middle age or later, by the absence of a history of atopy, by blood and sputum eosinophilia, and by a bad prognosis. The principles of psychotherapeutic management are identical to those in extrinsic asthma. A search for allergic factors is usually unsuccessful, and the position of disodium cromoglycate in this form of asthma has not yet been fully determined, for although patients without apparent allergic factors have shown a response to the drug, the search for allergens has not usually been rigorous. A trial of the drug for one month is certainly reasonable.

Treatment with bronchodilators may be needed continuously, since the course of the disease is often progressive rather than episodic. This should be attempted with oral therapy, reserving inhalations for the treatment of the acute attack if posssible.

In the progressive form of the disease, steroid therapy will almost certainly be needed. If the patient presents with status asthmaticus, the aim should be to control airways obstruction by initial large doses (40–60 mg prednisone/day), for 4–5 days gradually reducing the dose over about 2 weeks to acceptable levels if possible. If however the course is one of gradually increasing airways obstruction, it is probably better to start with small doses of prednisone (2.5 mg daily) and gradually work up to the dose at which life becomes tolerable for the patient. Unfortunately, in this form of asthma it is frequently impossible to make life bearable for the patient without producing the side-effects of corticosteroids. Some physicians believe that in intrinsic asthma no attempt should be made to stop steroid therapy altogether, but rather that it should be continued at the lowest possible maintenance dose for the remainder of the patient's life. This is because an attempt to withdraw steroids, however gradual, may be followed by a relapse which is resistant to steroid treatment. Although there is no firm objective evidence for this view, in terms of controlled trials, it is compatible with the authors' experience.

STATUS ASTHMATICUS

We define this as an acute attack of asthma which is unimproved by sympathomimetic drugs given sublingually or by inhalation. This is a medical emergency. The view, once widely held, that patients never die in an acute asthmatic attack, is fallacious. The recent increase in deaths from asthma is discussed below.

The traditional drug of first choice is adrenaline, 1:1000 strength, 0.5 ml being given subcutaneously over 8 minutes and repeated if necessary in 30 minutes. This treatment may now deserve reconsideration. It was undoubtedly often effective when previous treatment consisted of an inhaled bronchodilator delivered from a hand nebuliser. Such devices may not create droplets in sufficient numbers, or of correct size to reach the relevant airways. The modern 'metered-dose' aerosol canisters are certainly more efficient. In the authors' experience in hospital practice, the patient has usually already received large doses of isoprenaline or another sympathomimetic, and may have a tachycardia of 150. In this situation, there seems little to be gained by giving another catecholamine, with risk of arryhthmias, and indeed adrenaline has rarely been effective. We therefore think that aminophylline is here the drug of first choice. However, in general practice, in milder cases where large doses of catecholamine have not been given, adrenaline should be used first. If adrenaline has no effect within 30 minutes, aminophylline, 0.25–0.5 g in 10–20 ml sterile water, should be given intravenously. Very rarely, sudden death has been reported after the drug has been given intravenously, and this is thought to be associated with rapid injection. It should therefore be given slowly, over 5–10 minutes. If there is no effect in 20 minutes, 200–300 mg of hydrocortisone should be given intravenously, and the patient transferred to hospital, for even if the patient rapidly improves, close observation will be needed for at least 24 hours. It may be necessary to repeat the dose of intravenous hydrocortisone 2–4 hourly. If only one or two doses are required there is no need to follow it with oral prednisone. If more than two doses are given, oral prednisone 20 mg t.d.s. should be prescribed for 2–3 days, and the dose then gradually reduced and stopped over 10–14 days. If the attack has been precipitated by a respiratory tract infection, this should be treated; usually a wide spectrum antibiotic such as tetracycline or ampicillin is suitable.

Hypoxia and acidosis predispose to lethal arrhythmias, especially in the presence of isoprenaline. Oxygen should be given if the arterial oxygen tension (P_aO_2) is less than 60 mmHg. Bronchodilatation is frequently followed by a fall in P_aO_2; oxygen should therefore be continued after the wheeze has disappeared. The hypoxic drive to breathe will thereby be removed, but in classical acute asthma this contributes only a little to the overall respiratory drive. Nevertheless the arterial CO_2 tension (P_aCO_2) should be measured during oxygen breathing to make sure that alveolar ventilation does not decrease. A rising P_aCO_2 may then be an indication for artificial ventilation, discussed below. Apart from the liability to arrhythmias, there is evidence that bronchodilators are less effective in the presence of acidosis; measurement of pH and P_aCO_2 will allow this to be assessed and corrected.

Many patients with status asthmaticus are dehydrated, probably because of increased water loss through the skin and in the expired air. Blood volume may be diminished. This should be treated by intravenous fluids, the rate and amount being controlled by observation of the central venous pressure. The jugular venous pulse may be a very difficult guide, for it may be obscured by the movements of accessory muscles of respiration, and it will certainly show wide pressure swings with respiration. It is therefore highly preferable to measure the right heart filling pressure with a right atrial catheter which may be introduced by the 'float' catheter technique.

Finally there remains the rare case which is intransigent to these measures, including intravenous steroids. The blood gases must then be measured frequently, for the main indication of impending death is a rising P_aCO_2, and this is a late sign. If the attack is prolonged, the patient will eventually become exhausted, alveolar ventilation will decrease, and the final outcome is death in respiratory failure, perhaps with a terminal arrhythmia. A P_aCO_2 which gradually rises to an abnormally high level (>45 mmHg) is therefore a sinister sign; at this stage preparation should be made for artificial respiration (intubation and intermittent positive-pressure respiration).

Although the precise indications for artificial

respiration are not yet agreed, they basically consist of

(a) a P_aCO_2 of more than 60 mmHg on admission,

(b) a P_aCO_2 of 50–60 mmHg on admission which does not fall after about 8 hours treatment,

(c) a P_aCO_2 which rises, despite treatment, to approach 50 mmHg,

(d) evidence of increasing exhaustion of the patient.

One useful piece of evidence of the latter is a decrease in the pulsus paradoxus which characteristically accompanies acute asthma. The magnitude of the paradoxical pressure swing in systolic pressure is dependent on the magnitude of the intrapleural pressure swings, and hence on the amount of respiratory effort which the patient can achieve. In a deteriorating patient, a fall in the amplitude of the paradoxical systolic pressure swings may then be a useful objective index of increasing exhaustion. It should be emphasised that the presence of exhaustion and of a rising, abnormally high, P_aCO_3 are late signs; if present, artificial respiration is urgently needed.

Post-mortem studies of lungs from patients who have died of acute asthma usually show small airways blocked by inspissated mucus. Any techniques for making these inspissated plugs less tenacious and therefore easy to expectorate would be welcome. Mucolytic drugs have been tried, but without convincing success. Bronchial lavage has been successful in some people's hands but is not without danger and should only be carried out in ITUs by those experienced in the technique. The new 'plate humidifiers' may well be the technique most useful in severe attacks of asthma. By adjusting the speed of vibration of the plate it is possible to produce droplets of the right size (100 μm) and in sufficient quantity. At present these humidifiers are too cumbersome and experimental to be used outside hospitals or special units.

Deaths from acute asthma

In the late 1960s, there was an increase in deaths from asthma. In many cases, there was circumstantial evidence of an over-dose of a sympathomimetic drug from a 'metered-dose' aerosol canister. This suspicion was partly confirmed by demonstration of a correlation between deaths due to asthma and prescription of such preparations. One cause of the increased death rate therefore appeared to be misuse of drugs in this form. Possibly the too frequent use of a sympathomimetic drug, in circumstances where airways obstruction is unrelieved, and in the presence of anoxia, has caused lethal arrhythmias. It is therefore of the greatest importance that on prescription of a metered-dose canister, the patient should be first told never, under any circumstances, to exceed the recommended dose, and secondly instructed to seek medical help urgently should the attack not respond to the drug. For the same reason, we have suggested that these preparations should not be prescribed to patients with chronic bronchospasm where a satisfactory effect can be achieved with oral therapy.

CHRONIC BRONCHITIS

The main aims of treatment in chronic bronchitis are:

(a) to remove factors which cause bronchial irritation;

(b) to treat infection;

(c) to alleviate airways obstruction.

Factors which cause bronchial irritation

It is of primary importance for the patient to give up smoking. Occupations which involve exposure to dust should be avoided, but loss of earnings may make this impossible.

Treatment of infection

There is no satisfactory method for assessing the pathogenic significance of bacteria in the sputum of chronic bronchitics. An organism which can be shown to be present significantly more often in patients with purulent sputum can be assumed to be related to the infection though not necessarily causative. An organism found as frequently in patients with mucoid sputum as in those with purulent sputum can be concluded to be a nonpathogen. The pathogenic significance of organisms can be assessed by determining the clinical response to chemotherapy, e.g. the disappearance or reduction of purulent sputum, or by measuring the plasma antibody levels against the bacteria, but this is again circumstantial rather than direct evidence.

Haemophilus influenzae can be cultured from about 80% of patients in remission but with purulent sputum. There is a close correlation between the presence of this organism and of sputum purulence, and specific serum antibodies are found more frequently in patients with purulent sputum (69%) than those with mucoid sputum (25%) and are only found in 6% of normal controls. *H. influenzae* is probably pathogenic in about half of the acute exacerbations in chronic bronchitics but is rarely a cause of pneumonia.

Str. pneumoniae may be a cause of exacerbations of bronchitis, but is more commonly the cause of pneumonia in bronchitics.

Bacteria which are rarely pathogenic

Coliform bacilli, *Haemophilus parainfluenzae, Klebsiella pneumoniae, Pasteurella septica,* Proteus, *Staph. aureus, Pseudomonas pyocyanea* and *Str. pyogenes.* These organisms are more likely to be pathogenic in patients who are receiving steroids or suffering from debilitating diseases such as carcinomatosis or leukaemia.

Non-pathogenic bacteria

Diphtheroid bacilli, *N. catarrhalis, Staph. albus, Str. non-haemolyticus* and *Str. viridans.*

Bacterial sensitivity

The pattern of sensitivity of *H. influenzae* and of the pneumococcus is sufficiently constant to justify 'blind' chemotherapy. The sensitivity of other organisms, especially *Staph. aureus,* is variable, and should always be determined if considered pathogenic.

The ideal goal in chemotherapy would be to attain a bactericidal concentration of antibiotic in the bronchial mucous membrane, in the micro-abscesses in the walls of the bronchioles, in the macrophages within the lung and in the sputum. The concentration of an oral antibiotic is higher in the blood than the sputum, and probably at an intermediate level in the tissues. Thus the attainment of a bactericidal concentration of antibiotic in the plasma does not imply that a bactericidal level has been reached in tissues or sputum. It is generally true that a higher antibiotic concentration can be achieved in purulent than in mucoid sputum. This is certainly true for ampicillin, and almost certainly for streptomycin and the tetracyclines.

We may now outline some broad principles for the chemotherapy of chronic bronchitis.

(a) The bacterial pathogens most likely to be encountered in chronic bronchitics are: in remission, *H. influenzae;* in acute exacerbations, *Str. pneumoniae* and *H. influenzae;* in pneumonia, *Str. pneumoniae* or *Staph. aureus.*

(b) In the majority of patients chemotherapy may be undertaken 'blind' without a sputum culture. If there is pneumonia, or a failure to respond to treatment, or the patient is very ill,

the sputum should be cultured; if there is time and there is no danger to the patient, three separate cultures should be taken before chemotherapy begins.

(c) In general chemotherapy is unlikely to benefit a patient whose sputum is mucoid (non-purulent), especially if no pathogens are isolated on sputum culture.

(d) Acute exacerbations should always be treated with antibiotics or chemotherapeutic agents.

Treatment of acute exacerbations

These are usually recognised by an increase in purulence and/or volume of sputum, usually with fever and a deterioration in the patient's general clinical condition. In some patients however sudden deterioration may occur without any immediate change in the sputum. In patients who are not severely ill ampicillin (500 mg 6-hourly), tetracycline (500 mg 6-hourly), or co-trimoxazole (2 tablets twice daily) may be given immediately without sputum culture. Again, the recent isolation of a few strains of *Str. pneumoniae* resistant to tetracycline should be noted. In patients who are severely ill both sputum and blood should be taken for culture before beginning treatment, and a more potent bactericidal combination should be used. The approach is exactly that of the treatment of a severe pneumonia (see page 131); a combination of ampicillin (1 g 6-hourly) and cloxacillin (500 mg 6-hourly) is probably the best initial choice, while awaiting the results of sputum and blood culture.

Treatment of chronic bronchitis in remission, but with purulent sputum

Although histological examination of the lungs in patients with chronic bronchitis suggests that bacterial infection is responsible for much of the damage, there is no direct evidence that it can be prevented by efficient bacterial suppression. However many clinical trials have shown that there is a clinical improvement in patients treated with ampicillin or tetracycline.

If the patient is in remission and has purulent sputum then the infecting pathogen is almost always *H. influenzae.* It is then reasonable to try bactericidal therapy, to eliminate the organism from the infected sites in the lungs and from reservoirs of infection in the upper respiratory tract. Ampicillin should be given (1 g 6-hourly) for 4 days. There is no point in continuing this high dosage beyond 4 days for either the sputum will become non-purulent and bactericidal concentrations will no longer be obtained, or if purulent sputum continues it means that bactericidal concentrations have not been obtained in any case in the sputum or in the infected sites which form the reservoirs of organisms.

If bactericidal therapy is successful it can be repeated as necessary; if it fails or is followed by a rapid relapse then bacteriostatic therapy should be considered; here the aim is to suppress organisms sufficiently to allow inflammation to subside. A 1- or 2-week course of ampicillin (500 mg 6-hourly) or tetracycline (250 mg 6-hourly) should be given. If the patient improves, a decision has then to be made whether antibiotics should be given continuously, or intermittently as required. This problem will now be considered.

Prophylaxis against acute exacerbations

It is likely that viral infections are responsible for starting most exacerbations and that *H. influenzae* and/or *Str. pneumoniae* are responsible for subsequent bacterial damage. Immunological prophylaxis against viruses or the above bacteria is either impracticable or ineffective, except before an influenza epidemic, when active immunisation may diminish the severity of the illness or prevent it.

Prophylaxis against bacterial infection following viral infection can be intermittent or continuous. By intermittent prophylaxis we mean the the patient is given a supply of antibiotics to start taking immediately an upper respiratory infection starts or the sputum become purulent. This has been shown to decrease the severity and length of the acute exacerbation.

Continuous antibiotic prophylaxis has been shown in most trials to decrease the severity of acute exacerbations but not their number. One recent trial has shown that treatment from October to April also decreases the number of exacerbations, but that this decrease was only significant in those patients who had several exacerbations every winter. The argument is therefore not settled. In view of the disadvantages of continuous antibiotic therapy, particularly the acquisition of drug resistant organisms, it is probably best to give continuous prophylaxis only to those patients who have three or more exacerbations per winter, and intermittent prophylaxis to the rest.

The choice of drugs again lies between tetracycline, ampicillin, and co-trimoxazole. The tetracyclines, particularly oxytetracycline, are the cheapest, and therefore to be preferred in long-term treatment. For continuous or intermittent prophylaxis bacteriostatic doses (tetracycline 250 mg q.d.s.) should normally be used. In intermittent prophylaxis each course should last 10–14 days.

Other drugs

Cough suppressants should be avoided if possible but may occasionally be needed to allow a patient to sleep. They should never be given in respiratory failure.

There are several 'mucolytic' drugs available (e.g. methylcysteine, bromhexine), which certainly alter the viscidity, quantity and microscopic structure of sputum. It is theoretically attractive to decrease the tenacity of sputum in chronic bronchitis and indeed in status asthmaticus, but there is little objective evidence of benefit from such drugs.

Breathing exercises are a traditional part of the treatment of chronic airways obstruction of any cause. The aim of the treatment is to educate the subject to breathe in such a way that adequate ventilation is achieved at less energy cost, i.e. more efficiently. This is normally attempted by teaching the patient to breathe with a different rhythm from that which he would naturally maintain, and to try, at first consciously, to relax certain respiratory muscles which he would normally use. It is not clear how far these habits persist in the absence of the teacher. Moreover, electromyographic recordings have shown that the relevant muscles are not relaxed; a study of the work of breathing showed no increase in efficiency; and a controlled trial has shown no systematic change either in symptoms or lung function. We do not dispute that there may be a powerful psychotherapeutic effect.

EMPHYSEMA

The aetiology of emphysema is unknown, although a few patients have a congenital deficiency of α1-antitrypsin. There is no specific treatment. However, many patients also have chronic bronchitis, and some have airways obstruction which is partially reversed by bronchodilators. The treatment outlined in the last section again applies.

RESPIRATORY FAILURE

We define this as failure of the respiratory system to maintain the arterial P_aO_2 above 60 mmHg and/or the P_aCO_2 below 48 mmHg in a patient breathing air and at rest.

There are two sorts of respiratory failure. In the first type, alveolar ventilation is diminished because total ventilation is insufficient, as in some cases of poliomyelitis, acute infective polyneuritis, or drug overdose. Some form of artificial respiration may be required to increase both total and alveolar ventilation. The lungs are normal. If the alveolar hypoventilation is slight and temporary, hypoxia may be relieved by O_2 administration.

In the second type, gas exchange is impaired although total ventilation may be normal or increased. The lungs are usually abnormal. The impairment of gas exchange may be characterised by an increase in venous admixture within the lung (e.g. following myocardial infarction). Arterial hypoxia will then occur without significant CO_2 retention: the treatment is to correct the hypoxia with as high a concentration of oxygen as is needed; for the removal of the hypoxic drive to breathe will rarely cause any rise in P_aCO_2 without a significant rise in P_aCO_2. measurement. The precipitating cause, such as infarction or pneumonia, should be treated on its merits. It should be remembered that patients with apparently minor lung disease may be tipped into respiratory failure by morphine or any drug which is a respiratory depressant.

In severe chronic airways obstruction an increase in venous admixture initially leads to a fall in P_aO_2 without a significant rise in P_aCO_2. In some patients, as the disease progresses, alveolar hypoventilation occurs with an increase in P_aCO_2. These patients are relatively insensitive to CO_2 and their chemical drive to ventilation is in part due to hypoxia. The principles of treatment of this common form of respiratory failure are as follows:

(a) to relieve hypoxia without causing severe respiratory depression
(b) to treat any precipitating infection and clear respiratory secretions
(c) to relieve airways obstruction
(d) to treat fluid retention (cor pulmonale)
(e) to avoid drugs which decrease the drive to breathe
(f) to avoid artificial respiration if possible

Treatment of hypoxia

The main question centres around the degree of hypoxaemia that is acceptable in these patients. All would agree that a P_aO_2 of 30 mmHg or less is unacceptable. A level of 50 mmHg (saturation 70–75%) will almost certainly avoid any serious tissue hypoxia. The aim then should be to maintain the arterial P_aO_2 at about 50 mmHg; the P_aO_2 should only be permitted to rise above this level if alveolar hypoventilation is absent or slight (P_aCO_2 <50 mmHg).

Usually an inspired oxygen concentration of 28% will maintain the P_aO_2 at the required level, but occasionally it may be necessary to start with 24% O_2 to avoid severe alveolar hypoventilation. Oxygen at these concentrations may be given by Ventimask or by an Edinburgh mask. If oxygen therapy is to lead to CO_2 narcosis it usually does so within the first few hours of treatment. The warning signs are: first, onset of mental confusion or unconsciousness; second, failure of the patient to cough and co-operate with the physiotherapist; and third, a rising arterial P_aCO_2. It is a changing P_aCO_2 rather than its absolute level which is the best indication that the patient is improving or deteriorating. A P_aCO_2 of more than 70 mmHg may be acceptable if the patient is alert, able to cough effectively, and can co-operate with the medical staff.

Once oxygen therapy has been started it should not be discontinued abruptly until the patient's condition has improved. The danger of stopping oxygen arises because of the different capacity of the stores for O_2 and CO_2; the capacity for O_2 is small, but that for CO_2 immense. When oxygen is given to a severely ill patient there is normally some alveolar hypoventilation and CO_2 retention. When oxygen is discontinued the increased store of oxygen is rapidly washed away and alveolar P_aO_2 falls, sometimes to levels below those which preceded O_2 therapy. The abrupt termination of O_2 should therefore be avoided in patients with severe respiratory failure.

Treatment of infection and clearance of secretions

Bronchitis or pneumonia should be treated with antibiotics according to principles outlined above. Prompt treatment of acute exacerbations of pneumonia may stop the patient going into respiratory failure. When respiratory failure is present, it is essential for the patient to be encouraged to cough up secretions, for accumulation at the lung bases may lead to atelectasis, abscess formation and further pulmonary damage. If the patient is too drowsy and confused to co-operate with the physiotherapist, an intravenous injection of 2 ml of nikethamide may wake the patient up sufficiently to obtain this co-operation.

Bronchospasm

Bronchospasm, if present, should be treated by bronchodilators.

Edema

If there is congestive heart failure (cor pulmonale), diuretics should be given. There is some evidence that the use of diuretics alone produces an improvement in gas tension. Digitalis is frequently used; there is little evidence that it is beneficial in 'pure' cor pulmonale, but these patients often have coexisting ischaemic heart disease. If there is any suggestion of a double etiology for the congestive failure, it is certainly reasonable to digitalise the patient.

Other drugs

Cough suppressants or sedatives should never be given, as they all interfere with the clearance of secretions, and produce some degree of respiratory depression. We do not consider respiratory stimulants (analeptics) to be of sufficient benefit to justify their use, for the following reasons:

(a) they produce no useful change in P_aCO_2 or P_aO_2 in patients with chronic airways obstruction;

(b) the difference between the toxic and therapeutic dose is small (the toxic symptoms of the analeptics are apprehension, extreme fear, sweating, skin irritation, fits, nausea and vomiting);

(c) to produce any respiratory effect it is necessary to give the drug intravenously under continuous observation, with usually frequent changes in infusion rate.

The use of nikethamide when the patient is too drowsy to co-operate with the physiotherapist has been already mentioned.

Artificial ventilation

The need for tracheostomy and IPPR* is decreased by precise control of oxygen therapy. If despite all previous measures severe alveolar hypoventilation and CO_2 narcosis develops, artificial respiration may be unavoidable. The decision to employ it rests on the following factors.

Indications: (a) failure to attain a satisfactory relief of hypoxaemia without severe hypoventilation leading to CO_2 narcosis.

(b) Severe alveolar hypoventilation on admission to hospital.

Occasionally through neglect, delay in treating an acute exacerbation, or the injudicious use of oxygen, immediate resuscitation is necessary. It may be possible to improve matters by temporary ventilation through an endotracheal tube, so that tracheostomy is avoided.

Contraindications: (a) severe panacinar emphysema; the most important practical diagnosis aid

*Intermittent Positive Pressure Respiration.

is a good quality chest X-ray film. By the time a patient with severe panacinar emphysema develops respiratory failure during a chest infection, their lung destruction is so far advanced that a successful outcome of treatment by tracheostomy and IPPR is unlikely. Usually it is difficult or impossible to wean the patient from the respirator; even if this can be done such a patient is likely to be a respiratory cripple and succumb shortly to further infection.

(b) severe limitation of the patient's activities before the acute exacerbation. A patient who was working before the exacerbation is likely to have an adequate respiratory reserve to justify tracheostomy, while a bed ridden respiratory cripple is unlikely to benefit.

BRONCHIECTASIS

Respiratory infections in childhood, especially whooping cough and measles, may lead to blockage of small airways by secretions with subsequent atelectasis and infection. Bronchiectasis may follow. Active immunisation has already markedly decreased the incidence of pertussis, and will probably do the same for measles in the near future.

Whether in childhood or in adult life, atelectasis with or without suppurative pneumonia should be treated with physiotherapy and antibiotics, as previously outlined.

The treatment of the established disease involves

(a) postural drainage of the affected lobes, and

(b) antibiotic therapy, the aims being exactly as in chronic bronchitis.

Occasionally if the disease is localised to one lobe, surgical excision is indicated. Emphysema is always a contraindication to surgery.

SPONTANEOUS PNEUMOTHORAX

A tension pneumothorax should be drained immediately via a catheter in the second anterior intercostal space with an underwater seal.

If the pneumothorax is not under tension, the exact management is debatable, ranging from the conservative to the aggressive. The following regime lies somewhere between the two extremes.

(a) If the patient is less than 40, and has no coexisting respiratory disease, he may rest at home. If an X-ray film at one week shows no re-expansion at all, he should be admitted for the lung to be expanded by suction. If an X-ray at one week shows some expansion but a repeat film at 3 weeks shows the lung not fully expanded, again he should be admitted.

(b) If the patient is over 40, or has coexisting respiratory disease, he should be admitted to hospital. If there is no expansion at 3 days, or the lung is not fully expanded in 2 weeks, the lung should be expanded by suction.

(c) Once committed to mechanical expansion, the patient should have a daily chest X-ray. If the lung fails to expand because of a broncho-pleural fistula, surgery will be needed. If it expands completely, suction should be maintained for 48 hours thereafter; if expansion is still complete, the tube should be clamped for 24 hours; if all is still well, it may then be removed. The maintenance of full expansion should be checked by subsequent X-rays.

(d) Recurrent pneumothorax. The occurrence of two pneumothoraces on the same side is usually an indication for surgical measures, such as pleurodesis by the instillation of talc, or over-sewing of bullae. A full discussion of the various surgical measures which have been employed is beyond the scope of this chapter.

SARCOID

Lung disease is rarely an indication for treatment in sarcoidosis. The common hilar lymphadeno-pathy usually regresses spontaneously. The only indication for steroid therapy is progressive pulmonary fibrosis. This may be recognised by one or more of the following features: increasing dyspnea; progression (or failure to regress) of chest X-ray changes; falling vital capacity, and decreasing transfer factor. Steroid therapy is then indicated to try to prevent further progression of fibrosis. It is reasonable to give prednisone in high doses (40–60 mg/day) for 3 weeks followed by a gradual reduction to about 7.5 mg/day for 6–12 months.

CARCINOMA OF THE BRONCHUS

Radical treatment may be attempted by surgical excision or by radiotherapy. Recent evidence has suggested that for oat-cell carcinoma radiotherapy is preferable to surgery. Operability was assessed without recourse to the more recently developed techniques of mediastinoscopy and mediastino-tomy, and therefore surgery was attempted in cases where mediastinal spread had already occurred. Our view is that if a tumour is thought to be operable, surgery should be attempted, provided that a thorough search is made for media-stinal and other metastatic spread. Radiotherapy should be used for the inoperable case, may be used post-operatively, and is particularly indicated

in palliative treatment of pain, cough, haemopty-sis, or superior vena caval obstruction.

PULMONARY EMBOLISM

The treatment of pulmonary embolism is un-satisfactory and will probably continue to be so. It is far more logical to direct therapeutic effort at the prevention, detection and treatment of peripheral venous thrombosis, especially in the legs. Certain surgical operations (particularly on the legs and in the pelvis) are known to carry a particular risk of deep venous thrombosis (DVT) and it has been shown that prophylactic anticoagulants decrease the incidence of DVT and emboli. Recent work has shown firstly that the incidence of post-operative deep vein thrombosis is diminished if the calf muscles are stimulated mechanically or electrically during the operation, and secondly that, in general surgery, the incidence may be diminished by prophylactic sub-cutaneous heparin in low doses. Elderly and immobile patients who are confined to bed are likely to get DVT, especially post-operatively. Although prophylactic anticoagulants are not indicated, regular physiotherapy and firm bandaging of the calves are reasonable pre-cautions.

Clinical detection of DVT is notoriously un-reliable, and this has made previous studies of treatment difficult to assess. Recent techniques such as phlebography, the fibrogen ^{131}I scan, and the use of the Doppler velocity probe to detect patent venous channels, provide more exact diagnosis.

Anticoagulants should not be invariably pre-scribed for DVT. If the patient can be mobile, shows no evidence of pulmonary embolism, and has no thrombus except in the calf vein, treat-ment may be restricted to rapid mobilisation, bandaging the calf, and raising the foot of the bed. If however the patient is immobile, or if there has been a pulmonary embolus, or if there is extension of thrombus beyond the calf, anti-coagulants should be prescribed. It is customary to start with intravenous heparin and to continue with an oral anticoagulant such as warfarin. It is not known how long heparin should be con-tinued, nor whether a higher dose would be preferable to those normally employed. Surgical removal of thrombi may be indicated if large un-attached clots are seen on phlebography.

If a pulmonary embolus occurs, treatment de-pends on the clinical state of the patient. A large embolus may completely or nearly occlude the pulmonary artery and cause asystole or ventricular fibrillation. Theoretically resuscitation by cardiac massage might preserve the patient long enough for surgical removal of the clot, though such cases must be excessively rare. At the other end of the scale is the small embolus with no embarrassment to the circulation. Here anticoagulants should be started if not already given. In all cases, if a pulmonary embolus has occurred when the patient is already anticoagulated an attempt to prevent further embolism by surgery should be considered. Guided by phlebography, which will demonstrate the extent of the thrombi, the relevant veins may be tied above the level of the clot, or the inferior vena cava plicated.

Between these two extremes lie a range of cases where there is evidence of circulatory embarrassment, namely raised central venous pressure, low blood pressure, tachycardia, a right sided fourth heart sound, a loud or widely split pulmonary second sound or a cardiogram showing right heart strain. The management of such cases is extremely debatable, the main reason being the extreme difficulty in setting up proper trials.

The possibilities are:

(a) Low dose heparinisation (25–40 000 units/day).
(b) High dose heparinisation (about 100 000 units/day).
(c) Fibrinolytic therapy (streptokinase).
(d) Surgical removal of clots from the pulmonary arteries.

It is now clear that fibrinolytic therapy with streptokinase increases the rate of lysis of the embolus, whereas heparin does not. However it has not yet been shown that mortality is reduced by streptokinase as opposed to heparin therapy. Fibrinolytic therapy is then based on the reasonable assumption that it is better to reduce the obstruction to pulmonary blood flow as quickly as possible. High-dose heparin therapy has the theoretical advantage that it should oppose the effect of local release of serotonin at the site of the embolus, which has been shown to occur in animal experiments, but not convincingly in man.

It is reasonable to give low-dose heparin to patients with pulmonary emboli with absent or minimal signs of circulatory embarrassment. Phlebograms should be done to detect the presence of free-lying clots which require thrombectomy. In patients with definite right heart overload who appear to be slowly deteriorating, streptokinase should be given, if there are no contraindications such as recent surgery, systemic hypertension or peptic ulcer. Surgical removal of the embolus may then be reserved for cases which show definite evidence of rapid deterioration (e.g. falling blood pressure, rising pulse rate and central venous pressure) despite full medical treatment, or before medical treatment has begun.

13

INFECTIOUS DISEASES

J. C. TAYLOR

MALARIA

Standard therapy

Malignant tertian (*P. falciparum*) malaria responds to the prompt administration of a 4-aminoquinoline, e.g. chloroquine or amodiaquine. Delay increases the risk of serious complications. A routine course of treatment consists of oral chloroquine (expressed as base) 600 mg, 300 mg 6 hours later and 300 mg daily for 2 or 3 days. Total dose 1.5–1.8 g. An alternative is amodiaquine of which 600 mg (as base) is given on the first day and 400 mg daily for the next two or three days. Mepacrine and quinine are also effective though relatively more toxic. Mepacrine hydrochloride 900 mg on the first day is followed by 300 mg daily for 7 days. Quinine bisulphate or dihydrochloride is given for 7 days in a dose of 650 mg orally thrice daily. These drugs will also eradicate *P. falciparum* since there is no persistent exo-erythrocytic phase of this parasite.

Benign tertian (*P. vivax, P. ovale*) and quartan (*P. malariae*) malarias in overt form also respond to the above therapy but relapse can only be avoided by the concurrent administration of an 8-aminoquinoline, e.g. primaquine, to eradicate the exo-erythrocytic phase of these species. Primaquine (base) 15 mg is given daily for 14 days during which the patient should remain under supervision in case toxic effects should appear. These effects include cyanosis due to the formation of methaemoglobin, and anaemia with intravascular haemolysis in those patients who have red cells deficient in glucose-6-phosphate dehydrogenase.

Eradication therapy should be reserved for those who are leaving an endemic area. The alternative, suppressive therapy, will prevent clinical relapse but, except when it includes an 8-aminoquinoline, will not prevent the establishment of the exoerythrocytic phase of plasmodia other than *P. falciparum*.

An indigenous semi-immune patient in an area of endemic malaria should receive single dose therapy, e.g. chloroquine 600 mg, except where a malaria eradication programme is in progress.

Therapy of complications

The most serious complications of malaria are seen in the non-immune subject with *P. falciparum* infection and these constitute a real medical emergency since, failing treatment, death is likely within 24 hours. Indications for strenuous therapy include jaundice, a falling haematocrit, prostration, hypotension, oliguria and signs of cerebral involvement such as coma or mental abnormality. When there has been a possibility of exposure to malaria these clinical features call for antimalarial treatment while investigation proceeds.

In this situation chloroquine 200–300 mg (base) (5 mg/kg) should be given intramuscularly and repeated every 8 hours to a total of 900 mg (15 mg/kg) in 24 hours. Quinine dihydrochloride 600 mg (10 mg/kg) can be diluted to 20 ml and given intravenously very slowly (10 minutes), or injected equally slowly into a continuous i.v. infusion. Alternatively, the dose can be added to the fluid reservoir and given over 1 hour. On very rare occasions chloroquine 200 mg can be administered i.v. in the same careful manner. The parenteral dosage is repeated in 8 hours if necessary but the drug should be continued orally as soon as the patient's condition allows. Quinine should be used in patients with chloroquine resistance and in children as parenteral chloroquine should not be given under the age of 5 years.

In addition to specific treatment concurrent measures must be taken to deal with such complications as shock, haemolysis and oliguria. Blood transfusion is essential when the haematocrit is falling and steroids may help to halt haemolysis. Haemodialysis and peritoneal dialysis have much to offer in malaria with oliguria, and the patient should be moved to such facilities as soon as possible. Peritoneal dialysis should be employed if the patient cannot be moved. In the presence of oliguria a reduced dose of quinine of 600 mg/day has been recommended even when the patient is undergoing dialysis. Steroid therapy is thought to be of benefit in cerebral malaria and comatose patients should receive dexamethasone 4–10 mg 8-hourly.

The problem of resistance

In considering the choice of antimalarial therapy the geographical origin of the infection is important. Since 1960, *P. falciparum* infections have been recognised which do not respond to the 4-aminoquinolines (chloroquine). Areas which are widely affected include Malaysia, Phillipines, Thailand, Cambodia, Laos, Vietnam and, in South America, Brazil, Colombia, Venezuela, Guyana, Surinam and Panama. Africa and Asia west of Burma are not affected by chloroquine resistance. Clinical malaria due to these resistant strains of *P. falciparum* is refractory to treatment with chloroquine, pyrimethamine, mepacrine and rarely, quinine, i.e. fever and parasitaemia are unaffected. When an initial response is obtained a very high rate of recrudescence of parasitaemia and symptoms follows within four weeks. A number of successful solutions to this problem have evolved.

The treatment of acute malaria due to resistant plasmodia is satisfactory using quinine but is accompanied by a greater degree of toxicity than standard chloroquine therapy. Standard dosage is not sufficient and a 14-day course of quinine sulphate 650 mg thrice daily must be given. The recrudescence rate is high and a better regimen is required. However, it is vital to appreciate that parenteral quinine is the treatment of choice in a seriously ill patient where resistance is suspected. In less urgent cases or to accompany quinine the following have been found effective. Regional specialist help should be obtained in complicated or resistant cases.

(a) Quinine sulphate 2 g daily in divided doses for 14 days
Pyrimethamine 50 mg daily for 3 days
Dapsone (DDS) 25 mg daily for 28 days
(b) Quinine sulphate 2 g daily for 14 days
Sulfametopyrazine (Sulfalene) 1 g in divided doses on first day only
(c) Quinine sulphate 2 g daily for 7 days
Tetracycline 1–2 g daily for 7 days
(d) Pyrimethamine 50 mg daily for 3 days
Sulphadiazine 2 g daily for 5 days
(e) Pyrimethamine 50 mg single dose
Dapsone (DDS) 100 mg daily for 5 days

The shortest course is:

(f) Pyrimethamine 50 mg single dose
Sulphormethoxine 1 g single dose

Prophylaxis

Two drugs are active not only against the erythrocytic phase of all species of plasmodia (suppression) but also against the pre-erythrocytic phase of *P. falciparum* (causal prophylaxis). These are proguanil usually 100 mg daily and pyrimethamine usually 25 mg once weekly. These drugs are ineffective against the pre-erythrocytic phase of plasmodia other than *P. falciparum* and should be continued for four weeks after leaving endemic areas.

Suppression of all types of malaria in the erythrocytic asexual phase is possible with any antimalarial. As an alternative to proguanil and pyrimethamine, chloroquine 300 mg once weekly can be used but is increasingly being held in reserve. Relapse can occur on cessation of the suppressive regimen unless eradication of species other than *P. falciparum* is carried out with an 8-aminoquinoline, e.g. primaquine 45 mg once weekly for 8 weeks.

In areas where plasmodia are resistant to pyrimethamine and proguanil either double doses of proguanil, i.e. 200 mg daily can be used or chloroquine prophylaxis can be employed. When chloroquine resistance and multiple resistance are rife as in S.E. Asia the matter is complex and regimens like dapsone 100 mg daily with chloroquine 300 mg and primaquine 45 mg once weekly are required.

Anti-malarials in children

Chloroquine (base)

	Initial dose	6 hours	Day 2–5
Under 1 year	75 mg	75 mg	75 mg
1–3 years	150 mg	100 mg	75 mg
3–6 years	300 mg	150 mg	75 mg
6–12 years	300 mg	150 mg	150 mg
12–15 years	450–600 mg	150–300 mg	150–300 mg

Primaquine (base)

4–8 years	5–7.5 mg daily for 10 days
8–15 years	11.5–15 mg daily for 10 days

Proguanil

Birth–1 year	25–50 mg daily
2–5 years	50–100 mg daily
5–adult	100 mg daily

Pyrimethamine

Birth–12 years	12.5 mg once weekly
12 years–adult	25 mg once weekly

AMOEBIASIS

There are a number of effective drugs for the therapy of amoebiasis and they have been combined in various ways which have not been exhaustively compared. Two important principles are that intestinal parasites must be eliminated and that signs of systemic invasion indicate the need for a systemic amoebicide. Treatment has been simplified by the acceptance of metronidazole as the drug of choice.

Acute amboebic dysentery

Metronidazole is both a systemic and an intestinal amoebicide, and chloroquine need not be given in addition. As treatment for the more severe case it can replace emetine. Toxicity is very low and the dose is 800 mg thrice daily for 5–10 days. (Children 50 mg/kg in three divided doses daily.) It is effective in amoebic dysentery and in non-dysenteric bowel infection where that condition is thought to require treatment. The use of metronidazole, as of emetine, constitutes a therapeutic trial and in the event of failure, the diagnosis should be reconsidered.

Acute amoebic dysentery also responds to the administration of a tetracycline, an indirect amoebicide which acts through its effect on the bowel flora; and di-iodohydroxyquinoline, a direct amoebicide active in the lumen of the bowel. The addition of chloroquine, a systemic amoebicide is necessary to protect the liver from invasion. These three drugs are given simultaneously in the following dosage:—

Chlortetracycline 1 g daily for 5 days

Di-iodohydroxyquinoline 600 mg t.d.s. for 20 days

Chloroquine (base) 600 mg loading dose
300 mg 6 hours later
150 mg 12 hourly for 14 days

More severely ill patients require in addition, emetine hydrochloride 60 mg daily i.m. until symptoms subside or for not longer than 5 days. An alternative compound is dehydroemetine given in a dose of 80 mg daily i.m. for up to 10 days. The emetine compounds are given either along with or preceding the basic regimen for intestinal amoebiasis presented above and chloroquine may be omitted.

A less toxic alternative to emetine in seriously ill patients is metronidazole in conjunction with a tetracycline and di-iodohydroxyquinoline or diloxanide furoate.

In an urgent situation, emetine may be used to supplement metronidazole therapy until the condition of the patient improves.

Some practitioners in this field prefer to use emetine bismuth iodide (EBI) to obtain the intestinal amoebicidal effect, substituting it for tetracycline, di-iodohydroxyquinoline and chloroquine following the administration of emetine hydrochloride or dehydroemetine in the severely ill patient. The dose of EBI is 200 mg daily for 10 days. In the moderately ill patient EBI in this dosage may be combined with chlortetracycline 1 g daily for 7 days as a sole treatment.

Niridazole can replace di-iodohydroxyquinoline and chloroquine and, given with chlortetracycline, is effective in acute amoebic dysentry. This drug is an orally effective intestinal and systemic amoebicide which should be given in a dose of 500 mg thrice daily (25 mg/kg) for 10 days. It is, however, toxic especially to the nervous system, causing hallucinations and occasional convulsions, particularly when there is liver disease. Its use in amoebiasis is diminishing.

Asymptomatic intestinal amoebiasis

In circumstances where this state requires treatment, metronidazole 800 mg thrice daily for 5–10 days may be administered with excellent prospects of eradication.

Already alluded to for its lumenal effect in acute dysentery, is di-iodohydroxyquinoline in a dose of 600 mg thrice daily for 21 days.

An alternative drug with a lumenal amoebicidal action only is diloxanide furoate which is suitable for a symptomless cyst excretor in a dose of 500 mg thrice daily for 10 days.

Amoebic liver abscess

Amoebic liver abscess requires an amoebicide which is active systemically and again, metronidazole is effective in a dose of 800 mg thrice daily for 10 days.

Emetine compounds and chloroquine are in this class and in practice are usually given together. Emetine hydrochloride 60 mg/day for 4 days or dehydroemetine 90 mg/day for 10 days should be given along with chloroquine and di-iodohydroxyquinoline or diloxanide furoate.

Medical treatment alone will not suffice for large liver abscesses (more than 100 ml of pus) and diagnosis and localisation have been aided by the development of radioisotope scanning, at least in the more advanced centres. Therapeutic aspiration is then performed as an adjunct to the administration of amoebicidal drugs.

Certain amoebicidal drugs have toxic effects. Emetine compounds have cardiovascular actions such as bradycardia, hypotension, arrhythmias, and ECG abnormalities. EBI orally causes nausea and vomiting to such a degree as to require anti-emetics and sedatives to be administered. Niridazole also causes ECG T-wave changes, but without cardiovascular symptoms. It should not be combined with emetine compounds in adults.

Amoebiasis in children

Amoebic dysentery or liver abscess in a child especially one who is malnourished has a higher morbidity and mortality than in an adult.

In acute amoebic dysentery metronidazole 50 mg kg/day in divided doses (maximum 800 mg t.d.s.) is as effective as combined therapy.

Dual therapy is preferred in liver abscess and consists of metronidazole as above and dehydroemetine 2 mg kg/day, both for 10 days.

Paedriatric dosage: —

Metronidazole 50 mg/kg/day (maximum 800 mg t.d.s.)

Niridazole 25 mg/kg/day (maximum 1500 mg daily)

Emetine hydrochloride 1 mg/kg/day (maximum 60 mg daily)

Dehydroemetine 2 mg/kg/day (maximum 90 mg daily)

Diloxanide furoate 25 mg/kg/day (maximum 500 mg t.d.s.)

TUBERCULOSIS

In countries where the attack on tuberculosis has been continued for many years it is increasingly a problem of the old who are more susceptible to the toxic effects of drugs. The pool of patients, often unco-operative, with drug-resistant disease remains to be eliminated, but, with current methods, co-operative new patients should not relapse with drug-resistant disease. An effective regimen correctly administered should result in cure of almost all newly diagnosed patients.

Standard methods of therapy have two objectives:

(a) To render and maintain the patient non-infectious

(b) To avoid creating drug resistance

Primary therapy

For many years primary treatment of tuberculosis has consisted of a standard triple regimen of streptomycin, sodium PAS and isoniazid. After 3 months of satisfactory progress, with sensitive organisms on pre-treatment tests, the initial phase is complete and streptomycin is withdrawn. The maintenance phase of treatment is managed with two drugs, PAS and isoniazid. The total duration of the course varies from 18 months to 2 years. This regimen is very effective and, if faithfully followed, leads to cure in almost every case. Occasional failure is due to irregularity in drug taking brought about by the toxicity of unpalata-

bility of the drugs. Standard triple therapy for adults:

Streptomycin 0.75 g over 40 years. 1.0g under 40 years.

Isoniazid 300 mg one or two divided doses
Sodium PAS 12 g daily

The advantages of a supervised regimen may be continued into the maintenance phase by employing the twice weekly administration of streptomycin 1 g and isoniazid 15 mg/kg body weight with pyridoxine 10 mg.

Persistent positivity of the sputum with a report of pre-treatment resistance will require a change of therapy. The standard triple regimen is associated with a considerable incidence of toxicity and hypersensitivity. In these circumstances in the past there was no triple therapy of equal power and second-line drugs were less effective or more toxic. The introduction of two drugs, ethambutol and rifampicin, has brought a new flexibility to management and means that, in the event of problems, more than one line of effective treatment is available. The particular group of drugs chosen as primary therapy depends on availability and cost as well as on efficacy and convenience.

An injectable drug offers an opportunity for close supervision during the initial phase whether at home or in hospital. Streptomycin and isoniazid remain in the triple regimen but the third drug may be ethambutol or rifampicin. For the maintenance phase the two oral drugs are continued. A modern triple regimen consists of:

Streptomycin 0.75–1.0 g i.m.
Isoniazid 300 mg
Ethambutol 20 mg/kg for 60 days, then 15 mg/kg   one daily dose
or, in place of ethambutol,
Rifampicin 450–600 mg

This regimen avoids the gastric and sensitization problems of PAS but hypersensitivity to streptomycin and vestibular toxicity remain. When both PAS and streptomycin are displaced by rifampicin and ethambutol the triple regimen with isoniazid is both effective and of low toxicity. Treatment is later maintained with isoniazid and either ethambutol or rifampicin.

The drug responsible for a hypersensitivity reaction should be identified by testing with low doses but it is rarely necessary now to undertake desensitisation which can lead to the emergence of drug resistance. A change of therapy is better and reactions to daily administration of isoniazid, ethambutol or rifampicin are rare.

Ethambutol rarely causes retrobulbar neuritis and, after a pre-treatment ophthalmic assessment, patients should be advised to report any deterioration in vision and stop ethambutol at once.

Rifampicin therapy may alter liver function values, particularly the serum oxalacetic transaminase. The slight abnormality is usually temporary but a record of pre-treatment values should be obtained.

Differing opinions are held about the advisability of initial regimens consisting of two drugs only but several are now available which have been shown to be very satisfactory. Isoniazid can be combined with ethambutol or rifampicin in both initial and maintenance phases of treatment. The improvement in acceptability has rendered PAS obsolescent. An example of a two-drug regimen is:

Isoniazid 300 mg plus
Ethambutol 20 mg/kg for
60 days, then 15 mg/kg   one dose daily
or in place of ethambutol,
Rifampicin 450 mg under
50 kg; 600 mg over 50 kg

One objective of contemporary drug trials is to shorten the duration of chemotherapy for tuberculosis. There are hopeful signs but for the present it would be wise to adhere to 18 months course for mild to moderate non-cavitatory disease and 2 years for severe or cavitatory disease.

Re-treatment

Failure of treatment should now be exceptional and the incidence of relapse should be low but the necessity for re-treatment will remain. The failures of previous therapy are presently being rescued and many excrete resistant organisms. Fresh failures and newly resistant organisms are generated in those areas where anti-tuberculosis therapy cannot be rigidly controlled. Awareness of resistant infection does not begin with receipt of the first sensitivity report but with the all-important interrogation of the patient. This is directed towards assessing whether or not resistant bacilli are likely to be present. A pointer to resistance is a history of irregular or inadequate therapy. At least two effective drugs should have been included in any combination and a history of hypersensitivity is indicative of irregularity of treatment.

A recent report of fully sensitive organisms allows the patient to be managed normally, with the closest possible supervision. If resistance is suspected or proved at least three effective drugs should be administered. At present these should include ethambutol and rifampicin and, if streptomycin and isoniazid are excluded, one of the reserve drugs, ethionamide, pyrazinamide or cap-reomycin. Good results in the intensive initial phase have been obtained with capreomycin 15 mg/kg i.m. Attention is required to monthly serum potassium estimations, renal function and ototoxicity. Pyrazinamide is a potent drug but can be hepatotoxic and cause hyperuricaemia. The principal difficulty with ethionamide and prothionamide is gastrointestinal intolerance so that the patient may tolerate only 500 mg or 750 mg daily.

Reserve drugs; dose/24 hours:
Ethionamide 0.5–0.75 g in divided doses
Prothionamide 0.5–1.0 g in one or two doses
Pyrazinamide 40 mg/kg (up to 1.5 g twice daily)
Capreomycin 15 mg/kg i.m. (up to 1.0 g daily)

Corticosteroids

Provided adequate anti-tuberculous cover is simultaneously administered, corticosteroids are of value in severe tuberculous meningitis, tuberculous pleural effusion and in advanced pulmonary tuberculosis. An adult dose of 30 mg of prednisone daily may be reduced by 5 mg/day at weekly intervals.

Therapy with limited resources

In countries with limited resources to devote to the treatment of tuberculosis, ideal chemotherapy has to be modified to that which is possible economically. Three developments would help such countries: cheaper drugs, shorter courses and intermittent therapy. In such circumstances only essential hospital accommodation should be provided and most effort should be concentrated on the development of a clinic service. Finance and trained personnel for domiciliary supervision of therapy are not usually available and some believe that a supervised oral intermittent regimen is required.

In a dual regimen with isoniazid, PAS may be replaced by cheaper thiacetazone in countries where the latter has been shown to be effective and well tolerated. The dose must be thiacetazone 150 mg and isoniazid 300 mg in one tablet daily. The addition of streptomycin 1 g daily for the first eight weeks markedly strengthens this regimen. Alternatively, intermittent supervised therapy with streptomycin 0.75 g, isoniazid 15 mg/kg, pyridoxine 10 mg given twice weekly is effective and can be augmented by a preliminary period of 4 weeks of daily streptomycin and isoniazid. An intermittent oral regimen would be less demanding on scarce skills and one consisting of twice weekly PAS 200 mg/kg and isoniazid 15 mg/kg with pyridoxine 10 mg has given encouraging results when administered under supervision in one dose. An initial period of daily therapy with streptomycin, PAS and isoniazid for four weeks would strengthen this regimen.

Administration

Both established tuberculosis services and those in a formative state should concentrate on the supervision of out-patient treatment and not on the creation of expensive hospital beds. Sensitivity testing other than pre-treatment is of limited value and smear examination without routine culture will suffice in underdeveloped areas. Resources should not be devoted to following-up patients who have completed treatment but to detecting defaulters.

Therapy of children

As in adult disease a severe case should have triple therapy in the following dosage:
   Streptomycin 40 mg/kg/day in one dose
   Isoniazid 10 mg/kg/day in one dose
   PAS 300 mg/kg/day in divided doses
   or
   Ethambutol 15 mg/kg/day in one dose.
Rifampicin might be used to avoid the necessity for injections of streptomycin and the rate of dosage is 20 mg/kg/day in one dose. (Rimactane 100 mg in 5 ml) PAS should not be included in a regimen with rifampicin.

As soon as the organism is known to be sensitive to three drugs or after three months satisfactory progress in a severe case, streptomycin or another of the three may be discontinued.

Life-threatening forms of tuberculosis should be treated with four drugs, isoniazid, streptomycin, rifampicin and ethambutol until the sensitivity of the patient's or source-case strain is known.

Children with mild symptomatic primary tuberculosis, the source of whose organisms is known to be fully sensitive, may be managed as out-patients with dual therapy, i.e. isoniazid and PAS (or ethambutol) or isoniazid and rifampicin.

Asymptomatic primary tuberculosis is one indication for the use of 'disease' or 'secondary' chemoprophylaxis which is intended to prevent an infected individual from developing disease. Isoniazid is used alone in a dose of 10 mg/kg/day not exceeding 300 mg/day for 1 year.

GASTRO-ENTERITIS IN INFANTS

At present this condition, with one recent exception (*E. coli* 0 114), is generally mild in developed societies but is responsible for much

mortality and morbidity in less hygienic surroundings. It is a syndrome in which infection with known enteropathogenic types of *E. coli* contributes less than a third of the cases.

Whilst it is probable that in many countries the malnourished child with gastro-enteritis will present with isotonic or hypotonic dehydration, his better nourished contemporary may develop hypertonic (hypernatraemic) dehydration. Many infants are conditioned to develop this complication of diarrhea by a high calorie, high solute-load diet which permits the excretion of little free water. When fever, diarrhea and anorexia supervene, water intake falls while the high solute intake may continue. These increased extra-renal losses of water mean that through excreting a high solute load the infant passes into negative water balance.

Clinical picture

In the early stage of isotonic (or hypotonic) dehydration the infant is restless, cross and pale with slightly sunken eyes ($2\frac{1}{2}$–5% loss of weight). Next the eyes, with dry conjunctivae, are more sunken, the fontanelle is depressed and the skin loses its turgor and elasticity (5–10%). An infant with cold extremities, tachycardia, cyanosis and pallor has lost more than 10% of its body weight and is in a perilous condition.

By contrast, in hypernatraemic dehydration certain features of the classical picture which are attributable to sodium deficiency may be less prominent. Tachycardia, coldness, pallor and loss of skin turgor may be absent, the eyes and fontanelle less sunken. The skin may be warm and turgid but the mucous membranes are dry and the infant's thirst may be obvious. The positive features are related to the nervous system. The infant is lethargic and listless until touched when marked irritability becomes evident. Reflexes are often very brisk and there may be muscle twitching. Both types of dehydration may lead to coma and in both hyperventilation due to acidosis may be mistaken for evidence of a respiratory infection.

Management

When the infant's condition permits of a period of observation, treatment should begin in the home. Milk feeds are withdrawn and in their place is offered an electrolyte solution produced by dissolving two tablets of sodium chloride compound effervescent NF in 250 ml of water. Advice which should be countermanded includes total starvation and the administration of boiled water or sugar solutions of any type. Proprietary glucose solutions of strengths approaching 25% are particularly dangerous.

If a mother is not competent to notice further deterioration of her child by its lethargy or refusal to accept saline solution then the infant is better admitted to hospital at once. It is not necessary to admit every case of gastro-enteritis.

If domiciliary support fails and dehydration is developing, measurement of the serum electrolytes and acid base status is highly desirable as a guide to management in hospital. Whenever possible, fluid should be offered orally in the first instance. The quantity required is calculated on the basis of the recent pre-dehydration weight or of an estimate based on the dehydrated weight. The basic daily requirement from 5 days to 1 year old is 150 ml/kg (1–2 years 120 ml/kg) and a supplementary 25, 50 and 100 ml/kg is added when the loss of weight due to dehydration is estimated at 21%, 5% or 10% of body weight.

If the serum sodium is less than 150 mEq/1 the supplementary fluid should be added to the basic for the first 24 hours. A suitable fluid is half-strength Darrow's solution for acidosis*. If severe acidosis requires more bicarbonate than is present in the Darrow's solution this can be obtained in 8.4% sodium bicarbonate (1 mEq/l) solution (see below). When the deficit has been replaced, maintenance fluids are continued until normal feeding is resumed. For this purpose quarter-strength Darrow's solution or 1/5 physiological saline or Hartmann's lactated Ringer's solution, or dextrose are appropriate and should have potassium chloride 20 mEq/l added.

If the serum sodium exceeds 150 mEq/l (hypernatraemia) the basic maintenance volume only should be given in the first 24 hours and restoration of the deficit accomplished in 48 hours. This is to avoid too rapid expansion of cerebral intracellular volume with the attendant danger of convulsions. There is controversy concerning the composition of fluid for hypertonic cases. It is agreed that it should not be electrolyte-free and it should probably contain about 40 mEq/l (30–50) of sodium which over the first 48 hours should replace the sodium deficit. These patients are often severely acidotic and that sodium concentration may be exceeded by the required amount of 8.4% sodium bicarbonate (1 mEq/l)

---

*Full-strength Darrow's Solution for Acidosis:

KCl	2.70 g	Na	120 mEq/l
Na lactate	5.80 g	K	36 mEq/l
NaCl	4.00 g	Cl	140 mEq/l
Aqua dest.	to 1000 ml	HCO₃ equiv.	51 mEq/l (lactate)
		Osmolarity	313 mmol/l

in 5% dextrose. Some authorities advocate that provided urine is being formed potassium up to 40 mEq/l (20–40) should be added. It will be noticed that third-strength Darrow's solution with added potassium would often meet these requirements but on certain occasions special solutions will have to be produced. There is a temptation to indulge in pseudo-accuracy and much reliance can be placed on renal mechanisms to correct the disturbance.

The following formulae give an approximation of the amounts of bicarbonate required.

0.3 (weight in kg) × BE (base excess) = mEq of bicarbonate required, or from a measure of the serum bicarbonate or alkali reserve:

ECF (litres) × (normal HCO₃ − measured HCO₃) × 2 = mEq bicarbonate required.

Parenteral therapy

Intravenous fluids are required for the severely hypertonic infant and for both types of patient in circulatory failure. In the event of persisting diarrhea and failure to suck, attempts at oral intake should not be prolonged. If the infant shows signs of shock the best treatment is an infusion of plasma, correction of acidosis and administration of oxygen. Plasma 20 ml/kg is infused rapidly with sodium bicarbonate 10 mEq and 100 mg of hydrocortisone.

While oliguria persists and a period of rapid rehydration is required no potassium should be given intravenously until the serum level is known. A solution containing sodium (75–80 mEq/l) in 2.5% dextrose with 25–35% as bicarbonate (e.g. half-strength Hartmann's or half-strength saline—1/6 M lactate 2:1) may be administered at the rate of 25–50 ml/kg in 4 hours until urine flow is established. In the case of hypernatraemia this rapid phase must be terminated as soon as possible in accord with the replacement of volume and sodium deficit over 48 hours. In confirmed severe isotonic dehydration this initial hydrating solution could be isotonic, e.g. lactated Ringer's (Hartmann's) or saline—1/6 M lactate 2:1.

After the restoration of the circulation and urine formation, or omitting that phase, intravenous therapy follows the same principles as described for oral therapy, employing glucose/electrolyte fluids which are isotonic with plasma.

As soon as the infant is able to drink, replacement should begin by mouth using small volumes at first. The infusion may be discontinued when the basic requirement can be taken orally and there is no longer profuse diarrhea.

As recovery continues and the infant can take reasonable volumes (60 ml) at intervals of 2 hours, milk feeds are introduced beginning with half or even quarter strength, half-cream feeds. The volume and the intervals are gradually increased until normal feeding with full strength, full-cream milk is resumed. If diarrhea recurs clear fluids should be resumed and the process repeated in another 24–48 hours.

The place of antibiotics is controversial. They do not appear to be required in the sporadic mild forms currently prevalent and in occasional severe cases their effect is hard to judge. In an institutional outbreak of serious disease it is claimed that appropriate antibiotics not only prevent further spread but save those infants who receive them. If this is true it is likely to be a brief respite owing to the rapid acquisition by *E.coli* of transferable drug resistance and the routine use of antibiotics in the enteritis ward is neither necessary nor desirable.

Bacillary dysentery

Dysentery has not presented in a uniform manner throughout the world and its aetiology and epidemiology have not remained constant with the passage of time. In some circumstances it is a mild illness with little more than a nuisance value to the patient, in others a severe febrile illness; it is not surprising that therapeutic trials, few of them adequate, have failed to resolve the differences of opinion which exist. Where the disease is mild the symptoms abort in 48 hours and spontaneous bacteriological cure follows in 50–70% of patients within 7 days. There is no unequivocal evidence that antimicrobial treatment alters the clinical course nor that withholding it brings an hygienic disadvantage to the community. Consequently the approach to the mild case should be expectant and the patient may remain at home if the sanitary arrangements are suitable. Simple health education should not be neglected at this stage.

When the disease presents in a severe form and rapid symptomatic relief is desired an absorbable antimicrobial such as ampicillin 50–100 mg/kg/day for 5 days should be used. In the most severe cases the parenteral route should be employed. Alteration in bowel flora occurs when this drug is administered orally, towards colonisation by *Candida* and the *Klebsiella–Aerobacter* group but no undesirable consequences have been attributed to this when the course has been restricted to 5 days.

Sulphonamides have been rendered ineffective by the development of widespread resistance and should not be used. Resistance to the tetracyclines has restricted their use which had been attended in several instances by the development of staphy-

lococcal enterocolitis. Some British workers have claimed that non-absorbable streptomycin and kanamycin assist bacteriological clearance though neomycin does not. Others doubt the value of streptomycin.

The shigellae in common with other members of the enterobacteriaciae can acquire and transmit both transfer factor and resistance determinants and this in the present state of our knowledge should lead to caution in their exposure to antimicrobials.

Even in the brief period of illness when shigellosis is mild, symptomatic relief is desired and many substances such as starch, chalk, kaolin and pectin have been incorporated in antidiarrheal remedies. There seems to be no evidence that these have any effect.

Salmonellosis

Salmonella food poisoning without evidence of invasiveness is a self-limiting condition and likely to be cured before the results of bacteriological investigation become available. The exhibition of antibiotics in this condition does not improve on the spontaneous cure rate; indeed there is mounting evidence that the (convalescent) carrier state is thereby prolonged. Except in the very ill, febrile, septicaemic patient, antibiotics should be withheld and an expectant policy followed; this implies treatment of dehydration and electrolyte imbalance. When an antibiotic is thought to be indicated the choice should be made with the help of the bacteriology laboratory but either ampicillin or chloramphenicol in a dose of 500 mg 6-hourly may be started while waiting for sensitivity reports. If a patient has been given one course of appropriate antibiotic treatment and his faeces remain positive he should not be subjected to further courses of treatment.

Typhoid and paratyphoid fevers

These diseases generally present as severe systemic illnesses and require a more positive approach than salmonella enteritis which is self-limiting.

In the acute phase specific therapy should be with chloramphenicol orally or parenterally. The dose for adults should be not less than 2 g daily and should be continued for at least 10 days but extended according to response. In children the dose is 100 mg/kg with a maximum dose of 2g daily. Longer courses or higher doses than the above will not influence the incidence of relapse or complications.

Fluid and electrolyte balance must be measured and i.v. fluids may be required if oral intake fails

F

or is not being absorbed. If hypotension develops, plasma is the best treatment but if there has been significant haemorrhage, blood will be required. When intestinal dilatation is observed oral intake should not be trusted even if there is not a complete paralytic ileus I.v. fluids and gastric suction may be required for many days and should not be suspended until there is good evidence of returning intestinal function. Perforation in a toxic patient is difficult to diagnose and surgery carries a high mortality. A surgeon should be consulted but operation is best avoided and the complication treated conservatively. If obstruction follows perforation, surgery will be unavoidable.

The patient who relapses usually responds to a second course of 2 g of chloramphenicol daily for seven days.

Measles

No specific treatment is available for the primary effects of this virus infection. In the average case prophylactic antibiotics should have no place. Observation is all that is required during the first few days and defervescence can confidently be expected. A darkened room is not necessary and the child should be allowed up when, as his temperature falls, he requests it. In these early days generalised adventitious sounds in the chest and cough are attributable to the effects of the virus. If later complications due to bacteria are suspected they should be treated as described in the section on pneumonia. Encephalitis is a rare complication requiring specialised therapy. In an uncomplicated case the child will be up and about seven days from the onset of the rash and since he is by then non-infectious no restrictions are necessary.

Mumps

The manifestations of this disease are due exclusively to the mumps virus and there are no complications which could be avoided by the use of prophylactic antibiotics. A child or adult with salivary involvement needs only careful oral hygiene and sufficient fluid intake. Analgesics may be required, rarely morphine, especially in mumps orchitis. Rest in bed with support for the scrotum will be desired by the patient with acute orchitis. In severe cases of orchitis a short course of steroids may lead to more rapid resolution of pain.

Upper respiratory tract infections

These infections are complex in their aetiology but in all cases except for a minority with pharyn-gitis or tonsillitis they are due to viruses. Clinical examination alone does not allow separation of the few due to Str. pyogenes. If the throat is inflamed a throat swab is required to exclude streptococcal infection and, if the appearance is suspicious of pyogenic infection, penicillin can be administered while awaiting the result of the swab. In most cases however antibiotics should be withheld because there is no evidence of their efficacy against viruses nor as prophylaxis against bacterial superinfection. This is true whether the signs and symptoms are classified as a cold, a febrile cold, influenza, pharyngitis, tonsillitis or laryngitis or croup. If a report is received of the presence of Str. pyogenes a course of penicillin should be given which should continue for 10 days. Oral penicillin 250–500 mg 6-hourly is adequate for adults, 125–250 mg for children and in severe cases penicillin should be given i.m. for the first 24–48 hours. Infants with coryza may feed better after being given nasal drops of 1% saline solution of ephedrine 15 minutes before feeds. Secondary infection of sinuses or middle ear may occur and penicillin should be tried first in these cases. If i.m. penicillin does not control the temperature or the local signs in 24–48 hours the possibility of infection by H. influenzae or a penicillinase producing Staph. pyogenes should be considered and ampicillin 500 mg 6-hourly and cloxacillin in the same dosage should be added. Adequate courses i.e. 10 to 14 days should be given in otitis media and the ear carefully examined for healing if the tympanic membrane had ruptured.

Most cases of croup of viral origin recover rapidly with humidification and without antibiotics but the dangerous condition of acute epiglottitis has to be remembered especially in the older child or adult. The onset is acute with fever, leucocytosis and there is rapidly increasing respiratory difficulty. The patient is prostrated, has a painful throat and the epiglottis is inflamed and swollen. There is usually a septicaemia. When this diagnosis is made tracheotomy should be performed and chloramphenicol given at once. Severe cases of croup where the epiglottis cannot be seen and those with lower respiratory tract signs may be given ampicillin 125–250 mg 6-hourly.

Whooping cough

This distressing illness is unaffected by antibiotics active against B. pertussis, unless they are given as early as possible in the catarrhal stage. If there is a history of contact tetracycline or ampicillin or erythromycin should be given at the first sign of catarrhal symptoms. After the disease has been recognised by its characteristics it does not respond to drug therapy but it is customary to give a short 5-day course to eliminate persistent organisms. A mild case is best nursed at home and only severe or complicated cases admitted to hospital. A new-born infant should not be introduced into a home where his siblings are suffering from whooping cough.

Diet and fluid intake are often a problem and require a great deal of patience to manage. Secretions sometimes require to be aspirated from the oral pharynx and humidified oxygen may be required during spasms. If clinical or radiological examination reveal collapsed lung of segmental or lobar distribution physiotherapy may help the older child. However, re-expansion of the collapsed area can be expected in up to one year and surgery should not be contemplated earlier. When secondary infection of collapsed areas is recognised antibiotics should be given and continued if necessary until the lung re-expands.

Convulsions and other cerebral manifestations require more intensive care as a consequence of depressed reflexes, sedation, anticonvulsants and tube or parenteral feeding.

All cases, including those mild cases who have not previously had one, should have a chest radiograph just prior to dismissal or on complete recovery if they have been at home.

14

OPHTHALMOLOGY

P. FELLS

INFECTIONS

1. BACTERIAL

Hordeolum is a staphylococcal infection of the lid glands with a localised red, swollen and tender area. The more superficial glands are involved in the common stye, and the deeper Meibomian glands in the internal hordeolum. Treatment is by warm compresses and antibiotic ointment four times daily.

Chalazion is a chronic granulomatous inflammation of a Meibomian gland which often, but not necessarily, follows an internal hordeolum. Usually incision and curettage are necessary for their removal. Beware of multiple recurrences at the same site which may mean a rare adenocarcinoma of the Meibomian gland.

Blepharitis is a chronic, persistent bilateral inflammation of both upper and lower eye lids with associated low grade conjunctivitis. Although staphylococcal (ulcerative) and seborrheic forms are described both types are usually present. The eyes are itching and burning with red margins. Scales are seen along the eye lash roots. Ulcerated areas may be present. Often seborrhea of the scalp, eye brows and ears is associated. Treatment is by meticulous cleaning of lid margins daily with a moistened cotton applicator before applying antibiotic ointment e.g. chloramphenicol or neomycin to the lid margin. Selenium sulphide shampoo to the scalp helps in the seborrheic form. Although cure is rare, a mixture of antibiotic and corticosteroid ointment to the lid margins will usually keep it under control. Beware of overtreating and making an allergic blepharitis to one of the medicaments used.

Lacrimal sac infection is a common acute or chronic unilateral disease occurring in infants or in adults over 40, and is secondary to obstruction of the nasolacrimal duct. Usually it is a staphylococcal infection with pain, tenderness and swelling just below the inner canthus. In infants the dacryocystitis is secondary to delayed canalisation of the nasolacrimal ducts. Treatment is by massage to empty the tear sac followed by antibiotic drops four times daily. If there is no improvement by 6 months of age, then probing of the nasolacrimal duct may be done under general anaesthesia.

In adults acute dacryocystitis responds to warm compresses and systemic broad spectrum antibiotics, e.g. tetracyclines or the newer penicillins. The chronic form in adults rarely responds to syringing of the lacrimal passages and dacryocystorhinostomy is required.

Conjunctivitis is the commonest eye disease, usually caused by pyogenic bacteria or by viruses. In general, organisms pathogenic for the genitourinary tract are also pathogenic for the conjunctiva.

Bacterial conjunctivitis is usually acute, with a red eye, copious tears and sticky discharge, soon becoming bilateral. It is generally self limiting, lasting 10–14 days without treatment, but only 2–3 days in the pyogenic forms with treatment.

A stained conjunctival smear usually allows bacterial identification, but cultures are necessary for study of antibiotic sensitivities. Treatment is by chloramphenicol drops 2-hourly with ointment at night to both eyes. Extra care must be taken with personal hygiene to prevent the spread of 'pink eye' through the family.

2. VIRAL

Viral conjunctivitis

Trachoma affects approximately 20% of the world population mainly in the Middle and Far East and is the commonest cause of blindness when complicated by secondary bacterial conjunctivitis. It affects mainly the upper tarsal conjunctiva and superior cornea, beginning with follicular and then papillary hypertrophy, being followed by scarring and eventually an inactive vascular pannus. Treatment is by tetracycline 250 mg tablets four times a day for 7 days combined with either tetracycline ointment or 10% sulphacetamide drops to the eyes five times daily for 4 weeks.

Corneal grafting may be needed later.

Adenovirus infections tend to cause unilateral follicular conjunctivitis, with varying degrees of corneal infiltration, and tenderness of the preauricular lymph node on the affected side. The symptoms go in 2 to 4 weeks, regardless of treatment, but often sulphonamide drops are given to prevent secondary bacterial infection.

Herpes simplex keratitis

Following initial infection with the herpes simplex virus, which may be on the lips or in the eye, the virus remains latent in the affected tissue. Various resistance lowering factors such as fevers, exposure to cold or emotional upsets may start a recurrence and liberation of active virus. An initial mild herpetic conjunctivitis may be followed by a dendritic ulcer of the cornea. If suspected a dendritic ulcer can readily be seen by staining with fluorescein which shows the typical branching pattern. Treatment is by idoxuridine ointment five times a day for at least 5 days which prevents the viral replication within the corneal epithelium. Other methods of treatment include carbolisation of the virus-laden epithelium, or its freezing with the cryoprobe. Steroid drops must NEVER be used in treating dendritic ulcers as they encourage deep stromal keratitis (disciform keratitis) which is followed by scarring and vascularisation and a corneal graft may be needed to restore vision.

Herpes zoster ophthalmicus is an acute neurotropic viral infection of the first division of the fifth cranial nerve. Severe unilateral facial and forehead pain may precede the vesicular eruption by several days. If the tip of the nose is also involved then usually, but not always, the eye will be involved too since the naso-ciliary nerve has been affected. Keratitis, iridocyclitis and secondary glaucoma may follow. Optic neuritis and ocular motor nerve palsies can occur. Treatment is by ointment containing corticosteroids and neomycin to the skin lesion, local steroid drops to the eye and a cycloplegic for iritis, and acetazolamide tablets 250 mg up to four times daily for the secondary glaucoma.

Pain can be very troublesome, particularly in the elderly, and adequate analgesics must be used. Even so, some patients are left with a severe post-herpetic neuralgia. The place of systemic corticosteroids for the acute phase is disputed but claimed to reduce the incidence of late pain.

TRAUMA

Ocular injuries are still common, particularly in children and in industry. Many are preventable by proper observation of safety precautions and the wearing of appropriate protective goggles. When injuries do occur their initial treatment may determine whether useful vision, or even the eye itself, can be saved.

If the patient, child or adult, is suspected of having a perforating injury it is safer to defer examination of the eye until the patient is under a general anaesthetic. A potentially salvageable eye may have its contents extruded by muscle spasm following attempts by the examiner to separate the lids.

Visual acuity should be recorded if possible in any injury as it may be important medicolegally. Reading vision, even with a horizontal patient, is usually obtainable.

NON-PERFORATING INJURIES OF THE EYE BALL

Abrasions of conjunctiva or cornea

If the patient complains of a foreign body sensation in the eye but none can be seen by bright, oblique illumination then instill a drop of sterile fluorescein 2% solution, ideally from a Minims individual disposable unit. Abrasions will show up as greenish-yellow areas. Local anaesthetic such as 0.5% amethocaine may be needed to permit full examination of the eye. Antibiotic ointment such as chloramphenicol, with an eye pad and bandage for corneal abrasions, hasten healing. Inspect corneal abrasions next day for infection or ulcer formation.

Contusions

Blunt trauma may cause mild to severe injuries and detailed examination and follow-up are required.

Haemorrhage and swelling of the eye lids ('black eye') mean orbital fractures must be looked for. See below. Subconjunctival haemorrhage and conjunctival edema will clear spontaneously in 2 to 3 weeks.

Haemorrhage into the anterior chamber (hyphaema) requires strict bed rest, preferably in hospital, and patching of one or both eyes. Usually the blood is absorbed uneventfully but secondary haemorrhage may follow 3 to 6 days after the injury causing secondary glaucoma and blood-staining of the cornea. Treatment by irrigation of the anterior chamber with fibrinolysin to remove the blood clot is the best so far available.

Traumatic iridocyclitis, particularly in heavily pigmented eyes, needs cycloplegia with atropine 1% drops and corticosteroids, e.g. guttae prednisolone three times a day.

Ocular contusion may paralyse the pupil, rupture the root of the iris, or detach the ciliary body with a later risk of glaucoma. The lens may be dislocated, or a traumatic cataract form. Vitreous or retinal haemorrhages can occur, there may be retinal edema especially at the macula. Traumatic retinal detachment and choroidal rupture may follow severe injuries. Treatment is mainly expectant but surgery is required for some traumatic cataracts, and the retinal detachments.

Conjunctival and corneal foreign bodies

Foreign bodies within the conjunctival sac are among the commonest injuries. A bright light and a ×10 magnifying glass are essential to find small particles. The eye lids must be everted as a foreign body often lodges beneath the upper tarsal plate. A moistened cotton applicator may be used to wipe it away, or gentle irrigation of the conjunctival sac with sterile saline solution.

Corneal foreign bodies may respond to similar treatment after instilling 0.5% amethocaine drops but if the particle is firmly embedded in the cornea then the patient must go to the ophthalmologist for careful removal under the microscope. Hyoscine 0.25% drops and chloramphenicol ointment and a firm pad are applied and the patient must be checked next day to see that healing is occurring.

Burns

1. *Chemical burns.* Any chemical splashed into the eye must be washed out *at once* as the damage depends on the nature of the chemical and the time it is in contact with the cornea and conjunctiva. Immediate and copious lavage with plain tap water for at least 10 minutes is essential.

The lids must be held apart to ensure adequate washing out of the eye. After the initial lavage then isotonic sterile saline or buffered solutions or chelating agents can be used later. Local antibiotics and corticosteroids are applied and atropine drops.

Corneal ulceration and opacities, and adhesions between the lids and globe may still follow, particularly after alkaline burns as from cement or lime, and surgery may be required later but the results are often disappointing.

2. *Ultraviolet irradiation* from exposure to electric arc welding causes extreme pain, watering and photophobia some 6 to 12 hours later. Widespread minute fluorescein-staining spots of the cornea are seen with magnification. Treatment is by local anaesthetic drops such as amethocaine 0.5%, a cycloplegic such as homatropine 2% and a firm pad and bandage for 24 hours.

3. *Eclipse burns* of the macula from viewing the sun directly may cause permanent impairment of visual acuity. No treatment of any avail. Prevention is paramount.

4. *Thermal burns* of the eye lids are treated as are skin burns elsewhere. Full thickness eyelid burns require emergency skin grafting within 24 hours.

PERFORATING INJURIES OF THE EYE BALL

In *any* perforating ocular injury always suspect, look for and X-ray for an intra-ocular foreign body.

Lacerations or ruptures without prolapse of tissue

Rupture of the eye ball from direct blunt trauma may occur around the limbus with intact conjunctiva overlying the rupture. Posterior ruptures may also occur around the optic nerve.

Lacerations of the globe may follow glass or knife injuries. Direct suturing by the eye surgeon of such wounds under general anaesthesia is required. Local and systemic antibiotics are given, plus appropriate protection against tetanus infection.

Lacerations with prolapse of ocular contents

A small puncture wound of the cornea may be plugged by iris prolapse and simulate a corneal foreign body. If iris or ciliary body prolapse is small this may be abscissed and the wound sutured as described above. Any wound involving uveal tissue means that the patient must be followed closely to detect sympathetic ophthalmitis which may develop in the *un*injured eye. Sympathetic ophthalmitis can be prevented by enucleation of a severely injured eye within 10 days of the injury. This means that it is not an emergency measure to enucleate a badly damaged eye but it should first be repaired and observed for up to 10 days before making this decision.

Intra-ocular foreign bodies

If an intra-ocular foreign body is suspected, and in particular if there is a history of striking a hammer upon a cold chisel followed by pain and blurred vision in one eye, X-rays must be taken.

Specialised X-rays are essential to confirm and also localise any radio-opaque foreign body. Slit-lamp microscopy, or ophthalmoscopy may reveal the site of penetration and sometimes the particle itself. Iron or copper particles must be removed from the eye because of later disorganisation of the eye by electro-chemical changes. Detailed surgical management is highly specialised.

LACERATIONS OF EYE LIDS

Eye lid lacerations should be repaired early but only after lacerations of the globe have been excluded. Small superficial lid lacerations parallel to the lid margin may be sutured directly.

Lacerations involving the lid margins may form a notch if incorrectly sutured. Lacerations of the medial ends of the lid margins may sever the canaliculi and these must be repaired to avoid constant watering. Lacerations of the upper lid must be examined carefully for associated damage to the levator muscle of the upper lid with resultant ptosis. These three types of injury need specialist repair. Finally penetration of the thin orbital roof with frontal lobe damage may be found.

ORBITAL INJURIES

Bony injury

Direct trauma can fracture the orbital rim, e.g. inferior orbital rim fracture with a sprung fronto-zygomatic suture from injury over the zygoma. Emphysema of orbital tissues may follow blowing the nose if the fracture extends into a sinus.

Blunt trauma to the globe by a fist or similar sized convex object can cause a blow-out fracture of the thin orbital floor and leave the rim intact. These patients may present with just a 'black eye' but have paraesthesia in the upper lip on that side from infra-orbital nerve involvement, and diplopia, particularly on trying to look up or down. This is due to trapping of the inferior rectus muscle or its fascial attachments within the fracture, or to haematoma of the muscle. As edema of the lids settles then enophthalmos may become evident. Properly aligned X-rays along the plane of the normal orbital floor will confirm the herniation of orbital contents into the antrum. Surgical intervention is necessary if any of the following conditions are found: (i) retraction of the globe on attempted up-gaze (ii) *large* herniation of orbital contents (iii) enophthalmos of 3 mm or more. The majority of cases do not need operation. The decision to intervene need not be taken for up to 10 days by which time the diplopia is usually resolving spontaneously. If operation is necessary a direct approach can be made along the orbital floor, or a Caldwell–Luc approach to the antral roof and the prolapse and fracture reduced. Various materials can be used to reinforce the orbital floor, such as silicone rubber.

Penetrating injuries

Any penetrating injury of the orbit may involve the sinuses or anterior cranial fossa too. Foreign bodies must be localised carefully to distinguish them from intra-ocular ones. Many intra-orbital foreign bodies are best left alone.

Pulsating exophthalmos may result from a fracture involving the cavernous sinus and causing a direct arterio-venous shunt which transmits the pulse to the orbital contents.

Differential diagnosis of the red eye

	Acute conjunctivitis	*Corneal trauma or keratitis*	*Acute iritis*	*Acute glaucoma*	*Spontaneous sub-conjunctival haemorrhage*
Symptoms	slightly gritty, sore eye	irritation and pain	aching eye	severe pain, nausea and vomiting	none
Vision	normal	slightly blurred	slightly blurred	marked blurring	normal
Discharge	sticky	watery	none	none	none
Conjunctival infection	generalised	mainly around the cornea	mainly around the cornea	generalised	localised patch of blood
Cornea	clear	abrasion patch, or dull, opaque area of ulceration	clear, with keratic precipitates	steamy	clear
Pupil, size	normal	small	normal, or small, irregular	dilated, irregular	normal
Pupil, light reaction	normal	normal	sluggish	minimal	normal
Tension to palpation	normal	normal	normal	rock hard	normal
Management	smear for microscopy and culture, local antibiotics	investigation antibiotics mydriatics	full medical investigation mydriatics cortiscosteroids	emergency treatment, miotics, acetazolamide, surgery	check blood pressure, blood film and for bleeding tendency

NEVER USE CORTICOSTEROID EYE DROPS UNTIL THE DIAGNOSIS HAS BEEN MADE

GLAUCOMA

Glaucoma is a disease in which the intra-ocular pressure is elevated to levels that cause loss of vision by pressure damage on the optic nerve. More than 2% of the population over 40 years have glaucoma and it is a common cause of blindness.

Open-angle glaucoma

The normal intra-ocular pressure of 14 to 18 mmHg is necessary to keep the eye ball a constant shape to that its optical focusing properties remain stable. This pressure is maintained by the production of aqueous humour by the ciliary body which flows forwards through the pupil into the anterior chamber and drains through the angle between iris and cornea into the canal of Schlemm and eventually into the venous system. If the outflow resistance is increased then the intra-ocular pressure will rise and if this pressure stays high then vision will be insidiously lost.

Early diagnosis is difficult. All patients over the age of 40 years should have the intra-ocular pressure measured and this can be done by the general practitioner with a Schiøtz tonometer. If the pressure is 25 mmHg or higher the patient should be referred to the ophthalmologist. The optic disc appears cupped, with a grey rim and nasal displacement of the retinal vessels. Careful measurement of visual fields is essential in making the diagnosis and in evaluating the effect of treatment. Medical treatment comprises pilocarpine 1–4% drops four times daily. In addition, eserine 0.25% or neutral adrenaline 1% may be used. These drops increase aqueous outflow. Acetazolamide tablets 250 mg up to four times daily may also be required to control the pressure by reducing aqueous production. Only if control cannot be adequately maintained by these means will surgical methods of increasing aqueous drainage be used.

Angle closure (acute) glaucoma

This is an ophthalmic emergency. The patient has blurring of vision in one eye with severe ocular pain, headache and even nausea and vomiting. This is due to the iris being pushed forwards peripherally so that the drainage angle is completely blocked and intra-ocular pressure rises rapidly. Many of these patients give a history of slight blurring of vision in the dark and of seeing coloured haloes around lights due to mild corneal edema. These mild attacks usually subside during sleep. Contributing factors to the development of angle closure are a shallow anterior chamber, high hypermetropia, a large lens within the eye and pupillary dilatation. For routine fundoscopy a short-acting mydriatic such as cyclopentolate 0.5% or phenylephrine 2.5% should be used, and a miotic instilled after the examination.

In the acute attack of glaucoma the eye is red, the cornea hazy, the pupil irregularly dilated and the eye feels rock hard to palpation.

Treatment is by intensive miotics, usually pilocarpine 4% every 15 minutes, intravenous acetazolamide 500 mg followed by oral acetazolamide. Orally 3 ml/kg bodyweight of 50% glycerol may be used as a dehydrating agent, provided the patient is not a diabetic. Morphine 15–20 mg for pain also helps with miosis.

Intravenous mannitol, 1.8 g/kg bodyweight may also be used to bring down the pressure as an immediate pre-operative step. Once the intra-ocular pressure has been lowered a peripheral iridectomy should be done to prevent further attacks. The second eye usually will be found to have a similar predisposition to angle closure glaucoma and many surgeons advocate later prophylactic peripheral iridectomy to this eye.

Infantile glaucoma is raised intra-ocular pressure occurring within the first three years of life. In this age group, the raised pressure causes haziness and enlargement of the cornea, with lacrimation and photophobia as prominent signs. The raised pressure is due to abnormal development of the anterior chamber angle, but once diagnosed early surgery can help up to 80% of these infants.

Secondary glaucoma may follow iritis, trauma to the eye, lens dislocation, etc. Treatment is aimed at the causative condition.

SUDDEN LOSS OF VISION

ACCIDENTALLY DISCOVERED POOR VISION

Poor vision in one eye may be accidentally discovered when the patient chances to cover one eye, or at a routine eye sight test such as school children have.

Refractive error in one eye may be responsible, e.g. marked myopia, hypermetropia or astigmatism. Measure the patient's visual acuity looking through a pinhole. If this improves vision to nearly normal it means that spectacles can do the same.

Strabismic amblyopia due to a squint is preventable provided if it is detected early enough. All children should have their visual acuity in each eye tested by 5 years of age, and preferably by their 4th birthday. If acuity is low on one side refraction under a cycloplegic should be done and the ocular media and fundi checked for any obvious cause of poor vision. If none is found then spectacles will be worn if indicated and the fixing eye patched to make the vision develop properly in the 'lazy eye'.

Once equal visual acuity has been obtained in the two eyes then the eyes must be made straight. Sometimes glasses alone suffice, or with the addition of miotic drops. In other patients surgery is needed to reposition the extra-ocular muscles.

Visual field loss affecting one eye severely may be due to glaucoma which has destroyed the sight on one side and already affected the other eye before being discovered. Lesions affecting the visual pathways may do the same, e.g. pituitary tumours. Confrontation testing of visual fields will indicate the degree of field loss in the remaining eye. Refer to the ophthalmologist or neurologist.

TRANSIENT LOSS OF VISION

Papilledema due to raised intracranial pressure may cause blackouts lasting 5 to 15 seconds only, or a patchy blurring of vision. Headaches, nausea and vomiting may be present and general examination is required since the prime causes are cerebral tumours and hypertension. Appropriate treatment is then instituted.

Carotid artery insufficiency causes unilateral blindness 'like a curtain coming down over the eye' and returning to normal in 4 or 5 minutes. It occurs as a warning symptom in 50% of cases of carotid occlusion. Transient contralateral limb pareses may occur. Listen along the course of the carotids for bruits. Examine the fundi for bright cholesterol embolic plaques in the arterioles. Refer the patient for assessment for possible surgical endarterectomy, or long-term anticoagulants.

Basilar artery insufficiency produces varied symptoms, including dysphagia, dysarthria, dysphonia and numbness of the lips. 80% of patients with basilar insufficiency have ocular signs including diplopia, usually from VIth nerve involvement. Scintillating scotomas and various field defects may be present. Horizontal or vertical gaze palsies can occur, as may vestibular nystagmus. Visual hallucinations and diplopia are never found in carotid insufficiency.

Migraine typically presents a zig-zag flashing before the headache develops. The visual loss may progress to a hemianopia lasting 15–30 minutes. Often migraine will be aborted by ergotamine tartrate taken at the first warning of an impending attack. Prolonged and even permanent hemianopia following migrainous symptoms means that arteriovenous anomalies must be suspected.

LONGER LASTING OR PERMANENT LOSS OF VISION

Central retinal artery occlusion causes sudden and often permanent loss of vision. A pale edematous area of the posterior pole is seen with a red patch at the macula. With branch occlusions of the retinal arterioles the embolus may be visible. Most emboli are atheromatous in older patients, but in young adults heart disease, particularly the rheumatic type, may be responsible. Treatment if it is to have any hope of success must be prompt. Methods of attempted vasodilation to allow the embolus to pass peripherally into the retina include intermittent globe massage with the fingers, breathing a 95% mixture of oxygen and carbon dioxide, intravenous acetazolamide 500 mg to soften the eye, and paracentesis of the anterior chamber. Retrobulbar injections of tolazoline or acetylcholine may also be tried.

Central retinal vein thrombosis may be complete or partial. A dramatic fundus picture of dilated and tortuous veins is seen. Causes of both primary and secondary polycythaemia must be searched for and treated. No treatment for the eye is effective but surprisingly good visual acuity sometimes returns after several weeks. Other cases progress to thrombotic glaucoma.

Ischaemic optic atrophy causes sudden visual loss, usually of the lower field with a pale and swollen optic disc, sometimes accompanied by splinter haemorrhages. Later neovascularization of the optic nerve head develops. Systemic corticosteroids may be tried.

Cranial (temporal) arteritis is followed by blindness in half the patients within a period of weeks. General malaise, weight loss and insomnia with severe headache and localised tenderness over the superficial cranial arteries may be found. Ophthalmoplegias occur in 15% of cases. Rarely is sudden blindness the first symptom. The erythrocytic sedimentation rate (ESR) is usually well over 40 mm in one hour and a temporal artery biopsy confirms the diagnosis. Emergency medical treatment with 60 mg of prednisolone a day is started but must be reduced and continued at least 6 months, the dosage being adjusted according to the ESR.

Optic neuritis may be due to a wide range of causes of which the commonest are multiple sclerosis and the toxic amblyopias. The latter include tobacco, methyl alcohol, quinine and salicylates.

The optic disc has blurred margins, filling of the physiological cup, distended veins and surrounding retinal edema. It must be differentiated from papilledema on the associated findings.

Retrobulbar neuritis means that the optic nerve is affected posteriorly so that no changes are visible ophthalmoscopically.

In retrobulbar neuritis, the patients present with sudden loss of vision, rarely total, and a central scotoma can be shown. There is pain on eye movement and the pupil shows a poorly sustained constriction to light. Visual improvement occurs in the ensuing 2 to 3 weeks and there is no conclusive evidence that treatment with systemic corticosteroids helps. Only 50% of patients with retrobulbar neuritis will develop later evidence of multiple sclerosis.

The toxic amblyopias all require drug withdrawal. In addition the tobacco amblyopia responds to vitamin B supplements and the use of intramuscular hydroxocobalamin. For methanol poisoning the acidosis must be controlled by alkali therapy with monitoring of the blood CO_2 combining power. Ethyl alcohol helps by inhibiting the toxic degradation of methanol to formaldehyde.

Vitreous haemorrhages cause sudden visual loss and may take weeks or months to clear. Often diabetic retinopathy or hypertensive retinopathy will be seen in the other eye. Treatment is for the systemic condition.

Retinal detachments may be preceded by sudden floating spots or flashes of light with later loss of visual field and then of visual acuity as the detachment spreads to include the macula. Only immediate specialist referral and surgical treatment can prevent permanent visual loss.

Drugs in Current Use

Edited by J. R. Trounce

Contents

Category 1

DRUGS USED IN NEUROLOGICAL DISEASE

M. D. O'BRIEN

THE TREATMENT OF EPILEPSY

Drugs used in the treatment of epilepsy fall clearly into three groups; those used in petit mal, those used in all other forms of epilepsy and those used in status epilepticus.

The measurement of the blood levels of anti-convulsant drugs has been a major advance in the management of patients with epilepsy. There is a very good correlation between blood levels and brain tissue concentrations with most drugs in common use. Many of the factors which determine blood levels have not been fully evaluated; these include variations in usage, absorption, metabolism, drug interaction and excretion, so that blood levels may vary considerably between patients and in one patient on a constant dosage. However it is now possible to monitor blood levels so that optimum dosage can be used.

DRUGS USED IN THE TREATMENT OF GENERALISED SEIZURES AND FOCAL EPILEPSY

Phenytoin sodium

Pharmacological action. Phenytoin appears to inhibit the spread of epileptic discharges, but it does not depress spontaneous discharge from an epileptic focus or cause general depression of the CNS in therapeutically effective dosage. It produces this effect by a stabilising action on excitable membranes without interfering with the normal functions of excitable cells and this may be related to a reduction of intracellular sodium.

Therapeutic use. The drug is the most effective and widely used anti-convulsant in the treatment of generalised convulsive disorders and focal epilepsy. The usual initial adult dose is 200 mg daily and this may be increased to 300 or 400 mg daily. Signs of toxicity often develop at higher doses and increases above 400 mg daily should be monitored with blood levels. The hydroxylation of phenytoin in the liver is a saturatable enzymatic process so that very small increments

at the higher dose levels can result in a considerable rise in the blood level. In patients where response to treatment is unsatisfactory, estimation of blood levels can be helpful. Children should start on about half the adult dose.

Contraindications and side effects. The drug is very safe with low toxicity. A number of side effects occur especially in larger dosage;

1. A few patients are hypersensitive to the drug and become intoxicated with relatively small doses. Some of these patients have genetically determined defective liver enzymes.

2. A reversible syndrome of principally cerebellar dysfunction with giddiness, ataxia, double vision, nystagmus, ptosis, slurred speech, dysequilibrium, drowsiness, confusion and headache are the commonest signs of intoxication and in most patients it is directly related to the serum concentration of phenytoin.

3. Neuro-psychiatric symptoms rarely occur and are usually associated with prolonged administration. These patients often have a low serum folate and may respond to treatment with folic acid. Although an increase in the seizure frequency has been reported following treatment with folic acid, this does not appear to be an important clinical problem. If sufficiently severe this folic acid deficiency may produce a megaloblastic anaemia.

4. Gingival hypertrophy is not uncommon in children on prolonged medication; the effects of this can be minimised by careful dental hygiene. Rashes, gastrointestinal upsets and lymphadenopathy are also occasionally reported.

5. Phenytoin is a powerful enzyme inducer and by increasing the rate of breakdown of vitamin D, may cause rickets or osteomalacia.

Primidone

Pharmacological action. This drug is closely related to phenobarbitone and much of its effect is due to its conversion to phenobarbitone in the body, however it also has an anti-convulsant effect of its own and this may account for the good results obtained in temporal lobe and psycho-motor epilepsy. Serial blood levels in a patient taking primidone alone show measurable phenobarbitone after about a week and after about three weeks there should be a ratio of phenobarbitone to primidone of 2:1.

Therapeutic use. The drug is of value in all forms of major epilepsy and is often preferred to phenobarbitone as an additional drug to phenytoin because it is less sedating. It must be introduced very gradually, starting with 125 mg at night and increasing to a therapeutic dose, which is usually about 750 mg daily in adults. Dose levels of up to 1500 mg a day may be tolerated but the higher dose levels should be monitored with blood level measurements.

Contraindications and side effects. The commonest side effects are vertigo, ataxia and sedation which commonly occur when treatment is initiated and may be minimised by starting with small doses. These side effects may be dose limiting, but sedation is much less of a problem than with phenobarbitone. A few patients are quite intolerant of this drug even in small dosage. Rashes may occur but these are rare.

Phenobarbitone

Pharmacological action. This drug is an effective anti-convulsant for generalised seizures and focal epilepsy. The major site of action appears to be the neural synapse and it is thought that the drug slows or blocks the transport of sodium and potassium across the cellular membrane; this action damps down both excitory and inhibitory post-synaptic potential generation. All barbiturates exert a markedly depressive effect on repetitive activity in CNS pathways; but phenobarbitone is almost alone in raising the threshold to seizure activity out of proportion to the degree of sedation.

Therapeutic use. Although very effective in the treatment of most major and focal epilepsy, it is often unsatisfactory in the treatment of temporal lobe and psycho-motor epilepsy. The usual initial daily dose for adults is 60–90 mg a day in divided doses. Dosage in excess of 150 mg a day usually causes intolerable sedation but the higher doses may be tolerated and measurements of blood levels are often helpful in determining the therapeutic level. The initial dose for children is about half the adult dose. Phenobarbitone should only be withdrawn very gradually because there is a small risk of withdrawal seizure.

Contraindications and side effects. The sedative effect of phenobarbitone is the most usual dose-limiting factor. Occasionally, phenobarbitone has a paradoxically exciting effect on children, particularly the mentally retarded. This may be due to suppression of the higher inhibitory cerebral function and amphetamines may have the opposite effect in these children. The drug should be used with extreme caution in hepatic insufficiency and blood levels should be monitored in these patients. In common with all barbiturates it is contraindicated in acute intermittent porphyria. It should be used with caution in status epilepticus because of its long action and respiratory depression. As with all barbiturates the development of a rash may require withdrawal of the drug.

Phenobarbitone is an enzyme inducer and interacts particularly with oral anticoagulants (see page 218).

Sodium valproate

Pharmacological action. This recently introduced drug is the salt of a branched chain fatty acid, chemically distinct from other anti-convulsants. It is thought to work by the inhibition of GABA-transaminase thus increasing the CNS levels of GABA, a largely inhibitory transmitter.

Therapeutic use. Valproate is effective in all forms of epilepsy, particularly idiopathic epilepsy and petit mal. It is also effective for myoclonus. The initial dose is 400 mg daily and this may be increased to 1400 mg daily in divided doses. It is well tolerated by children.

Contraindications and side effects. Valproate is usually very well tolerated but a few patients complain of drowsiness or gastrointestinal irritation on quite small doses. It should therefore be given after food.

Clonazepam

Pharmacological action. The mechanism of action of this recently introduced benzodiazepine drug is unknown but it has a marked anti-convulsant effect in oral doses which do not produce undue sedation, unlike diazepam.

Therapeutic use. Clonazepam is effective in all forms of epilepsy including petit mal. The initial dose is 0.5–1.5 mg daily and this may be increased to 12–16 mg daily. There is a very variable tolerance to this drug.

Contraindications and side effects. Drowsiness may be a prominent early side-effect but can be minimised by starting with a low dose; otherwise the drug is well tolerated.

Carbamazepine

Pharmacological action. This drug is an iminodibenzyl compound which is chemically related to both the trycyclic anti-depressants and the phenothiazines.

Therapeutic use. It is an effective anti-convulsant

in all forms of epilepsy except petit mal and is a valuable adjuvant to the more standard drugs. The initial dose is 200 mg daily and this may be increased to 800 mg/day in divided doses. Dose levels above 1200 mg/day are rarely tolerated.
Contraindications and side effects. The drug is usually well tolerated but rashes are a drug limiting idiosyncrasy. Giddiness, nausea and dysequilibrium are dose limiting side effects and in some patients occur after quite small doses.

Sulthiame

Pharmacological action. This drug is a sulphonamide congener with weak carbonic anhydrase activity. It enhances the blood levels of phenytoin, presumably because it competes with the same liver enzymes; this may be its most useful property.
Therapeutic use. The initial adult dose is 200 mg daily, and this may be increased to 600 mg daily.
Contraindications and side effects. As a weak carbonic anhydrase inhibitor it may produce features of metabolic acidosis such as overbreathing. Headaches, nausea, vomiting, dizziness, drowsiness, blurred vision and gastrointestinal disturbances may complicate its use.

Pheneturide and phenocetamide

Pharmacological action. These drugs are acetylurea derivatives, they are therapeutically effective in all forms of epilepsy and they appear to produce their effect by raising the threshold to seizure activity.
Therapeutic use. They may be useful as additional drugs in intractable epilepsy or as a substitute for one of the more established drugs when these cannot be tolerated. They have very little depressant effect. The adult dose is 400–1000 mg daily in divided doses.
Contraindications and side effects. Gastrointestinal upsets, rashes, drowsiness and psychoses have been reported but the drugs are usually well tolerated.

DRUGS USED IN THE TREATMENT OF PETIT MAL
Ethosuximide

Pharmacological action. This is the drug of choice in the treatment of petit mal and is also sometimes effective in myoclonus. It is the most effective of the three suxinamide derivatives.
Therapeutic use. It is most commonly used in children and the adult and child doses are the same. An initial dose of 500 mg/day may be increased to 1500 mg/day.

Contraindications and side effects. Gastrointestinal upsets, headaches and drowsiness may occur. There is no evidence that this drug exacerbates or induces grand mal attacks.

Troxidone

Pharmacological action. Troxidone is an antiepileptic drug with a specificity for the treatment of petit mal seizures. It probably produces its effect by blocking the propagation of an epileptic discharge between the cortex and the thalamus, while local cortical spread of seizure activity is unaffected. It therefore has little effect on major epilepsy.
Therapeutic use. The drug is no longer the treatment of choice for petit mal but it may be useful if ethosuximide is not tolerated or as an additional drug in intractable cases. In children the initial dose is 300 mg/day in divided doses and this may be increased to 900 mg/day. In adults an initial dose of 900 mg/day may be increased to 1800 mg/day.
Contraindications and side effects. A frequently observed side effect is hemeralopia (blurring of vision in bright light) this is probably due to an effect of the drug on the ganglion layer of the retina. Skin rashes may occur and indicate a sensitivity reaction. Bone marrow depression may occur with prolonged treatment. Nephrosis, hepatitis and lupus erythematosus have also been reported.

Valproate and clonazepam—see page 164

TREATMENT OF STATUS EPILEPTICUS
Diazepam

Pharmacological action. This drug is thought to exert an action on the limbic system or its connections. In addition it has an anti-epileptic effect when given in large doses parenterally, but has no effect in the usual oral dosage.
Therapeutic use. The only use of diazepam in the treatment of epilepsy is in the control of status epilepticus. The drug must be given parenterally and a combined dose of 10 mg intravenously and 10 mg intramuscularly is often effective; this may be repeated as necessary. The principal advantage of diazepam is the control of cortical activity without depression of the respiratory centre.
Contraindications and side effects. Caution should be exercised when this drug is used with phenobarbitone.

Chlormethiazole

Pharmacological action. Chlormethiazole is a sedative with anti-convulsant properties which is derived from the thiazole part of the thiamine (Vitamin B_1) molecule.

Therapeutic use. It is given in continuous intravenous infusion at about 500–700 mg/hour using a solution containing 8 g/litre.

Contraindications and side effects. The drug invariably produces sedation but this is not usually a problem in the treatment of status epilepticus. Sedation leading to coma and depression of the respiratory centre may occur with very large doses, particularly if the drug is given intermittently. It has a very short biological half-life so that accumulation is not a problem.

Paraldehyde

Pharmacological action. Paraldehyde is a polymer of acetaldehyde. It has no effect on the respiratory centres or blood pressure in normal dosage.

Therapeutic use. This may be a very useful drug in the initial control of severe status particularly when other drugs have been given and have failed to produce a response. The dose is 3–5 ml given by intramuscular injection.

Contraindications and side effects. Care must be exercised to place the injection in the upper and outer quadrant of the buttock to avoid possible damage to the sciatic nerve.

Short acting barbiturates (pentothal, thiopental, methohexitone)

These drugs may be useful in the treatment of status when given in a slow intravenous infusion, but very careful monitoring is required and this should only be done in an intensive care situation where artificial respiration is available if required.

THE TREATMENT OF MIGRAINE

Drugs used in the treatment of migraine fall clearly into two groups; those used in the acute attack and those used in prophylaxis.

DRUGS USED IN THE ACUTE ATTACK

Ergotamine tartrate

Pharmacological action. This drug is thought to exert its beneficial action by vasoconstriction of non-cerebral cranial vessels.

Therapeutic use. Ergotamine is often very effective in the treatment of the acute attack and it should be given as early as possible. There are a number of dose forms available;

1. By mouth. 1–2 mg of ergotamine tartrate is given as early as possible in an attack. This route of administration may be ineffective because of poor absorption, particularly in patients with nausea and vomiting.

2. By suppository. This is a satisfactory method of administration particularly in those patients with repeated vomiting during an attack. The absorption from the rectum is good.

3. By inhalation. This provides a very rapid absorption and some patients find this method of administration most useful. Usually one or two inhalations are sufficient. Each inhalation contains 0.36 mg of ergotamine tartrate.

4. By injection. If the above methods of administration fail then intramuscular injection of 0.25 or 0.5 mg of ergotamine tartrate early in the attack may be very effective. It usually has to be self administered.

Contraindications and side effects. The immediate toxic effects of ergotamine tartrate are nausea and vomiting. There is however considerable variability in tolerance and some patients are extremely sensitive; in a few patients the side effects of the drug are due to peripheral vasoconstriction and these include numbness, tingling and chilling of the extremities, a rise in blood pressure and painful uterine contractions. Contraindications to its use include peripheral vascular disease, hypertension, coronary, hepatic and renal insufficiency, pregnancy, sepsis and infection. Habituation occasionally occurs and in a few patients persistent headaches may be due to the continued use of the drug.

DRUGS USED IN PROPHYLAXIS

Methysergide

Pharmacological action. The precise pharmacological action of methysergide is not known. It is a powerful serotonin antagonist and acts by competitive inhibition. Serotonin is known to be involved in migraine since blood levels fall in an attack and high levels of its metabolite 5-hydroxyindolylacetic acid are found in the urine after an attack.

Therapeutic use. The drug may be very effective in the prophylaxis of migraine in a daily dose of 1–6 mg. Treatment should be started with 1–2 mg at night for a week to see whether the patient develops side effects. If these do not occur then the dose can be gradually increased until the migraine is controlled or until the dose reaches 6 mg/day. Continuous treatment for more than 6 months is undesirable without a drug-free interval of at least a month. The dosage should be gradually decreased for two or three weeks before withdrawing the drug to prevent rebound attacks.

Contraindications and side effects. There is considerable variability in tolerance to methysergide.

About 40% experience side effects and these are sufficiently severe to stop the use of the drug in 15%. The most common early side effects are a stimulant action on the appetite, nausea, vomiting, diarrhea and abdominal pain, peripheral edema, thrombophlebitis and tingling of the periphery. The most important side effect is the development of retroperitoneal fibrosis. This does not occur earlier than 4–6 months of continuous treatment and most patients have taken the drug for many years. The risk of developing this complication appears to be minimised by stopping treatment for a month or two every 4–6 months. Retroperitoneal fibrosis presents with a low grade fever, pain in the loins, oliguria, dysuria and symptoms of uraemia. The diagnosis is confirmed by pyelographic evidence of ureteric obstruction. This complication occurs in about 1% of patients on continuous treatment. Methysergide is contraindicated in pregnancy and arterial and venous disease of all types, valvular heart disease, chronic pulmonary diseases, impaired renal or hepatic function, peptic ulcer and any of the collagenoses.

Dihydroergotamine

Pharmacological action. This dihydrogenated ergot-alkaloid has the same pharmacological properties as ergotamine, although its effect is much weaker and more prolonged.

Therapeutic use. It may safely be used for prolonged periods and the initial dose is 1 mg daily which may be increased to 3 mg daily.

Contraindications and side effects. This drug is relatively non-toxic when used in this way, its effects are otherwise those of ergotamine.

Pizotifen

Pharmacological action. A recently introduced serotonin antagonist which is thought to have a similar mode of action to methysergide.

Therapeutic use. Treatment should be started with 1.5 mg daily in divided doses and this may be increased to 3 mg daily.

Contraindications and side effects. Drowsiness and increased appetite may limit the use of this drug.

Clonidine

Pharmacological action. This drug is an imidiazole derivative which has been widely used in the treatment of hypertension (see page 203). The precise pharmacological effect is unknown but it may act centrally on autonomic pathways.

Therapeutic use. It has been found empirically that small doses of this drug, about one tenth of that used for hypertension, has a prophylactic effect in some patients with migraine. The dose range is 0.075 to 0.15 mg daily.

Contraindications and side effects. At these dose levels side effects are negligible, but sedation may occur.

THE TREATMENT OF PARKINSON'S DISEASE

Parkinson's disease is a degenerative condition which results from a striatal deficiency of the neurotransmitter dopamine, although the dopamine receptors remain capable of responding if dopamine is made available. Dopamine does not cross the blood–brain barrier but the laevo-isomer of its immediate precursor, dopa, can be given orally and reaches the basal ganglia where it is converted to dopamine by the enzyme dopa-decarboxylase. This enzyme is also present in blood vessels, gastrointestinal tract and liver where it converts over 90% of an oral dose of L-dopa. Large oral doses are therefore required to give satisfactory levels in the brain and this is associated with a high incidence of non-cerebral side effects. These can be minimised by the coincident use of a decarboxylase inhibitor which does not cross the blood–brain barrier. Combinations of this type are now the standard treatment for Parkinson's disease.

There may also be a failure to produce dopa-decarboxylase in the brain and this may be one of the factors which limit the effect of L-dopa in the advanced stages of the disease. These patients may respond to a dopamine agonist which does not need the enzyme because it acts directly on the dopamine receptors. *Bromocryptine* is a dopamine agonist and may be the first of a new generation of drugs in the treatment of parkinsonism.

Anti-cholinergic drugs are also beneficial in Parkinson's disease and this is due to a central effect. Sudden withdrawal of these drugs usually results in a much greater deterioration in the patients' condition than might be expected. It is beneficial to combine anti-cholinergic drugs with L-dopa.

Levadopa (L-dopa)

Therapeutic use. L-dopa alone is now seldom used to start treatment, but there remains a large number of patients whose parkinsonism is under satisfactory control on L-dopa alone. The optimal dose for most patients lies between 2 and 6 g daily. Many patients are unable to tolerate larger dosage because of intolerable side effects. It is necessary to start treatment with a very small dose, sometimes as low as 125 mg at night and to increase this every few days until a therapeutic dose is achieved or side effects limit medication. It should be given in multiple divided doses and always after food. A beneficial response is usually seen very early and this most noticeably affects the bradykinesia and rigidity; tremor is affected rather variably and usually at higher dosage.

Continued improvement may occur after several weeks on a stabilised regime.

L-dopa with a decarboxylase inhibitor

Therapeutic use. Much smaller doses of L-dopa can be used in this combination since there is very little breakdown of L-dopa outside the brain. The dose is usually limited by central side effects.

Two combined preparations are available:

L-dopa and carbidopa in a ratio of 10:1, tablets are available containing 250 mg and 100 mg of L-dopa.

L-dopa and benzerazide in a ratio of 4:1, capsules are available containing 200 mg and 100 mg of L-dopa.

The initial dose is 200 or 250 mg of L-dopa daily in 2 doses and this may be quite quickly increased to 750–800 mg daily. Central side effects are very common at the larger doses, particularly dyskinesia, and this usually limits the dose.

Contraindications and side effects; central:

1. Dyskinesia. Involuntary movements occur in about 60–70% of patients at the higher dose range and are the most common dose limiting side effect. The commonest dyskinesiae are of the face, tongue and jaw with grimacing and choreoathetotic movements. Also seen are choreoathetotic movements of the arms and legs and repetitive movements such as foot tapping. These side effects are directly related to the dose of levodopa and will often disappear with a small reduction.

2. Psychiatric disturbances. These may occur at any dose level in susceptible patients, particularly post-encephalitic patients, and vary from restlessness, anxiety, agitation and insomnia to hypomania. In these circumstances the drug should be withdrawn completely for 24 hours and then re-introduced gradually in lower dosage. Levodopa should be used with extreme caution in patients with a previous history of psychiatric disturbance and is contraindicated in dementia.

3. A long term complication is the so called "on/off" effect with fairly rapid changes from bradykinesia to marked abnormal movements which may occur several times a day. This side effect is rarely seen during the first two years of continuous treatment.

Contraindications and side effects; peripheral:

4. Gastrointestinal symptoms. These are the most commonly experienced side effects of L-dopa alone and may occur in 70–80% of patients during the initial stages of therapy, particularly if there has been a rapid increase in dose. These symptoms of nausea and vomiting may persist in as many as 30% of patients and become either dose or drug limiting. Patients may be helped over the initial phase with an anti-emetic drug such as cyclizine; phenothiazine derivatives should of course be avoided. This side effect can be minimised by taking multiple divided doses after food.

5. Cardiovascular. Postural hypotension is very common but is only disabling in a very small proportion of patients. Cardiac arrhythmias may occur in those patients with heart disease and it is therefore wise always to obtain an ECG before commencing treatment. L-dòpa should not be used in the period immediately following a myocardial infarct.

Benzhexol hydrochloride

Pharmacological action. The peripheral actions of benzhexol resemble atropine and the central actions are those of the belladonna alkaloids. Its central effect is probably produced by blocking acetylcholine.

Therapeutic use. This is the most effective of the anti-cholinergic drugs in the treatment of parkinsonism. Rigidity, bradykinesia and tremor are all favourably affected in some degree. The initial dose is 1–2 mg twice a day and this may be gradually increased. A total daily dose in excess of 15–20 mg/day is rarely tolerated.

Contraindications and side effects. The side effects resemble those of atropine and may be very troublesome in about 10% of patients. Most patients complain of a dry mouth and some of blurred vision. Overdosage produces mental confusion, delirium, agitation and hallucinations.

Other anti-cholinergic drugs

These drugs all act in a similar way to benzhexol and have similar side effects. Sometimes a patient will tolerate one of these preparations better than another.

Drug	Initial dose	Maintenance dose
Methixene	2.5 mg b.d.	Up to 30 mg/day
Procyclidine	2.5 mg t.d.s.	Up to 30 mg/day
Biperiden	2 mg b.d.	Up to 8 mg/day
Benztropine	0.5 mg b.d.	Up to 6 mg/day
Orphenidrine hydrochloride	50 mg t.d.s.	Up to 300 mg/day
Ethopropazine	50 mg/day	Up to 800 mg/day

Benztropine, biperiden and orphenidrine are available for parenteral administration and may be useful in this form in the treatment of drug induced dystonias.

Amantadine

Pharmacological action. The mode of action of this anti-viral agent in parkinsonism is unknown. Like L-dopa, it is more effective in relieving the bradykinesia and rigidity than tremor, but it is much less effective than L-dopa.

Therapeutic use. It is a useful addition to L-dopa in those patients who are unable to tolerate an effective dose because of side effects. The dose is 200 mg daily.

Contraindications and side effects. There are no side effects.

THE TREATMENT OF TRIGEMINAL NEURALGIA

Carbamazepine

For a description of this drug see page 164 in the section on the treatment of epilepsy. It has a specific effect on this condition and controls the pain in more than 70% of patients. The initial dose in the treatment of trigeminal neuralgia is 300 mg daily and this may be increased gradually to 1200 mg daily.

Category 2

HYPNOTICS

J. R. TROUNCE

HYPNOTICS AND SLEEP

There is no doubt that hypnotics are overprescribed. Although there may be occasions when the use of hypnotics for a short period is desirable, their use over long periods by patients with a sleep problem is generally to be deplored.

Normal sleep consists of a series of cycles each lasting about ninety minutes. The cycle starts with 'orthodox' sleep which deepens with slow pulse and respiration rate. This period is associated with the release of growth hormone. It is followed by a shorter period of rapid eye movement (REM) sleep when the subject is more restless and dreams occur.

In old age the normal sleep pattern may become deranged so that although the total time asleep during 24 hours remains unaltered, the night may be broken up by short periods of wakefulness.

Hypnotic drugs shorten the period of REM sleep to a greater or lesser degree. Whether this is of any serious significance is not known, and the brain appears to return towards a normal pattern with continued use of hypnotics. If however, the hypnotic is stopped, the duration of REM sleep is increased for a time and this may be the reason for the period of restlessness which occurs when a hypnotic is withdrawn.

The effect of hypnotics is usually said to last about 8 hours or less, but it has been shown that some depression of skilled activities persists well into the next day. Finally, it cannot be said too often that insomnia may be a symptom of depression.

THE BARBITURATES

Pharmacological action. The group of barbiturate hypnotics have the general formula

Substitution can occur in the R_1 and R_2 positions, producing a large number of compounds. For example:

	R_1	R_2
Quinalbarbitone	$CH_2CH=CH_2$	C_5H_{11}
Amylobarbitone	CH_2H_5	C_5H_{11}
Phenobarbitone	C_2H_5	Phenyl

The introduction of a phenyl group confers anticonvulsant properties and also decreases conjugation in the liver, and thus prolongs action.

This group of drugs is well absorbed from the intestinal tract and penetrates widely through the tissues. They are largely conjugated in the liver and only phenobarbitone is excreted to any degree (30%) unchanged in the urine. Renal excretion of phenobarbitone is enhanced in an alkaline urine; this increases the ionised fraction in the urine and decreases back diffusion from the tubules to the blood. With repeated dosage tolerance will develop, and it has been shown that barbiturates will induce enzymes in the liver which metabolise the drug. The enhanced production of glucuronyl transferase by barbiturates has been used in treating neonatal jaundice.

The effect of the very short-acting barbiturate is terminated by redistribution of the drug — a short while after administration a major portion passes from the brain to fat and muscle.

Barbiturates produce sleep by depressing both the cortex and reticular activating systems. In larger doses they produce unconsciousness, and the very quick acting ones can be used as anaesthetic agents.

In hypnotic doses the barbiturates have no effect on perception of pain, and in those suffering pain they must be combined with an analgesic.

Barbiturates lower the blood pressure by reducing cardiac output. This is partially due to venous pooling and perhaps also to a direct effect on the myocardium.

The respiratory centre is depressed, especially with large doses, and this is an important feature of overdosage.

Therapeutic use. Barbiturates can be classified in terms of their duration of action:

1. Long acting group. Phenobaritone is the most important. Its action is generally considered too long for a hypnotic but unlike other barbiturates it is an anticonvulsant and is used in grand mal epilepsy. The usual anticonvulsant dose is 30–60 mg two or three times daily, but the top range of dose may well produce drowsiness. The sodium salt is also available for intramuscular injection in doses of 60–200 mg in status epilepticus. It is also used as a sedative in doses of 30 mg twice daily.

2. Medium acting group. This includes the commonly used hypnotics. Various members of the group vary a little in their speed of onset and duration of action, but generally they produce sleep in about half an hour, which lasts about six hours.

Most commonly used are:

	Dose	
Pentobarbitone	100–200 mg	} very
Quinalbarbitone	50–200 mg	} rapidly
Heptobarbitone	200–400 mg	} metabolised
Amylobarbitone sodium	100–200 mg	} less
Butobarbitone	100–200 mg	} rapidly metabolised

The actual dose of barbiturate used will depend on the size of the patient and on any complicating factors which may modify the patient's sensitivity to the drug (see below).

3. Short acting group. This group includes thiopentone sodium and hexobarbitone sodium.

They are used for short duration anaesthesia and also for induction of anaesthesia.

Contraindications and side effects. Barbiturates should not be given to those who have previously had a hypersensitivity reaction to them. Barbiturates will precipitate an acute attack of porphyria in those with this disease.

They should be used with great care if at all in those with decreased liver function or with chronic respiratory disease. In the elderly, barbiturates may produce confusion rather than sleep.

Skin rashes are the commonest side effect with barbiturates and may take a variety of forms from irritating erythemas to bullous eruptions.

The most important side effects are overdosage and dependence.

Overdosage of barbiturates produces coma with respiratory depression. With very large doses there is also a falling blood pressure with circulatory, and ultimately, renal failure. The lethal dose is very variable, as is the fatal blood level.

In general, a blood level of more than 3.0 mg/ 100 ml with a short acting barbiturate or 10 mg/ 100 ml with phenobarbitone, suggests a seriously ill patient. Blood levels are, however, a poor guide to prognosis. It must be remembered that the effects of barbiturates will be enhanced by other CNS depressant drugs, in particular alcohol.

Dependence on barbiturates is now recognised as a serious problem. Continued taking of barbiturates in doses of 600 mg daily or more causes chronic intoxication with psychological dependence, weakness, dizziness, slurred speech, nystagmus and sometimes orthostatic hypotension. Withdrawal symptoms can be severe and include anxiety, weakness, and in particular, convulsions.

Although barbiturates are still widely used there are very few patients for whom a safer hypnotic is not available.

NON-BARBITURATE HYPNOTICS

Glutethimide

Pharmacological action. Glutethimide is related to the barbiturates but is usually called a 'non-barbiturate' hypnotic. It is fairly well absorbed from the intestinal tract and is entirely metabolised in the body. It produces sleep lasting about 6–8 hours.

Therapeutic use. Glutethimide is a useful hypnotic in doses of 250–500 mg before retiring.

Contraindications and side effects. Contraindications are similar to those for the barbiturates. Side effects are skin rashes and nausea. Rarely it may produce convulsions. Glutethimide has some cholinergic blocking effect and may interfere with bowel or bladder function. Dependence can occur.

Overdosage differs from barbiturates in that although there is some respiratory depression failing circulation with low blood pressure is a prominent feature – the pupils are also widely dilated due to the drug's anticholinergic action.

Methyprylon

Pharmacological action. Methyprylon is a piperidinedione compound related to glutethimide. Its hypnotic action is very similar to that of the barbiturates and it is almost entirely metabolised by the liver. The usual hypnotic dose is 200–400 mg.

Contraindications and side effects. Death can occur from overdosage and as with the barbiturates, dependence and tolerance can develop.

Carbromal

Pharmacological action. Carbromal is a bromine-containing derivative of urea. It is a mild, short-acting hypnotic (about 4 hours) and is given in doses of 300–900 mg. It can however, cause rashes which may be purpuric, and bromism can occur after prolonged use.

Chloral hydrate

Pharmacological action. Chloral hydrate is well absorbed from the intestine. In the body it is rapidly converted to trichlorethanol which is the main active substance. Trichlorethanol is inactivated by conversion to the glucuronide, and to trichloracetic acid. These products are excreted in the urine. Chloral produces sleep lasting about 8 hours.

Therapeutic use. Chloral is a gastric irritant and is therefore usually given well diluted in a solution such as chloral mixture BNF (10 ml contains 1.0 g) or as syrup of chloral hydrate USP. It has an unpleasant taste. The usual adult dose is 1–2 g but some adults may require a larger dose. It is particularly useful and safe as a hypnotic or sedative in children when the dose is 15–30 mg/kg bodyweight. It is also said to be less liable than the barbiturates to cause confusion in the elderly.

Contraindications and side effects. Chloral should not be used in patients with peptic ulcer, in those with severe liver disease or in renal failure. Chloral can occasionally cause rashes. Overdosage is rarely a serious problem.

There are a number of chloral compounds which are similar in action and uses to chloral. Unlike chloral however they are stable in tablet form and less liable to cause gastric irritation and are more palatable:

	Dose
Dichlorphenazone	0.65–2.0 g
Triclofos	1.0–2.0 g
Chloral betaine	870 mg–1.7 g
Chloralhexadol	0.8–1.6 g

The phenazone moiety of dichlorphenazone, which itself is a mild analgesic, can cause skin rashes and rarely agranulocytosis.

Ethchlorvynol

This mild hypnotic has a particularly rapid and short hypnotic effect. It has no special advantages but it is metabolised rather than excreted by the kidneys and might therefore be useful in renal failure. The dose is 500 mg–1.0 g orally.

Occasionally its use may be associated with some hangover and confusion.

Methylpentynol

This drug is a mild, short acting hypnotic with no particular advantages. It is a liquid and is given in capsule form and may produce a rather unpleasant tasting belch. The usual dose is 250–500 mg and large doses produce a state resembling alcoholic intoxication. Rashes may occur. Methylpentynol carbamate is similar but has a more prolonged action.

Paraldehyde

Pharmacological action. Paraldehyde is a fairly powerful and rapidly acting hypnotic. It is well absorbed from the intestinal tract and from the rectum and also after intramuscular injection. It produces sleep lasting about eight hours, and is also an anticonvulsant. It is largely metabolised in the liver but about 10% is excreted unchanged by the lungs.

Therapeutic use. Paraldehyde can be used as a hypnotic in doses of 3–8 ml orally, or as a 10% solution in normal saline rectally. It has however largely gone out of use for it tastes unpleasant, and the patient emits a particular smell for hours after administration, from the breath, urine and sweat.

It can also be given intramuscularly in doses of 4.0 ml and repeated as required to quieten noisy patients, or in status epilepticus. By this route however it is painful, and may lead to abscess formation, so again has been largely discarded.

Contraindications and side effects. Paraldehyde is nevertheless a safe drug and side effects are rare. However, dependence can occur. Paraldehyde also changes slowly to acetic acid when stored, and bottles more than six months old should be thrown away.

THE BENZODIAZEPINES

This group of drugs all have hypnotic properties although some are used primarily as tranquillisers and others primarily to induce sleep. Whether there is much to choose between them as hypnotics is open to some doubt.

Nitrazepam

Pharmacological action. Nitrazepam is a fairly quick-acting hypnotic. It is believed to depress the reticular activating system rather than the cerebral cortex and its effect on REM sleep is minimal. It is relatively non-toxic and considerable overdosage can occur without serious effects.

Therapeutic use and side effects. Nitrazepam is a useful hypnotic, as effective as the short acting barbiturates. The hypnotic action of the drug usually lasts about six hours; rarely, patients complain of some drowsiness persisting into the next day. Nitrazepam is said to be less liable to cause confusion in the elderly. The oral dose is 5–10 mg at night. In old people 2.5 mg may be sufficient.

Flurazepam

Flurazepam appears very similar to nitrazepam and has no outstanding advantages over that drug. The dose is 15–30 mg.

OTHER HYPNOTICS

Methaqualone

Pharmacological action. Methaqualone is a hypnotic similar in effectiveness to the barbiturates. Its action may last for 6–12 hours. The usual dose is 150–300 mg and toxic side effects are rare, but sleep may sometimes be preceded by transient paraesthesia. It is contraindicated in liver disease.

A combination of methaqualone 250 mg and diphenhydramine 25 mg per tablet is an effective hypnotic. Dependence, however, is not uncommon. Larger doses produce a distinctive clinical picture with coma, combined with hypertonia, myoclonia and increased tendon reflexes.

Propiomazine

Pharmacological action. Propiomazine is related to the antihistamine promethazine but differs in that it has greater sedation and hypnotic properties. The usual dose is 200 mg.
Contraindication and side effects. Propriomazine is of low toxicity but dry mouth and rashes can occur.

Chlormethiazole

Pharmacological action and therapeutic use. Chlormethiazole is a sedative and hypnotic being related structurally to Vitamin B_1. It probably acts by producing cortical depression. It can be used as a hypnotic but has proved particularly valuable in treating withdrawal symptoms in alcoholics. It has been tried with success in pre-eclamptic toxaemia, when it produces minimal fetal depression, and in status epilepticus.

As a hypnotic the dose is 2–4 tablets or capsules (500 mg of chlormethiazole). In the elderly it can be used as a sedative in doses of one capsule three times daily. In acute alcoholic withdrawal symptoms, three capsules four times daily and reduced as necessary, is usually satisfactory. Chlormethiazole can also be given by intravenous infusion.
Contraindications and side effects. The most obvious side effect is an unpleasant tingling in the nose a few minutes after administration. Occasionally it can also cause nausea. Toxicity is generally low but the action is additional with other CNS depressants.

Category 3

THE ANALGESICS

W. G. REEVES and P. AMLOT

These can be subdivided into (i) MAJOR or narcotic analgesics and (ii) MINOR or antipyretic analgesics. For certain kinds of pain other more specific measures may be indicated, e.g. carbamazepine for trigeminal neuralgia and ergot for migraine. Details will be found in the relevant sections. Certain diseases may present initially with pain as the major or only symptom, e.g. hyperparathyroidism, myxedema and depression, and prompt diagnosis and relevant treatment may give relief. The presence and nature of a pain is frequently of diagnostic help, and the administration of an analgesic should not, wherever possible, precede or overshadow history-taking, examination and diagnosis.

THE MAJOR OR NARCOTIC ANALGESICS

Opium was the earliest source of all narcotic analgesics. All the analgesic alkaloids (e.g. morphine, codeine and thebaine) were found to be phenanthrene derivatives, whereas other alkaloids (e.g. papaverine and narcotine) were inactive as analgesics (see Table 1). Other semi-synthetic and synthetic substances have since been developed and used as analgesics, yet despite wide chemical differences the pharmacological actions of all the major analgesics are very similar. For this reason morphine will be taken as the central drug of this group and discussed in some detail; the actions of the other drugs being described in relation to it.

The narcotic antagonists will also be included in this section as they are closely related to the narcotic analgesics.

Morphine

Pharmacological action. A powerful analgesic and narcotic having various stimulating and depressant actions on the nervous system. Centrally it produces euphoria and depresses the cortex, thalamus, cerebellum, respiratory and cough centres. It stimulates the vagus, vomiting centre and spinal cord and also causes constriction of

Table 1. The opiates

Useful analgesics	Related drugs with other uses
Phenanthrene derivatives	
Morphine	Apomorphine (emetic)
Diamorphine	Ethyl morphine (eye-drops)
Papaveretum	Nalorphine*
Hydromorphone	Thebaine (not used)
Oxymorphone	
Metopon	
Codeine	
Pholcodine	
Dihydrocodeine	
Hydrocodone	
Oxycodone	
Benzylisoquinoline alkaloids	
	Papaverine (vasodilator)

* Narcotic antagonist.

the pupil. Increased ADH secretion reduces the urine output and if hypercapnia develops intracranial pressure may be increased. Peripherally, morphine reduces secretions and increases tone in involuntary muscle. The latter effect is most marked in the muscle and sphincters of the gastrointestinal and biliary tracts and similar effects have been described in the urinary tract. Skin vessels are dilated and there is increased sweating.

Tolerance develops with 2–3 weeks of continuous use, chiefly in relation to its depressant actions. Physical dependence may begin even earlier leading to a withdrawal syndrome on stopping the drug. If use of the drug is prolonged overt addiction may develop.

Morphine is metabolised in the liver and excreted chiefly into the urine but also into the gut via the bile. Its analgesic effect is maximal at about 1 hour and lasts for 3–4 hours.

Therapeutic use. Morphine sulphate is the most frequently used preparation for oral or parenteral use but other salts are available:

Oral preparations: Morphine sulphate
Morphine hydrochloride
Parenteral preparations: Morphine sulphate
Morphine tartrate
Morphine acetate

The dose for all these preparations is roughly the same and is usually 10–15 mg. Absorption from the gastrointestinal tract is often unreliable and subcutaneous or intramuscular injection is more effective. Morphine can also be given as a slow intravenous injection.

It is used to relieve pain which is not amenable to the milder analgesics and is of particular value when this is associated with anxiety and restlessness. Its use in patients suffering from haemorrhage, trauma or shock, who are not troubled by pain, is of doubtful merit in view of the well-documented tendency for morphine to lower the blood pressure. However, it is difficult to deny its good effect when given to patients with gastrointestinal haemorrhage and other factors may play a part here. It relieves the dyspnea of cardiac asthma and is also used to suppress unwanted coughing, to control diarrhea and as a premedication (with hyoscine or atropine) before surgery.

The euphoriant effect is used in the management of terminal disease and where this is associated with severe pain, chlorpromazine produces a useful synergistic effect as well as having a mild anti-emetic action. In cases where respiratory depression or undue somnolence becomes a problem an analeptic such as amiphenazole (q.v.) may be used with morphine to good effect.
Contraindications and side effects. Morphine should not be used in the presence of respiratory depression, cyanosis, obstructive airways disease, hepatic insufficiency, acute alcoholism, toxic confusional states, convulsive disorders or raised intracranial pressure. It is unwise to give it alone for cholecystitis, biliary disorders, pancreatitis or diverticulitis, but increased smooth muscle activity can be offset by combination with propantheline. It is badly tolerated by patients with myxedema and the elderly and debilitated. Its action is enhanced by monoamine oxidase inhibitors, neostigmine, chlorpromazine, barbiturates and alcohol. Potentiation occurs with hypotensive agents.

Side effects include: nausea and vomiting (especially if not resting in bed), constipation, tremors, restlessness, insomnia and rarely convulsions. The nausea and vomiting can be readily prevented by the co-administration of an anti-emetic such as cyclizine tartrate (50 mg). Itching and urticaria occur as well as other rashes. Hypotension which may be postural is usually mild but is often pronounced when the drug is given to patients following myocardial infarction. Toxic doses produce respiratory depression, cyanosis, hypotension, pin-point pupils and coma. These effects are best treated by an injection of one of the specific antagonists nalorphine or levallorphan (see later).

Diamorphine (heroin)
Pharmacological action. Slightly more potent than morphine. It has an earlier onset and shorter duration of action (about 2 hours). It more readily produces euphoria, is a powerful anti-tussive and respiratory depressant but is probably less likely to cause vomiting or constipation.
Therapeutic use. It may be given as an elixir or linctus in a dose of 5–10 mg or by injection in a dose of 3–6 mg initially. It is not available in some countries because of the problem of addiction. It is favoured by some for the pain of acute myocardial infarction. It is most often used for terminal disease and occasionally for post-operative analgesia and sedation.
Contraindications and side effects. As morphine; it has often been thought to be more addictive than morphine but this point is still debated.

Papaveretum (total extract of opium)
Pharmacological action. Very similar to morphine which forms most of the active part of this preparation. However it is better tolerated and is said to cause less respiratory depression and vomiting.
Therapeutic use. As morphine. Dose: 10–20 mg orally or i.m.
Contraindications and side effects. As morphine.

Hydromorphone
Pharmacological action. Very similar to morphine, being slightly more potent and having a shorter duration of action.
Therapeutic use. As morphine. Dose: 2–5 mg orally; 2 mg by injection.
Contraindications and side effects. As morphine.

Oxymorphone
Pharmacological action. Slightly more potent than morphine and producing more euphoria, respiratory depression, nausea and vomiting.
Therapeutic use. Dose: 5–10 mg orally; 1.5–5 mg i.m. or s.c.

Metopon
Pharmacological action. A narcotic analgesic about twice as potent as morphine but in all other respects the same. Dose: 3–6 mg.

Codeine
Pharmacological action. Analgesic but much less potent than morphine. It is a mild hypnotic but

does not depress the respiratory centre or constipate as much as morphine. It is an effective cough suppressant. Little of it is metabolised in the body, most appearing in the urine.

Therapeutic use. It is used as the hydrochloride, phosphate or sulphate and the dose for all three salts is 10–60 mg. It is taken as a tablet, linctus or i.m. injection. It is most useful for the control of less severe pain, unwanted cough and diarrhea. It does show a synergistic action with aspirin and is often prepared in combination with the antipyretic analgesics.

Contraindications and side effects. Less than morphine. Overdosage gives a different picture consisting of narcosis often preceded by exhilaration and excitement and followed by convulsions. Nausea and vomiting are prominent, the pupils constrict and there is a tachycardia.

Pholcodine

Pharmacological action. A derivative of morphine with almost no analgesic action. It does not suppress respiration but is an effective cough suppressant.

Dihydrocodeine

Pharmacological action. It has a shorter duration of action and is less potent than morphine. Is as good a cough suppressant as codeine.

Therapeutic use. Preparations:
Dihydrocodeine phosphate – dose 10–30 mg
Dihydrocodeine bitartrate – dose 10–60 mg
It can be given as a linctus, tablet, i.m. or s.c. injection. It has few side effects; contraindications as morphine.

Hydrocodone

Pharmacological action. Intermediate in action between morphine and codeine. It is chiefly used as a cough suppressant.

Therapeutic use. It is used as the phosphate, hydrochloride or acid tartrate. The dose for each is 5–15 mg orally but it can also be given as a s.c. injection.

Oxycodone

Pharmacological action. A moderately strong analgesic, slightly more potent and possibly more addicting than codeine.

Therapeutic use. Preparations:
Oxycodone hydrochloride – dose 5–30 mg orally; 5 mg by injection
Oxycodone pectinate – dose i.m. 10–20 mg
The latter acts for much longer (up to 10 hours).

Contraindications and side effects. As morphine.

Nalorphine

Pharmacological action. It is a specific narcotic analgesic antagonist reducing or abolishing most of the actions of morphine and all the major analgesics. It does not antagonise the depressant effect on the cough centre and hence there is little evidence of antagonism with pholcodine and other anti-tussives which have little analgesic effect. It acts within a few seconds of intravenous injection, increasing the rate and volume of respiration and can awaken a patient from a narcotic state. It reverses the rise in biliary pressure and miosis but has similar analgesic properties to morphine. It is not effective in reversing depression produced by barbiturates, cyclopropane or ether.

Therapeutic use. Dose: 5–10 mg i.v. as either the hydrochloride or hydrobromide. It is used particularly to treat overdosage with narcotic analgesics and in severe cases much larger doses may be required. It has also been used in a test for narcotic analgesic addiction in which the reversing effect on pupil size is noted. If given to an addict it will precipitate withdrawal symptoms.

It is also used to prevent respiratory depression in the newborn. It can be given i.v. 10 mg to the mother 10 minutes before delivery or injected directly into the umbilical vein immediately after birth (0.25–1 mg).

Contraindications and side effects. If given on its own it may cause respiratory depression and disturbing psychotic effects. In addicts to morphine and its derivatives it will produce withdrawal symptoms. Side effects include drowsiness, irritability, miosis, nausea, pallor, sweating and hypotension.

Table 2.   Phenylheptylamine derivatives

Useful analgesics	Related drugs with other uses
Methadone	
Phenadoxone	
Propoxyphene (d-propoxyphene)	l-Propoxyphene (anti-tussive)
Dextromoramide	
Dipipanone	

Methadone

Pharmacological action. A potent analgesic similar to morphine but with less sedative effect and a longer duration of action. It is more reliably absorbed from the gastrointestinal tract.

Therapeutic use. Dose: orally 5–10 mg; i.m. 5–10 mg; linctus 1–2 mg doses. It is not used intravenously. It is useful for severe pain and unproductive cough. It is not suitable as a premedication unless combined with a short-acting barbiturate or hyoscine. It has been used in the rehabilitation of morphine and heroin addicts as withdrawal from it is less unpleasant, probably because of its longer duration of action. *Contraindications and side effects.* As with morphine nausea, vomiting, dizziness, respiratory depression and constriction of the pupils occur, although it less readily produces constipation. It may lower the blood pressure and children tolerate it poorly. It is not recommended for use in obstetrics as it significantly depresses fetal respiration.

Phenadoxone

Pharmacological action. An effective analgesic with a mild hypnotic effect. It reduces smooth muscle activity and does not cause constipation in normal doses. Orally it acts within 15–30 minutes and lasts for 1–3 hours. When used parenterally there may be considerable irritation at injection sites. It is not used intravenously.
Therapeutic use. Dose: orally 10–30 mg; i.m. or s.c. 5–15 mg.
Contraindications and side effects. As for methadone.

Propoxyphene

Pharmacological action. It is chemically similar to methadone but is only a mild analgesic having a similar onset, duration of action and potency to codeine. It is not anti-tussive.
Therapeutic use. Dose: 30–60 mg orally. It is used for mild to moderate pain associated with chronic and recurrent disease. It is often combined with aspirin or paracetamol for this purpose.
Contraindications and side effects. Nausea and vomiting occur less than with codeine although it does cause constipation. In large doses it causes drowsiness, dizziness, general excitement, mental confusion, twitching, respiratory depression, convulsions and coma. Local irritation occurs if given subcutaneously. It is only mildly addictive but can block the withdrawal effects of morphine and is antagonised by nalorphine.

Dextromoramide

Pharmacological action. A strong analgesic, slightly more powerful than morphine and with a similar duration of actions. It is well absorbed by mouth.
Therapeutic use. Preparations: alone or as the acid tartrate (5 mg dextromoramide ≡ 6.9 mg D-acid tartrate). Dose: 5–20 mg orally or i.m. It may also be given by s.c. or i.v. injection or administered rectally.
Contraindications and side effects. As for morphine but respiratory depression is not evident with oral therapeutic doses.

Dipipanone

Pharmacological action. A potent analgesic of similar strength to morphine with a more rapid onset but a similar duration of action. There is less respiratory depression and it is effective orally.
Therapeutic use. Dose: 25–50 mg s.c. or i.m. Oral tablets of 10 mg are usually combined with cyclizine 30 mg.

Table 3. Phenylpiperidine derivatives

Useful analgesics	Related drugs with other uses
Pethidine	Diphenoxylate (costive)
Alphaprodine	
Anileridine	
Piminidone	
Fentanyl	
Phenoperidine	
Ethoheptazine	

Pethidine

Pharmacological action. An effective analgesic but less potent and with about half the duration of action of morphine. It is only a mild sedative, euphoria is less marked and dysphoric sensations are more likely to occur. It does not affect the size of the pupil in therapeutic doses and is a poor cough suppressant. It does not cause constipation but its effect on smooth muscle is similar to morphine. It reduces the severity of labour pains without diminishing the force of uterine contraction but like most other major analgesics it prolongs labour.
Therapeutic use. Dose: orally 50–100 mg; s.c. or i.m. 25–100 mg and i.v. 25–50 mg. It is used as an alternative to morphine to relieve pain; for obstetric analgesia and in conjunction with barbiturates or hyoscine to produce obstetric amnesia. It is also used commonly for pre- and post-operative medication. Pethidine (50 mg) has been combined with levallorphan tartrate (0.625 mg) as an injection. This was primarily designed for use in obstetrics but is only of marginal benefit. In view of its effect on smooth muscle it should be given with propantheline for the treatment of visceral colic.
Contraindications and side effects. Nausea and

vomiting are as frequent as with comparable doses of morphine but constipation is less. The blood pressure may fall after i.v. administration and this is especially noticeable in patients with acute myocardial infarction. Pethidine can cause excitement and dysphoria especially with over-dosage when incoordination, tremor, convulsions, respiratory depression and coma may supervene. Its action is potentiated by mono-amine oxidase inhibitors and phenothiazines. There is a danger of addiction.

Alphaprodine

Pharmacological action. It has similar potency and action to pethidine but is more rapid in onset and of shorter duration. Given subcutaneously and with an adequate peripheral circulation it will have an analgesic effect within 5 minutes lasting for about 2 hours.
Therapeutic use. Dose: s.c. 20–60 mg and i.v. 20–30 mg. It is used chiefly in obstetrics and for premedication and minor surgical procedures.
Contraindications and side effects. Dizziness, itching and sweating occur but nausea, vomiting and respiratory depressions are less likely than with morphine. However, it will cause depression of fetal respiration if given within 2 hours of delivery.

Anileridine

Pharmacological action. Similar but less potent than morphine. It is rapidly absorbed by mouth and acts more quickly and for a shorter time than morphine.
Therapeutic use. Preparations: orally anileridine hydrochloride dose 25 mg; s.c. or i.v. anileridine phosphate dose 25–50 mg. It is used as a shorter acting analgesic especially as a premedication and in obstetrics.
Contraindications and side effects. Similar to morphine but it tends to cause more restlessness and less nausea, vomiting and constipation.

Fentanyl

Pharmacological action. A very potent analgesic with a rapid onset and brief duration of action. It causes respiratory depression and has an emetic effect.
Therapeutic use. Dose: 0.1–0.6 mg i.v. It has been primarily used in association with tranquillizers such as triperidol and droperidol to produce brief surgical anaesthesia especially in young, old and debilitated patients. They block the emetic effect and the general effects are antagonised by nalorphine.
Contraindications and side effects. As morphine.

Phenoperidine

Pharmacological action. A potent analgesic which in large doses produces sedation and respiratory suppression.
Therapeutic use. I.m. or i.v. 0.5–1 mg for analgesia; 2–5 mg where respiratory depression is desired. It is used in similar situations to fentanyl in combination with a 'neuroleptic' agent, e.g. droperidol (q.v.) to produce surgical anaesthesia. It is of particular value for sedation during artificial ventilation.
Contraindications and side effects. As morphine.

Ethoheptazine

Pharmacological action. An analgesic of equivalent strength to codeine. It is not anti-tussive or a respiratory suppressant and does not sedate. It acts within 30 minutes and lasts for 4–5 hours.
Therapeutic use. Dose: 75–150 mg orally. It is used chiefly in conjunction with aspirin or paracetamol.
Contraindications and side effects. Similar to morphine but appears not to be addictive.

Table 4. Morphinans and benzmorphans

Useful analgesics	Related drugs with other uses
Morphinans	
Levorphanol (l-methorphan)	d-Methorphan (anti-tussive) Levallorphan *
Benzmorphans Phenazocine Pentazocine	

* Narcotic antagonist.

Levorphanol

Pharmacological action. A potent analgesic similar to morphine but causing less drowsiness. It is as effective by mouth as it is by injection.
Therapeutic use. Dose: orally 1.5–4.5 mg; i.m. or s.c. 2–4 mg and i.v. 1–1.5 mg. It is used as an alternative to morphine and can be used for premedication (2 mg s.c.) with atropine or hyoscine.
Contraindications and side effects. As morphine.

Levallorphan

Pharmacological action. A narcotic antagonist having similar effects to nalorphine but with a greater potency and longer duration of action. Small doses antagonise the respiratory depression of narcotic drugs—larger doses also antagonising the analgesic effect.

Therapeutic use. Dose: 1–2 mg i.v. with further doses as necessary. It is often used to reverse respiratory depression in the newborn when it is given to the mother (1–2 mg) 10 minutes before delivery or directly into the umbilical vein (0.05–0.25 mg) of the infant.

Contraindications and side effects. As for nalorphine.

Phenazocine

Pharmacological action. An analgesic of similar potency and actions to morphine. It is less sedative but may cause more respiratory depression.

Therapeutic use. Dose: orally 5 mg i.m. or i.v. 1–4 mg. It may be superior for obstetric use but otherwise has been used as an alternative to morphine.

Contraindications and side effects. Similar to morphine but usually less marked. Facial pruritus may follow i.v. injection.

Pentazocine

Pharmacological action. This drug was developed as an antagonist to phenazocine and was found to be a powerful analgesic itself of a similar potency to morphine. It is also a sedative and depresses respiration when given parenterally. However, it appears to be much less addictive and does not lower the blood pressure unlike most of the other strong analgesics.

Therapeutic use. Dose: orally 25–100 mg; s.c. or i.m. 30–60 mg and i.v. 20–30 mg. It can be used as an alternative to morphine and in a comparison with morphine, diamorphine, methadone and pethidine it was the only drug which did not tend to lower the blood pressure, other side effects being much the same for all these drugs. However, a significant rise in pulmonary artery as well as aortic pressure has been recorded after the administration of 30–60 mg i.v. and a similar effect is seen with intramuscular doses. In view of this pentazocine would seem not to be the drug of choice for acute myocardial infarction despite its other advantages. There is no reason to suppose that these effects can cause harm in patients with a normal cardiovascular system.

It also has a shorter duration of action than morphine, being effective for around 4 hours.

Pentazocine has been shown to be equivalent to pethidine for the management of labour.

Contraindications and side effects. Similar to morphine apart from its low addiction potential. There have been several reports of transient but disturbing hallucinations. It is not antagonised by nalorphine and it is recommended that methyl phenidate (see later) be given as an antidote instead.

Table 5 Equivalent doses of the major analgesics* (in mg)

Morphine	10	Dextromoramide	5–7.5
Diamorphine	5	Dipipanone	20–25
Hydromorphone	2	Pethidine	75
Oxymorphone	1	Alphaprodine	40–60
Metopon	3.5	Anileridine	30–40
Codeine	120	Piminidone	7.5–10
Dihydrocodeine	60	Phenoperidine	1.5
Oxycodone	10–15	Levorphanol	3
Methadone	10	Phenazocine	2–3
Phenadoxone	10–20	Pentazocine	30

*These doses represent that dose which when given subcutaneously produces an analgesic effect approximately equivalent to 10 mg subcutaneous morphine.

THE MINOR OR ANTIPYRETIC ANALGESICS

Nearly all share analgesic, antipyretic and antirheumatic (anti-inflammatory) properties. These drugs are free of addiction potential, although patients can become habituated to their use. Their exact site of action is still not entirely clear. Vasodilatation, whether produced centrally or peripherally, causes much of the antipyretic activity. The salicylates and probably most other drugs in this group are believed to exert their analgesic action by preventing the release of prostaglandins. In the case of salicylates this is thought to occur both peripherally where it reduces inflammation, and in the brain where it prevents the perception of pain. The action of paracetamol is believed to be confined to the brain and thus it has no anti-inflammatory action.

THE SALICYLATES

Acetylsalicylic acid (aspirin)

Pharmacological action. An effective minor analgesic with considerable antipyretic and anti-inflammatory properties. In large doses it is uricosuric. In smaller doses it causes uric acid retention. It also has a mild hypoglycaemic and hypoprothrombinaemic action. It is rapidly metabolised to salicylic acid which is probably responsible for most of its effects. Both acids are excreted rapidly in the urine and the more so if this is kept alkaline. Its effect lasts for about 4 hours.

Therapeutic use. Doses: 300–1200 mg orally. It is the most effective and useful of the minor analgesics and is used for all kinds of less severe pain, e.g. headache, neuralgia, rheumatic and muscle pains. It is of particular use for acute and chronic rheumatism. In these conditions doses of up to 4–8 g a day are used, although in the chronic situation much less will often suffice. It has been used for gout but is inferior to the other uricosuric agents.

Contraindications and side effects. Gastric irritation is the commonest problem and may be accompanied by occult blood loss. Occasionally frank haematemesis and melaena occur. With larger doses, dizziness, tinnitus, deafness, sweating, nausea and vomiting may develop. In sensitive patients salicylates may precipitate attacks of asthma, angio-neurotic edema and other allergy. Therapeutic doses produce minor platelet abnormalities and long-term use has caused pancytopenia. Toxic doses cause hyperthermia, hyperventilation, excitement, coma and convulsions. Complex and changing acid–base disturbances also accompany overdosage. Salicylates should not be given to patients having a history of dyspepsia or peptic ulceration, known sensitivity, asthma or severe renal disease.

Other preparations have been made to try and overcome the irritant effect on the stomach, e.g. aluminium acetylsalicylate and calcium acetylsalicylate. The latter is more soluble, better absorbed and less irritant than acetylsalicylic acid. It is the usual form of 'Soluble Aspirin', containing acetylsalicylic acid, calcium carbonate and citric acid, which on dissolving gives a solution of calcium acetylsalicylate. Aloxiprin is a polymeric condensation product of aluminium hydroxide and acetylsalicylic acid and is also better tolerated.

Various forms of buffered aspirin have been developed but they have little advantage over calcium aspirin. Absorption of aspirin in the small intestine does not appear to cause the irritation and bleeding seen in the gastric mucosa, thus enteric coated and esterified forms of aspirin have been produced which reduce chronic blood loss considerably. These preparations are valuable in patients requiring chronic therapy. Examples are Safapryn in which the aspirin is coated with paracetamol, and benorylate which is an ester of paracetamol and aspirin.

Sodium salicylate

Pharmacological action. Similar to aspirin but less analgesic and a more effective antipyretic. It is more irritant to the stomach.

Therapeutic use. Dose: 600–2000 mg. It has been used for acute rheumatic fever in doses of 5–10 g daily, but aspirin is more suitable for rheumatoid arthritis in view of its greater analgesic activity.

Contraindications and side effects. As aspirin.

PARA-AMINOPHENOL DERIVATIVES

Paracetamol

Pharmacological action. An effective analgesic and antipyretic of similar potency to aspirin. It has little anti-inflammatory activity, less side effects and does not cause gastric irritation. It is not uricosuric.

Therapeutic use. Dose: 500–1000 mg as tablets or elixir. It is used widely for all kinds of mild pain and is the drug of choice when aspirin is contraindicated. It is contained in many combined analgesic preparations.

Contraindications and side effects. These are few and rarely troublesome. Overdosage causes severe hepatic damage and death occurs as a result of liver failure. Unfortunately paracetamol is largely metabolised by the liver so that with overdosage its metabolism is delayed. Recent work suggests that hepatic toxicity can be blocked by cysteamine.

Phenacetin

Pharmacological action. Similar to paracetamol. Most of its action is due to the formation of paracetamol *in vivo*.

Therapeutic use. Dose: 300–600 mg. It is a common constituent of analgesic combinations.

Contraindications and side effects. Its toxic effects are similar to acetanilide (see later) and are due to small amounts of aniline being formed. This may cause methaemoglobinaemia and a haemolytic anaemia.

Analgesic nephropathy. Renal damage consisting of interstitial nephritis and papillary necrosis was first described in Sweden, where patients had been taking large amounts of phenacetin over long periods. Since then the disorder has been reported from all over the world, although there are differences in incidence between countries. Large quantities of phenacetin are needed to cause this damage and most of these patients have taken well over a kilogram of phenacetin over the years.

There is considerable difference of opinion as to whether other mild analgesics, particularly aspirin and paracetamol, can also produce similar changes in the kidney. Although it is possible with these analgesics to produce renal damage in animals, studies in rheumatology clinics, where aspirin and paracetamol are used in high dosage over long periods, suggest that they do not affect the kidneys.

Acetanilide

Pharmacological action. As with the case of phenacetin its action is very largely due to the formation of paracetamol by the liver.

Therapeutic use. Dose: 120–300 mg. It used to be included in most headache powders but has latterly been replaced because of its toxicity.

Contraindications and side effects. Toxicity is chiefly due to the liberation of aniline which causes methaemoglobinaemia. Large doses produce cyanosis, cardiovascular depression and collapse.

PYRAZOLONE DERIVATIVES

Phenazone

Pharmacological action. An effective minor analgesic having a more rapid and transient action than phenacetin, although like the other drugs in this group it is more potent than the salicylates. It is antipyretic and anti-inflammatory and in large doses uricosuric. Like the other uricosuric agents it may cause uric acid retention in low dosage.

Therapeutic use. Dose: 300–600 mg. It is used as an alternative to aspirin and forms part of many combined remedies.

Contraindications and side effects. Rashes are common and some types of erythematous eruption leave residual pigmentation. Methaemoglobinaemia and cyanosis is a rare complication. Toxic doses produce nausea, fainting and collapse. Prolonged administration has led to agranulocytosis. It is nevertheless one of the least toxic drugs of this group.

Aminopyrine

Pharmacological action and side effects. In action in resembles phenazone but this drug has been withdrawn from general use because of the high incidence of agranulocytosis.

Phenylbutazone

Pharmacological action. It is analgesic, antipyretic, anti-inflammatory and uricosuric. It is hydroxylated *in vivo* to form oxyphenbutazone.

Therapeutic use. Dose: orally 200–400 mg daily in divided doses, taken with food or milk. It can also be given i.m. in a dose of 600 mg (prepared with xylocaine) and rectally as 250 mg suppositories. It is used particularly for arthritic pain in association with rheumatoid arthritis, osteoarthritis, ankylosing spondylitis, psoriasis and gout.

Contraindications and side effects. Untoward reactions are common. They include nausea, stomatitis, epigastric pain, diarrhea, vertigo and edema. The latter is due to sodium retention and may be offset by a low salt diet or a diuretic. Reactivation of peptic ulcers with perforation, haematemesis and melaena may occur. Less often agranulocytosis, thrombocytopenia, aplastic anaemia and a macrocytic anaemia responding to folic acid have occurred and a possible link with leukaemia is still uncertain. Hepatitis, acute renal failure and skin rashes have also been described.

Severe hypoprothrombinaemia occurs in people who are also being treated with coumarin anticoagulants and this may give rise to serious complications. This effect is due to competitive binding of these drugs to plasma albumin.

Phenylbutazone should not be given to patients with known cardiac, liver or renal disease, or to those with a history of peptic ulceration, blood dyscrasia or allergy. It should not be used with gold salts.

Oxyphenbutazone

Pharmacological action and therapeutic use. A derivative of phenylbutazone with similar effects and uses. It is less effective in relieving stiffness or pain in rheumatoid arthritis or ankylosing spondylitis, but it is better tolerated. Dose: 300–600 mg daily in divided doses, taken with meals.

Contraindications and side effects. Similar to phenylbutazone but less severe.

Sulphinpyrazone (see page 41)

Pharmacological action and therapeutic use. A marked uricosuric agent with little direct analgesic or anti-inflammatory effect. It has been used for chronic gout in an initial dose of 50 mg q.d.s. with meals. This is increased to 500 mg daily over a period of a week and reduced to about 200 mg daily when controlled.

Contraindications and side effects. Gastrointestinal symptoms occur but are less severe than with phenylbutazone and blood dyscrasias are rare. It should not be used in the presence of impaired renal function or peptic ulceration. Salicylates reduce its effect.

Nifenazone

Pharmacological action and therapeutic use. A pyrazolone chemically resembling aminopyrine, having analgesic, antipyretic and anti-inflammatory effects. It is inferior to phenylbutazone or oxyphenbutazone. Dose: orally 250–500 mg 1, 2 or 3 times daily. 400 mg suppositories are available for rectal use.

Contraindications and side effects. Gastrointestinal symptoms may occur and in view of its chemical relationships blood dyscrasias are a possibility.

Phenyramidol

Pharmacological action, therapeutic use and side effects. A moderate analgesic which like phenylbutazone can cause serious hypoprothombinaemia in patients on anticoagulant therapy. Dose: 200–400 mg. It may also cause nausea, dyspepsia, drowsiness, pruritus and skin rashes. It is contraindicated in patients having salicylate sensitivity.

QUINOLINE DERIVATIVES

Cinchophen and neocinchophen

Pharmacological action and therapeutic use. Both these extracts from quinine or cinchona bark are analgesic and antipyretic and of similar potency to the salicylates. Neocinchophen is more uricosuric and they were both used for chronic gout although more effective agents are now available. Dose: 200–500 mg.

Contraindications and side effects. Similar to the salicylates. In addition even therapeutic doses can cause hepatitis.

COLCHICINE DERIVATIVES

Colchicine

Pharmacological action. An alkaloid from meadow saffron which is analgesic for acute gout. It is also anti-mitotic but has little effect in leukaemia, although demecolcine (see later) has been used for leukaemia.

Therapeutic use. Doses for acute gout: 1 mg stat. followed by 0.5 mg 2-hourly until pain ceases or vomiting or diarrhea develops.

Contraindications and side effects. Stomatitis, nausea, vomiting, abdominal pain, and diarrhea. It should be avoided in the old and feeble and in those with gastrointestinal disorders.

INDOLE DERIVATIVE

Indomethacin

Pharmacological action. This indole derivative is an effective analgesic, antipyretic and anti-inflammatory agent of value in acute gout and various forms of arthritis. It is not recommended as a general analgesic.

Therapeutic use. Dose: orally starting with 25 mg daily and increasing to 25 mg three times daily. It can also be used as 100 mg suppositories. Its chief route of elimination is via the kidneys and the dose will therefore require modification in the presence of renal insufficiency. For acute gout 50 mg is recommended orally followed by 25 mg 6-hourly.

Contraindications and side effects. These are frequent but usually less serious than those found with phenylbutazone. They include dizziness, headache, vertigo, drowsiness, confusion, psychiatric disturbances, anorexia, nausea, vomiting, dyspepsia, diarrhea, gastrointestinal bleeding and

corneal and retinal changes which are usually reversible. Pruritus, rashes and edema also occur and a reversible leucopenia has been described in patients with rheumatoid arthritis. Deaths have occurred in children treated with indomethacin and it is now only recommended for adult use.

THE FENAMATES
Mefenamic acid

Pharmacological action. A derivative of anthranilic acid which is analgesic, antipyretic and anti-inflammatory. Its analgesic effect is greater than aspirin or paracetamol and roughly equivalent to codeine. Its anti-inflammatory activity is less powerful than phenylbutazone. Its effect comes on 1 hour after an oral dose and lasts for up to 6 hours.

Therapeutic use. Dose: 250–500 mg q.d.s. It is used as a general analgesic as well as supplementing other measures used for arthritic pain.

Contraindications and side effects. Diarrhea is the most common side effect but is usually reversible. It occurs in 10–20% of cases. Reversible leucopenia, haemolytic anaemia and maculopapular rashes have been described. Gastric irritation occurs but is much less frequent or troublesome than with aspirin. Elevation of the blood urea may occur and renal papillary necrosis has been described in animal studies.

Flufenamic acid

Pharmacological action. Similar to mefenamic acid but less analgesic and antipyretic and more anti-inflammatory.

Therapeutic use. Dose: 100–120 mg t.d.s. It is most useful for arthritic pain.

Contraindications and side effects. It also tends to cause diarrhea in some patients and occasionally produces dyspeptic symptoms.

OTHER ANTI-INFLAMMATORY AGENTS

These are a new group of substances derived from aryl substitution of esters, phenols, or enols. They all have anti-inflammatory activity which is thought due to a prostaglandin inhibitory effect. They are indicated in the treatment of chronic inflammatory diseases particularly rheumatoid arthritis.

Propionic acid derivatives

Pharmacological action and therapeutic use. All these drugs have a similar potency comparable at the above dose ranges to 4 g of aspirin daily. Naproxen has the advantage of a longer duration of action requiring only b.d. dosage.

	Dose
Ibuprofen:	100–200 mg t.d.s.
Ketoprofen:	50 mg q.d.s.
Fenoprofen:	400–600 mg q.d.s.
Naproxen:	250 mg b.d.

Contraindications and side effects. They all cause less gastric irritation than aspirin but severe gastrointestinal bleeding has been reported in a number of patients so they should probably be avoided in patients giving a history of peptic ulceration.

They displace warfarin from its protein binding sites so care should be taken in patients receiving anticoagulants.

Alcofenac (arylacetic acid)

Pharmacological action and therapeutic use. Preliminary data suggest that this drug may be slightly more potent than the previous group. Its potency at a dosage of 1.5–3.0 g is equivalent to 300 mg of phenylbutazone and whereas the previous group of drugs do not appear to affect joint size in rheumatoid arthritis, alcofenac is as effective as phenylbutazone.

Side effects. It likewise causes less gastric irritation. Transient morbilliform rashes at the beginning of treatment have been recorded in a number of patients.

GOLD

Sodium aurothiomalate, aurothioglucose and aurothioglycanide

Pharmacological action and therapeutic use. These three preparations will be considered collectively. Their action is uncertain but they have a long-lasting effect on rheumatoid arthritis especially in the early stages. Gold is ineffective in other kinds of arthritis.

Dose: after a test of 10 mg i.m., weekly injections increasing by an increment of 10 mg up to 50 mg are given, usually up to a total dose of

1 g although injections may be continued indefinitely, preferably at a reduced dose. The dosage required with aurothioglycanide may be a little higher.

Contraindications and side effects. Toxic effects occur in at least 30% of cases and include pruritus, urticaria, purpura, dermatitis which may exfoliate, stomatitis which may ulcerate and less commonly thrombocytopenia, aplastic anaemia, hepatic and renal damage, peripheral neuropathy and an encephalopathy may develop. The urine should be examined for protein before each injection and blood counts made every 2–3 weeks. Gold therapy should be stopped as soon as any toxic effect appears. Serious toxic effects should be treated with dimercaprol (q.v.). Corticosteroids may be useful, especially for a severe dermatitis.

Gold should not be used in the presence of known renal or hepatic damage, anaemia, blood dyscrasias, skin diseases or any serious illness.

ANTIMALARIALS

Chloroquine phosphate and hydroxychloroquine sulphate

Pharmacological action. Their mode of action is unknown. They have a beneficial effect in up to 50% of cases of rheumatoid arthritis.

Therapeutic use. Doses:

Chloroquine phosphate—orally 250–750 mg daily initially, and 150 mg daily for maintenance.

Hydroxychloroquine sulphate—orally 800–1200 mg daily initially and 200 mg daily for maintenance.

Contraindications and side effects. Toxic effects include nausea, vomiting, dizziness, diarrhea and blurring of vision. After continued use bleached hair, rashes, corneal opacities and retinal degeneration may develop. The latter may be irreversible.

During treatment a six-monthly ophthalmic examination is mandatory in order to detect presymptomatic corneal or retinal damage. Eighth nerve damage also occurs. These drugs should not be given during pregnancy.

CORTICOSTEROIDS

Some of these agents have a powerful anti-inflammatory effect which is discussed later.

Category 4

DRUGS AFFECTING THE AUTONOMIC NERVOUS SYSTEM AND MOTOR END-PLATE

W. G. REEVES and J. R. TROUNCE

When considering the drugs which affect the autonomic nervous system and motor end-plate, it is useful to think in terms of four basic kinds of neuronal connection between the central nervous system and the end-organ. These are displayed diagrammatically below. The chemical transmitter at the first synapse in each case is acetylcholine. All these sites are 'nicotinic' as the effects of transmission can be mimicked by

Table 1

α *Effects*	β *Effects*
VASOCONSTRICTION particularly in skin and gut producing a rise in systolic and diastolic blood pressure with reflex slowing of the heart MYDRIASIS ADRENERGIC SWEATING	β_1 increased rate and force of contraction of the HEART β_2 BRONCHODILATATION VASODILATATION particularly of coronary vessels and vessels in skeletal muscle

The drugs affecting the autonomic nervous system and motor end-plate will be discussed under the following headings:

1. Sympathomimetic drugs.

2. Anti-adrenergic drugs:
   (a) Post-ganglionic neurone blockers.
   (b) α- and β-receptor blocking agents.

3. Parasympathomimetic drugs.
   (a) Choline esters.
   (b) Choline-esterase inhibitors.
   (c) Pilocarpine.

4. Anti-cholinergic drugs:
   (a) Ganglion-blocking agents.
   (b) Neuromuscular-blocking agents.
   (c) Drugs blocking muscarinic sites (atropine and related drugs).

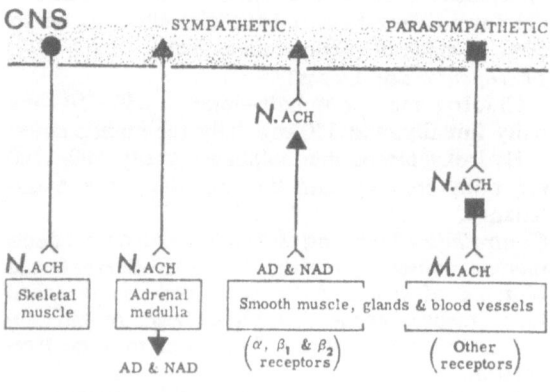

N=nicotinic; M=muscarinic; ACH=acetylcholine;
AD=adrenaline; NAD=noradrenaline

nicotine-like substances. The second synapse in the parasympathetic pathway is rather different and although dependent on acetylcholine as transmitter it is also stimulated by muscarine-like substances. In the sympathetic pathway adrenaline and noradrenaline are the second synapse transmitter and the various end-organ receptors have been classified into α and β chiefly according to whether their effect is an excitatory or inhibitory one. This classification has proved useful but has required a little modification.

SYMPATHOMIMETIC DRUGS

Adrenaline

Pharmacological action. Both α and β receptors are stimulated, its action resembling the activity of the sympathetic nervous system itself. Its α effects are to constrict blood vessels in skin and viscera, dilate the pupil and release glucose from the liver. The β effects are to increase the rate and force of contraction of the heart, dilate blood vessels in muscle and heart and dilate the bronchi.

Like noradrenaline, it is inactive by mouth but has a rapid onset and short duration of action after subcutaneous injection.

Therapeutic use. It is generally used as the acid tartrate or the hydrochloride. Dose: s.c. or i.m. 0.4–1 mg. It is often used locally in dilute solutions of varying strengths from 1 : 200 000 to 1 : 1000 depending on the situation. It is not given intravenously. It is used to stop or reduce capillary bleeding both during and after surgery; to reduce nasal congestion; in combination with local anaesthetics (e.g. procaine) to prolong their action; to produce bronchodilatation in asthma; to counteract anaphylactic shock and other less serious allergic manifestations, e.g. urticaria, hay fever and angioneurotic edema and to reverse heart block with syncope or even cardiac arrest. In the latter case it is often given as an intra-cardiac injection. It is also used in eye drops for retinoscopy and for open-angle (chronic simple) glaucoma in which situation it lowers the intra-ocular pressure. In narrow angle glaucoma it may increase the pressure.

Contraindications and side effects. It may produce feelings of anxiety, restlessness, palpitations, tachycardia, tremors, weakness, dizziness, headache and cold extremities. In excess it can cause cardiac arrhythmias and gangrene of extremities. It should not be used in very nervous or anxious patients or those with hypertension, ischaemic heart disease, hyperthyroidism, or in conjunction with trichlorethylene, halothane or cyclopropane. It is best avoided in patients who are receiving monoamine oxidase inhibitors.

Noradrenaline

Pharmacological action. It has a predominant effect on α receptors causing vasoconstriction in muscle, skin and viscera, dilatation of the pupil, reduced muscular activity in the gastrointestinal and urinary tracts and glucose release from the liver. Both systolic and diastolic blood pressures rise and there is reflex slowing of the heart. It causes less cardiac stimulation than adrenaline.

Therapeutic use. The acid tartrate is usually used, the dose being 2–20 μg/minute intravenously. Its chief use has been to treat hypotension in association with peripheral circulatory failure complicating myocardial infarction, the removal of phaeochromocytomas, the use of ganglion-blocking agents and many other conditions. The intense vasoconstriction usually restores the blood pressure but at the expense of adequate perfusion, especially of the kidneys. Latterly the trend has been to attach more significance to blood flow than pressure and to try and improve the former by using a combination of an α-adrenergic blocking agent and intravenous infusion of fluid. Noradrenaline infusions should be stopped slowly as otherwise an abrupt fall in blood pressure may follow.

Contraindications and side effects. Gangrene of the extremities may follow prolonged infusions and severe phlebitis and necrosis around the site of injection has often been a sequel.

Isoprenaline

Pharmacological action. This is almost entirely on β-receptors, producing a marked increase in the rate and force of contraction of the heart and relaxation of peripheral blood vessels, bronchi and most of the smooth muscle of the gut.

Therapeutic use. It is usually given as the sulphate in a dose of 5–20 mg sublingually or by inhalation in an atomiser or as a pressurised aerosol. The hydrochloride is also used in a dose of 10 mg sublingually; or by inhalation as a 1 : 2 solution. It can also be given i.m. or i.v. as an infusion. It is used widely in the control of bronchial asthma but has the disadvantage of stimulating the heart often to a considerable degree. It also produces ventilation/perfusion imbalance in the lungs and a fall in arterial oxygen tension. The pharmacological separation of the β effects on heart and bronchial muscle and the advent of drugs which have predominantly a β_2 effect, eg. salbutamol, reduces this problem. It has been suggested that the combination of isoprenaline with phenylephrine will prevent the reduction in arterial oxygen levels. However, such a manoeuvre does not get round the other untoward effects of isoprenaline. It is only given by injection in the management of complete heart block and for long-term control it is best given as an oral sustained-release preparation, e.g. saventrine.

Contraindications and side effects. These include tachycardia, praecordial pain, hypotension, dizziness, headache, tremor and weakness. It should not be given in the presence of acute coronary insufficiency, heart failure and only with caution in hyperthyroidism.

Orciprenaline

Pharmacological action. An analogue of isoprenaline having similar β_1 and β_2 effects and which is fully active when swallowed.

Therapeutic use. It is used almost entirely as a bronchodilator. Dose: orally 10–20 mg; as a 5 % solution by inhalation or 0.5 mg s.c. or i.m. *Contraindications and side effects.* As isoprenaline but usually less troublesome.

Salbutamol

Pharmacological action. A drug which stimulates β_2 receptors in bronchial muscle but which has little or no effect on β_1 receptors in the heart.
Therapeutic use. This has considerable advantages over isoprenaline in the management of bronchial asthma as it is both longer acting and does not have the risk of precipitating untoward cardiac effects, e.g. arrhythmias. It is given as a pressurised aerosol discharging puffs of 100 μg or as an 0.5% solution by a Wright's nebuliser. Dose 100–400 μg. It can also be used as tablets in a dose of 2–5 mg b.d. or t.d.s. given by subcutaneous or intravenous injection.
Contraindications and side effects. So far remarkably few side effects have been seen although tremor is occasionally noticeable.

Terbutaline

Pharmacological action. Like salbutamol this new agent is chemically very similar to isoprenaline but also has the distinction of being a selective β_2 receptor stimulator.
Therapeutic use and side effects. As salbutamol. Dose 2.5–5.0 mg t.d.s. It can also be given subcutaneously (0.25 mg) up to four times a day.

Ephedrine

Pharmacological action. This is similar to adrenaline as it has both α and β effects, although its effect is slower and more sustained. It acts partly on the receptor directly but also by releasing noradrenaline from stores at adrenergic nerve endings. It may also work partly by inhibiting amine-oxidase. It has a greater stimulating effect on the central nervous system in adults although children may be sedated. It is effective orally.
Therapeutic use. Dose: 15–60 mg orally or subcutaneously as the hydrochloride or sulphate. It is also used as a 1% spray. Its chief use is as a bronchodilator. It is sometimes used to increase conduction in complete heart block, to alleviate narcolepsy and cataplexy and to augment the effect of neostigmine in myasthenia. It is also useful in the management of enuresis.
Contraindications and side effects. Large doses may cause headache, nausea, vomiting, palpitations, difficulty in micturition, muscular weakness, tremors, anxiety, restlessness and insomnia. It should not be given to elderly men and those in whom prostatism is suspected. It should not be used in the presence of ischaemic heart disease, hypertension and thyrotoxicosis.

Amphetamine

Pharmacological action. A sympathomimetic drug with a marked stimulating effect on the central nervous system. It lessens fatigue, gives a feeling of well-being and can easily produce a state of habituation or addiction, especially following indiscriminate use. It also suppresses appetite.
Therapeutic use. Dose: orally 5–10 mg. It has been used in the management of narcolepsy and occasionally in epilepsy and parkinsonism. Other agents have now largely replaced it in all these situations in view of the very real danger of dependence. It should not be used as a tonic, to reduce appetite or to treat depression. It should not be given with MAO inhibitors.

Dexamphetamine

Pharmacological action and therapeutic use. This has the same effects, uses and disadvantages as amphetamine.

Methylphenidate

Pharmacological action and therapeutic use. This has a similar action to amphetamine but is the recommended antidote for pentazocine (q.v.) overdosage as nalorphine is ineffective.

Hydroxyamphetamine

Pharmacological action and therapeutic use. This has an effective vasopressor action without the central effects of amphetamine. It also has a direct stimulating action on the heart. It has been used to correct hypotension, bradycardia and as a nasal decongestant and mydriatic. Dose: orally 20–60 mg; i.m. 10–20 mg and i.v. 5–10 mg.

Methylamphetamine

Pharmacological action and therapeutic use. These are the same as for amphetamine with the exception that i.m. or i.v. it is an effective α-stimulator and produces a vasopressor effect in a dose of 10–30 mg. Its central stimulant effects are marked even in small doses and this has led to its vogue as a drug of addiction.

Methoxyphenamine

Pharmacological action and therapeutic use. This drug has little vasopressor activity but does dilate bronchi and is used in the control of asthma. Dose: orally 50–100 mg every 3 or 4 hours.

There are many other sympathomimetic drugs which have been used as vasopressor agents. These include:

Cyclopentamine/mephentermine/metaraminol/ methoxamine/phenylephrine/phenylpropranolamine

Most of them are α stimulators although metaraminol has both α and β effects and mephentermine has almost entirely a β-stimulating effect.

ANTI-ADRENERGIC DRUGS

POST-GANGLIONIC NEURONE BLOCKERS

These are discussed in the section on HYPOTENSIVE DRUGS (see page 204).

α-BLOCKING AGENTS

Phentolamine

Pharmacological action. This is similar to tolazoline (q.v.) although it is rather more potent and has a shorter duration of action. It acts by competing with α-stimulating agents for the α receptors and its effects can be reversed by giving large amounts of these drugs. It is not reliably effective when given orally.

Therapeutic use. Dose: orally 40–100 mg 4–6-hourly as the hydrochloride or i.v. 5–10 mg as the mesylate. The latter is used chiefly in the diagnosis of phaeochromocytoma. In this situation a fall in blood pressure of at least 32/25 mmHg should occur within 2 minutes of giving 5 mg i.v. Orally, phentolamine has been given for the control of hypertension in phaeochromocytoma prior to surgery.

Parenterally it can also be used as an antidote to adrenaline or noradrenaline.

Contraindications and side effects. Orally it may cause nausea, vomiting, diarrhea and gastrointestinal disturbances. Less often tachycardia, praecordial pain and postural hypotension are troublesome.

Phenoxybenzamine

Pharmacological action. A powerful α-blocker which acts for longer than phentolamine, its effect lasting for several days. It probably alters the receptor in some way rather than acting by competition and its effects cannot be reversed by noradrenaline. The maximum effect of an i.v. injection may take an hour to develop.

Therapeutic use. Dose: orally 10–20 mg initially, subsequent doses to be determined according to the patient's response. It has been used for peripheral vascular disease but is not suitable for the control of hypertension, other than that due to phaeochromocytoma, because of side effects which usually develop with the dose levels required. Latterly it has been used in the management of peripheral circulatory failure in combination with the intravenous infusion of fluid

and central venous pressure monitoring. This is in preference to the previous vogue of giving α-stimulators, e.g. noradrenaline, which produces marked vasoconstriction but at the cost of a severe reduction in flow and tissue perfusion. I.v. a total daily dose of 0.5–1 mg/kg bodyweight is given in 250–500 ml normal saline or dextrose injection over a period of at least 1 hour.

Contraindications and side effects. It should not be given where a fall in blood pressure would be dangerous. A single large dose can cause postural hypotension lasting for 2 days or more. Other side effects include nasal congestion, dry mouth, pupillary constriction, drowsiness, fatigue and weakness. Anorexia, nausea, vomiting and other gastrointestinal disturbances tend to occur more with oral therapy.

Thymoxamine

Pharmacological action. This is a potent and fairly specific α-blocking agent having a marked vasodilator effect. It produces its effect by a competitive and reversible blockade of the α-receptors.

Therapeutic use. Dose: orally 5–10 mg 3 or 4 times daily; or 5–30 mg daily s.c. or i.m. or by slow i.v. injection. Its chief use is as a peripheral vasodilator.

Contraindications and side effects. These include nausea, diarrhea, facial flushing, vertigo and headache, but are less severe than those seen with phentolamine.

Some phenothiazines, e.g. chlorpromazine hydrochloride, also have an α-blocking effect, which is strong enough to cause hypotension. Some ergot alkaloids have α-blocking activity but this is usually masked by their powerful direct vasoconstrictor effect.

β-BLOCKING AGENTS

This group of drugs block the β adrenergic receptors. They vary somewhat in their selectivity.

The results of β-blockade are:—

(1) *Cardiac.* The loss of adrenergic drive leads to a fall in cardiac output and a reduction in heart rate. This is seen particularly when the adrenergic drive is increased as in exercise. There is also a reduction in blood pressure. This may not be seen for some weeks after starting the drug and the cause is obscure, although one factor is probably the fall in cardiac output. In addition β-blockade may lead to a fall in plasma renin but this does not appear to be related to its hypotensive action. Loss of adrenergic stimulation

reduces the excitability of the heart and in addition a number of β-blockers also have a direct membrane stabilising effect on heart muscle similar to that of quinidine.

(2) *Bronchial*. β-blockade causes some bronchial constriction which is of little importance except in patients with asthma, where a severe attack can be precipitated. The bronchial constriction is less marked with selective β-blockers which affect predominantly β_1 receptors.

(3) *Metabolic*. β-blockade inhibits the release of glucose by the liver, and this is potentially dangerous in patients receiving insulin. It also prevents the release of triglycerides and free fatty acids following an emotional episode.

Therapeutic uses

(1) *Hypertension*. β-blockers are widely used in treating hypertension, they are frequently combined with other hypotensive agents, for details see page 202.

(2) *Angina of effort*. The damping down effect on cardiac function produced by β-blockers makes them invaluable in angina, for details see page 197.

(3) *Cardiac arrhythmias*. For details see page 198.

(4) *Thyrotoxicosis*. In this condition there is marked adrenergic activity which can easily be reduced by β-blockers until the underlying disease is brought under control.

(5) *Phaeochromocytoma*. To reduce β-stimulation which is particularly liable to occur during operation.

Individual β-blockers. Details of the individual β-blockers are given in the table below.

	Selectivity	Intrinsic sympathetic activity	Membrane stabilising
Propranolol	$\beta_1 + \beta_2$	−	+
Oxprenolol	$\beta_1 + \beta_2$	+	+
Timolol	$\beta_1 + \beta_2$	−	+
Metoprolol	$\beta_1 > \beta_2$	−	∓
Sotalol	$\beta_1 + \beta_2$	−	−
Practolol	$\beta_1 > \beta_2$	+	−
Pindolol	$\beta_1 > \beta_2$	+	+
Atenolol	$\beta_1 > \beta_2$	−	−
Acebutalol	$\beta_1 > \beta_2$	+	+

There is no evidence as yet that any particular blocker is to be preferred in the treatment of hypertension or angina. If there is a history of asthma it would be better to use one of the more selective β-blockers and proceed with care, but it must be remembered that cardio-selectivity is only a matter of degree and the categories in the table are a rough approximation.

Intrinsic sympathetic activity and membrane stabilising effect have yet to be shown to be of any practical importance, although those with some intrinsic sympathetic activity do not produce so much bradycardia.

Practolol, because of side effects (see later) should be avoided in long term treatment.

Their use in cardiac arrhythmias is considered on page 198. Dosage is usually three times daily, although twice may sometimes be suitable particularly for metoprolol and sotalol. Acebutolol differs from the others in that it is recommended only for cardiac arrhythmias and angina.

Contraindications and side effects. Cardiac failure. Patients in or nearly in cardiac failure will be made worse by β-blockers which should therefore be avoided if possible. Heart block will be made worse.

Intravenous administration of β-blockers will be followed by marked bradycardia and should generally be preceded by atropine.

Asthmatics will be made worse by β-blockers, and these drugs should be avoided if possible. One of the selective β-blockers would be the least troublesome.

Insulin hypoglycaemia may be difficult to control as the normal release of glucose by the liver is inhibited by β-blockers.

Other side effects include bradycardia, cold extremities, tinnitus, abdominal discomfort and diarrhea or constipation.

Prolonged use of practolol has been followed by thickening of the skin of the palms and xerosis. A retroperitoneal fibrosis like syndrome has also been reported.

Pindolol has been reported as being associated with disturbing dreams.

PARASYMPATHOMIMETIC DRUGS

CHOLINE ESTERS

Methacholine

Pharmacological action. Like acetylcholine it stimulates the parasympathetic nervous system but has predominantly a muscarinic effect. It chiefly affects the cardiovascular system causing bradycardia and dilatation of peripheral blood vessels. It increases salivation, sweating and bronchial secretion.

Therapeutic use. Dose: orally 10–500 mg; s.c. 10–25 mg. It is not given intravenously. Methacholine bromide is sometimes used and has a similar action. Dose: orally 200–600 mg. Methacholine has been used to stop supraventricular tachycardias and to stimulate the bowel and bladder, although carbachol is probably better for the latter.

Contraindications and side effects. These include nausea, vomiting, flushing, increased salivation, involuntary defaecation, bradycardia, transient heart block, hypotension, dyspnea and substernal discomfort. If given by injection it may give rise to a terrifying feeling of choking. It should not be given to patients with asthma, hypertension, ischaemic heart disease, Addison's disease or peptic ulceration. Serious reactions have resulted from the combined use of methacholine and neostigmine.

Carbachol

Pharmacological action. It has both muscarinic and nicotinic effects but chiefly affects the gastro-intestinal tract.

Therapeutic use. Dose: s.c. 0.25 mg repeated up to 2 or 3 times at 30-minute intervals. It is also used in a 0.8% aqueous solution as eye drops. Its most frequent use is for post-operative intestinal atony and retention of urine. It has also been used for supraventricular tachycardias and is occasionally used as a miotic. Unwanted side effects can be reversed with atropine 0.6 mg s.c.

Contraindications and side effects. It may cause sweating, nausea, faintness, colic and diarrhea. It should not be used in the presence of mechanical obstruction in the gastrointestinal or urinary tracts or after gastrointestinal anastomosis. It is less safe in the elderly.

Bethanechol

Pharmacological action. This is similar to methacholine but it is not destroyed by choline-esterase. It is less toxic and less active than methacholine.

Therapeutic use. Dose: orally 5–30 mg up to 3 times a day; s.c. 2.5–5 mg at no less than four-hourly intervals. It is the best tolerated of these three drugs for the treatment of postoperative intestinal stasis (e.g. after vagotomy) and distension, and is also useful for postoperative urinary retention.

Contraindications and side effects. As carbachol but less troublesome.

CHOLINE-ESTERASE INHIBITORS
Physostigmine

Pharmacological action. It potentiates the action of acetylcholine by inhibiting choline-esterase. It thus produces muscarinic and nicotinic effects as well as acting on the central nervous system. It is particularly useful as a miotic acting within 10 minutes of local application, the effect lasting for about 12 hours.

Therapeutic use. It is now only used as eye-drops. It is useful for the relief of glaucoma and to counteract the dilation produced by atropine or cocaine.

Neostigmine

Pharmacological action. This has a similar action to physostigmine although the nicotinic effects are more and the muscarinic effects less prominent. It is thus used chiefly for its effect on skeletal muscle.

Therapeutic use. Preparations: N. bromide—orally, N. methyl sulphate—by injection. It is still the mainstay of treatment for myasthenia gravis and is used in a dose of 15–30 mg orally three or four times daily. It can be given by i.m. or i.v. injection 1–2.5 mg several times daily up to a total of 3 mg/day. It has also been used as a diagnostic aid for myasthenia in a dose of 1–1.5 mg i.m. or i.v. Increase in muscular power with improvement in symptoms should be noticeable within 15 minutes. Neostigmine is also used as an antidote to the muscle relaxants tubocurarine and gallamine. 2.5 mg is given i.v. after 0.5–1 mg atropine i.v.

Contraindications and side effects. Toxic effects include restlessness, weakness, nausea, vomiting, diarrhea and abdominal pain. Increased sweating, salivation and lachrymation occur, and if excessive doses are given generalised muscular twitching convulsions and collapse may ensue. The muscarinic effects can be controlled with atropine. Neostigmine should not be used in patients with asthma, ischaemic heart disease, parkinsonism, epilepsy, bradycardia, hypotension, and intestinal or urinary tract obstruction. Its use during operation involving intestinal anastomosis is associated with an increased incidence of leaking from the intestinal suture line. This effect seems to be considerably reduced if halothane is used as the general anaesthetic.

Pyridostigmine

Pharmacological action. Similar to neostigmine but with a quarter of the potency. It is slower in onset, acting within 30–45 minutes and lasting for 4–6 hours.

Therapeutic use. It is used, often in association with neostigmine, for myasthenia gravis, in a dose of 60–240 mg orally and 1–5 mg s.c. or i.m.

Contraindications and side effects. As neostigmine.

Ambenonium

Pharmacological action and therapeutic uses. Similar to neostigmine but longer lasting. It is used for myasthenia gravis especially when neostigmine is poorly tolerated. Dose: 5–25 mg three or four times daily.

Contraindications and side effects. As neostigmine but less marked.

Edrophonium

Pharmacological action. Similar to neostigmine but its effect on skeletal muscle is much more marked and most of its effect is probably due to a direct action on the muscle receptor rather than inhibition of choline-esterase. It has a rapid onset and short duration of action.

Therapeutic use. It is particularly useful in the diagnosis of myasthenia gravis. A test dose of 2 mg is given i.v. and if there has been no untoward effect after 30 seconds a further 8 mg is given. With myasthenia there is immediate improvement and increase in muscle power which disappears within 5 minutes. It is therefore not suitable for routine use. It is also suitable for deciding in a myasthenic patient between weakness due to too much or too little neostigmine.

Contraindications and side effects. As neostigmine but very short-lived.

Dyflos (DFP)

Pharmacological action. Causes prolonged inhibition of choline-esterase as do many of the organophosphates. Its effect may last for two weeks and thus it is not suitable for systemic use. Its action resembles neostigmine and physostigmine and its particular value is as a miotic.

Therapeutic use. Eye drops are made up as a 10% solution in arachis oil. Dose: 1 drop t.d.s. It is used as a miotic for glaucoma.

Contraindications and side effects. Ocular pain often occurs initially and there may be a transient rise in intra-ocular pressure. After prolonged medication iris cysts may develop which usually regress after treatment has ceased. DFP can be absorbed through the skin, conjunctiva and respiratory and gastrointestinal tracts. Its vapour is very toxic and thus eye drops are made up in an oily substance. Systematic administration via one or more of these routes leads to ciliary and iris spasm, transient bronchial constriction, muscle fibrillation, salivation, diarrhea, urinary retention, restlessness, headache, convulsions, and collapse.

Most of these effects of poisoning can be controlled by i.m. or i.v. injections of 1–2 mg atropine sulphate. This may be repeated every 10–30 minutes until signs of atropinisation appear. 20 mg or more may be required. A specific choline-esterase reactivor, e.g. pralidoxime should be given (dose: 1–2 g daily, i.m. or i.v.) and repeated as necessary. Artificial ventilation may be required.

Contraindications are as for neostigmine, with the additional exclusion that it should not be used for acute congestive (narrow angle) glaucoma as here it may cause a further rise in pressure; neither should it be used in the presence of retinal damage.

Ecothiopate

Pharmacological action and therapeutic use. Very similar to dyflos. It is used as a miotic. It is usually used as an 0.25% aqueous solution. Dose: from 1 drop alternate days to twice a day.

Contraindications and side effects. As dyflos.

PILOCARPINE

Pilocarpine

Pharmacological action. An alkaloid having the muscarinic effects of acetylcholine with little of its nicotinic effects. It is used chiefly as a miotic and has about half the activity of physostigmine and acts for a shorter length of time. It has also been used to counteract the side effects of ganglion-blocking agents.

Therapeutic use. As a miotic it is used as a 1% solution; orally it is given in a dose of 2.5–12 mg.

Contraindications and side effects. Increased salivation, sweating and production of tears predominate. With excessive doses nausea, vomiting, diarrhea, dyspnea, confusion, tremor and convulsions may occur.

ANTI-CHOLINERGIC DRUGS

GANGLION BLOCKING AGENTS

Hexamethonium/pentolinium/mecamylamine/pempidine/trimetaphan

These are now rarely used for the rapid control of an elevated blood pressure and are discussed in the section on HYPOTENSIVE DRUGS (see page 204.

NEUROMUSCULAR-BLOCKING AGENTS

Depolarising agents

Suxamethonium

Pharmacological action. This drug acts by depolarising voluntary muscle in a similar way to acetycholine but as suxamethonium is destroyed less quickly the depolarisation temporarily persists. The onset of relaxation is preceded by a short period of contraction which causes pain if the patient is conscious, and probably causes the muscle pain which occurs for up to 3 days after its use. The effect of this drug is not reversed by cholinergic drugs. It is destroyed by plasma pseudo-choline-esterase.

Therapeutic use. Dose: 30–50 mg i.v. It is used as a short-acting muscle relaxant in conjunction with major and minor surgical and manipulative procedures.

Contraindications and side effects. Prolonged apnea will occur in those with a low or atypical plasma pseudo-choline-esterase. The former may occur with liver disease, severe anaemia, malnutrition or after treatment with anti-choline-esterases, e.g. neostigmine. The latter is an hereditary defect. A prolonged effect may also follow if streptomycin or neomycin is given soon after the administration of suxamethonium. Repeated doses can cause bradycardia and arrhythmias. Generalised muscle pain is a common after effect and can be prevented by giving a small dose of a competitive blocking agent before the suxamethonium.

Non-depolarising agents

Tubocurarine

Pharmacological action. This drug acts by competing with acetylcholine for the receptors on the motor end-plate. It does not cause depolarisation but prevents its occurrence due to acetylcholine. This causes a flaccid paralysis. It develops within a minute of i.v. injection and lasts for 20–45 minutes. Tubocurarine also has a ganglion-blocking effect and causes tissue histamine to be released. These effects explain the occasional occurrence of a fall in blood pressure and the development of bronchospasm.

The action of tubocurarine is reversed by anti-choline-esterase drugs, e.g. neostigmine methyl-sulphate 2.5–5 mg i.v. preceded by 0.5–1 mg atropine i.v. to prevent the parasympathetic effects of the neostigmine.

Therapeutic use. Dose: initially 5 mg i.v. as a test dose followed in 5 minutes by 10–20 mg i.v. Additional doses of 2–4 mg can be given at 30 minute intervals up to a total dose of 45 mg.

Dimethyltubocurarine bromide, chloride or iodide can be used instead of tubocurarine chloride and these drugs are all roughly three times as potent requiring about a third of the above dose. This drug is used to produce muscular relaxation during surgery and is also used to control muscle spasm and convulsions in tetanus.

Contraindications and side effects. It is rarely toxic but may occasionally lower the blood pressure and cause bronchospasm. Administration of tubocurarine before or after the use of suxamethonium can cause a state of neostigmine-resistant curarisation. This will require continued

ventilation but usually settles after a few hours. It tends to occur in patients who are dehydrated, hypokalaemic or otherwise metabolically disturbed. Tubocurarine should not be used in patients with myasthenia or those with respiratory, hepatic or renal disease. Patients with carcinomatous neuromyopathies often give abnormal and prolonged responses to muscle relaxants. Potentiation occurs with ether, chlorpromazine and some antibiotics (e.g. streptomycin, neomycin and polymyxin).

Gallamine

Pharmacological action. It is similar to tubocurarine but has little effect on autonomic ganglia. It does not produce histamine release and is less potent and shorter-acting. Relaxation starts within 2 minutes and lasts for about 20 minutes. *Therapeutic use.* Dose: 80–120 mg i.v. Up to half of the initial amount can be given as a second dose. It is used to obtain shorter periods of muscular relaxation during surgery and to minimise the convulsions of shock therapy. Premedication with atropine is necessary to prevent excessive salivation.

Contraindications and side effects. As tubocurarine. In addition it may produce allergic reactions in people sensitive to iodine and occasionally causes a tachycardia which persists for a while after the relaxant effect has disappeared.

DRUGS BLOCKING MUSCARINIC SITES (ATROPINE AND RELATED DRUGS)

Atropine (dl-hyoscyamine)

Pharmacological action. Centrally it initially stimulates and later depresses the nervous system. It reduces tremor and muscular rigidity especially in people with parkinsonism and may help oculogyric crises although the mechanism is unknown. Peripherally it blocks the muscarinic effects of acetylcholine and thus antagonises all the effects of acetylcholine except for those at autonomic ganglia and the neuro-muscular junction. It has an anti-spasmodic action on smooth muscle and decreases secretions. It depresses vagal activity causing slowing of the heart. It is also an anti-emetic.

It has both a mydriatic and cycloplegic action on the eye and may cause a rise in intraocular pressure.

Therapeutic use. Dose: 0.25–2 mg orally, s.c. or i.m. Its effect on the gut is utilised in the treatment of peptic ulceration and pylorospasm. In congenital hypertrophic pyloric stenosis it is usually given as atropine methonitrate in a dose of 2–6 ml of a 0.1% aqueous solution half an hour before feeds. The methonitrate has less effect on the central nervous system and is less toxic to infants. It is also used to control bronchial asthma in a compound adrenaline and atropine spray or as the methonitrate alone in a pressurised aerosol. However atropine may make bronchial secretions extremely viscid and sympathomimetic agents are often preferred.

Atropine is often used for its effect on the heart, e.g. to prevent vagal syncope and to correct the bradycardia due to digitalis, opiates, choline-esters, pilocarpine or anti-choline-esterases. It has also been used for partial heart block. It is used as a premedication in view of its ability to reduce secretions and protect the heart from vagal inhibition. It has been used in parkinsonism and will also reduce the sialorrhea, but other atropine-like agents, e.g. benzhexol are probably more suitable.

Atropine has an anti-emetic effect but other drugs, e.g. cyclizine, meclozine, etc. cause less side effects. As a mydriatic and cycloplegic it is used as 1% eye drops. Dilatation occurs within 30 minutes and may last 2 weeks. For this reason homatropine is usually preferred.

Contraindications and side effects. These include dry mouth, thirst, dilatation of pupils with loss of accommodation and photophobia, flushing, difficulty with micturition and constipation. Toxic doses cause restlessness, excitement, confusion and hallucinations, tachycardia and hyperpyrexia. Later drowsiness, stupor and generalized central depression may occur. Side effects may even occur with eye drops. Atropine must not be used on patients with a narrow angle between the iris or cornea or those who have developed glaucoma. It should be used with care in those with prostatic enlargement, ischaemic heart disease or cardiac failure, and should not be used in paralytic ileus. The danger of hyperpyrexia should be considered in unduly hot weather or climates.

Hyoscine (scopolamine)

Pharmacological action. Similar to atropine although its effect on the central nervous system is between 3 and 10 times as potent. This is usually a depressant effect although excitement can occur especially in the elderly.

Mydriasis is quicker in onset and of shorter duration.

Therapeutic use. Dose: as atropine. It has been used for acute mania, parkinsonism and as an hypnotic. It is also used as a premedication, usually in combination with an opiate, and as a mydriatic.

Contraindications and side effects. As atropine but it should be avoided in the elderly.

Hyoscine hydrobromide

Pharmacological action. Very similar actions and uses to hyoscine.
Therapeutic use. Dose: 0.3–0.6 mg s.c.

Hyoscine butylbromide

Pharmacological action. It is often ineffective orally but parenterally it is an effective smooth muscle relaxant and is used for this effect on the cardia, stomach, colon and biliary and renal tracts. It does not have much effect on gastric secretion and unlike hyoscine it also has a ganglion blocking action. Dose: 20–40 mg s.c. or i.m.; 10–20 mg i.v.

Hyoscine methobromide

Pharmacological action. A quarternary amine which thus lacks the central action of atropine and is a more selective inhibitor of gastric secretion. It is longer acting than hyoscine.
Therapeutic use. Dose: orally 2.5–5 mg 8-hourly; 0.25 to 1 mg s.c. or i.m. three or four times a day.

Homatropine hydrobromide

Pharmacological action. Similar to atropine but rather weaker. As a mydriatic its action is more rapid and less prolonged although it may last for 24 hours. The dilatation is easily reversed with physostigmine. It is rarely used systematically although the methobromide has been used for its effect on the gastrointestinal tract.
Therapeutic use. Dose: 0.5–2 mg as a 1 or 2% solution.

Cyclopentolate

Pharmacological action and therapeutic use. A mydriatic and cycloplegic agent quicker and shorter-acting than homatropine. Mydriasis develops within 10–20 minutes and cycloplegia soon after; the effect lasting for 6–12 hours. Dose: 1–2 drops of a 0.5 or 1% solution. Its effect is best reversed by pilocarpine.

Lachesine

Pharmacological action and therapeutic use. A mydriatic and cycloplegic agent having a slower onset of action which is less prolonged than atropine, achieving a maximum at 1 hour and disappearing within 6 hours. It does not cause conjunctival irritation and is a useful alternative for those patients who show a sensitivity to substances of the atropine group. Usual dose is 2 drops of a 1% solution.

Propantheline

Pharmacological action. It is one of many synthetic anti-choline drugs and has a marked peripheral atropine-like effect with little effect on the CNS. It is also a weak ganglion-blocker and at very high doses has a curare-like effect on the neuromuscular junction.

Therapeutic use. Dose: 15–30 mg orally, i.m. or i.v. Its more frequent use is to reduce gastric intestinal secretion and motility. It is an effective antispasmodic and may be given with an opiate for visceral colic to reduce the stimulating effect of the former on smooth muscle.

Contraindications and side effects. As for atropine with the additional hazard that in toxic doses paralysis of voluntary muscle may occur.

There are many more anticholinergic agents which have been developed for systemic use, chiefly for their effects in reducing spasm, motility and secretion in the gastrointestinal tract. Four further drugs will be mentioned by name, although they differ little from propantheline in their actions, uses and side effects.

Poldine

Pharmacological action and therapeutic use. This is a potent inhibitor of gastric secretion with a prolonged action. Dose: 2–4 mg orally, 6-hourly, but this often requires adjustment as atropine-like side effects are common at the higher dose levels.

Dicyclomine

Pharmacological action and therapeutic use. It is an anti-spasmodic similar to but weaker than atropine. It has also a mild local anaesthetic action. Dose: 10–20 mg orally, three or four times daily.

Tricyclamol

Pharmacological action and therapeutic use. Similar to atropine. It also has ganglion blocking activity in large doses. Dose: 50–100 mg orally four- or six-hourly before meals.

Isopropamide

Pharmacological action and therapeutic use. Similar to tricyclamol except that it has a more prolonged action. Dose: orally 5 mg 8–12-hourly.

Category 5

DRUGS USED IN CARDIAC DISEASE

D. C. DEUCHAR

Digoxin

Pharmacological action. Digoxin is a pure glycoside obtained from the leaves of *Digitalis lanata*.

The action of the digitalis glycosides at the cellular level is uncertain, but it is possible that they affect the movement of ions across the cell membrane in such a way as to reduce the sodium and potassium gradients, whilst conserving calcium within the cell. The result of the former is to lead to an increased ease of depolarisation of the cell membrane – this could explain the toxic effects on the heart – and of the latter is to improve the contractility of the muscle fibre. In addition to these direct cellular actions the cardiac glycosides are known to increase vagal control of the heart.

The effects of digitalis glycosides are most readily seen in patients with cardiac failure and tachycardia, in whom they lower the venous pressure and slow the heart rate. Part of this slowing can be blocked by atropine but part is due to a direct action on the SA node. A greater slowing effect can be produced in patients with atrial fibrillation due to diminished conduction from the atria to the ventricles; it has recently been shown that digitalis increases the normal delay in the activation of the AV node by the atrial action potential. A more indirect effect is the occurrence of diuresis which is due to the improvement in the circulation. There is no useful action on the healthy myocardium and digitalis is of no benefit, therefore, where the impediment to the circulation is a mechanical one (e.g. valve stenosis or regurgitation) unless this is complicated by secondary myocardial failure. Unfortunately, the margin between the dose required to achieve the desired therapeutic response and that which leads to toxic effects is small.

Therapeutic use. Digitalis glycosides have their greatest use in the patient with myocardial failure and atrial fibrillation. It is of value also in the management of either of these disorders alone. When used in patients with atrial fibrillation the response of the ventricular rate is usually a convenient index as to the adequacy of treatment. In patients with sinus rhythm it is necessary to give the drug until the desired therapeutic result is obtained or until evidence of toxicity necessitates reduction of dosage.

Digitalis is also of value in the management of other arrhythmias particularly as a prophylaxis against paroxysms of supraventricular tachycardia in young subjects. In atrial flutter it may convert the rhythm to atrial fibrillation and then control the ventricular rate; sometimes it may succeed in increasing the degree of atrioventricular block without change of rhythm, thereby controlling the tachycardia, but more often this is not achieved before serious toxic effects are apparent. Rather surprisingly digitalis may also abolish ventricular or supraventricular ectopic beats, even though in toxic doses it may stimulate them. Digitalis is often ineffective in slowing the heart rate when infection, hyperthyroidism or anxiety are responsible for the tachycardia.

In general, older patients require less digitalis than younger ones; impairment of renal function reduces excretion and therefore the required dose; potassium depletion, most commonly the result of diuretic therapy, potentiates the toxicity of digitalis and this must be watched for in patients on diuretics.

Digoxin has the same actions as digitoxin or prepared digitalis but it is absorbed more rapidly and has a quicker onset of action. It is also available for intramuscular or intravenous injection; the latter is to be preferred as the preparation is irritating and absorption from an intramuscular site is less reliable. By mouth it takes effect in about an hour and peak activity is reached in 6–7 hours; by injection onset of effect may be detected in 10–15 minutes and the full effect is obtained by 2 hours. After stopping the drug the effect lasts for several days.

Because of its more rapid onset of action digoxin has especial value in the urgent treatment of left heart failure with uncontrolled atrial fibrillation. It is also particularly useful in the management of infants in heart failure where its greater flexibility of use is an advantage.

For rapid effect the usual adult oral loading dose is 1.0–1.5 mg followed by 0.25–0.5 mg every 6 hours until the desired therapeutic response is achieved. Maintenance usually requires

0.25 mg 1–3 times daily. Intravenously 0.5–1.0 mg may be given, provided no digitalis preparation has been given in the previous two weeks; if digitalis has been given, not more than 0.25 mg should be given at any one time and at least two hours should elapse between each injection for its effect to be assessed.

Attention has recently been drawn to considerable differences in the biological availability of digoxin tablets of differing manufacture. These differences are related to absorption rates which in turn depend on the rate of dissolution of the tablets and the particle size of the material of which they are composed. It is desirable therefore to prescribe the same known brand of digoxin each time for any one patient.

For children the loading dose can be calculated on the basis of 0.025 mg per kg bodyweight, either by mouth or injection every 6 hours, adjusted to an appropriate maintenance dose when the desired response is achieved. The administration of small fractional doses is facilitated by the availability of tablets of 0.0625 mg, i.e. one-quarter of the normal 0.25 mg tablet.

Contraindications and side effects. Although theoretically digitalis should not be given to patients with ectopic beats, ventricular arrhythmias or early after myocardial infarction, because of its known potentiating effect on depolarisation, in practice it should not be withheld on these grounds if its use is otherwise indicated.

Gastrointestinal disturbances, anorexia, nausea, vomiting, and sometimes diarrhea, are usually the first manifestations of digitalis toxicity. Other, less common, non-cardiac manifestations include headache, facial pain, drowsiness, mental confusion, and blurring of vision and, rarely, disturbances of colour vision, so that objects seen by the patient take on a yellow or green hue.

The more serious toxic effects of digitalis are related to its action on the heart. Ectopic beats, usually ventricular and characteristically coupled to the preceding normal beat are common. In some cases they occur so regularly that they produce pulsus bigeminus which can be readily recognised clinically. When this is not so it is important in patients with atrial fibrillation to ensure that the increased rate and irregularity of the heart beat is not misinterpreted as indicating a lack of control of the atrial fibrillation necessitating an increased dose. Patients previously in sinus rhythm may develop paroxysmal atrial tachycardia with varying atrioventricular block; and in patients with atrial fibrillation the occurrence of a regular ventricular rhythm due to AV junctional rhythm is usually an indication of toxicity; the continued or increased administration of digitalis in these situations is likely to

be fatal. Ventricular tachycardia and later ventricular fibrillation are the usual fatal disturbances of rhythm. Other effects are sinus bradycardia and increased atrioventricular block, at first only detectable on the electrocardiogram but later leading to slowing of the ventricular rate. The use of recently developed techniques for estimating plasma digoxin indicates that toxicity is related to plasma levels; levels of less than 1.5 ng/ml are unlikely to be associated with toxic effects.

Prepared digitalis (digitalis leaf)

Pharmacological action. As for digoxin.

Prepared digitalis is the dried leaf of the foxglove, *Digitalis purpurea*, adjusted by dilution to a standard activity ascertained by biological assay. It contains a number of glycosides.

Therapeutic uses. The usual initial leading dose for an adult is between 1.0 and 1.5 g given in divided doses over 24 hours; maintenance usually requires 100–200 mg daily. It is readily absorbed but its full effect takes some hours to develop; it is slowly excreted and once established the effect may take several days or even weeks to wear off. Now that pure glycoside preparations, which do not require biological assay, are readily available, prepared digitalis is little used.

Contraindications and side effects. As for digoxin.

Digitoxin

Pharmacological action. As for digoxin.

Digitoxin is a crystalline glycoside obtained from the leaves of several species of *Digitalis*.

Therapeutic use. Digitoxin has properties which are almost identical with those of prepared digitalis, including its slow onset of action and the persistence of its effect. Digitoxin is the most potent (weight for weight) of the cardiac glycosides and the most persistent in its effect; accumulation with prolonged administration may therefore be a problem. There is some clinical evidence that the gastrointestinal side effects are less pronounced than with some other glycosides. In general, however, its slow onset of effect and persistence outweigh this slight advantage and, although widely used in some countries, it would seem to be less convenient than digoxin.

Owing to its high potency the initial loading dose is about 1.0 mg in divided dose and the maintenance dose is between 0.05 and 0.2 mg daily. Preparations for intravenous administration are available but the onset of the effect when given by this route is no faster than when it is given by mouth.

Contraindications and side effects. As for digoxin.

Lanatoside C

Pharmacological action. As for digoxin.

Deslanoside is desacetyl-lanatoside C and is the active material used for intravenous preparations corresponding to the orally administered lanatoside C. Their properties are virtually identical. Lanatoside C is a glycoside obtained from the leaf of *Digitalis lanata.*

Therapeutic use. These preparations have virtually the same uses as digoxin but have a more rapid onset of action (10 minutes) and a more rapid clearance. They are also reputed to have a larger margin between the therapeutic and toxic dose. For these reasons the intravenous preparation particularly is sometimes of use in rapidly changing situations.

The initial loading dose of lanatoside C given by mouth is about 1.0–1.5 mg with a daily maintenance dose of 0.25–0.75 mg daily for adults and a loading dose of 0.025–0.05 mg/lb bodyweight for children. For deslanoside the corresponding intravenous doses are, for adults 0.8–1.2 mg followed by 0.4 mg doses every 2–4 hours as required and, for children 0.01 mg/lb bodyweight.

Contraindications and side effects. As for digoxin.

Aminophylline

Pharmacological action. Aminophylline is a mixture of theophylline and ethylenediamine; the latter helps to improve the solubility of the theophylline and also increases its pharmacological activity. The principal effect of aminophylline is to relax the tone of involuntary muscle, especially of the bronchial tree. It lowers the venous pressure in patients with congestive heart failure. It has a weak diuretic action and also appears to increase the sensitivity of the respiratory centre to increasing carbon dioxide tension.

Therapeutic use. When administered by intravenous injection it has a very rapid beneficial effect on bronchospasm. It is probably most often used for severe bronchial asthma but because of its combination of effects it is of great value in the management of cardiac asthma. The usual dose is 250 mg in 10 ml of solution injected *slowly.*

Aminophylline is not satisfactorily given by mouth because it is a gastric irritant. Several proprietary preparations of aminophylline or closely related substances have been developed to permit oral use; in general they do not have the same potency as the injected drug. It is well absorbed through the rectal mucosa so that, in the form of suppositories, patients can use it for the prevention or relief of attacks of paroxysmal nocturnal dyspnea. These suppositories normally contain 360 mg.

Contraindications and side effects. Side effects have been most commonly associated with too-rapid injection; this may lead to restlessness, palpitation, dizziness, nausea, or hypotension. Sudden death has been reported following intravenous injection in normal doses and again this has been associated with rapid injection.

Serious toxic effects appear to have been reported most frequently in children, which suggests that in them its use requires greater caution than in adults.

Quinidine

Pharmacological action. Quinidine is the dextrorotatory stereo-isomer of quinine. Its principal therapeutic effect is prolongation of the refractory period of cardiac muscle, thereby reducing the rate at which successive contractions can occur. It does, however, have a powerful general depressive action on the myocardium, reducing excitability, contractility and conduction, and it also has some atropine-like action, reducing vagal tone. It has recently been shown that its effect on atrioventricular conduction is due to prolongation of the conduction of the impulse from the AV node to the ventricular myocardium (compare action of digoxin on conduction).

Therapeutic use. Quinidine is a potent cardiac-depressant anti-arrhythmic drug, although considered by many to be too toxic for common use. The recent introduction of other less dangerous substances and the advent of the electric-shock correction of arrhythmias have now reduced its usefulness. It does, however, still have a place in the management of some patients with rhythm disturbance, especially if these are supraventricular. It is often effective in correcting or preventing atrial or ventricular tachy-arrhythmias and in abolishing atrial or ventricular ectopic beats. When used for the treatment of supraventricular tachycardias (e.g. atrial flutter) with some degree of atrioventricular block, digitalis should be given first to avoid a sudden, possibly dangerous, increase in ventricular rate which can result from one-to-one conduction developing as the rate of the supraventricular focus is slowed.

Although quinidine may be given intravenously with the protection of electrocardiographic control in urgent cases, e.g. to stop ventricular tachycardia when the patient's life is threatened, it is usually given by mouth. The desired therapeutic response is commonly obtained with a blood level of about 6–8 mg/l. Blood levels above 10 mg/l are associated with a high incidence of toxic effects. The effects of the drug are not, however, uniformly related to the blood level and electrocardiographic monitoring of the response is an alternative way of controlling the dose; the drug may be given until some prolongation of the PR interval and QT time are apparent and changes in the ST segment and T waves occur. An increase in these effects and a widening of the QRS complex are evidence of excessive dosage. Various dose schedules have been described using repeated doses at short intervals to build up higher blood levels each day on top of the residue left from the previous day; a common one uses 0.3 g or 0.4 g every 2 hours for 5 doses on successive days for about 3 or 4 days; if necessary the individual dose may be increased to 0.5 g on the fourth or fifth day and to 0.6 g on the sixth day. Before starting full therapeutic doses a test dose of 0.2 g should be given to detect any hypersensitivity. The introduction of slow release tablets containing 250 mg of quinidine bisulphate (equivalent to 200 mg of sulphate) allows for a simpler twice daily regime. It is also claimed to diminish the risks of quinidine therapy but this has not been well established.

Contraindications and side effects. Quinidine is absolutely contraindicated by a history of serious reaction to the drug and is given with an increased risk to patients with heart block, or bundle branch block, severe congestive cardiac failure and renal failure, especially in the presence of hyperkalaemia. Individuals may show hypersensitivity to the drug by developing tinnitus, vertigo, blurring of vision or blindness, headache, confusion, rashes, bronchospasm, gastrointestinal disturbances, fever, collapse with hypotension or death from ventricular fibrillation. These reactions may also occur as dose-related side-effects; thrombocytopenic purpura has also been reported. Increase of the width of the QRS complex by more than 25% of its control value, the development of bundle branch block, of second degree or complete heart block, of ventricular ectopic beats, or atrial standstill are all indications of cardiac toxicity and call for withdrawal of the drug before ventricular tachycardia, fibrillation or asystole occur.

Disopyramide

Pharmacological action. Disopyramide prolongs the refractory period of the AV node and slows myocardial and Purkinje fibre conduction. It also reduces atrial and ventricular myocardial excitability and prolongs the ventricular myocardial refractory period. Its actions are therefore very similar to those of quinidine (see above). It has some anticholinergic activity.

Therapeutic use. It has been used for the control of arrhythmias following myocardial infarction and for the control of paroxysmal supraventricular tachycardia. In general its uses are similar to those of quinidine and it appears to have the advantage of lesser toxicity. It is given by mouth, the basic dose being 100 mg which may be given three or four times a day; up to double this dose may be used if needed.

Contraindications and side effects. Disopyramide is contraindicated in patients with complete heart block and should be used with caution in the presence of lesser degrees of block or of myocardial failure. In the last situation a digitalis preparation should be given at the same time. Because of its anticholinergic activity it should not be used for patients with glaucoma or urinary retention; the commonest side effects (dryness of the mouth, blurred vision and difficulty with micturition) are related to this activity. Gastrointestinal irritation may occur and individual sensitivity to the drug is a rare possibility.

Procainamide

Pharmacological action. Procainamide hydrochloride has a depressant action on the myocardium, diminishing the excitability, conductivity and contractility of both atrium and ventricle, and prolonging the refractory period of the atrium. It has been shown that, like quinidine, its action on atrio-ventricular conductivity is distal to the AV node.

Therapeutic use. It is chiefly of use in suppressing ventricular ectopic beats or arrhythmias; it has some effect on atrial arrhythmias and may even convert atrial fibrillation to sinus rhythm, but it is less successful in the management of supraventricular arrhythmias. For the rapid correction of serious arrhythmias, such as ventricular tachycardia, it may be given intravenously but caution is required as it can precipitate depression of myocardial activity with severe hypotension and sometimes the initiation of ventricular fibrillation. It is more safely given by mouth and, when used for the correction of a rhythm disturbance, the dose is 1.0 g followed by 0.25–1.0 g every 4–6 hours. For the long-term prevention of ectopic beats the usual dose is 500 mg every 4–6 hours. Larger doses are sometimes required. (A slow release preparation is now available but experience is limited.) When used intravenously the dose for the control of ventricular arrhythmias is 0.2–1.0 g injected slowly in dilute solution.

Contraindications and side effects. Procainamide antagonises the action of sulphonamides. It should be avoided in patients subject to bronchial asthma and those known to be hypersensitive to it, in patients with renal failure and those with conduction defects of the heart.

Reported side effects include anorexia, nausea, vomiting and diarrhea, with large oral doses, and severe hypotension when given intravenously. Prolonged or repeated administration has been shown to lead to a high incidence of drug-induced systemic lupus erythematosus; this incidence increases steadily with continuing administration so that it is probably undesirable to use this drug except on a short term basis. Long term administration may also induce leucopenia, granulocytopenia or, rarely, fatal agranulocytosis. Abdominal pain, hepatomegaly with evidence of liver damage, confusion, pruritus and hypersensitivity with fever and urticaria have also been described.

Lignocaine

Pharmacological action. Although primarily used for its local anaesthetic action, lignocaine decreases cardiac excitability. It differs, however, in having little or no depressant effect on myocardial contractility.

Therapeutic use. Lignocaine like procainamide is more useful in the treatment of ventricular rhythm disorders. It is not effective when given by mouth but given intravenously it is used to suppress ventricular ectopic beats or to arrest and prevent ventricular tachycardia, especially after myocardial infarction or cardiac surgery. It may be given as a single dose of 1–2 mg/kg of bodyweight or by continuous intravenuous infusion at a rate of 1–2 mg/minute.

Contraindications and side effects. Lignocaine should be used with caution in the presence of heart block as it can give rise to asystole. The development of serious tachycardia due to the development of 1:1 conduction has been reported as may happen with quinidine (see above) when used in the presence of atrial flutter. The earliest side effects are drowsiness, euphoria and muscular fasciculation; larger doses may produce hypotension, apprehension, confusion, nausea, vomiting, convulsions and ultimately respiratory and circulatory collapse.

Phenytoin sodium

Pharmacological action. In addition to its anticonvulsant action, phenytoin has been shown to have some anti-arrhythmic effect on the heart. The precise mode of action of phenytoin is uncertain, although it appears to have a depressant effect on pacemaker tissue and on myocardial function; unlike other anti-arrhythmic drugs it does not appear to delay activation of the AV node or slow conduction from the node to the ventricles.

Therapeutic use. It is said to be most effective in correcting supraventricular and ventricular arrhythmias resulting from digitalis intoxication and to be of use in preventing paroxysmal arrhythmias. It is not effective in the correction of atrial flutter or fibrillation. The true value of this drug as an anti-arrhythmic agent still remains to be determined.

It may be administered intravenously as a single dose of up to about 250 mg (or 5 mg/kg bodyweight), injected slowly, followed by maintenance doses of 200–400 mg orally, or by intramuscular injection.

Contraindications and side effects. As it may itself produce bradycardia or atrioventricular block it should not be used when either of these are already present; it probably has an additive effect with procainamide or lignocaine in depressing pacemaker tissue so should be used with caution in patients who have recently received these drugs. Sinus arrest has been reported after administration of 250 mg intravenously.

Intravenous injection can produce hypotension. Prolonged administration can, of course, produce the toxic effects which are better known in relation to its use as an anti-convulsant.

β-ADRENERGIC BLOCKING AGENTS
Propranolol

Pharmacological action. These are a series of compounds with structures related to that of the natural catecholamines, synthesised in a search for substances which would block the effect of the stimulation of the β-sympathetic receptors (see page 207). It slows the sinus rate and reduces myocardial contractility to some extent in the resting state but has a more obvious effect in reducing the tachycardia and increase in cardiac output which normally occurs in response to exercise. The subsequent demonstration that propranolol was a racemic mixture of stereoisomers, each of which has slightly different effects, and the preparation of other pharmacologically related substances, each with its own differing spectrum of effects, suggests that the hypothetical concept of β-receptor blockade is an over-simplification; nonetheless, the observed effects mentioned above remain true. In addition, propranolol seems to have an action on the myocardial cell membrane resembling that of quinidine. Apart from its cardiac action it also blocks the bronchodilator sympathetic action.

Therapeutic use. Propranolol found its first application as an anti-arrhythmic agent; it is effective in abolishing ectopic beats occurring during anaesthesia and, with digitalis, will often reduce the ventricular rate in atrial fibrillation when digitalis alone fails to do so. It is very effective in controlling sinus tachycardia related to anxiety. It has also been found useful in controlling arrhythmias induced by digitalis intoxication and in hyperthyroidism, where the cardiovascular disturbance is mediated by sympathetic over-activity. It is an effective antidote to tachycardia or rhythm disturbance induced by sympathetic amines therapeutically administered or produced endogenously by a phaeochromocytoma.

Its effect of impairing myocardial contractility led to its trial in the management of patients with hypertrophic obstructive cardiomyopathy (muscular subaortic stenosis) and of patients with Fallot's tetralogy subject to cyanotic attacks, whose right ventricular outflow obstruction was presumably variable due to a muscular mechanism at infundibular level; in both groups it has proved of value in some cases.

For the above purposes it is usually given orally three or four times a day in doses from 10 to 40 mg each; initially the full desired effect is often obtained by a small dose but it is commonly necessary subsequently to increase this to maintain the response. In acute situations, and when used under anaesthesia, it may be given by intravenous injection; the initial dose then should be only 1–2 mg given *slowly*, followed by further doses, if required, as the effect of the drug can be assessed; it is recommended, particularly in patients with recent myocardial infarction, that intravenous administration should be preceded by 1–2 mg atropine injected intravenously or bradycardia may occur.

The reduction by propranolol of the normal increase in the cardiac output on exercise suggested that it might be of value in the treatment of angina pectoris by limiting the myocardial demand for oxygen. It has been found to be of considerable value in this respect but maintenance of the response is usually dependent upon considerable increases in the dose up to levels of over 80 mg four times a day. Initial reports that it is of value in the treatment of hypertension have been confirmed by subsequent studies (see page 208).

Contraindications and side effects. Because of its action on the sympathetic nervous control of the bronchiolar musculature it should not be used for patients subject to asthma or bronchospasm of any cause. Because of its myocardial depressant effect, it should not be used in patients with myocardial failure or heart block. Even in patients with no clinical evidence of myocardial failure beforehand, propranolol administration has been held responsible for its development subsequently, especially when given on a long term basis in high doses, usually for the control of angina pectoris. Intravenous administration, especially if the initial dose is rather large (10 mg or more), has been followed by hypotension, extreme bradycardia and occasionally the precipitation of ventricular fibrillation.

Propranolol may also cause nausea, vomiting, diarrhea, lassitude, depression or insomnia; these effects are reduced by initial low dosage. Less commonly it has produced rashes, non-thrombocytopenic purpura, hallucinations and paraesthesiae.

Practolol

Pharmacological action. Practolol is another of the compounds which can block β-sympathetic activity. It differs from propranolol (q.v.) in not having direct myocardial depressant activity, in having some intrinsic sympathetic stimulant activity and by having a far lesser degree of blocking action on the sympathetic innervation of bronchial muscle.

Therapeutic use. Because it has no direct myocardial depressing effect and does not enhance bronchospasm, practolol is to be preferred to propranolol when treating patients with left heart failure or a tendency to bronchospasm. It is very effective in controlling supraventricular tachycardia and the ventricular rate in atrial fibrillation or flutter; for this it is used in an oral dose of 100 mg two or three times a day or it can be given intravenously in a dose of from 5–25 mg. In considerably larger doses (e.g. 1200 mg a day) it has been used for the management of angina pectoris. It has also been recommended for the treatment of hypertension.

Contraindications and side effects. In large doses it may give rise to diarrhea. It is contraindicated in patients who already have bradycardia or who have atrioventricular block.

Unfortunately practolol has been found to have other more serious side effects, It can induce a systemic lupus-like syndrome or a variety of psoriaform, ecxemoid or hyperkeratotic skin rashes all of which appear to be reversible. More importantly however, it can induce xerophthalmia leading sometimes to corneal scarring, and also sclerosing peritonitis, which may develop some time after stopping the drug. These complications appear to be specifically related to practolol and as there are alternatives there seems little reason for its continued use.

Oxprenolol

Pharmacological action. Oxprenolol hydrochloride has actions similar to propranolol and practolol. It differs from propranolol, however, in possessing intrinsic sympathetic stimulating activity and it differs from practolol in being less cardio-selective so that it also has some blocking action on bronchiolar sympathetic endings.

Therapeutic use. It is of value in the treatment of arrhythmias, particularly those of supraventricular origin or due to digitalis intoxication. The oral dose is 20–40 mg two or three times a day. It appears to be useful after myocardial infarction, having less myocardial depressant activity, and may suppress ventricular ectopic activity when lignocaine fails to do so; for this purpose it may be given by intravenous injections of 2 mg followed by infusion at a rate of 0.25 mg/ minute. It has proved to be effective in the management of angina pectoris. The dose for angina pectoris starts with 40 mg twice daily, increasing after a few days to 120–200 mg daily (in divided doses); up to 800 mg daily has been used. It is also widely used in the treatment of hypertension.

Contraindications and side effects. As with other β-blocking agents it is contraindicated in patients with atrioventricular block or bradycardia. Like propranolol, though not to so great a degree, it should be used with caution in patients with a tendency to bronchospasm. It may produce gastrointestinal disturbances and a feeling of lassitude, but these can usually be avoided by starting with small doses and increasing the dose gradually. Hypertension and ventricular fibrillation have been recorded after intravenous administration in acute situations (e.g. ventricular tachycardia after myocardial infarction). Aggravation of angina pectoris or the development of status anginosus has been described following withdrawal of treatment with oxprenolol.

A number of other β-blockers are now available (see page 208). They appear similar to those described above.

Verapamil

Pharmacological action. Originally thought to act by blockade of β-sympathetic receptor activity verapamil has now been shown to have a unique anti-arrhythmic action thought to be mediated through interference with the movement of calcium ions within the myocardial cells. It produces an atropine-resistant bradycardia and has a strong negative inotropic action. It has been shown also specifically to slow conduction through the AV node. In higher concentrations it produces total cardiac asystole.

Therapeutic use. Because of its action on the AV node it is useful in the management of supraventricular tachycardia, especially when this is associated with anomalous accessory conduction

(e.g. the W.P.W.* syndrome), and in the control of atrial flutter or fibrillation. A slow intravenous injection of 2.5–10 mg will abort the majority of attacks of supraventricular tachycardia. It may be given orally in a dose of 40–160 mg three times a day, usually in combination with a digitalis preparation, for the longer term control of paroxysmal tachycardia.

Contraindications and side effects. Verapamil should not be used in patients with conduction disturbances and only with caution in patients with impaired myocardial function. Sudden death due to refractory cardiac asystole has been reported after intravenous administration; this hazard may be related to concurrent digitalization.

Bretylium tosylate

Pharmacological action. Bretylium tosylate acts presynaptically and blocks all sympathetic nervous activity but does not block the effect of circulating catecholamines. It has a positive inotropic action on heart muscle but it is not clear how this is mediated. In animals it has been shown to raise the threshold for the electrical induction of ventricular fibrillation.

Therapeutic use. Originally introduced for the treatment of hypertension but since superseded by more satisfactory agents, bretylium tosylate has recently been advocated for the management of ventricular arrhythmias after myocardial infarction. It is reported to suppress ventricular ectopic beats and to prevent ventricular fibrillation whilst at the same time improving cardiac performance. Administered intravenously during cardiac massage, it may revert ventricular fibrillation to normal rhythm. Intravenous administration may cause nausea or vomiting so it is better to administer by intramuscular injection 300 mg, unless the situation is urgent; the dose can be repeated every 6–12 hours and supplementary doses of 100 mg may be given according to need at hourly intervals.

Contraindications and side effects. By all routes of administration it tends to produce loose stools. Its pharmacological action produces postural hypotension but this is not a problem in recumbent patients; supine hypotension occurs only occasionally. Nasal stuffiness is also reported but is not a serious problem.

Glyceryl trinitrate

Pharmacological action. Several organic nitrites and nitrates have a direct action in involuntary muscle, producing relaxation; this effect results in widespread vasodilatation. The distribution and

---

*Wolff Parkinson-White.

degree of this varies with different compounds but in the case of glyceryl trinitrate is widespread and includes the coronary arterial vessels, but with relatively little effect on the skin vessels. Recent studies have demonstrated that it produces a reduction in the resistance of the coronary circulation but that this is offset by the fall in blood pressure which results from the more generalised vasodilatation so that the myocardial blood flow is diminished; the fall in systemic blood pressure, however, is such that the myocardial work is decreased by a proportion which is greater than that of the reduction of myocardial blood flow. The net result is an increase in myocardial blood flow relative to its work.

Therapeutic use. Glyceryl trinitrate, in the form of 0.5 mg tablets allowed to dissolve in the mouth so that it is absorbed through the oral mucosa, is used for the prevention and relief of angina pectoris. It acts within two or three minutes and the effects lasts for 15–30 minutes. Repeated use leads to the development of tolerance but a cessation of use for a few days re-establishes the normal effect.

Contraindications and side effects. Glyceryl trinitrate causes a rise in intraocular tension, so should be avoided in patients with glaucoma. It also causes widespread dilatation of the blood vessels of the head and neck and in some individuals this results in distressing headache or throbbing in the head; it should be used with caution in patients with cerebrovascular disease, intracranial lesions or recent head injury. In some patients the hypotensive effect produces a sensation of syncope which may be accompanied by nausea or vomiting.

Amyl nitrite

Pharmacological action. Similar to glyceryl trinitrate but with a greater effect on the skin vessels, especially of the face and neck.

Therapeutic use. Amyl nitrite is a highly volatile liquid administered by inhalation of the vapour released by crushing a glass capsule containing 0.2 ml of the liquid. It has an effect in about 10 seconds which lasts only 2–3 minutes. Its penetrating odour and the abruptness and intensity of the vasodilatation of the head and face make it objectionable to many patients.

Contraindications and side effects. As for glyceryl trinitrate.

Sorbide nitrate

Pharmacological action. As for glyceryl trinitrate.

Therapeutic use. When given as a 10 mg tablet dissolved in the mouth its effect is produced in about 10–15 minutes and lasts up to 4 hours.

With this slower, but more prolonged action it is of little use for the immediate relief of angina pectoris but is recommended as a prophylactic. Acute experiments show that it can increase exercise tolerance before the onset of anginal pain but well-controlled trials of its chronic use have failed to show convincing evidence of its effectiveness on a long term basis.

Pentaerythritol

Pharmacological action. As for glyceryl trinitrate. *Therapeutic use.* When given by mouth pentaerythritol tetranitrate produces some fall in the blood pressure after about an hour, which lasts for about 5 hours. It is therefore of no value in the treatment of the acute attack of angina pectoris. Its activity is similar to sorbide nitrate (see above) and it is commonly used as a prophylactic agent although many trials have failed to show any statistically significant benefit. The dose is 20–30 mg.

Dipyridamole

Pharmacological action. Extensive studies in experimental animals and in man have established that dipyridamole has a remarkably selective, but powerful, vasodilator action on the coronary blood vessels, leading to a significant increase in coronary blood flow. It also appears to have an effect in inhibiting platelet clumping.

Therapeutic use. The pharmacological action of dipyridamole led to the expectation that it would be of value in the treatment of ischaemic heart disease; so far no study has shown that it is of any symptomatic benefit in that condition. Its effect on platelet clumping has led to its use, sometimes in combination with aspirin, as a thrombus-formation inhibitor in coronary artery disease and in patients with prosthetic heart valves. It can be given by mouth in a dose of 25–50 mg two or three times daily or by slow intravenous injection in a dose of 10–20 mg.

Contraindications and side effects. There do not appear to be any contraindications to its use; it may cause anorexia or nausea, headache, dizziness, or faintness and occasionally, after intravenous injection, facial flushing or some fall in the blood pressure.

Prenylamine

Pharmacological action. Like dipyridamole, prenylamine lactate has been shown to have a powerful coronary vascular dilating effect. It also has a slight hypotensive action which is probably mediated by an antagonistic effect against sympathetic activity.

Therapeutic use. The combination of coronary vasodilatation and sympathetic blockade suggests that this drug should be of value in the treatment of angina pectoris. Several trials have reported its successful use as a prophylactic agent in a dose of 60 mg two to four times a day.

Contraindications and side effects. Prenylamine is contraindicated in the presence of conduction defects, heart failure, or hepatic disease. Patients already receiving hypotensive agents may require some reduction in the dose whilst receiving prenylamine. Gastric intolerance has been reported occasionally when the drug is first administered; rashes rarely occur.

Cholestyramine

Pharmacological action. Cholestyramine is a basic anion-exchange resin which binds bile acids in the intestine and thereby prevents their reabsorption and interferes with the absorption of other lipids.

Therapeutic use. In total daily doses of 12–15 g cholestyramine has been shown to reduce the blood-cholesterol levels especially in patients with Type IIA hyperlipidaemia and has been used to correct this biochemical deviation in the hope of reducing the risk of development of atheroma. It is also said to be effective in relieving itching in obstructive jaundice.

Contraindications and side effects. It may produce gastrointestinal discomfort.

Polidexide

Pharmacological action. Polidexide is an anion-exchange resin with similar actions to cholestyramine.

Therapeutic use. Taken as one sachet (containing 3.0 g) three to five times daily it is used as an alternative to cholestyramine. It is however more palatable so patients are more likely to find it an acceptable form of treatment. Combination with clofibrate has been reported as enhancing its blood cholesterol lowering effect.

Contraindications and side effects. Treatment with anticoagulants may be affected, so that more frequent monitoring may be required and the dose of anticoagulant increased. It may also cause constipation and abdominal distension.

Clofibrate

Pharmacological action. Clofibrate lowers elevated serum triglyceride and cholesterol levels by its effects upon low-density β-lipoproteins. These effects appear to result from the binding of clofibrate to specific sites on the plasma proteins which in turn leads to a redistribution between the plasma and liver of several factors which affect the blood/lipid pattern. It also seems to correct a number of factors which produce the hypercoagulability often associated with atherosclerotic disease.

Therapeutic use. Prolonged administration is used in patients with atherosclerosis, especially if this is manifest by clinical evidence of coronary heart disease, cerebral or peripheral vascular disease and those with type IV hyperlipidaemia or diabetic arteriopathy in the hope of reducing progression of vascular disease. Recent reports suggest that in patients with angina it may reduce the risk of myocardial infarction and early death from coronary disease but these have not been confirmed. The drug is introduced gradually and is then maintained at 20–30 mg/kg bodyweight daily in divided doses.

Contraindications and side effects. Clofibrate should not be given during pregnancy or to patients with impaired renal or hepatic function. It potentiates the action of anticoagulant drugs and, in some patients, of insulin so that it should be introduced cautiously to patients receiving these. It may cause nausea, gastrointestinal discomfort, drowsiness or produce rashes; a gain in weight frequently follows its administration. A rise in serum transaminases and a fall in alkaline phosphatase levels may occur but are probably related to the action of the drug rather than to hepatotoxicity.

Isoprenaline

Pharmacological action. Isoprenaline is a potent stimulator of the β-receptors of the sympathetic nervous system. It increases the heart rate, improves atrioventricular conduction, increases myocardial contractility and produces predominant vasodilation in the systemic circulation.

Therapeutic use. It is of considerable value in improving myocardial function in patients who have had recent myocardial infarction or undergone major cardiac surgery and thereby leads to improved tissue perfusion. For this purpose it is infused intravenously as 2–5 mg diluted in 500 ml of 5% dextrose at a rate of 2–50 drops/minute, carefully controlled and adjusted according to the response of the patient whose electrocardiogram should be under continuous oscilloscope observation. In the form of tablets of 30 mg contained in a slow release base it can be given by mouth to increase the idioventricular rate or improve the conduction in patients with complete heart block, but this treatment is often ineffective or attended by intolerable side effects.

Contraindications and side effects. Isoprenaline should not be given to patients with hyperthyroidism or who have any form of ventricular arrhythmia. It can provoke tachycardia, ectopic beats and ventricular fibrillation. Headache, palpitations, anginal pain, flushing, apprehension, tremor, nausea and weakness are common side effects of overdosage.

Atropine

Pharmacological action. In relation to the cardiovascular system atropine blocks the inhibiting effect of vagal activity on the sinus and atrioventricular nodes. If the heart is affected by increased vagal tone atropine increases the heart rate and reduces the atrioventricular conduction time.

Therapeutic use. It is the specific treatment for vagally mediated bradycardia with or without atrioventricular conduction defects such as may occur from digitalis intoxication or reflexly after myocardial infarction, DC shock correction of arrhythmias, or in response to procedures such as aortic catheterisation or cardiac puncture. For this purpose it can be given by intravenous injection of between 0.25 and 1.5 mg. Its use in acute myocardial infarction to prevent cardiac slowing, and the reputed risk of severe arrhythmias following this, has been advocated, but recent reports have failed to establish significant benefit from this.

Calcium chloride

Pharmacological action. In relation to the cardiovascular system it is a powerful stimulator of myocardial contractility.

Therapeutic use. The effect of calcium chloride is transient so that it is of no value for long term treatment but a slow injection of 0.5–2 g intravenously will often restore the contractility of an asystolic ventricle or improve that of a fibrillating ventricle so as to permit successful electrical defibrillation.

Contraindications and side effects. Calcium chloride should not be used if digitalis intoxication is a possible cause of the arrhythmia. Calcium chloride is irritating to the tissues so that care must be exercised during intravenous injection.

Category 6

DRUGS USED IN THE TREATMENT OF HYPERTENSIVE AND VASCULAR DISEASES

J. R. TROUNCE

AGENTS ACTING DIRECTLY ON ARTERIOLES

Hydrallazine

Pharmacological action. Hydrallazine produces a widespread vasodilatation with a fall in blood pressure which is not usually affected by posture. The greatest fall is in the diastolic pressure. This is accompanied by a rise in pulse rate and cardiac output which to some extent neutralises the hypotensive action of the drug. How this rise in cardiac output is achieved is not known but it is possible that hydrallazine reflexly augments the actions of the adrenergic nervous system.

Hydrallazine is well absorbed and the drug is largely metabolised.

Therapeutic use. Hydrallazine is a mild blood pressure lowering agent and its use is limited by the high incidence of side effects. The initial dose is 10 mg four times daily, and this is gradually increased to a total of 100–200 mg daily. In order to prevent the rise in pulse rate and cardiac output which accompanies its use hydrallazine may be combined with a β-blocker (see below). It increases renal blood flow and is therefore said to be particularly useful in hypertension complicating renal disease.

Contraindication and side effects. Headaches are particularly common at the start of treatment, but usually disappear after a week or so of continued treatment. They may be accompanied by nausea and diarrhea. In the higher dose range (over 400 mg daily) and after prolonged treatment about 10% of patients show a rheumatoid-like syndrome, sometimes accompanied by a positive LE phenomena. This may take a considerable time to subside after stopping the drug.

Hydrallazine may also produce skin rashes and rarely a peripheral neuropathy.

The rise in pulse rate and output caused by hydrallazine may precipitate anginal pain in those with coronary disease. Under these circumstances it should be combined with a β-blocker.

Prazosin

Pharmacological action. Prazosin lowers the blood pressure by a direct relaxing effect on the walls of the arteries. It is probably also a mild α-blocker. It appears to have no central effect. The fall in blood pressure is little affected by posture.

Therapeutic use. Prazosin used alone produces a moderate fall in blood pressure. This action may take several weeks to reach a maximum. The initial dose is 1–2 mg three times daily, and may be increased. Twice daily dosage may be sufficient. It seem that prazosin will be particularly useful if combined with a diuretic or a β-blocker.

Contraindications and side effects. Dizziness and sometimes headaches may occur, and the dizziness does not appear to be related to the fall in blood pressure. The most important is a transient loss of consciousness. This occurs at the start of treatment but the exact mechanism is not known. The risk can be minimised by starting with a small dose (1.0 mg) and thereafter keeping the patient under observation for a few hours.

Diazoxide

Diazoxide is related to the benzothiadiazine diuretics. It is a powerful agent for lowering the blood pressure when given intravenously, reducing peripheral resistance by a direct action on the arterial walls. It has no diuretic action and may in fact cause salt and water retention. It is used in the treatment of acute hypertensive crises, the dose being 5 mg/kg intravenously and it must be given undiluted as it is ineffective if given by slow intravenous infusion. A single dose lasts up to 6 hours.

Diazoxide inhibits insulin release and causes a rise in blood sugar levels. Although it is also effective orally, it is not usually given for more than a week or two to bring a severely hypertensive patient under control. It is also used in the treatment of hypoglycaemia due to tumours of the β-cells of the pancreas.

THE GANGLION BLOCKERS

Pharmacological action. The ganglion blockers were the first effective blood pressure lowering agents. They interfere with transmission at the relay ganglia of both the adrenergic and cholinergic nervous systems. At these sites they compete with acetylcholine and thus prevent depolarisation of the membrane of the postsynaptic nerve cells.

The actions of these drugs can be grouped according to the system involved:
1. Cardiovascular system. Loss of adrenergic tone leads to arterial and venous vasodilatation. This causes pooling of blood with a decreased venous return to the heart and a fall in cardiac output. The drop in cardiac output and the arteriolar dilatation are responsible for the fall in blood pressure which is largely postural (i.e. only seen on standing and abolished by lying flat).
2. Gastrointestinal. Loss of cholinergic activity causes a dry mouth, slows intestine transit, and leads to constipation and occasionally ileus.
3. Genito-urinary. Retention may occur especially if there is some bladder neck obstruction and impotence is an occasional complication.
4. Eyes. Pupils may dilate with paralysis of accommodation.

These drugs are largely excreted by the kidney and with impaired renal function, accumulation will occur.

Therapeutic use. Although they are potent hypotensive agents, the widespread pharmacological effect of these drugs, and the fact that the fall in blood pressure is postural, has led to their being replaced by other agents and they are now rarely used.

The chief individual ganglion blockers available are:

Hexamethonium bromide was the prototype drug. It is irregularly and poorly absorbed from the intestine and was not therefore very satisfactory for the long-term treatment of hypertension.

Pentolinium tartrate is slightly better absorbed orally, but is now largely used in hypertensive crises when it is given by subcutaneous injection. The initial dose is 2.5 mg (1.25 mg in the elderly) and then a further 1.0 mg is given every fifteen minutes until a satisfactory fall in blood pressure is produced. (Note; the blood pressure must be taken sitting or standing.)

Mecamylamine is well absorbed from the intestine and the initial oral dose is 2.5 mg twice daily. This is increased every four days until a satis-factory fall in blood pressure is produced. Mecamylamine is only slowly excreted in an alkaline urine and because of this should not be combined with acetazolamide. In addition to the side effects of ganglion blockade, mecamylamine may produce tremor and weakness due to an action on voluntary muscle.

Pempidine is also absorbed and the initial dose is 2.5 mg three times a day and increased as required.

Trimetaphan is a very rapidly acting ganglion blocker. It is given by intravenous infusion in a 1:1000 solution. Its effects pass off rapidly after stopping infusion. It is largely used to produce controlled postural hypotension.

Contraindications and side effects. Ganglion blockers should be used with care or not at all in patients where a sudden fall in blood pressure could be dangerous. This will include those with severe myocardial or cerebral ischaemia.

In patients with renal failure a blood urea of over 100 mg% usually contraindicates as a large fall in blood pressure may cause a further disastrous deterioration in renal function and there is also the problem of impaired excretion.

Patients on these drugs are unduly sensitive to sympathomimetic amines.

THE ADRENERGIC BLOCKERS
THOSE BLOCKING THE POST GANGLIONIC NERVES

This group of drugs is quite widely used to lower blood pressure. They all produce this effect by interfering in some way with the release of noradrenaline at the adrenergic nerve ending. In general, they also cause a fall in blood pressure, which is largely postural. This is largely due to loss of vasomotor tone causing peripheral pooling of blood with decreased venous return and a lowered cardiac output. Prolonged treatment may result in some increase in blood volume and thus some decrease in efficiency of the hypotensive agent.

They all have side effects which are referable to adrenergic blockade. There are however minor differences in both the duration of action and in the incidence of side effects.

The main drugs of this type in use at present are:

Guanethidine

Pharmacological action. Guanethidine decreases a release of noradrenaline at adrenergic nerve endings. If injected intravenously it causes a transient rise in blood pressure, because it inhibits re-uptake of noradrenaline by nerve endings.

Guanethidine also causes some depletion of peripheral noradrenaline stores. It is only moderately well absorbed from the intestines and is only slowly excreted by the kidneys, and it is several days before a single dose is cleared from the body. This means that one dose daily is adequate.

Therapeutic use. Guanethidine is given initially in a dose of 10 mg in the morning. The dose is increased at weekly intervals until a satisfactory control of blood pressure is produced, usually with around 20–60 mg daily. The rather prolonged action of guanethidine makes it difficult to control the blood pressure if it varies widely throughout the day. Tolerance does not usually develop to any marked extent with guanethidine, but can be due to sodium and water retention and is controlled by using a diuretic.

Contraindications and side effects. Diarrhea is the most troublesome side effect but can be controlled with codeine phosphate or with the addition of a ganglion blocking agent. Bradycardia is usual but is not important. Other results of adrenergic blockade are failure of ejaculation and parotid pain.

As with the ganglion blockers guanethidine must be used with great care in those with marked cerebral or myocardial ischaemia or in renal failure.

Guanoxan

Pharmacological action. Guanoxan is a combination of the guanethidine ring with benzodioxane. It blocks release of noradrenaline and also depletes peripheral stores. In addition, presumably due to its benzodioxane moiety, it has some direct blocking action on circulating adrenaline and noradrenaline. The fall in blood pressure is postural but less markedly so than guanethidine.

Therapeutic use. Guanoxan is administered in an initial dose of 20 mg daily and increased every four days as required.

Contraindications and side effects. Guanoxan causes diarrhea and failure of ejaculation. In addition it may cause drowsiness, particularly early in treatment. Changes in liver function tests are not uncommon and occasionally they may be followed by jaundice.

It would seem that the risk of liver damage should limit the use of the drug.

Guanochlor

Pharmacological action. Guanochlor interferes with noradrenaline release and storage and may also interfere with the conversion of dopamine to noradrenaline. It produces a postural fall in blood pressure.

Therapeutic use. Guanochlor is given in an initial dose of 10 mg twice daily and this is increased every third day until a satisfactory fall in blood pressure is produced.

Contraindications and side effects. In a few patients guanochlor causes some urea retention but there does not appear to be any interference with overall renal function. It may also cause salt and water retention and may have to be combined with a diuretic. Guanochlor causes pain in skeletal muscle in a small number of patients; the reason for this is unknown. Other side effects are similar to those of the adrenergic blocking group as a whole.

Bethanidine

Pharmacological action. Bethanidine lowers blood pressure by blocking noradrenaline release from the adrenergic nerve endings. It has no peripheral depleting action and no blocking action on circulating noradrenaline. It is rapidly and well absorbed producing a peak effect within 4–5 hours. It is excreted via the kidneys and entirely eliminated within about 12 hours.

Therapeutic use. The relatively short action of bethanidine enables the blood pressure to be controlled more flexibly as the dose can be modified to meet fluctuation during the day.

The initial dose is 10 mg twice daily and this is increased by adding 5 or 10 mg to each dose until adequate control is obtained. If the blood pressure is very variable during the day bethanidine can be given three or four times daily. Some tolerance may develop.

In severe hypertension it appears to have some synergistic action with methyldopa.

Contraindications and side effects. The fall in blood pressure is markedly postural. However, diarrhea is unusual.

Other side effects are similar to guanethidine, but it occasionally causes depression. It should not be used when a phaeochromocytoma is suspected and should not be combined with the amphetamine group of drugs.

Debrisoquine

Pharmacological action. Debrisoquine prevents release of noradrenaline at adrenergic nerve endings without depleting peripheral stores and produces a postural fall in blood pressure. It is relatively rapid in action and is very similar to bethanidine.

Therapeutic use. The initial dose is 10 mg twice daily and this is increased every three or four days until a satisfactory fall in blood pressure results.

Contraindications and side effects. Debrisoquine is fairly free of side effects. When they occur they include diarrhea, failure of ejaculation, muscle weakness and tiredness. Contraindications are the same for any agent which can cause a considerable fall in blood pressure.

THOSE ACTING ON SEVERAL SITES

Methyldopa

Pharmacological action. Methyldopa differs from all the other drugs which inhibit the adrenergic nervous system. It is believed to be converted to methylnoradrenaline at the adrenergic nerve endings and this substance which is only a weak vasoconstrictor acts as a 'false mediator'. It seems that the peripheral action of methyldopa cannot entirely explain its blood pressure lowering properties and it is probably that there is a central component to its action. The important result of these is that with methyldopa the fall in blood pressure is almost as great lying as standing.

Methyldopa is well absorbed but its hypotensive effect is delayed for 4–6 hours. It is excreted via the kidneys and about half the dose is cleared from the body in 12 hours, and excretion is complete in 48 hours.

Therapeutic use. Methyldopa is very widely used in the treatment of hypertension. The initial dose is 250 mg twice daily and this is increased every fourth day until a satisfactory response is obtained. The usual dose is 250 mg four times daily. It is not worth giving more than 2.0 g daily as further increases in dose will not usually increase the hypotensive effect. Methyldopa has a tendency to provoke sodium and water retention and its action can be augmented by combining it with a diuretic.

Contraindications and side effects. Methyldopa produces drowsiness in 20–30% of patients, although this may diminish with continued treatment. Other side effects include dry mouth, nasal congestion and lactation. Marked water retention is rare but can cause edema. It responds to a diuretic.

Methyldopa can also provoke hypersensitivity phenomena. About 20% of those on long term treatment at high dosage levels develop a positive direct Coombs test and occasionally a frank haemolytic anaemia. Other hypersensitivity phenomena have been described, including drug fever, skin rashes and rarely, liver damage. In patients with renal failure, retention of the drug can give rise to a Parkinson-like state.

Methyldopa should therefore not be used in liver disease, and with care in those with impaired renal function.

Clonidine

Pharmacological action. In acute experiments clonidine causes a fall in blood pressure associated with a drop in cardiac output. With long term administration, however, the fall in blood pressure is probably due to a central action and it is not related to posture.

Resistance to the hypotensive action of clonidine can develop. It appears to be due to associated sodium retention and can be reversed by a diuretic.

Therapeutic use. Clonidine will lower blood pressure effectively in hypertensives. The lack of postural fall is an advantage and impotence is not a feature of its action. However, side effects are rather common. Its place in treating hypertension is probably as a substitute for methyldopa when that drug for some reason is unsatisfactory. The initial dose is 200 μg daily and increased as required.

It has also been found useful in preventing attacks of migraine. The initial dose should be small and it may take several weeks to become effective.

Contraindications and side effects. The most frequent are sedation and a dry mouth. Peripheral vasoconstriction with 'cold hands' has been reported. It should be avoided in those with manic or depressive tendencies as it may cause psychological disturbances. Too rapid withdrawal of the drug may cause 'rebound' hypertension which can be controlled with propranolol and phentolamine.

β-ADRENERGIC BLOCKING AGENTS

Pharmacological action (See page 198).
Therapeutic use. β-blockers cause a fall in blood pressure which is largely unrelated to posture. The reduction in blood pressure may be delayed for several weeks after starting the drugs and persists for some weeks after the drug is stopped.

How the fall in blood pressure is brought about is not known but β-blockers certainly produce a fall in cardiac output which could be contributory. It has been suggested that inhibition of the angiotensin–renin mechanism which certainly occurs with most β-blockers is a factor, but this has not been confirmed and the fall in blood pressure does not seem to be related to the level of plasma renin or to its fall as a result of treatment.

There are now many β-blockers available for

the treatment of hypertension. The more cardio-selective ones appear to be as useful as those affecting both β_1 and β_2 receptors. At the time of writing there is no evidence that any particular β-blocker is to be preferred. Practolol, because of its side effects should be avoided in long term treatment.

Drug	Daily dose	
	Initial	Maximum
Propranolol	80 mg	1000 mg
Oxprenolol	120 mg	800 mg
Sotalol	80 mg	800 mg
Pindolol	360 mg	1080 mg
Metoprolol	200 mg	400 mg
Timolol	15 mg	45 mg

One interesting point is whether β-blockers will decrease the incidence of ischaemic heart disease in hypertensive patients. This complication of hypertension is not affected when the blood pressure is lowered by other types of hypotensive agent, but there is some evidence that β-blockers may reduce the incidence of coronary episodes and sudden death. Confirmation is however required.

It is best to start with a low dose of β-blocker and work up slowly until optimal results are obtained. In practice, maximum doses given above have sometimes been exceeded. One practical problem of high dosage is the number of pills the patient may have to consume.

β-blockers may be combined with advantage with other hypotensive agents, in particular diuretics, or directly achieving vasodilations such as hydrallazine or prazosin.

Contraindications and side effects (see page 199).

α-ADRENERGIC BLOCKING AGENTS (see above)

Phentolamine/Phenoxybenzamine

MONOAMINE-OXIDASE (MAO) INHIBITORS

Pargyline

Pharmacological action. The drug is a mono-amine-oxidase inhibitor and also lowers blood pressure, probably by blocking the post-ganglionic part of the adrenergic nervous system. The fall in blood pressure is partially postural.

It is only slowly excreted and one dose daily is adequate.

Therapeutic use. Pargyline is given in an initial dose of 25 mg orally. It takes about two weeks to produce its full effect and the dose is there-after increased by 10 mg at two-weekly intervals. *Contraindications and side effects.* Pargyline has all the side effects and dangers of other MAO inhibitors (see above). The inherent dangers limit its use as a hypertensive agent. It is also contraindicated in liver or kidney failure, in thyrotoxicosis and in pregnancy.

RAUWOLFIA ALKALOIDS

This group of alkaloids are mild hypotensive agents. They may be used either as various crude fractions or as the pure alkaloids (reserpine, rescinnamine, deserpidine, etc.). Reserpine is the most widely used.

Reserpine

Pharmacological action. Reserpine lowers blood pressure by reducing the activity of the sympathetic nervous system and also by a tranquilising and depressing action on the brain. Reserpine depletes catecholamines in both the peripheral sympathetic nervous systems and in the brain and it seems probable its effects are due to this depletion.

Therapeutic use. Reserpine in doses of up to 0.25 mg twice daily has a moderate blood pressure lowering action which is unrelated to posture, and which is due to fall in peripheral resistance. It is well absorbed from the intestine but it is usually four or five days before it begins to lower the blood pressure and it may be a week or two before it becomes fully effective. Likewise its activity will continue for several days after stopping the drug. At this dosage level side effects can be troublesome and a lower dose (0.25 mg daily) may be used, combined with a diuretic.

There are a number of other preparations available which contain reserpine or related alkaloids. They include:

Methoserpedine, 10 mg ⎫
Rescinnamine, 0.35 mg ⎬ equivalent to 0.25 mg
Deserpedine, 0.5 mg ⎭ of reserpine

There is no evidence that they have any advantage over reserpine.

The other actions of reserpine can be grouped:

1. Sympatholytic effects: including brady-cardia, nasal stuffiness and extrasystoles. There may also be increased gastrointestinal motor activity with a raised gastric acid secretion and occasionally peptic ulceration and diarrhea.

2. Central effects can be troublesome. Some drowsiness and general lack of 'go' with decreased libido is common, and occasionally a psychotic depression develops. With large doses a Parkinson-like state can be produced.

In addition, patients may show weight gain due to fluid retention.

Contraindications and side effects. Reserpine should not be used in depressed patients and should be used with care in those with intestinal disease, particularly peptic ulcer and ulcerative colitis. Recently it has been reported that there is a higher incidence of carcinoma of the breast in patients taking reserpine than can be accounted for by chance. Although this observation requires confirmation it would seem unwise to start a patient on reserpine when there are so many other hypotensive agents available.

DIURETICS

Pharmacology. A wide variety of diuretics will lower blood pressure. In the early stages of treatment this appears related to the decrease in circulating blood volume which follows natriuresis. However, after some weeks' treatment both blood volume and cardiac output return to normal but the hypotensive action continues.

Therapeutic use. The fall in blood pressure produced by diuretics is relatively small but they are particularly useful when combined with other hypotensive agents when they increase and smooth out the hypotensive action of these drugs. In addition some hypotensive agents (particularly methyldopa) may cause sodium and water retention which can be reversed by diuretics. They may also prevent the development of resistance to some hypotensive drugs, in particular the adrenergic blocking agents.

In theory, the longer-acting diuretics, such as chlorthalidone should be most suitable in hypertension, but in practice any of the benzothiadiazines, or even the relatively short-acting frusemide are satisfactory. The choice of diuretics and side effects are considered later (see page 210).

Spironolactone (page 212)

Pharmacological action and therapeutic use. Spironolactone is a steroidal lactone which blocks the action of aldosterone. Spironolactone produces a significant fall in blood pressure in hypertensive patients with high plasma aldosterone levels and low plasma renin levels, whether or not they have an adrenal adenoma. The exact cause of the fall is not known but it is associated with a return of the body sodium and potassium content towards normal. High doses of spirono-

lactone (up to 400 mg daily) are usually required, but this drug does appear to offer an alternative to surgery in this small group of hypertensive patients.

PERIPHERAL VASODILATORS

Tolazoline

Pharmacological action. Tolazoline produces peripheral vasodilatation, mainly of skin vessels. This is largely due to a direct action on the vessel wall but it is also a weak α receptor blocker. Tolazoline also increases both heart rate and output, and so may actually increase blood pressure. It also stimulates gastric secretion. It is well absorbed and rapidly excreted via the kidneys.

Therapeutic use. Tolazoline is used in doses of 25–50 mg three times a day in the treatment of peripheral vascular disease. There is no good evidence that it has any benefit in atherosclerotic disease but may help in Raynaud's phenomena.

Contraindications and side effects. Tolazoline may cause tachycardia and cardiac arrhythmias, flushing and diarrhea. It may also exacerbate peptic ulceration.

It should not be used in heart failure, angina of effort, or in those with peptic ulceration.

Cyclendelate

Pharmacological action and therapeutic use. The drug produces vasodilatation by acting directly on the arterial wall. It has been used for peripheral vascular disease and is also claimed to increase cerebral blood flow. There is little evidence that it is of benefit in vascular disease of the limbs or the brain.

The usual dose if 400 mg three times daily. Side effects include flushing, dizziness and headaches.

Inositol nicotinate

A mild vasodilator. The initial dose is 200 mg four times daily and it can be increased. It appears free of ill effects.

Isoxsuprine

This drug causes a combination of peripheral vasodilatation with an increase in cardiac output. The dose is 10 mg four times daily. Its efficiency in peripheral vascular disease is doubtful.

Category 7

DIURETICS AND CATION EXCHANGE RESINS

C. S. OGG

DIURETICS

Diuretics are indicated in any patient who has adequate renal function and who has edema arising from a central rather than a local cause. They play a major part in the management of cardiac failure and of edema attributable to a low plasma protein level whether this arises on a nutritional, hepatic or renal basis. In addition they have a valuable supplementary role in the treatment of hypertension and are sometimes useful in the treatment of renal calculi and of some cases of poisoning.

The power of modern diuretics has diminished the therapeutic value of dietary sodium restriction. This still has a place, however, and its effect may be increased by the oral administration of a cation exchange resin in the potassium, ammonium or calcium phase.

Benzothiadiazines and related drugs

Pharmacological action and therapeutic use. There are at least eleven drugs of this type in use (Table 1). They differ in their intestinal absorption and diuretic potency and in their solubility in fat which determines their rate of excretion, and duration of action.

Table 1. The benzothiadiazines

Approved name	Duration of action (hours)	Dose (mg)
Chlorothiazide	12	500–2000
Cyclopenthiazide	12	0.25–2.0
Cyclothiazide	24	1.0–6.0
Bendrofluazide	18	2.5–10.0
Benzthiazide	12	25–200
Hydrochlorothiazide	14	25–200
Hydroflumethiazide	14	25–200
Methyclothiazide	24	2.5–10.0
Polythiazide	48	1.0–8.0
Trichlormethiazide	24	1.0–8.0

In addition there are a number of closely related drugs (Table 2) which have a different heterocyclic moiety but common side chains, similar actions and identical side effects.

Table 2. Diuretics which resemble the benzothiadiazines

Approved name	Duration of action (hours)	Dose (mg)
Chlorthalidone	72	50–200
Clorexolone	48	10–50
Quinethazone	24	50–200
Clopamide	24	20–80
Mefruside	24	25–100
Metolazone	18	10–20

All these drugs increase the urinary excretion of sodium and have secondary effects on the excretion of water, chloride and potassium. They are weak inhibitors of carbonic anhydrase and may impair the ability to excrete an acid urine.

Some doubt exists concerning their sites of action on the kidney. Stop-flow studies indicate an effect on the proximal convoluted tubule but micropuncture work suggests that the most important action is on the proximal part of the distal convoluted tubule. They are all given orally and, in addition, there is a preparation of chlorothiazide that is suitable for intravenous injection (dose: 500 mg). The shorter acting drugs are given daily, usually in the mornings, but the longer acting ones need be given only on alternate days.

In addition to their conventional uses, the benzothiadiazines have been shown to lower the urinary excretion of calcium and may prove to be of value in the prevention of renal caculi.

Contraindications and side effects. The benzothiadiazines and related drugs are all fairly safe but have a number of well recognised side effects.

Early in treatment, potassium excretion rises due to the increased amount of sodium available for exchange in the distal tubule. Later, relatively less sodium and more potassium ions appear in the urine and, eventually, potassium may become the major urinary cation with the development of potassium depletion and an extracellular alkalosis. Ultimately edema may be completely resistant to treatment and the serum sodium concentration falls. Intracellular potassium depletion contributes to this state and it is advisable to stop the diuretic and replace potassium while restricting the intake of sodium and water. Although the serum potassium level is a poor index of potassium depletion, it is worth measuring it regularly in those on prolonged treatment especially with large doses of diuretic. In such patients supplements of potassium chloride are indicated (see later). Possibly because it is not an inhibitor, carbonic anhydrase metolizone appears to produce less potassium depletion than other drugs in this group.

Frusemide

Pharmacological action and therapeutic use. Frusemide has some chemical similarity to the benzothiadiazines but produces a substantially greater diuretic effect. This is not increased by the addition of a benzothiadiazine suggesting that frusemide acts at the same sites in the tubule plus another site which is thought to be the ascending limb of Henle's loop. Absorption from the gut is rapid and complete, and excretion is by the kidney.

A diuresis begins within two minutes of intravenous administration (dose: 20–60 mg) and lasts only 2 hours. This makes it ideal for the treatment of acute pulmonary edema.

After oral administration (dose: 40–120 mg) the diuretic effect lasts about 4 hours. This transient action makes it relatively unsuitable for maintenance therapy unless weaker drugs have proved ineffective. Its great power makes it useful in the treatment of patients with impaired renal function when very large doses (500–2000 mg daily) may be given. Recently it has been suggested that similar large doses may be of value in the treatment of patients with acute renal failure due to acute tubular necrosis. Under these circumstances, frusemide can be given intravenously at a rate which should not exceed 4 mg/minute.

Contraindications and side effects. The main problems derive from its potency, and it is easy to produce acute hypovolaemia and chronic electrolyte depletion. It is logical to start treatment with a small dose and to take particular care when the edema is associated with hypoproteinaemia and hypovolaemia. In these circumstances it may be necessary to maintain the blood volume by the intravenous administration of salt poor albumin or an osmotic diuretic (see later). Apart from this, the drug is fairly safe; potassium depletion and hyperuricaemia occur frequently but

carbohydrate intolerance is seen less often than with the benzothiadiazines. Leucopenia, thrombocytopenia and diarrhea have been reported. There is some evidence that the simultaneous administration of frusemide enhances the nephrotoxicity of cephaloridine and this combination of drugs should be avoided.

Ethacrynic acid

Pharmacological action and therapeutic use. Chemically this drug differs substantially from frusemide and the benzothiadiazines. It has a powerful diuretic action which is not increased by frusemide and which lasts about 8 hours. It is well absorbed from the gut (dose: 50–400 mg) and may also be given intravenously (dose: 50 mg). Excretion is via the kidneys and liver.

Contraindications and side effects. Electrolyte depletion and hypovolaemia are real hazards and it is essential to start treatment with small doses. Potassium supplements are necessary during maintenance therapy. Hyperuricaemia, thrombocytopenia and skin rashes may also occur and there is a rather high incidence of gastrointestinal symptoms. Patients have been reported who developed deafness when treated with large doses of ethacrynic acid in the presence of renal failure.

Bumetanide

Pharmacological action and therapeutic use. This drug is similar to frusemide but differs chemically and is more powerful on a weight for weight basis. It is well absorbed from the intestine and the oral dose is 1–4 mg. Its diuretic effect lasts about three hours. It can also be given intravenously when the dose is 0.5–4.0 mg.

Contraindications and side effects. Hypokalaemia occurs commonly and as with other powerful diuretics hypovolaemia is a definite hazard. The drug also causes uric acid retention.

Organic mercurials

Pharmacological action and therapeutic use. These drugs were the first effective diuretics and remain among the most powerful. Unfortunately they are poorly absorbed from the gut and are usually given by intramuscular injection; in view of this inconvenience they have been largely replaced by oral diuretics. Excretion is via the kidneys. They inhibit sodium and chloride reabsorption in the proximal convoluted tubule but also act on the distal part of the nephron. Chlormerodrin and mercurophylline may be given orally but are not as powerful as mersalyl and mercaptomerin which are given by injection. Mersalyl

Inj. B.P. (dose: 2 ml i.m.) contains a small amount of theophylline which is itself a weak diuretic (see later) but which is included because it improves absorption from the injection site. The action lasts 24 hours and it is usual to repeat the dose every 2–4 days. Diuresis is enhanced by the administration of ammonium chloride (dose: 2–6 g daily). This may be attributable to the chloride ion but it is possible that the acidifying effect releases active mercuric ion within the tubular cell.

Contraindications and side effects. Intravenous injection is rarely followed by circulatory collapse and this route of administration should never be used. However even after intramuscular injection some patients develop hypersensitivity reactions with bronchospasm and urticaria. Stomatitis and anorexia may also occur with prolonged courses. Other side effects are rare but include proteinuria, the nephrotic syndrome and acute renal failure. Mercurials are not given to patients with established renal disease and it is advisable to test the urine regularly during treatment. If a patient becomes resistant to mersalyl there is a risk of mercury poisoning and therapy should be reviewed; if there is a severe alkalosis responsiveness can be restored with ammonium chloride but if this fails treatment should be stopped. Significant potassium depletion is rare and it is unnecessary to give supplements routinely although it is wise to measure the plasma potassium level occasionally.

Triamterene

Pharmacological action and therapeutic use. This drug has a relatively weak action and is not given alone. It inhibits sodium/potassium exchange in the distal convoluted tubule and supplements the effect of diuretics which act higher up the nephron. It is given orally, the usual dose being 100–300 mg daily. Excretion is via the kidneys.

Contraindications and side effects. Potassium retention and hyperkalaemia occur frequently, and reversible impairment of renal function may also be seen. Plasma levels of urea and potassium should be measured regularly and the drug should not be given to patients with renal failure. Other side effects include anorexia, abdominal discomfort and skin rashes.

Amiloride

Pharmacological action and therapeutic use. Chemically it has a minor resemblance to triamterene, and like it acts on the distal convoluted tubule to produce a sodium and water diuresis with conservation of potassium. It is a more powerful diuretic but is most useful for its effect of potentiating the actions of ethacrynic acid, frusemide and the benzothiadiazines and in removing the need for potassium supplements. The oral dose is 10–40 mg daily and the action is complete within 24 hours, the drug being excreted in the urine.

Contraindications and side effects. Occasional patients develop gastrointestinal disturbances. However the only important problem is the development of severe hyperkalaemia in some patients with renal functional impairment in whom the drug may accumulate.

Spironolactone

Pharmacological action and therapeutic use. The majority of edematous patients, particularly those with hypoproteinaemia, have evidence of hyperaldosteronism. Spironolactone is a competitive inhibitor of the action of aldosterone and has a weak diuretic effect with conservation of potassium. It is used in combination with drugs acting higher up the nephron and has a definite place in the treatment of resistant edema when its effect on potassium excretion is particularly valuable. The original preparation was poorly absorbed from the gut and has been replaced by a microcrystalline form which is absorbed better. The dose is 25 mg q.d.s. and it is common to observe a delay of two or three days before the diuretic effect appears. In the treatment of primary hyperaldosteronism very large (100 mg q.d.s) doses must be used.

Contraindications and side effects. These are rare but include gynaecomastia, hirsutism, headache, mental confusion and drowsiness. Hyperkalaemia may develop and spironolactone should not be given to patients with renal failure.

Carbonic anhydrase inhibitors

Pharmacological action and therapeutic use. As diuretics these drugs (which include acetazolamide, ethoxzolomide, methazolomide, and dichlorphenamide) are now only of historic interest. They prevent bicarbonate reabsorption and the excretion of hydrogen ions, leading to an increased excretion of sodium and potassium ions. However, the effect is transient as the development of a metabolic acidosis leads to a fall in the filtered bicarbonate.

Contraindications and side effects. These include potassium depletion, renal calculi, drowsiness, paraesthesiae, thrombocytopenia and skin rashes.

Xanthines

Pharmacological action and therapeutic use. The xanthines are weak diuretics and are not used alone. Caffeine, theophylline and amino metradine act when given orally but aminophylline, the most effective, is inactivated by gastric acidity and is given either as suppositories (360 mg) or intravenously (250–500 mg). Aminophylline increases the cardiac output and may be given at the peak of a diuresis produced by other diuretics when it produces a further increase in urine flow.

Contraindications and side effects. Cardiac arrest has been observed following rapid intravenous injection of aminophylline and this drug must therefore be given slowly over several minutes. Despite this precaution vomiting and hypotension may occur.

OSMOTIC DIURETICS

Mannitol

Pharmacological action and therapeutic use. Osmotic diuretics are believed to act by increasing the solute load–nephron, which in turn decreases the tubular transit time and the time available for reabsorption of water and electrolytes. In addition sodium and water reabsorption in the proximal convoluted tubule is limited by the relative hypertonicity of the tubular contents.

Mannitol may be used in the treatment of resistant edema associated with hypoproteinaemia and hypovolaemia. It is given at the same time as a conventional diuretic and leads to a further increase in urine flow while the patient is protected from the expected fall in blood volume. It also has a place in the treatment of poisoning with drugs such as phenobarbitone and the salicylates, which are filtered at the glomerulus and partially reabsorbed by the tubules. The usual dose is 25–50 g followed by continuous intravenous administration of 10–20 g/hour, the rate being adjusted according to the response observed.

There is good evidence that under certain circumstances, the pre-operative prophylactic administration of mannitol protects patients from the development of acute renal failure. However, the value of mannitol therapy in the treatment of patients with incipient acute renal failure is not yet proved. Providing there are no signs of circulatory overload a formal trial of mannitol is justified; occasionally there is a dramatic response but if there is none, the treatment must be stopped.

Contraindications and side effects. Two principal dangers arise from treatment of this type. Circulatory overload may be avoided by regular observation, careful fluid balance, and the cessation of treatment in the absence of a diuresis. The second danger is of fluid and electrolyte depletion; the composition of the urine passed must be measured and any losses which are not required must be replaced intravenously.

POTASSIUM SUPPLEMENTS

The majority of diuretics produce significant potassium loss and, unless spironolactone, triamterene or amiloride are being used, the administration of potassium supplements should be considered. This is particularly important when the patient has liver disease or is receiving digoxin. A high potassium intake in the form of fresh fruit is advisable. However, many potassium rich foods such as milk and meat extracts are also rich in sodium and may be contraindicated. Potassium depletion is usually associated with chloride depletion and it is therefore essential to replace potassium as the chloride salt. Solutions of potassium chloride are unpalatable and the salt is usually given as a capsule or tablet. The administration of simple tablets of potassium chloride, particularly in combination with a benzothiadiazine, has been associated with the development of jejunal ulceration. There are three commercial preparations from which the salt is released slowly available in the U.K.; these are Slow K (Ciba) and Kloref (Cox-Continental) which contain 600 mg (8 mEq of potassium) and 500 mg (6.5 mEq of potassium) of potassium chloride respectively. Tablets of Sando K (Sandoz) may be dissolved in water immediately before use and yield a solution containing 12 mEq of potassium and 8 mEq of chloride. Usually the patient requires 25–50 mEq of potassium daily.

CATION EXCHANGE RESINS

These are synthetic polymers which act as weak, insoluble acids and bind cations relatively loosely according to their relative concentrations and the pH of the medium. Generally speaking, they have an affinity in decreasing order for calcium, potassium, sodium and ammonium ions. They are given in a particular phase with the object of removing other cations present in excess.

Ammonium polystyrene sulphonate

Pharmacological action and therapeutic use. This is used in the treatment of resistant edema. It is usually given orally in a dose of 15 g three times a day but may be given as an enema in doses of 50–100 g in 10% dextrose. It is unpalatable and may be partially disguised if given in a flavoured drink or mixed with honey. Sodium ions exchange for ammonium ions and the patient may be spared rigorous dietary sodium restriction.

Contraindications and side effects. The resin may aggravate a severe acidosis and is therefore contraindicated in the presence of renal failure. Potassium ions will be removed along with sodium ions and potassium depletion should be anticipated. This may be overcome with the help of potassium supplements or by giving some of the resin in the potassium phase. Katonium contains 75% ammonium polystyrene sulphonate and 25% potassium polystyrene sulphonate. Minor gastrointestinal disturbances are common.

Sodium polystyrene sulphonate

This resin is used in the treatment of hyperkalaemia in renal failure and is given in the same way as ammonium polystyrene sulphonate. Potassium ions exchange for sodium ions and there is a risk of sodium overload. This has led to the introduction of resin in the calcium phase (calcium polystyrene sulphonate) but hypercalcaemia has been reported after prolonged use and it has been suggested that resin in the aluminium phase is used if prolonged administration becomes necessary.

Category 8

DRUGS USED IN HAEMATOLOGY

P. BARKHAN

IRON

Iron is commonly administered orally and less often parenterally. Therapeutically, the important consideration is the elemental iron content of the preparation and not simply the total weight of the iron complex in the dose. To achieve a complete response in most cases 1000–2000 mg elemental iron must enter the body.

ORAL IRON THERAPY

On average about 20% of the oral dose of an iron preparation is absorbed. Thus to ensure the absorption of 2 g iron a course of therapy must supply 10 g iron—the amount of the iron salt used to provide this dose will depend on its iron content. These iron preparations are taken daily and a course should last at least six months.

Ferrous sulphate

Pharmacological action. Haemoglobin biosynthesis.
Therapeutic use. The preferred iron preparation for the treatment of iron-deficiency anaemia. Each tablet contains 200 mg ferrous sulphate of which 60 mg is elemental iron. The usual dose is 1–2 tablets taken three times a day by mouth after meals. For children and those who have difficulty in swallowing tablets, liquid preparation in the form of syrups or elixirs are used: 5 ml contains 45 mg elemental iron and the dose is 5–10 ml three times a day after meals. Used prophylactically in pregnancy in a dose of 200 mg daily.
Contraindications and side effects. Like other oral iron preparations, it may irritate the bowel and so exacerbate symptoms in patients with ulcerative colitis or with regional ileitis or in those with a colostomy and is therefore generally contraindicated in these conditions. In some patients oral iron produces nausea and dyspeptic symptoms which can often be avoided or lessened by taking the tablets after meals with a drink of water and by halving the dose. Constipation is not uncommon but if the dose is excessive there may be diarrhea. Exceptionally an itchy skin

rash may develop. All iron preparations blacken the faeces. Patients who are intolerant of ferrous sulphate may do better on either ferrous gluconate or ferrous fumarate or a slow release preparation (see below).

Other iron preparations are only used in those intolerant to ferrous sulphate. Contraindications and side effects are the same as for ferrous sulphate.

Preparation	Elemental iron per tablet	Dose
Ferrous fumarate	65 mg	1–2 tabs t.d.s. after meals
Ferrous gluconate	36 mg	1–2 tabs t.d.s. after meals
Slow Release Preparations		
Ferrogradumet	105 mg	1 tab daily before breakfast
Feospan	45 mg	2–3 caps before meals
Slow Fe	50 mg	1–2 tabs daily

PARENTERAL IRON THERAPY

This form of therapy is reserved for those few patients who fail to respond to adequate doses of oral iron because of intestinal malabsorption or who are intolerant of oral preparations, or for those who are unwilling or cannot be relied on to take tablets regularly for a period of several months. Oral iron should be discontinued at least 48 hours before an injection of iron is given to minimise the danger of generalised reactions.

Iron dextran

Pharmacological action. Haemoglobin biosynthesis.
Therapeutic use. Used intramuscularly usually but can also be given intravenously. 1 ml contains 50 mg elemental iron. Intramuscular injections should be deep and should be confined to the upper outer quadrant of the buttock. A test dose of 0.5 ml should be injected first to detect hyper-

H

sensitivity. Not more than 100 mg (2 ml) should be injected at any one time and to avoid local pain the injection should be made slowly and smoothly. Injections are given at intervals of 1–2 days, alternating the buttocks, until a dose of 1–2 g (20–40 ml) has been given. The total dose required can be calculated from the haemoglobin deficit—for every gram of haemoglobin/100 ml in deficit 300 mg iron is given.

Alternatively the total dose of iron dextran can be given as a single intravenous infusion over about 8 hours. The calculated dose of iron-dextran is added to 500 ml normal saline: the infusion rate should not exceed 5–10 drops/minute for the first 30 minutes since reactions will usually be evident in this time and if there is no reaction the infusion rate is increased to 20–30 drops/minute.

Contraindications and side effects. Iron dextran should not be used in patients with a history of allergy or asthma. The skin around the injection site may be stained, sometimes permanently. Intramuscular injections may produce severe local pain if given rapidly. If administered intravenously there may be thrombophlebitis at the infusion site; leakage outside the vein causes intense local pain and an inflammatory reaction follows. Occasional side effects are fever, allergic reactions, enlargement of lymph nodes and arthralgia. Although local sarcomata have been produced in rabbits by the long-term intramuscular injection of large doses of iron dextran there is no evidence that its use in the recommended clinical dosage carries any such risk for man.

Iron-sorbitol

Pharmacological action. Haemoglobin biosynthesis.

Therapeutic use. Used intramuscularly only and the method of administration is similar to that described for iron dextran. About 36% of the injected dose is excreted in the urine and the calculated total dose should be increased by that amount.

Contraindications and side effects. Iron-sorbitol injections may be followed by fever, vomiting, disorientation, a metallic taste and local urticarial reactions. It should not be used if there is a history of allergy or asthma.

Vitamin B_{12}

Pharmacological action. Vitamin B_{12} is an essential co-factor in DNA and protein synthesis and is required for cell division and growth, particularly in rapidly proliferating tissues such as bone marrow and gastrointestinal epithelium. The synthesis and preservation of myelin in nerve tissue is also dependent on an adequate supply of vitamin B_{12}.

Therapeutic use. Used in megaloblastic anaemias due to vitamin B_{12} deficiency, pernicious anaemia, post-gastrectomy states, diseases involving the terminal ileum, small intestinal blind loops, infestation with the fish tape worm and in strict vegetarians (vegans). Vitamin B_{12} in the form of hydroxocobalamin is preferred to cyanocobalamin because of better retention and is given by intramuscular injection. For initiating therapy 1000 μg is given on alternate days for the first week. Thereafter maintenance therapy is essential (except when the cause can be eliminated), and consists of 1000 μg hydroxocobalamin every two months.

Contraindications and side effects. Vitamin B_{12} should not be used in megaloblastic anaemias due to folic acid deficiency and it is of no value in anaemias not due to vitamin B_{12} deficiency. Very occasionally hypersensitivity reactions may occur.

FOLIC ACID

Pharmacological action. Folic acid is converted in the body into its biologically active form tetrahydrofolic acid by the enzyme folic acid reductase. Its prime role is to accept and transfer 1–carbon fragments, such as methyl groups, for biosynthesis of purines and thymine and thus of DNA, RNA and proteins. The methyl group is transferred to homocysteine to form methionine and this step requires vitamin B_{12}.

Therapeutic use. It is used in megaloblastic anaemia due to folic acid deficiency. Folic acid is usually administered orally in tablet form. For the treatment of established anaemia a daily dose of 5 mg is given until the blood picture is normal or until the dietary deficiency or malabsorption has been corrected. In pregnancy it is used prophylactically in a daily dose of 400 μg in combination with an iron salt. Folic acid is given by intramuscular injection in a dose of 15 mg if there is vomiting. The reduced form of folic acid, folinic acid, is used to treat toxicity due to folic acid antagonists and a dose of 15 mg is given by intravenous injection.

Contraindications and side effects. Folic acid should not be used in pernicious anaemia. Nor should it be used in other anaemias associated with B_{12} deficiency unless there is also a superadded folic acid deficiency: side effects are almost unknown.

Pyridoxine

Pharmacological action. Pyridoxine is one of the forms of vitamin B$_6$. It is required for the biosynthesis of haemoglobin. Synthesis of haem is reduced in its absence and consequently utilisation of iron and thus haemoglobin synthesis is impaired.

Therapeutic use. Some cases of congenital and of idiopathic acquired sideroblastic anaemia respond to pyridoxine. It is given by mouth in doses of 500 mg daily and treatment is continued indefinitely. Folic acid deficiency may also be present in such cases if there are associated megaloblastic changes when folic acid and pyridoxine are given together.

ANABOLIC STEROIDS

Methendienone

Pharmacological action. Anabolic steroids increase the sensitivity of erythropoietic stem cells to the action of erythropoietin.

Therapeutic use. Testosterone or a non-virilising anabolic steroid such as methendienone may sometimes stimulate erythropoiesis in hypoplastic anaemia and in myelofibrosis and are worth a trial. The dose of methendienone is 5 mg t.d.s. daily.

ANTICOAGULANT DRUGS

Heparin

Pharmacological action. In conjunction with a plasma co-factor heparin exerts a direct and immediate anticoagulant effect, both *in vitro* and *in vivo*, by suppressing the activation of prothrombin and inhibiting the action of thrombin. Heparin also has a lipaemia-clearing action via activation of lipoprotein lipase but this effect occurs only *in vivo*.

Therapeutic use. Heparin is used in the prevention and treatment of intravascular thrombosis and embolism, either alone or combined with oral anticoagulant drugs. It cannot be given by mouth since it is destroyed in the gastrointestinal tract and is administered parenterally, usually intravenously. For preventing intravascular coagulation as in cardiac-bypass surgery heparin is used alone in a dose of 300 u/kg and supplemental doses of 150 u/kg are given every 45 minutes during the period of bypass. For treating established thrombosis an initial intravenous dose of 15 000 u is given followed by 10 000 u every six hours through an indwelling catheter or needle with a diaphragm. Heparin is also given by continuous infusion: 40 000 u are added to 500 ml saline and infused over 24 hours. Continuous infusion gives a uniform but relatively low level of heparin in the blood and it is important to ascertain that a satisfactory anticoagulant effect is obtained by doing whole blood clotting times on several occasions during the day – the clotting time should be about twice normal. In established thrombosis heparin is usually used in combination with oral anticoagulant drugs which are started at the same time: the heparin is given for five days by which time the oral anticoagulant will have reached a therapeutic level. Heparin has been given by deep subcutaneous injection using a concentrated solution of heparin (25 000 u/ml): a priming intravenous dose of 15 000 u is given followed by 25 000 u subcutaneously every 12 hours. Intramuscular administration is not recommended because of the danger of formation of large painful haematomata.

Prevention of postoperative venous thrombosis. The prophylactic use of heparin in small doses commencing pre-operatively appears safe and effective in preventing post-operative deep-vein thrombosis: the dose is 5000 u subcutaneously, given 12 hours and then immediately pre-operatively, followed by 5000 u b.d. for 7 days.

Contraindications and side effects. Heparin in therapeutic doses should not be used in the immediate postoperative period because it may cause serious bleeding from the operation site. Otherwise there is little or no danger of serious haemorrhage when the period of heparin administration does not exceed 7 days. Treatment for longer periods carries a definite risk of haemorrhage which increases with the duration of treatment. Side effects due to hypersensitivity are rare: local wheal formation, erythema, urticaria, macular skin rashes, facial flushing, fever and bronchospasm have been reported. Severe itching and burning of the feet coming on about a week after starting treatment with heparin has also been described. Long-term heparin therapy extending over weeks, although not generally used now has produced alopecia and osteoporosis. Arterial punctures should not be performed in patients on therapeutic doses of heparin.

Neutralisation of heparin. This can be rapidly accomplished by giving protamine sulphate intravenously: 1.5 mg of protamine sulphate will neutralise 100 units of heparin. Protamine sulphate is supplied as a solution containing 10 mg/ml and the appropriate volume diluted in isotonic saline is injected slowly over a period of 10 minutes. Rapid injection or excessive doses may cause hypotension. If possible the amount of heparin to be neutralised and the effectiveness of neutralisation should be checked by appropriate tests.

ORAL ANTICOAGULANTS

Apart from different dose requirements their pharmacological actions and therapeutic uses are similar and much of what is written about phenindione is applicable to the other preparations as well.

Phenindione

Pharmacological action. Phenindione decreases the coagulability of the blood by depressing the synthesis in the liver of the four vitamin K dependent plasma clotting factors (prothrombin and factors VII, IX and X). It acts as a competitive inhibitor of vitamin K. With suitable doses of phenindione the plasma concentration of these clotting factors is reduced to the therapeutic level of 5–15% in 48–72 hours. Unlike heparin, phenindione is inactive *in vitro*. It is rapidly and completely absorbed from the bowel within three hours of ingesting the dose. It also has a uricosuric effect.

Therapeutic use. Phenindione is used for the prevention and treatment of thrombosis and embolism. The drug is taken by mouth and dosage is regulated by appropriate tests, usually Quick prothrombin time test or the Thrombotest, both tests being carried out on citrated plasma. For safe and effective therapy the prothrombin complex of factors should be maintained between 5 and 15% of the normal level: levels below 5% increase the risk of haemorrhage while levels above 15% are less effective. Very ill patients, those in the early postoperative period or in congestive cardiac failure, those with liver or renal failure and old patients in general, tend to be more sensitive to the anticoagulant action of these drugs than do patients in good general condition. Large and overweight patients usually require higher doses than small and thin patients. The prothrombin time is done before starting treatment. To initiate therapy in patients whose general condition is reasonably good a single dose of 200 mg is given on the first day followed by 100 mg (50 mg b.d.) on the second day. No further doses are given until the results of the 'prothrombin' test, which is done on the third day, are known. The size of subsequent doses for maintenance therapy is dependent on this result: most patients will require a maintenance dose of 50–100 mg daily, given in divided doses in the morning and evening, but some may require doses as high as 175 mg. For patients who may be unduly sensitive the induction doses are halved and daily maintenance doses may be as low as 10 mg: as their general condition improves these patients will require higher doses to keep them in the therapeutic range. If heparin has also been used it is important to ensure that the blood sample for the prothrombin test is taken not less than 8 hours after the last dose of heparin – the presence of heparin will itself prolong the prothrombin time. Some patients can be maintained on a constant daily dose while others are more easily controlled by varying the dose, e.g. alternating doses of 50 mg and 75 mg, or a constant dose for 5 days during the week with a lower or higher dose on the remaining days. Tests are done frequently until a stable anticoagulant level has been achieved: thereafter, for patients in hospital, tests are done once or twice a week, and, for out-patients on long term therapy, once or twice a week for the first two weeks after discharge and then monthly. Patients on long-term treatment should be advised not to vary their diets too much since the amount of vitamin K in the diet will vary with its composition.

Barbiturates and tranquillising drugs tend to reduce sensitivity to oral anticoagulant drugs. Clofibrate, phenylbutazone, tetracycline, cholestyramine, quinidine and anabolic steriods tend to increase the sensitivity. In general patients on anticoagulant drugs should not take aspirin or drugs like phenylbutazone. Some preparations, e.g. Pernivit used for chilblains contain vitamin K and depress the anticoagulant response.

For elective surgery in patients on long term anticoagulant therapy, the drug is stopped 48 hours before the operation and restarted on the third postoperative day. Postpartum prophylaxis can also be started on the third day.

Contraindications and side effects. Oral anticoagulant drugs should not be used in patients who cannot be relied on to take the prescribed dose or to attend for control. Because of the danger of bleeding anticoagulant therapy is potentially dangerous in patients with peptic ulceration or other gastrointestinal lesions which may bleed. Most patients tolerate phenindione very well but a few (1–2%) develop a skin rash which in occasional cases take the form of a severe exfoliative dermatitis. Haematuria is not uncommon and can usually be brought under control by reducing the dose temporarily. Recurrent haematuria may be due to local lesions of the kidney or bladder. Patients who are otherwise well controlled may develop melaena or rectal bleeding and this should prompt a search for a local lesion in the gastrointestinal tract. Haemorrhage into the wall of the bowel may give signs of intestinal obstruction and retroperitoneal haemorrhage may lead to ileus. A very occasional side effect of phenindione is agranulocytosis and there are isolated reports of hepatic and of renal damage. Occasionally patients develop diarrhea during phenindione therapy. Drug fever has been reported.

The urine may be coloured pink during phenindione therapy and this should not be mistaken for haematuria.

Intramuscular injections should be avoided in patients on anticoagulant therapy since they may cause painful haematomata.

Oral anticoagulant drugs, but not heparin, cross the placenta and are excreted in the breast milk. They should therefore not be used in pregnancy or when breast feeding. Heparin is used instead in these circumstances.

Warfarin

Pharmacological action. See phenindione. The drug has a longer action than phenindione.

Therapeutic use. See phenindione. For starting treatment a single dose of 20–50 mg, depending on weight and clinical condition, is given by mouth. No further doses are given until the third day when the prothrombin time is done. Maintenance doses are usually from 5–10 mg taken as a single dose at about the same time each day. Very ill patients tend to be difficult to stabilise on warfarin but can be controlled more easily with phenindione. For long term therapy, however, warfarin is preferable to phenindione. Warfarin is also used in those patients who have developed hypersensitivity or other reactions to phenindione. Warfarin can be administered intravenously if a patient is vomiting: the intravenous dose is the same as the oral dose.

Contraindications and side effects. See phenindione. Warfarin appears to cause fewer side effects than phenindione and is the preferred drug. A few patients may develop nausea, vomiting, or diarrhea. Occasionally patients are completely resistant to the anticoagulant effect of warfarin but they will respond if changed to another drug such as phenindione or nicoumalone.

Nicoumalone

Pharmacological action. See phenindione.

Therapeutic use. See phenindione. The drug is administered orally and the induction dose is about 12 mg given in a single dose. Therapeutic levels are reached in 36–96 hours. The results of the prothrombin test on the third day will determine the maintenance dose, which is usually about 4 mg.

Contraindications and side effects. See phenindione. Skin rashes have been reported.

Vitamin K$_1$

Pharmacological action. An essential co-factor in the biosynthesis of four plasma clotting factors: prothrombin, and factors VII, IX and X.

Therapeutic use. An antidote to the action of oral anticoagulant drugs. Used to treat bleeding due to excessive hypoprothrombinaemia. An intravenous dose of 10–20 mg will usually be effective in stopping the bleeding and reducing the prothrombin time in 12–24 hours. Excessive doses should be avoided in patients in whom anticoagulants are to be resumed since they may then be temporarily refractory to treatment. Vitamin K$_7$ is also used in treating the hypoprothrombinaemia associated with obstructive jaundice or severe intestinal malabsorption—in these cases intravenous doses of 5–10 mg are given. For preventing haemorrhagic disease of the newborn 1.0 mg is injected intramuscularly.

ε-Aminocaproic acid (EACA)

Pharmacological action. EACA is a competitive inhibitor of plasminogen activation.

Therapeutic use. EACA has been used in the treatment of bleeding associated with severe fibrinolysis. Major surgical operations, particularly on the heart and lungs, may be complicated by serious bleeding associated with marked fibrinolysis which leads to digestion of fibrinogen and other clotting factors. In such cases intravenous injection of 5 g EACA may improve haemostasis but fibrinogen may also have to be administered at the same time if the plasma fibrinogen concentration is below 50 mg/100 ml. Menorrhagia, in the absence of a local lesion in the uterus, has been reported to respond to oral EACA therapy. EACA has been of value in severe haematuria following prostatic surgery, the dose being 5 g given orally or intravenously and repeated for not more than 1–2 doses at 6-hourly intervals if necessary. EACA is also used prophylactically in conjunction with AHG concentrates in haemophiliac patients undergoing dental surgery.

Contraindications and some side effects. EACA should not be used in chest surgery after closure of the chest since blood clots formed in the pleural or pericardial cavity may be unlysable and then become organised. It should also not be used in bleeding from the upper renal tract because the unlysed clots may lead to permanent obstructive nephropathy. The use of EACA in surgical patients carries the risk of subsequent thrombosis in the postoperative period. EACA is contraindicated in fibrinolysis secondary to disseminated intravascular coagulation. Oral EACA therapy may produce diarrhea in some patients.

FIBRINOLYTIC AGENTS

Fibrinolytic agents provide the most effective treatment of venous thrombosis and pulmonary embolism. They are used systemically or regionally. The fresher the thrombus, the more readily can it be lysed. Thus, early fibrinolytic therapy, preferably within 24 hours, will produce the most effective thrombolysis. Two agents, streptokinase and urokinase, are of established value.

Streptokinase

Pharmacological action and therapeutic use. Streptokinase, a streptococcal exotoxin, converts a plasma proteolytic enzyme, plasminogen, to its active form, plasmin, which degrades and solubilizes the fibrin component of a thrombus, thus leading to thrombolysis and the formation of fibrinogen degradation products. Plasmin is not specific for fibrin but will attack other proteins, e.g. fibrinogen and coagulation factors V and VIII. Furthermore, the fibrin degradation products to which it gives rise interfere with fibrin polymerization and with platelet function, thus impairing haemostasis. The object of therapy is to produce almost complete depletion of plasminogen, thus avoiding hyperplasminaemia which can impair haemostatic function.

Streptokinase is given intravenously via an antecubital vein, or intra-arterially. A dose of 250 000 u is given initially to overcome the action of streptokinase antibodies (due to previous streptococcal infections) and antiplasmins. Thereafter, it is infused continuously at a rate of 100 000 u/hour for 5–7 days. Thrombolysis is assessed by phlebography or pulmonary angiography. For pulmonary embolism, streptokinase is infused via a catheter directly into the pulmonary artery. Systemic fibrinolysis can be monitored by the thrombin time which should be kept at about twice the control time, longer thrombin times indicating insufficient plasminogen

depletion and therefore the need to increase the dose of streptokinase. After successful thrombolysis, streptokinase is stopped and anticoagulant therapy continued with heparin for seven days and then oral anticoagulants for at least 6 months to prevent recurrence of thrombosis.

Streptokinase can also be used for de-clotting arterio-venous shunts, e.g. in patients with renal failure on dialysis, by direct instillation into the shunt.

Contraindications and side effects. Successful use of streptokinase systemically inevitably involves the risk of haemorrhage, especially in the first 10 days after major surgery. Arterial puncture should not be performed in patients on thrombolytic therapy unless for local thrombolysis. As streptokinase is a foreign protein it can cause allergic reactions such as chills, fever, bronchospasm and skin rashes. It is contraindicated in anyone with a history of allergy or asthma. The antigenicity gives rise to antibodies which produce resistance to streptokinase, this effect lasting many months and making successive courses ineffective.

Urokinase

This is extracted from human urine. As it is of human origin, it is, unlike streptokinase, not antigenic, but is more expensive.

Pharmacological action and therapeutic use. This is similar to streptokinase. An important theoretical advantage of urokinase over streptokinase is its much higher gel phase/soluble plasminogen ratio, i.e. it has a greater affinity for plasminogen in a thrombus than for plasminogen in the circulating plama. Thus urokinase produces less systemic hyperplasminaemia and consequently less impairment of haemostasis.

Contraindications and side effects. The major hazard of urokinase therapy, like that of streptokinase, is haemorrhage (see above).

Category 9

ANTIMICROBIALS

R. K. KNIGHT

Benzylpenicillin

Pharmacological action. Like all penicillins benzylpenicillin acts upon dividing bacteria by interfering with cell-wall synthesis; it is bactericidal. Inactivated by gastric acid its absorption from the intestine is incomplete. Injected parenterally it is distributed throughout all tissues except bone, nervous tissue and serous spaces. Optimal blood levels are obtained 30–60 minutes after injection, very little being detectable after 6 hours. Sixty per cent is excreted by the kidneys—mainly via the tubules. This route of excretion can be inhibited by probenecid, increasing the blood level for a given dose.

Therapeutic use. Benzylpenicillin is highly effective against infections caused by susceptible organisms principally the Gram-positive cocci (pneumococcus, *Streptococcus pyogenes*, and non-penicillinase producing staphylococcus), Gram-negative cocci (meningococcus and gonococcus), Gram-positive bacilli (clostridia and actinomyces) and *Treponema pallidum*. Resistance to benzylpenicillin has become a serious problem with penicillinase-producing *Staphylococcus aureus*.

Ideally it should be given 6-hourly to maintain optimal blood levels. For most infections the dose is 150 mg to 600 mg (250 000–1 000 000 units) intramuscularly every 6 hours until the infection is controlled. In subacute bacterial endocarditis where the organism is less sensitive and relatively inaccessible high doses of 6–18 g daily may be required and this is best given via continuous intravenous infusion. It may be injected into the pleura, pericardium or joints for infections at these sites. Intrathecal injections (not more than 12 mg) have been used in meningitis but inflamed meninges probably allow enough to pass from the blood into the cerebrospinal fluid.

Contraindications and side effects. Benzylpenicillin is virtually free from toxic effects when given intramuscularly in the usual doses although pain at the site of injection is common. Convulsions can follow intrathecal injection and very large intravenous doses in the presence of renal failure may cause encephalopathy. Since benzyl-penicillin is supplied either as the sodium or potassium salt, retention of these cations will be important in, for example, bacterial endocarditis or severe renal disease.

The combination of benzylpenicillin with a bacteristatic antibiotic may greatly reduce its efficacy by preventing the former from acting upon dividing bacteria.

Hypersensitivity reactions occur most often in patients with a history of allergy such as eczema and asthma, and when repeated courses of treatment are given. Patients should not, except in extreme illnesses (and then only with suitable precautions), be given penicillin if they have a history of hypersensitivity to it. The common manifestations of this are urticaria, other rashes (including erythema multiforme) and drug fever. Less frequent but more serious effects are wheezing, laryngeal edema and shock. Others include exfoliative dermatitis, haemolytic anaemia and thrombocytopenia. The Jarisch–Herxheimer reaction should be anticipated in the treatment of tertiary syphilis. Penicillin should not be used topically because of the risk of sensitising the patient and producing resistant organisms.

Procaine penicillin

Pharmacological action. Procaine penicillin differs from benzylpenicillin only by the addition of procaine, thereby slowing absorption and maintaining blood levels for 12–24 hours.

Therapeutic use. It is useful where fewer injections are desired or required on grounds of expediency as in domiciliary practice or in children. The dose is usually 900 mg (1 500 000 units) once a day or 600 mg (1 000 000 units) 12-hourly. In order to achieve an optimal blood level quickly it is wise to give with the first injection a dose of benzylpenicillin.

Contraindications and side effects. As for benzylpenicillin. The duration of its effect makes procaine penicillin potentially more dangerous in hypersensitivity reactions. Rare psychotic reactions have been reported after administration of procaine penicillin possibly due to inadvertent intravenous injection.

Phenoxymethylpenicillin

Pharmacological action. Phenoxymethylpenicillin is resistant to gastric acid so absorption from the intestine is more reliable and complete than with benzylpenicillin. Furthermore its excretion is slower.

Therapeutic use. The oral route possesses obvious advantages, particularly in children. For most susceptible infections phenoxymethylpenicillin can be given instead of benzylpenicillin although some clinicians prefer to begin a course of treatment with 'priming' injections of the latter. Tablets are of 125 or 250 mg which should be given 6-hourly on an empty stomach. A flavoured oral suspension is available containing 125 mg in 5 ml. Oral penicillin is appropriate in pneumococcal and streptococcal infections of the upper respiratory tract and middle ear. It is also useful in prophylaxis against recurrence of rheumatic fever and glomerulonephritis—the dose being 125 or 250 mg daily.

Contraindications and side effects. These are similar to those mentioned for benzylpenicillin although allergy is less frequent. Looseness of the bowels is often encountered and, owing to alteration of the bacterial status quo in the alimentary tract, oral and perineal monilia infection may arise.

Phenethicillin

Phenethicillin is another orally active derivative of 6-amino-penicillinic acid which has no therapeutic advantage over phenoxymethylpenicillin. It is more expensive.

Cloxacillin

Pharmacological action. Cloxacillin is a synthetic penicillin unaffected by penicillinase which is resistant to gastric acid and can therefore be taken by mouth.

Therapeutic use. It is much less active than benzylpenicillin against most organisms except penicillinase-producing staphylococci. It should be reserved exclusively for serious systemic infections caused by these organisms which are usually acquired in hospital. It is expensive.

The dose is usually 500 mg every 4 to 6 hours until the infection is under control. It can be given by intramuscular injection when 250 mg 4-6-hourly is usually adequate.

Contraindications and side effects. It is free from direct toxicity. Allergic reactions occur as with other penicillins. Looseness of the bowels and oral or perineal monilia overgrowth are common.

Flucloxacillin

Pharmacological action. Flucloxacillin is closely related to cloxacillin. It is well absorbed from the gut and higher free serum levels are achieved than with cloxacillin.

Therapeutic use. It has the same range of antibacterial activity as cloxacillin. Its place is therefore in the treatment of infections caused by penicillin-resistant organisms. The oral dose is 250 mg 6-hourly. For serious infections the parenteral route is preferable when 250–500 mg 4–6-hourly should be given.

Contraindications and side effects. These are similar to those mentioned for cloxacillin.

Methicillin

Methicillin has a similar range of anti-staphylococcal activity to cloxacillin and flucloxacillin but since it is not acid stable it must be given parenterally. Some strains of staphylococci resistant to methicillin have emerged in hospitals. Large doses intramuscularly are painful.

Ampicillin

Pharmacological action. Ampicillin is a derivative of 6-amino-penicillanic acid which is resistant to gastric acid and therefore effective by mouth although absorption from the intestine is variable. Sustained blood levels are usually obtained and it is concentrated in the bile and urine. It is rapidly destroyed by penicillinase.

Therapeutic use. Ampicillin differs from most other penicillins by being bactericidal to some Gram-negative bacilli including *E. coli,* some proteus strains, salmonellae and *Haemophilus influenzae.* Urinary tract infections due to susceptible organisms are treated with 500 mg 6-hourly for 10–14 days. In acute exacerbations of chronic bronchitis (frequently associated with *Haemophilus influenzae*) 500 mg 6-hourly is usually effective, but a very high dose of 1 g 6-hourly for a week reduces the likelihood of subsequent relapse. Typhoid and paratyphoid organisms are very susceptible *in vitro* but infections need to be treated with 1 g 6-hourly for 14–28 days. Certain coliform organisms produce penicillinase making them resistant to ampicillin.

Contraindications and side effects. Sensitivity rashes are more frequent than with other penicillins and may appear 4–5 days after withdrawal of the drug. Nausea and heartburn are often experienced. Looseness of the bowels may occur and oral and perineal monilia is encountered.

Amoxycillin

Amoxycillin is a new penicillin derivative very similar to ampicillin. The only practical difference is that somewhat higher blood levels are achieved with doses given 8-hourly (rather than 6-hourly). The range of activity and side effects are the same for these two antibiotics.

Telampicillin

This is very similar to amoxycillin.

Carbenicillin

Pharmacological action. Carbenicillin is a semi-synthetic penicillin active against *Ps. aeruginosa* and certain Gram-negative organisms including strains of proteus. It is inactivated by penicillinase. Parenteral administration is necessary. High blood and urinary levels are obtained.
Therapeutic use. Carbenicillin may be used in the treatment of severe systemic infections (septicaemia, endocarditis), meningitis and urinary tract infections caused by susceptible organisms, which are usually Gram-negative. It may also be used in the treatment (or prophylaxis) of infection in burns. The intramuscular dose is 1–2 g 6-hourly but it may be given by slow intravenous injection (3–4 g) 4-hourly. The dose is smaller for children and when renal function is impaired. Higher blood levels are obtained by the concurrent use of probenecid.
Contraindications and side effects. Pain is common at the site of intramuscular injection and may be relieved by adding a local analgesic. It should not be given to patients known to be hypersensitive to penicillin.

Carfecillin

This is a pherylester of carbenicillin. It can be taken orally but is otherwise similar to carbenicillin.

Cephaloridine

Pharmacological action. Cephaloridine is a semi-synthetic preparation related to penicillin. Injection is necessary since it is not absorbed from the intestine. After intramuscular injection adequate blood levels are obtained for 8 hours and it is excreted unchanged in the urine.

Therapeutic use. It is highly active against certain streptococci (pneumoniae, pyogenes and viridans) and *Staphylococcus aureus* even when penicillin resistant. It is also active against *E. coli, Proteus mirabilis* and some shigella species. The dose is 250 or 500 mg 6-hourly for 5–14 days. The intravenous dose is 250 mg. It may be given intrathecally, diluting 25 mg in 10 ml of fluid.
Contraindications and side effects. It is not toxic in usual dosage although intrathecally it may cause drowsiness. Skin rashes may occur and caution is required in patients known to be hypersensitive to penicillin since cross sensitivity occurs between these related substances. Renal damage may occur with doses exceeding 6–8 g daily.

Cephalothin

Cephalothin is similar to cephaloridine in its action and range of antibacterial effect. Nephrotoxicity is not a problem in man so that cephalothin is preferable to cephaloridine in the presence of impaired renal function. The usual dose for susceptible infection is 0.5 to 1.0 g 6-hourly by intravenous or intramuscular injection. For serious and more resistant infections 4–12 g daily may be required intravenously.

Cephalexin

Cephalexin is a cephalosporin which is well absorbed from the gut. The oral dose is 0.5–1.0 g 4 times daily.

It has a wide antibacterial activity similar to cephaloridine.

Cephradine

Cephradine is a new semi-synthetic cephalosporin very similar to cephalexin.

Sodium fusidate

Pharmacological action. Sodium fusidate is well absorbed from the intestine and becomes widely distributed in most tissues though not the cerebrospinal fluid. It is active (bactericidal) against penicillinase-producing staphylococci.
Therapeutic use. Its use is virtually confined to the treatment of infections due to penicillin resistant staphylococci. Combined with benzylpenicillin it may be more effective but the result is unpredictable. The dose for appropriate infections is 500 mg three times daily with or before meals. For children a suspension is available and the dose 23–33 mg/kg daily. Resistance to its action may occur during therapy. It is available for topical application.

Contraindications and side effects. No serious toxic effects have been reported. Nausea, heartburn and diarrhea may occur. It is extremely expensive.

Tetracyclines

Tetracycline   Oxytetracycline
Chlortetracycline   Demethylchlortetracycline
Lymecycline   Methacycline
Chlormethylencycline   Tetracycline-phosphate
                          complex.

Pharmacological action. The antibacterial activity of the various tetracyclines is virtually identical. They are bacteriostatic against a wide range of organisms including most of the pathogenic Gram-negative and Gram-positive bacteria (except some strains of proteus and *Ps. aeruginosa*), certain rickettsiae, large viruses and *Entamoeba hystolytica*. Absolute cross resistance exists between members of the tetracycline group.

Tetracyclines are usually given by mouth, absorption from the intestine is good and diffusion takes place through most tissues though not well into the cerebrospinal fluid. The liver partly inactivates them by producing protein binding and some metabolic breakdown. Concentration and excretion is high in the bile; the kidneys excrete appreciable amounts.

Good blood levels are obtained for up to 6 hours with tetracycline, oxytetracycline and chlortetracycline. Because of slower excretion demethylchlortetracycline gives adequate blood levels for up to 12 hours.

Therapeutic use. In hospitals there is a growing population of tetracycline resistant organisms, particularly some Gram-negative species and *Staphylococcus aureus*. Outside hospital the widest use for tetracyclines is in acute exacerbations of chronic bronchitis where the organism is usually either *Haemophilus influenzae* or *Streptococcus pneumoniae*. They are the first choice in rickettsial and certain viral infections and the most effective form of therapy for brucellosis. Although effective against *E. coli* they are not the most appropriate choice for urinary tract infections as they are bacteristatic and resistance often develops.

Tetracycline, oxytetracycline and chlortetracycline are given orally in tablet or capsule form, the dose being 250 mg 6-hourly for most susceptible infections but for more serious ones 500 mg 6-hourly will be necessary. For children a flavoured suspension is available the dose being 30 mg/kg bodyweight daily in divided doses.

The dosage of demethylchlortetracycline is usually 300 mg 12-hourly, methacycline 150 mg 6-hourly and lymecycline 300 mg 6-hourly (100 mg four to six hourly i.m.).

Topical preparations are available for the treatment of skin infections.

Although there are many varieties of tetracyclines the minor differences in absorption and excretion do not offer significant therapeutic advantage.

Contraindications and side effects. Epigastric burning, anorexia, nausea and vomiting are sometimes experienced, Allergy and marrow dyscrasias have been very rarely encountered. Tetracyclines cross the placenta and are deposited in developing bones and teeth of the fetus giving yellow discoloration. They should therefore be avoided in pregnancy and preferably not given to children less than eight years old. Large parenteral doses given in pregnancy have also caused fatal hepatic damage. Infants developing hydrocephalus due to tetracyclines have been reported, and exacerbations of myasthenia gravis may occur when these are given. Serious catabolism with a rise in blood urea and glomerular damage is likely to occur in patients with chronic renal failure, who should not therefore be given tetracyclines. Patients with healthy kidneys may suffer renal damage with aminoaciduria if tablets are given which have deteriorated through age. Phototoxicity is frequent with demethylchlortetracycline and occasionally seen with others.

The most frequent side effects are due to the overgrowth of potentially pathogenic organisms in the alimentary, respiratory and genitourinary tracts. Many patients develop candidiasis of the mouth and gut. In hospital severe staphylococcal infection of the bowel or lung may ensue. Looseness of the bowels is commonplace. Pain at the site of injection is relieved by concurrently giving procaine.

Doxycycline

Doxycycline is very similar to the other tetracyclines except that once daily dosage is sufficient. It is also perhaps less liable to exacerbate renal failure. The usual dose is 200 mg on the first day followed by 100 mg daily.

Minocycline

Minocycline is similar to tetracycline with much the same antibacterial range. There is some evidence that organisms which have become resistant to tetracycline may not be resistant to minocycline.

The initial dose for an adult is 200 mg followed by 100 mg twice daily.

Chloramphenicol

Pharmacological action. Chloramphenicol is prepared synthetically. It is well absorbed when given by mouth, readily diffusable into tissues and body fluids including the cerebrospinal fluid. Good blood levels are obtained for up to six hours. It is bacteriostatic.

Therapeutic use. The use of chloramphenicol is governed by the fact that it can cause fatal damage to the bone marrow although this is rare. Its range of activity is similar to the tetracyclines but it is particularly effective against salmonellae and other Gram-negative organisms. It is the antibiotic of first choice in typhoid fever when it should be given for 14 days, the dose usually being 500 mg 6-hourly. It is also used in *Haemophilus influenzae* meningitis in children when it can be given as the succinate parenterally if necessary. It is doubtful if its use can be justified in other infections except *Klebsiella pneumoniae*.

Contraindications and side effects. Blood dyscrasias include granulocytopenia, thrombocytopenia and aplastic anaemia. Many fatalities have occurred and are apparently related to the total dose or repeated courses. Circulatory collapse (the 'grey syndrome') causing death may occur in neonates and infants given large doses. Other toxic effects that have been noted are Jarisch–Herxheimer reactions, jaundice, optic neuritis and skin rashes.

Erythromycin

Pharmacological action. Several preparations of erythromycin exist which include the base, stearate, ethylcarbonate which are given orally and the lactobionate which is used parenterally. The range of activity is very similar to that of benzylpenicillin but the erythromycins are usually bacteriostatic. The differences between the preparations are mainly in the rate of absorption and the serum levels obtained. The estolate gives somewhat higher and more predictable blood levels and may be bactericidal.

Therapeutic use. With the discovery of newer antibiotics the role of erythromycin has diminished considerably. It is used in common Gram-positive infections in patients known to be allergic to penicillin. Some strains of staphylococci acquired outside hospitals are susceptible but resistance develops rapidly. The dose is 250 or 500 mg 6-hourly depending upon the severity of the infection. Infants and children require 4–11 mg/kg 6-hourly. The lactobionate is given by intramuscular injection 2–5 mg/kg three times daily.

Contraindications and side effects. Toxicity is low except with erythromycin estolate which may cause hepatitis, cholestatic jaundice and severe abdominal pain indistinguishable from biliary colic. Heartburn, nausea and looseness of the bowels are common. Allergic reactions are uncommon.

Lincomycin

Pharmacological action. Lincomycin resembles erythromycin in its properties although chemically it is unrelated. There is evidence that *in vivo* it readily penetrates bone and into the eye.

Therapeutic use. Its ability to penetrate bone makes it useful in the treatment of acute or chronic suppurative osteomyelitis or joint disease caused by penicillin resistant *Staphylococcus aureus*. It has the advantage that it can be given orally. For acute infections the dose is 500 mg 6-hourly by mouth, the duration of therapy depending on the response. In chronic infections the same dose may be given for 4–6 weeks and then reduced to 8-hourly for as long as a year if necessary.

Contraindications and side effects. Minor gastro-intestinal disturbances such as looseness of the bowels are common and occassionally severe and dangerous colitis. Other side effects are few but include skin rashes, granulocytopenia and headache.

Clindamycin

Clindamycin is similar to lincomycin in its range of action and effects. It is effective against *Bacteroides*. The adult dose is 150–450 mg 6-hourly before meals. It may cause looseness of the bowels and occasionally a pseudo-membraneous colitis (with some fatalities).

Streptomycin

Pharmacological action. Streptomycin is bactericidal to certain Gram-negative bacteria and particularly *Mycobacterium tuberculosis*. It is not absorbed from the intestinal tract and is given therefore by intramuscular injection. Maximum blood level is reached in 1–2 hours and this falls to low levels in about 6 hours. It is distributed in extra-cellular fluid (except the CSF) and excreted in the bile and the urine.

Therapeutic use. The principal role of streptomycin is in the treatment of tuberculosis where, to avoid the development of resistant organisms, it is always given in combination with other anti-tuberculous drugs. The usual dose is 1 g daily i.m., but it may be given 2 or 3 times per week.

It may be used in the treatment of urinary tract infections but many organisms are now resistant. It is more effective in alkaline urine. Combined with penicillin in the treatment of *Streptococcus viridans* endocarditis synergistic enhancement takes place with improved results. It is useful in the treatment of certain bowel infections namely the dysentery organisms and *E. coli*. A 5-day course of 1–2 g daily usually suffices.

Contraindications and side effects. Damage to the inner ear is the most common and serious toxic effect of streptomycin. Both vestibular function and hearing may be involved though the latter is less common. Some individuals are particularly susceptible and the risk is greater in the elderly or patients with impaired renal function. Dihydrostreptomycin is much more likely to produce hearing loss. Neuromuscular block leading to respiratory paralysis has been reported following injection of streptomycin into the pleural space.

Skin hypersensitivity reactions are common in persons handling the drug. Allergic reactions by patients are usually of the delayed type (although anaphylactic shock has been reported) manifested as fever, skin rash, arthritis and lymphadenopathy.

Kanamycin

Pharmacological action. Kanamycin is similar to streptomycin and neomycin in its antibacterial and pharmacological activity. Its use is usually confined to parenteral therapy. Peak serum levels are achieved one hour after i.m. injection and it is not detected after 6 hours. Appreciable quantities are excreted in the urine, very little in the bile.

Therapeutic use. Its main use is in Gram-negative infections. Almost all strains of *E. coli* and proteus are inhibited by 8 mg/ml or less *in vitro* and these levels are readily achieved *in vivo*. Many other micro-organisms are susceptible but resistance develops rapidly in staphylococci.

In adults the standard dose is 250 mg i.m. 6-hourly. For children it is 12.5 to 15 mg/kg bodyweight depending on the severity of the infection. Fulminating infections with septicaemia usually require intravenous therapy when the dose is the same as with i.m. injections. It can be given into the peritoneum (250 mg in 500 ml of saline twice daily for 2–3 days) for severe peritoneal infections.

Kanamycin should be reserved for serious infections such as septicaemia resulting from urinary tract infection in pregnancy or the puerperium, proteus septicaemia, *E. coli* meningitis

in the newborn or Gram-negative infections of the peritoneum.

Contraindications and side effects. Ototoxicity occurs particularly in the presence of renal insufficiency when the dose must be reduced. Estimation of the blood concentrations of the drug are useful in these circumstances. Nephrotoxicity in man is relatively low but albuminuria and urinary casts have been reported; tubular damage may occur if therapy is prolonged. Kanamycin shares with streptomycin and neomycin the ability to interfere with neuromuscular transmission particularly after intraperitoneal administration. Allergic reactions are rare.

Neomycin

Pharmacological action. Neomycin is closely related to streptomycin and has similar antibacterial activity. Highly toxic parenterally it is used in topical preparations for the eye, ear or skin and may be given by mouth since absorption from the intact intestine is generally low.

Therapeutic use. In tablet form or for children as an elixir it is used for so-called bowel sterilisation before colonic surgery, for the treatment of bacillary dysentery and for certain types of *E. coli* enteritis. For adults the dose is 500 mg 6-hourly for 5 days for infection and for 3 days preoperatively. The dose for infants and young children is 50 mg/kg bodyweight daily divided into four doses.

Numerous topical preparations are available for use in infections of the conjunctivae, external ear and skin. It is combined with bacitracin and polymixin in aerosols or fine powders for wounds or operation sites.

Contraindications and side effects. The high degree of ototoxicity precludes its use parenterally. Neomycin may damage the intestinal mucosa causing malabsorption. While usually hardly any of the drug is absorbed, in certain circumstances this may be important. Kidney damage has been reported after oral use. It shares with streptomycin a curare-like action enhanced by the use of muscle relaxants and certain types of general anaesthesia. Topical use of neomycin has led to an increasing incidence of skin hypersensitivity.

Gentamicin

Pharmacological action. Gentamicin is related to streptomycin chemically and in its range of action against Gram-negative organisms. It is also effective against *Ps. aeruginosa*. It is given by intramuscular injection and excreted by the kidneys.

Therapeutic use. Its use has been largely confined to urinary tract infections by susceptible organisms. Serious systemic infections have been successfully treated. The dose is 0.8–1.2 mg/kg daily given in three equal doses 8-hourly.

Contraindications and side effects. The main toxic effects are upon the inner ear and labyrinthine damage is more frequent when renal function is impaired. Hypersensitivity has so far been uncommon.

Polymixin B

Pharmacological action. Polymixin B is poorly absorbed from the alimentary tract and is therefore given parenterally when it is excreted in the urine. It is also used topically for ophthalmic and skin infections.

Therapeutic use. Polymixin B is active against *Ps. aeruginosa* and other Gram-negative organisms but is used when resistance to safe antibiotics has been demonstrated. Infections of the urinary tract or meningitis due to *Ps. aeruginosa* are the situations where it is most useful. The dosage is 50 mg (500 000 u) 8-hourly by intramuscular injection combined with procaine to relieve local pain. It is effective topically in the treatment of infected burns and otitis externa where it is often combined with bacitracin.

Contraindications and side effects. Topical therapy is safe and hypersensitivity uncommon. Parenterally it is toxic to the kidneys and neurological disturbances (paraesthesiae, neuromuscular block, convulsions) have been reported.

Colistin

Pharmacological action. Colistin which is identical to polymixin E is very similar in its pharmacological properties to polymixin B.

Therapeutic use. The indications for the use of colistin are the same as those for polymixin B, namely infections (particularly of the urinary tract) due to *Ps. aeruginosa*. The preparation for injection is called colistin sulphomethate and in the USA this is combined with a local analgesic. The dosage is usually 1 000 000 u 8-hourly.

Contraindications and side effects. These are similar to those with polymixin B.

Sulphonamides

Pharmacological action. Although there are numerous sulphonamide preparations with different properties certain generalisations can be made. Some are insoluble and when taken orally remain within the intestine but most are readily absorbed from the gastrointestinal tract. After absorption there is variable protein binding, acetylation and excretion by the kidney. The rate of excretion

and the degree of penetration into the cerebrospinal fluid are related to the amount of protein binding. Their action is to inhibit folic acid synthesis of bacteria by competing with its precursor *para*-aminobenzoic acid to which they are chemically related. This action is bacteriostatic.

Therapeutic use. Sulphonamides are active against Gram-positive and Gram-negative cocci and certain Gram-negative bacilli. They are inhibited by the presence of pus. Clinically they are most useful in treatment of infections of the urinary tract and meningococcal meningitis (although resistant meningococci have been reported. Formerly used in bacillary dysentery they are now less useful as resistant strains are common. Occasionally a particular sulphonamide may be useful in bacterial conjunctivitis, trachoma, toxoplasmosis, nocardiosis and dermatitis herpetiformis.

For systemic infections sulphadiazine or sulphadimide are used most often with a loading dose of 3–6 g followed by 1–2 g 4- or 6-hourly. For children a quarter or half this dosage applies. These preparations can be used for urinary tract infections, half the above adult dose is then adequate.

Other sulphonamides are used in urinary tract infections such as sulphamethizole (0.2 g then 0.1 g 4-hourly) or sulphafurazole. The choice is wide but the effect of the various preparations is similar. The long acting sulphonamides include sulphamethoxypyridazine and sulphadimethoxine the dosage of these being 1 g daily.

Sulphonamides are sometimes used parenterally in the treatment of bacterial meningitis particularly in the UK when sulphadiazine is usually chosen. Other soluble sulphonamides are equally effective. These are best given via an intravenous saline infusion since it is important to ensure adequate hydration. The dose is usually 6 g per 24 hours.

Contraindications and side effects. Numerous adverse effects have been described and the reported incidence varies between 1 and 15%. Hypersensitivity reactions are fairly common and include fever and a variety of mild or serious skin eruptions. Almost all types of haematological disorders can occur. Gastrointestinal disturbances are usually minor but are very common; jaundice may be encountered. Crystalluria may occur if the urine is acid and concentrated. Other effects include arteritis and certain neurological disturbances.

Co-trimoxazole

Pharmacological action. Co-trimoxazole is a combination of trimethoprim (80 mg) and sulphamethoxazole (400 mg). The sulphonamides are mentioned above. Trimethoprim has a similar range of action to the sulphonamides. It inhibits the enzyme which reduces dihydrofolic acid to tetrahydrofolic acid – a stage in purine synthesis which follows that arrested by sulphonamides. The combination of trimethoprim with a sulphonamide produces a synergistic action which is much more effective than either substance alone. Trimethoprim is well absorbed after oral administration. It is slowly excreted by the kidney and adequate blood levels are obtained by 12-hourly doses. It penetrates to the cerebrospinal fluid.

Therapeutic use. The combination of trimethoprim and sulphamethoxazole is active against most of the pyogenic cocci (but have no advantage over the penicillins in this respect) and many Gram-negative organisms. The principal use is in urinary tract infections and for acute exacerbations of chronic bronchitis. The dose is usually two tablets twice daily. Gonorrhea has also been effectively treated.

Contraindications and toxic effects. Toxic effects have so far been rare but leucopenia has been reported. Trimethoprim should not be given early in pregnancy as teratogenic effects have been observed in experimental animals.

Isoniazid (INAH)

Pharmacological action. Isoniazid (Isonicotinic acid hydrazide, INAH) is a synthetic substance very active against *Mycobacterium tuberculosis.* It is well absorbed after an oral dose and is distributed throughout body fluids including cerebrospinal fluid. The ability to acetylate (inactivate) the drug is genetically determined and varies considerably between racial groups.

Therapeutic use. Isoniazid is only used in the treatment of all forms of tuberculosis but since resistance develops if it is used alone it should always be used in combination with at least one other antituberculous drug. The usual dosage is 300 mg daily in two or three doses. It is presented in many forms either alone or in combination with PAS. It can be given intramuscularly and intrathecally but these routes are rarely required.

Contraindications and side effects. The incidence of side effects is low but allergic reactions have occasionally been reported. The most important toxic effect is peripheral neuropathy which is commonest among slow inactivators. Rare adverse reactions include jaundice, psychosis, endocrine disturbances and a lupus erythematosus-like syndrome.

Para-aminosalicylic acid (PAS)

Pharmacological action. PAS is usually administered as the sodium or calcium salt. It is active against *Mycobacterium tuberculosis* although less so than streptomycin or INAH. It is well absorbed from the alimentary tract and distributed throughout body fluids but with poor penetration into the cerebrospinal fluid. Excretion via the kidneys is rapid.

Therapeutic use. Its use is confined to the treatment of tuberculosis always in combination with at least one other drug since resistance develops if it is used alone. Many preparations are available in tablet, powder or granular form usually in combination with INAH. The daily dose should ideally be 20 g but in practice 12 g is usually the maximum that is tolerated. It should be given with food. The main purpose of combining PAS with INAH is to ensure that patients take both (or neither) to mitigate the risk of resistance developing to one drug alone.

Contraindications and side effects. Nausea, anorexia, and abdominal discomfort are common. Diarrhea may occur. Hypersensitivity in the form of fever, skin rashes and lymphadenopathy are encountered. Desensitisation is often possible. Other reactions include pulmonary infiltration with eosinophilia, goitre with hypothyroidism, jaundice and haematological abnormalities.

Rifampicin

Pharmacological action. Rifampicin is an antibiotic active against Gram-positive bacteria and some Gram-negative bacteria as well as *Mycobacterium tuberculosis.* It is well absorbed by the oral route and readily diffusable into the tissues. It is mainly excreted in the bile.

Therapeutic use. Rifampicin is probably the most potent antituberculous agent and it has establised itself as a first-line drug in this field. Optimum duration of therapy has yet to be determined. The dose is 450–600 mg daily as a single dose. It should be given in combination with at least one other drug to prevent emergence of resistant strains.

Contraindications and side effects. Toxicity in man has not yet been fully studied but hepatic function may be impaired. Eosinophilia and leucopenia have been reported. Nausea occurs occasionally. It causes red discoloration of the sputum and urine. Patients with hepatic disease should not be treated with rifampicin and until further information is available it should be avoided in pregnancy. Rifampicin is an enzyme inducing substance and by increasing the rate of inactivation of estrogens may interfere with the action of contraceptives.

Ethambutol

Pharmacological action. Ethambutol is well absorbed by the oral route and excretion is predominantly via the kidney.

Therapeutic use. This is a relatively new and very effective antituberculous drug. The dose is usually initially 25 mg/kg bodyweight daily, then after two months 15 mg per kg daily.

Contraindications and side effects. The most important toxic effect of ethambutol is optic neuritis producing diminished visual acuity and central scotoma. Patients should have complete ophthalmological examination before therapy and visual acuity should be checked regularly during treatment. Other effects include rare instances of gastrointestinal disturbance and allergy.

Pyrazinamide

Pharmacological action. Pyrazinamide is very active against *Mycobacterium tuberculosis*. It is well absorbed when taken orally, and diffuses into the body fluids. It is excreted by the kidneys.

Therapeutic use. Pyrazinamide is a second line drug for the treatment of tuberculosis. The dosage is 30 mg/kg bodyweight daily in four doses, but this should not exceed 3 g/day.

Contraindications and side effects. Liver damage is common and may be fatal. Estimations of the serum transaminases should accompany its use. It may precipitate gout and cause skin rashes.

Ethionamide

Pharmacological action. Ethionamide is chemically related to INAH but not as effective. Absorption by mouth is good and distribution takes place throughout body fluids including the cerebrospinal fluid.

Therapeutic use. Ethionamide is used in the treatment of tuberculosis when organisms are resistant to the safer and more effective drugs. The dose is 0.5 g twice daily.

Contraindications and side effects. Side effects are common and include vomiting, diarrhea, peripheral neuropathy, convulsions and hepatic damage.

Cycloserine

Pharmacological action. Cycloserine is well absorbed from the intestine and freely diffusable throughout tissue fluids including the cerebrospinal fluid. It is excreted by the kidneys.

Therapeutic use. It is used as a second line drug in the treatment of tuberculosis. The dosage is 1 g daily in two doses but therapy should begin with 250 mg twice daily, increasing slowly by increments of 250 mg each week.

Contraindications and side effects. Serious toxic effects are relatively common and include psychoses, depression and convulsions.

Nalidixic acid

Pharmacological action. Nalidixic acid, a synthetic preparation, is well absorbed after oral administration and largely excreted (80%) in the urine where it appears in high concentrations.

Therapeutic use. The role of nalidixic acid is confined to the treatment of urinary tract infections where it is effective against many Gram-negative organisms. It must be used in high dosage (at least 4 g/day) but resistance frequently occurs during therapy. Successful treatment is less likely in the presence of abnormalities of the urinary tract and deep seated infections of the kidney respond poorly.

Contraindications and side effects. Adverse effects are few and mild but include allergic reactions (rashes, fever) haemolytic anaemia, skin photosensitivity, respiratory depression, a variety of disturbances in the nervous system and occasional nausea or vomiting. It causes positive reactions in the urine to 'Clinitest'.

Nitrofurantoin

Pharmacological action. Nitrofurantoin is a synthetic preparation which is absorbed from the gut and excreted in high concentration in the urine. Excretion is enhanced if the urine is acid. Blood levels are low at the usual dosage. It is effective against a large number of Gram-negative and Gram-positive organisms.

Therapeutic use. Its use is confined to the treatment of urinary tract infections by susceptible organisms. It is often useful against *E. coli* and some proteus infections. The dose for adults is 100 mg 6-hourly after food or, for prophylaxis, 50 mg 12-hourly. In renal failure its efficacy is reduced since less is excreted.

Contraindications and side effects. Nausea and vomiting occur frequently. Pulmonary infiltration and asthma have been reported. Nitrofurantoin has caused megaloblastic anaemia, and haemolytic anaemia – particularly in glucose-6-phosphate dehydrogenase deficiency. Peripheral neuropathy has been encountered, chiefly where there is impaired renal function.

Amphotericin B

Pharmacological action. Amphotericin B is poorly absorbed from the alimentary tract. It is given by intravenous infusion. Urinary excretion is slow

and adequate blood levels persist for long periods. It is also used topically as a lozenge or ointment.
Therapeutic use. It is the drug of choice in systemic fungal disease and is indicated in serious infections due to candidiasis, histoplasmosis, coccidioidomycosis, cryptococcosis and blastomycosis. The dose is 1.0 mg/kg daily given by infusion over a period of 6 hours. The duration of therapy depends on severity of the infection and the response but it may be necessary to continue for several weeks.

Amphotericin B is available in tablet form (10 mg) for the treatment of oral candida infection.

For fungal meningitis 0.5 mg mixed with 20 mg of hydrocortisone can be given intrathecally.
Contraindications and side effects. Kidney damage occurs in nearly all patients given amphotericin B intravenously. The renal lesion, which may be permanent, consists of tubular swelling with calcification. Fever, nausea, vomiting, anorexia and severe malaise are common. They are to some extent mitigated by giving 50 mg hydrocortisone at the start of each infusion. Nearly all patients develop a normocytic normochromic anaemia. Intrathecal injection often produces severe headache.

Nystatin

Pharmacological action. Nystatin is an antifungal antibiotic which is poorly absorbed from the alimentary tract.
Therapeutic use. It is used principally in the treatment of infections by *Candida albicans.* Lesions in the mouth respond to 500 000 units in the suspension given 8-hourly. Monilial vaginitis is treated with pessaries (100 000 units) inserted once or twice daily. Candidiasis of the intestine is treated by tablets or the suspension. It may be given as an aerosol or inhaled in powder form for pulmonary candidiasis and aspergillosis.
Contraindications and side effects. Toxicity is low and side effects are few. It has an unpleasant taste and nausea, vomiting and diarrhea occasionally occur.

Griseofulvin

Pharmacological action. Griseofulvin is partly but adequately absorbed from the alimentary tract and is then selectively taken up by precursors of keratin. It is particularly effective against superficial fungal infections of the hair, nails and skin.
Therapeutic use. It is the treatment of choice in ringworm of the nails and hair. Treatment is usually necessary for weeks or months since new keratin, free from the fungus, may be reinfected by the old keratin before this has been shed.

Dosage for adults is 0.5 g daily either as one or two doses. Children require 125 to 250 mg daily. The course of therapy should be continued until after the fungus has disappeared from scrapings of previously infected tissue.
Contraindications and side effects. Nausea and abdominal discomfort are occasionally experienced. Depression of the white count has been reported and griseofulvin antagonises the action of warfarin. Skin rashes and, rarely, photosensitivity may occur. Other infrequent adverse effects include allergic reactions, transient proteinuria, mood change, gynaecomastia in children and disturbances in porphyrin metabolism. The drug should be avoided in porphyria.

Flucytosine

Pharmacological action. Flucytosine is an antifungal agent, probably acting as a uracil antimetabolite. It is absorbed from the intestinal tract and is excreted unchanged by the kidneys.
Therapeutic use. Flucytosine is effective against *Candida albicans, Cryptococcus neoformans* and *Torulopsis glabrata,* and is used to treat infections caused by these fungi. The usual dose is 200 mg/kg body weight per day divided into four doses. As it is excreted by the kidney, reduced dosage is required in patients with impaired renal function. Patients with a creatinine clearance of 10–20 ml per minute require only 50 mg every 24 hours.
Side effects include nausea and diarrhea and occasional depression of the blood count.

Category 10

DRUGS USED IN TROPICAL MEDICINE IN THE UK

R. L. PARSONS

THE TREATMENT OF MALARIA

4-AMINOQUINOLINES

Chloroquine

Pharmacological action. Chloroquine is a powerful suppressant of all types of human malaria being able to penetrate the red cell wall. It has a triple action, being *schizonticidal* against vivax, ovale, malariae and most falciparum strains. In addition chloroquine has a *gametocidal* action against the first three species, but not falciparum. It is also effective against the *exo-erythrocytic* stages of falciparum, but not the others. The bitter tasting tablets are rapidly absorbed, and slowly excreted. The phosphate and sulphate salts of chloroquine contain 63 and 73 mg of chloroquine base respectively.

Therapeutic use. Chloroquine is the best drug for acute malaria. It may be administered orally, by intramuscular injection or as an intravenous infusion. It should be given parenterally if there is severe diarrhea, vomiting, coma, or a parasitaemia of more than 10%. The doses are:—

1. *Treatment of acute primary attacks of malaria in non-immune subjects.* An initial loading dose of 600 mg (base) is given, followed by a 300 mg (base) dose 6 hours later, and 300 mg (base) on each of the next 2 days. Smaller doses may suffice to treat relapses.

2. In the *chemoprophylaxis of malaria*, either given alone or in combination with primaquine. 0.5 g of chloroquine phosphate is given on the same day of each week.

3. For *cerebral malaria*, chloroquine (the equivalent of 200–300 mg base) by intravenous or intramuscular injection, repeated in four hours and then followed by oral administration as above.

Side effects and contraindications are uncommon since chloroquine is non-toxic, provided the correct dose is given. Pruritus, erythema, urticaria, headache, giddiness, bleaching of the hair and weight loss may occur. Blurred vision may be caused by temporary paralysis of accommodation. Long term chloroquine therapy in large doses (i.e. 250–750 mg daily—for months or years) may produce keratopathy and optic neuritis. Doses of more than 5 mg of chloroquine base per kg may cause convulsions. The drug crosses the placenta and may lead to fetal damage.

Hydroxychloroquine

Pharmacological action. This is identical to chloroquine. Hydroxychloroquine is also used in the treatment of giardiasis, discoid lupus erythematosus and rheumatoid arthritis. 100 mg of hydroxychloroquine contains 78 mg of hydroxychloroquine base.

Therapeutic use. In the treatment of malaria, a daily dose of 0.4–1.2 g is used, after an initial dose of 800 mg followed by 400 mg 6–8 hours later, and a further 400 mg daily for 2 days. The usual suppressive dose is 400 mg weekly.

Side effects and contraindications. As for chloroquine.

Amodiaquine

Pharmacological action. This 4-aminoquinoline is more active than chloroquine against falciparum strains with multiple drug resistance. It is a powerful suppressant of all types of human malaria. Absorption is rapid and metabolism slow.

Therapeutic use. In the treatment of acute malaria, 600 mg of amodiaquine base is given on day 1 followed by 400 mg daily for 2 days, or until the fever and parasitaemia have subsided. The same dose should then be continued for a further month at weekly intervals. 400 mg of the base once weekly is sufficient for prophylaxis.

Side effects and contraindications. Like chloroquine, the tablets have a bitter taste, but "camoquin" used for infants has been made to taste pleasant. In adults who take the drug for more than 9 months, a reversible grey-purple pigmentation of the palate, nails, face and scar tissue may occur. Apart from diarrhea, nausea, vomiting and lethargy, amodiaquine is non-toxic at normal doses. However leucopenia, agranulocytosis, corneal deposits and retinopathy have been reported.

9-AMINO-ACRIDINE DYES

Mepacrine

Pharmacological action. Mepacrine is a good suppressive of malaria, having a rapidly schizonticidal action against the asexual forms of all species except falciparum. It also has a gametocidal action against vivax and malariae, but has been largely superseded by the 4-aminoquinolines in view of its toxicity. Mepacrine is also used in giardiasis and tapeworm infestation.

Therapeutic use. In the treatment of malaria, an initial dose of 300 mg t.d.s. is reduced to a thrice daily dose of 200 mg on day 2, and thereafter 100 mg t.d.s. for 5 days. From day 8 until 21 days later 100 mg t.d.s. must be given.

The suppressive daily dose is a single 100 mg tablet, but this must be started at least 14 days before exposure occurs.

Side effects and contraindications. Mepacrine is toxic. It stains the skin and conjunctivae yellow, and may cause occassional deaths from hepatitis. A lichenoid, eczematous, or exfoliative dermatitis may occur. Reversible psychosis and aplastic anaemia are other problems that may follow long continued use. In children injections are too toxic. The normal side effects include headache, dizziness, and gastrointestinal upsets. Mepacrine also enhances the toxicity of the 8-aminoquinolines.

Quinine salts

Pharmacological action. Quinine hydrochloride and dihydrochloride are preferable to the sulphate salt which is insoluble. Quinine is a highly active schizonticidal drug, but has no effect on the tissue forms. It is gametocidal for vivax and malariae, but not falciparum. Less toxic and more potent alternatives have largely superseded quinine. High doses are required every 6–8 hours, since quinine is rapidly metabolized and excreted.

Therapeutic use. Quinine still has a definite place in the treatment of cerebral and chloroquine resistant cerebral malaria. It is also combined with primaquine for the radical cure of relapsing vivax malaria.

In the treatment of acute cerebral malaria, 500–1000 mg is administered intravenously over 15–20 minutes either through a wide bore needle, or preferably through the side arm of a 500 ml infusion of saline, glucose or plasma. The rate of infusion must not exceed 50 mg/min. Not more than three such doses should be given every 24 hours.

A switch to the oral dose is made when the patient regains consciousness, usually within a few hours. Normally an initial oral dose of 650 mg b.d./t.d.s. is given during the first three days, and is followed by 650 mg b.d. for a further 7 days.

Side effects and contraindications. The local irritant effect of quinine is responsible for gastrointestinal side effects such as abdominal pain, nausea and diarrhea. Headache, giddiness, tinnitus and blurred vision are the main features of cinchonism. Idiosyncrasy may lead to edema of the face, mouth and lungs and skin rashes. Neurological symptoms include excitement, confusion, delirium, and syncope. Renal damage may lead to anuria and uraemia. Collapse, electrocardiographic abnormalities, abortion and subcutaneous haemorrhage may occur. Infusions that extravasate may cause sloughing and fibrosis.

Pregnancy is a relative, but not an absolute contraindication to quinine. In renal failure the dose of quinine should not exceed 600 mg daily, given in an infusion of 5% dextrose or normal saline.

8-AMINOQUINOLINES

Primaquine

Pharmacological action. Primaquine has a strong gametocidal action against all forms of the malarial parasite. It is effective against the exoerythrocytic forms of vivax and falciparum malaria, but has no schizonticidal action. Primaquine is used in the radical cure of relapsing vivax, ovale and malariae infection, when it is combined with a fast acting schizonticidal drug such as quinine or chloroquine. It is less effective in producing a cure of falciparum infection. Each 13.2 mg of primaquine phosphate (1 tablet) contains 7.5 mg of the base.

Therapeutic use. In the radical cure of malaria, 1 tablet containing 7.5 mg of primaquine base is given twice daily for two weeks immediately following a schizonticidal drug. A combination of 45 mg of primaquine base and 300 mg of chloroquine is given every week in the prophylaxis of malaria.

Side effects and contraindications. In Caucasians normal therapeutic doses are innocuous. Larger doses are responsible for abdominal cramps, vomiting, syncope, and hepatic damage. Cyanosis due to methaemoglobinaemia is not serious. Haemolytic anaemia occurs in coloured subjects with glucose-6-phosphate dehydrogenase deficiency. This is usually found in Africa, India, S.E. Asia and the Middle East. These and the toxic effects of the drug on the bone marrow are the most serious. The degree of haemolysis may be sufficiently severe to resemble the clinical picture of blackwater fever.

BIGUANIDES

Proguanil hydrochloride
Pharmacological action. Proguanil is an inhibitor of dihydrofolate reductase. It is a powerful suppressant of falciparum malaria being effective against both the erythrocytic and exo-erythrocytic parasites. It is schizonticidal against all species, but not gametocidal. Proguanil also prevents the sexual development of malarial parasites within the stomach of mosquitos. Absorption is rapid, but the action is slow since it is converted to an active metabolite. Excretion is rapid, so daily dosing is required.
Therapeutic use. A daily dose of 100–200 mg is started one day before and continued for one month after leaving a malarial area. Proguanil acts as a causal prophylactic against all species, but only effects a radical cure against falciparum malaria. Relapses of vivax may occur once the drug is discontinued, since it is ineffective against the tissue forms of this parasite. Proguanil should be taken after meals.
Side effects and contraindications. Proguanil is non-toxic; vomiting, anorexia, weight loss and malaise being the only side effects encountered. Renal irritation may occur leading to haematuria. Proguanil may be used during pregnancy.

DIAMINOPYRIDINES

Pyrimethamine
Pharmacological action. Pyrimethamine, like proguanil is a synthetic inhibitor of the enzyme dihydrofolate reductase. It is schizonticidal and a powerful suppressant of the tissue forms of all species of the malaria parasite. Since the drug has little effect upon immature schizonts within the red cell, it is slow to control an attack of malaria. Pyrimethamine also prevents sexual development of the parasite within the mosquito. Cross resistance with proguanil to resistant strains of falciparum occurs.

Absorption of pyrimethamine after oral administration is rapid, but excretion is slow. The drug is secreted into breast milk. Pyrimethamine has also been used in the treatment of toxoplasmosis.
Therapeutic use. Causal prophylaxis with a weekly dose of 25–50 mg is recommended. It is more acceptable to children because it is tasteless.

Pyrimethamine need not be taken until the day prior to exposure to infection, but like proguanil should be continued for one month after the last day of exposure. Combined therapy with Maloprim (pyrimethamine and dapsone) has successfully prevented malaria in regions where resistance has occurred.
Side effects and contraindications are unusual, but leucopenia and thrombocytopenia may occur with prolonged treatment. Very large doses cause vomiting, convulsions and respiratory failure. Macrocytic and megaloblastic anaemias, due to folate deficiency may occur.

THE TREATMENT OF SCHISTOSOMIASIS (BILHARZIA)

Niridazole
Pharmacological action. This nitro derivative of imidazolidinone is effective against all three schistosoma parasites, *Entameba histolytica* and guinea worm infestation. After oral administration, it is slowly absorbed being metabolised rapidly to metabolites which colour the urine and faeces dark brown, and are widely distributed to the tissues. Niridazole is incompatible with isoniazid.
Therapeutic use. An oral dose of 25 mg/kg is given as two daily doses for 5 days in *S. haematobium*, and 10 days for *S. mansoni* infestations. Guinea worm infestations should receive a 7–10-day course. The maximum adult dose is 2 g/day. 500 mg (adult) and 100 mg (children) tablets are available. In hepatosplenic schistosomiasis, the patient should be confined to bed because of the risk of neuropsychiatric disturbance, but this is not necessary in urinary and intestinal schistosomiasis.
Side effects and contraindications. Anorexia, nausea, vomiting, headache and drowsiness commonly occur. Neuropsychiatric disturbances including anxiety, confusion, hallucinations and convulsions are more likely in those with heavy infestations. Allergic reactions, eosinophilia, cardiographic and electroencephalographic abnormalities have been reported. Those with glucose-6-phosphate dehydrogenase deficiency may develop haemolysis.

This drug should not be given to epileptics, those with a history of heart disease, psychosis, or who have impaired hepatic function.

Sodium antimony tartrate
Pharmacological action. This organic trivalent antimonial must be administered intravenously

since absorption by mouth and per rectum is poor. Excretion into the bile and urine is slow so that antimony tends to accumulate. This drug is effective against all forms of bilharzia and has also been used in leishmaniasis, filiariasis and *Lymphogranuloma inguinale*. Given by mouth the drug has an emetic action. This drug was the mainstay in the treatment of schistosomiasis until the newer orally absorbed schistosomicidal compounds became available.

Therapeutic use. An initial dose of 30 mg i.v. is increased to 60 mg 2 days later. This is increased to 90 mg and 120 mg over the next four days. Injections are given every other day as a freshly prepared solution in 10 ml of saline until a complete course of twelve injections has been received. If extravasation may be followed by tissue necrosis, so great care must be taken when administering the drug intravenously.

Side effects and contraindications. Careful administration reduces the likelihood of coughing, vomiting, and joint pains. Whenever possible, the patient should be kept in bed for the whole of a course of treatment, since electrocardiographic changes, microemboli in the lungs, pulmonary edema and pneumonia have followed the use of sodium antimony tartrate. Since it is a cardiac depressant, bradycardia and hypotension may occur. Cardiac arrhythmias, exfoliative dermatitis, abdominal and thoracic muscular pains and herpes zoster may be produced by antimonials.

Contraindications include pyrexia, cardiac, respiratory, renal and hepatic disease. Intravenous injections should be given slowly and stopped immediately if coughing, vomiting or substernal pain occurs.

Lucanthone hydrochloride

Pharmacological action. Lucanthone is effective against *S. haematobium*, but less effective and against *S. mansoni* and valueless for *S. japonicum* infestations.

Therapeutic use. A daily dose of 0.5–1.0 g b.d. for 3 days is given. In children 25 mg/kg is given.

Side effects and contraindications. The skin and sclerotics are coloured orange yellow and the palms and soles a reddish brown colour. Nausea, vomiting, anorexia, epigastric or abdominal pain, headache and dizziness commonly occur. Convulsions, psychosis, depression, jaundice and acute hepatic necrosis has followed the use of lucanthone. Coloured individuals tolerate this drug better than whites. Caution in renal failure should be exercised. Lucanthone augments the effects of phenothiazines.

THE TREATMENT OF AMOEBIASIS

Emetine hydrochloride

Pharmacological action. Emetine is an ipecacuanha alkaloid which destroys any extraintestinal focus of infection. Although it rapidly and substantially depresses primary infection in the large gut, it rarely sterilises this infection completely even when treatment is prolonged. Other drugs must therefore be used to destroy any residual bowel infection.

Therapeutic use. The maximum dose is 60 mg daily by subcutaneous or intramuscular injection. Up to ten daily injections are given, the patient being confined to bed during a course of treatment. All strenuous activity is avoided for a further 3–4 weeks. A second course should not be started within 2 weeks of the first one.

Side effects and contraindications. Injections may produce tissue necrosis, which leads to sterile abscesses. Degenerative changes may occur in the myocardium, producing ECG changes, gut (diarrhea), nausea, vomiting, liver damage, peripheral neuritis, and hypotension. An acute degenerative myocarditis may lead to various arrhythmias, heart block, the last being a warning to stop the drug. Pain, tenderness and stiffness of the muscles may occur.

Emetine is contraindicated in cardiac and renal disease. It should not be given to children, the elderly, or during pregnancy. Daily ECGs should be performed after the fifth day of emetine, and the drug stopped if heart block occurs.

Emetine bismuth iodide

Pharmacological action. This emetine derivative is only partially absorbed and is used in the treatment of intestinal amoebiasis. It is released at high concentrations within the small intestine where it is lethal to the amoebae.

Therapeutic use. A daily dose of 60–200 mg is given last thing at night to reduce the inevitable nausea that follows its use. Since its effect on tissue amoebae is weak due to poor absorption of emetine bismuth iodide, a 3–4 day course of emetine injections should precede the 12-day course of emetine bismuth iodide. Activity should be restricted, and daily ECG and blood pressure recordings made. It is unnecessary to confine the patient to bed.

Side effects and contraindications. Gelatine or enteric-coated capsules are given to reduce the inevitable nausea and vomiting.

Contraindications: As for emetine hydrochloride.

Metronidazole

Pharmacological action. This imidazole derivative is active against *Trichomonas vaginalis*, giardiasis, *Entamoeba histolytica* and Vincent's infection. It is well-absorbed orally and widely distributed to all tissues, being active against both hepatic and intestinal amoebae, an advantage over other amoebicidal drugs. Metronidazole crosses the placenta and is secreted in breast milk.

Therapeutic use. Metronidazole is the safest, most effective and simplest treatment currently available for treating amoebic dysentery. 800 mg t.d.s. is given for 5–7 days. Children may be given 50 mg/kg in divided doses for 7 days. A single 2 g dose is given on 2–3 consecutive days in the treatment of hepatic amoebiasis. Alternatively 400 mg t.d.s. may be given for 3 days.

Side effects and contraindications. Metronidazole may cause a disulfiram like reaction after alcohol. Gastrointestinal side effects such as nausea, dry mouth, metallic taste, headaches, rashes, vertigo, depression, insomnia and drowsiness may all occur. Temporary leucopenia is not significant.

Metronidazole should not be given during the first trimester or to patients with blood dyscrasias, and they should be warned not to imbibe alcohol.

Chloroquine

Pharmacological action. Chloroquine is effective against intestinal amoebiasis complicated by metastatic infection. It is particularly useful in hepatic amoebiasis as it is concentrated in the liver.

Therapeutic use. An initial dose of 600 mg is followed by 300 mg in 6 hours. The maintenance dose is 150 mg b.d. for 14 days.

Side effects and contraindications. These have already been discussed in the section on malaria (see page 231).

Diloxanide furoate

Pharmacological action. Diloxanide is a safe and effective amoebicide acting within the bowel lumen. The furoate gives higher intestinal concentrations than the parent compound. It may be used alone, or to supplement emetine or chloroquine in the treatment of hepatic amoebiasis.

Therapeutic use. 500 mg is given t.d.s. for 10 days. Children are given 20 mg/kg daily in divided doses. The tablets should be protected from the light.

Side effects are insignificant. Flatulence, vomiting, pruritus and urticaria may occur. Albuminuria has been reported.

ANTHELMINTHICS

Niclosamide

Therapeutic action. The drug of choice in the treatment of tapeworm infestation. It can be given to outpatients without prior preparation. Two 0.5 g tablets are taken on waking and chewed well. The same procedure is repeated 1 hour later. Since the worm disintegrates following this treatment, there is no point in searching for the head, so follow up 6 months later is necessary. The dose for children is 0.25 g. If failure occurs the drug can be repeated for 2 days instead of one. A light meal may be taken three hours after starting the procedure. The cure rate is 90%.

Side effects and contraindications. Cysticercosis is a risk when this drug is used to treat *T. solium* infestations, due to disintegration of the worm.

Dichlorophen

Pharmacological action. This effective anthelminthic is active against human and animal tapeworms (*Diphyllobothrium latum*) and the dwarf tapeworm. Disintegration of the worm follows treatment with dichlorophen, so that the head does not appear in the stool. Niclosamide and dichlorophen are frequently given as combined therapy.

Therapeutic use. 6 g is given first thing in the morning on two successive days (children 2–4 g). There is no need for preliminary starvation, or subsequent purgation.

Side effects and contraindications. Intestinal colic usually occurs within 2–3 hours of administration and is followed by diarrhea. Vomiting increases the risk of cysticercosis. Urticaria, jaundice, and even death has followed the use of dichlorophen.

Mepacrine

Pharmacological action. This has already been considered (see page 232).

Therapeutic use. In treating cestode infestations 1 g in 40 ml of water is given via a duodenal tube, after a preliminary 48-hour fast in hospital. Alternatively 200 mg may be given every 10 minutes by mouth, but this is less effective and usually leads to vomiting. The stools should be examined during the ensuing 24 hours for the worm which is usually stained bright yellow.

Piperazine hydrate

Pharmacological action. This is one of the most effective anthelminthics against ascariasis. It is also effective against threadworms, but has no effect on tapeworms, hookworms or whipworms. Piperazine paralyses the roundworm producing narcosis, leading to expulsion of the worm by peristalsis. Piperazine salts (citrate, adipate, phosphate and tartrate) have little advantage over one another.

After oral administration, piperazine is absorbed and excreted in the urine.

Therapeutic use. Preliminary starvation and subsequent purgation are unnecessary. Piperazine is less effective against threadworms than viprynium and thiabendazole. For *Ascariasis* a single evening dose of 4 g is taken with the meal. Saline purgation should only be given if the patient is constipated. Divided doses are given in heavy infestations with ascaris. The dose in children is 120 mg/kg daily. Piperazine citrate or phosphate may be given as a syrup or as tablets. Threadworms are treated with 2 g daily for seven days. Children are given 1.5 g (7–12); 1 g (4–6); and 750 mg daily below the age of 3.

Side effects and contraindications are rare and usually due to over-dosage or renal failure. Headache, dizziness, paraesthesiae, muscular incoordination, nausea, vomiting, urticaria and blurred vision may all occur.

Viprynium embonate

Pharmacological action. This is an effective antihelminthic against *Enterobius vermicularis* (threadworm) and strongyloidiasis infestation. It is more effective than piperazine in threadworm infestation, but less effective in treating ascariasis. Tablets and a flavoured suspension are available, the latter containing 10 mg of anhydrous base per ml. The drug colours the stools red, and as many mothers know, staining occurs if the solution is spilt.

Therapeutic use. A single dose of 5 ml (containing 50 mg) of suspension or a single 50 mg tablet is given, being repeated in a week if necessary. All infected members of the family should be treated simultaneously to avoid reinfection.

Thiabendazole

Pharmacological action. Thiabendazole is effective against roundworm, hookworm, strongyloides and *Enterobius* species. It is also effective against *Trichinella* and animal nematodes. It is less effective against the whipworm. The drug is absorbed orally and excreted in the urine.

Therapeutic use. The drug should be taken immediately after food to reduce gastric irritation. The usual dose is 25 mg/kg after supper and again after breakfast the following morning, for

2–3 consecutive days. A single dose repeated in 7 days is sufficient for threadworms. 50% of patients with strongyloidiasis respond to the first dosage regimen.

Side effects and contraindications. Mild anorexia, nausea, vomiting, epigastric discomfort, vertigo, rashes, headache, fatigue and drowsiness commonly occur. Hypoglycaemia, bradycardia, hypotension, xanthopsia, bradycardia, lymphadenopathy, fever and chills are rare.

This drug should be avoided during pregnancy. Those with ascariasis may develop migration of their worms to other organs.

Bephenium hydroxynaphthoate

Pharmacological action. This anthelminthic is effective against roundworms, and hookworms of the species *Ankylostoma*, but less effective against *Necator* species and the whipworm. It is particularly useful for mixed roundworm and hookworm infestation, being non-toxic and more efficient than tetrachlorethylene in removing hookworms. 5 g contains 2.5 g of base.

Therapeutic use. 5 g daily for 4 days may achieve total eradication, but it is usually very difficult to get rid of the few residual worms. This drug should be taken on an empty stomach, a meal being taken 1 hour later. Children are given half the adult dose.

Side effects and contraindications. Mild anorexia, diarrhea, vomiting, headache and vertigo. The insoluble powder has a bitter taste.

Diethylcarbamazine citrate

Pharmacological action. This antifilarial is effective against *Wuchereria bancrofti, Loa loa* and tropical eosinophilia. If it is used for onchocerciasis or *Brugia malayi* infestations, allergic reactions may occur. The drug prevents the spread of infection to the vector by rapidly removing the microfilariae which remain in the reticuloendothelial system. It is effective against adult and microfilariae in *Loa loa.* In onchocerciasis the microfilariae are controlled, but the drug is less effective against adults. It is well absorbed from the gut and excreted in the urine.

Therapeutic use. A daily dose of 150–500 mg is given in *Wuchereria bancrofti* infestation for 21 days. A low initial dose should be given in *B. malayi* and *onchocerca volvulus* infestations to reduce the risk of severe local allergic reactions. In onchocerciasis a single daily dose of 50 mg is given for 3 days. This is then increased to 200 mg once daily (day 4), twice daily (day 5), and finally the usual dose of 200 mg t.d.s. is continued from day 6 for a further 14–21 days. An exacerbation of symptoms (itching and rash) may occur on the first day of treatment and be followed by transient fever, edema, dermatitis, severe pruritus, and eye symptoms (blepharitis, conjunctivitis and iridocyclitis). Antihistamines and corticosteroids may be used to treat these reactions.

Side effects and contraindications. Release of protein from the worms by drug is responsible for the exacerbations of filariasis already described. This may be treated with antihistamines and steroids. In onchocerciasis, diethylcarbamazine should be used cautiously, since allergic reactions may involve the eyes. Headache, anorexia, nausea and vomiting may also occur.

Pregnancy does not contraindicate diethylcarbamazine.

CYTOTOXIC DRUGS AND IMMUNOSUPPRESSION

J. R. TROUNCE

Although there is as yet no drug capable of entirely eradicating the common cancers, interesting developments are taking place in the strategy of managing neoplastic disease, in particular the lymphomas, acute leukaemias and chorionic carcinoma. In a number of patients with these conditions very long remissions can be induced; perhaps the word cure can be applied to some of them.

There are now quite a number of drugs which are partially effective against these neoplasms and research into how these drugs are best deployed is at present in progress. In the treatment of advanced Hodgkin's disease evidence is accumulating that repeated courses of combinations of these drugs is more effective than using them singly. In the acute leukaemias, drugs may again be used in combination; some drugs appear more useful for induction of a remission and others for maintenance therapy. *This means that in the text only approximate doses of individual drugs can be given as much will depend on whether the drug is used alone or as part of a combination regime.*

THE ALKYLATING AGENTS

These compounds have the general formula:

$$R—CH_2CH_2^+$$

They are capable of combining with a number of chemical groupings found in the cell. These include thiols, carboxyl, phosphate, amino and nucleic acid groups. Their effect on tumours is probably due to their linking with guanine in the DNA chain. It seems that cross-linkage between the DNA strands by alkylating agents is of particular importance. Alkylating agents thus interfere with mitosis and they may also produce abnormalities of the chromosomes.

The various alkylating agents, although having the same general action differ considerably in their solubility, absorption, penetration and speed of action. It also seems that certain alkylating agents are particularly effective in certain types of tumour; the reason for this is not known.

All this group of drugs damage normal cells, particularly those of the bone marrow and intestinal tract, and this is one of the main limitations of their use.

NITROGEN MUSTARDS

Mustine

Pharmacological action. Mustine is a highly reactive alkylating agent. It is rapidly transformed in solution into an ethyleneimmonium ion which is the active alkylating agent *in vivo*. Mustine is a highly irritant substance and can therefore only be given intravenously. After injection it rapidly combines with various groups and is cleared from the blood within a few minutes.

Therapeutic use. Mustine must be freshly made up before administration: it rapidly combines with water in solution. It is important to avoid extravasation of the drug around the vein and it is safest to set up an intravenous infusion of 5% dextrose and to inject the dose of mustine through the tubing with the drip running rapidly.

Mustine often causes nausea and vomiting for some hours after administration. The patient will suffer less upset if it is given in the evening combined with chlorpromazine 50–100 mg i.m. and an hypnotic.

The usual total dose of mustine is 0.4 mg/kg. It can be given as a single injection, or the course can be spread over several injections—usually 0.1 mg/kg on alternate days for four injections. Larger doses have been used but this causes a considerable increase in side effects. Mustine produces a rapid response in those with susceptible tumours.

Mustine can also be given intrapleurally or intraperitoneally in patients with recurrent malignant effusions. The usual dose is 20 mg as a single injection and the volume of the effusion should be reduced if possible to around 500 ml to produce optimal results. Some systemic absorption occurs but bone marrow depression is rare. Mustine may cause a temporary increase in the effusion but it should be effective within three weeks; if not it can be repeated.

Neoplasms which usually respond well to mustine are:

Hodgkin's disease
Lymphosarcoma
Reticulum celled sarcoma.

Neoplasms which sometimes show response to mustine are:

Carcinoma of the bronchus
Carcinoma of the ovary
Carcinoma of the breast
Seminomas.

Contraindications and side effects. Depression of the bone marrow is the most important toxic action of the drug. It affects the granulocytes and sometimes the platelets, and rarely it also causes erythrocyte depression. These effects are maximal about 10–14 days after giving the drug and they may clear up in 3–4 weeks.

Mustine usually produces severe nausea and vomiting (see above) and may also cause diarrhea and even ulceration of the gut. Rarely it causes rashes.

Great care must be taken if mustine is given to those with existing bone marrow depression. If it is essential to give the drug, a considerably smaller dose should be used and the bone marrow examined regularly. Facilities should also be available to nurse patients with severe leucopenia.

Mustine should also be avoided (as should all cytotoxic agents) in pregnancy. Although evidence from human sources is scanty, there is good experimental evidence that it can cause fetal abnormalities.

Degranol

Degranol is a mannitol–mustine compound. It is given intravenously and does not appear to have advantages over mustine.

Chlorambucil

Pharmacological action. Chlorambucil is a mustine–phenylbutyric acid compound. It is relatively non-irritant and is satisfactorily absorbed after oral admission.

Therapeutic use. The usual dose is 0.1–0.5 mg/kg daily as a single dose in the morning. It is usually two or three weeks before a response is seen and the course of treatment lasts 3–5 weeks. This may be followed by maintenance treatment at a dose of 2.0 mg daily.

Neoplasms which respond well to chlorambucil are:

Chronic lymphatic leukaemia
Hodgkin's disease
Reticulum-celled sarcoma

Neoplasms which occasionally respond to chlorambucil are:

Carcinoma of the ovary
Carcinoma of the testicles

Because of its predominant action on the lymphocyte series of cells chlorambucil has also been used as an immunosuppressive agent, and in the treatment of macroglobulinaemia.

Contraindications and side effects. Bone marrow depression can occur especially if the bone marrow is depressed or infiltrated. Weekly white cell counts are therefore required. Nausea occurs in about 10% of patients and it can rarely cause rashes.

Cyclophosphamide

Pharmacological action. Cyclophosphamide is inactive *in vitro*; in the body it is split by the enzyme phosphoramidase, liberating an alkylating agent. It was originally hoped that this would occur predominantly in tumours, but it is now realised that activation occurs throughout the body. It is well absorbed from the intestine and partially excreted in the urine where it may set up a chemical cystitis.

Therapeutic use. The dose of cyclophosphamide is between 3 and 6 mg/kg daily and it can be given orally or intravenously. The high dose level should not be continued for more than 5 days and this may be followed by an oral maintenance dose of 2.0 mg/kg/day. Sometimes doses of up to 15 mg/kg are given intravenously at weekly intervals in combination with other cytotoxics.

Neoplasms which often respond well to cyclophosphamide are:

Hodgkin's disease and other lymphomas
Multiple myeloma
Burkitt's tumour*
Maintenance therapy in acute lymphoblastic leukaemia.

Neoplasms which may show some response are:

Carcinoma of the breast
Carcinoma of the ovary
Neuroblastomas.

---

*Africans appear to tolerate cyclophosphamide very well and large doses are given (30 mg/kg for 5 days).

Cyclophosphamide in doses of around 100 mg/day can also be used as an immunosuppressive. *Contraindications and side effects.* Cyclophosphamide will produce leucopenia and regular white cell counts are required. However, it rarely causes platelet depression. About a third of the patients develop some degree of alopecia which is reversible. A few patients develop a chemical cystitis with haematuria and a high fluid intake is advisable. Other side effects include rashes and nausea.

Melphalan

Pharmacological action. Melphalan is a compound of phenylalanine and mustine. It was hoped that the combination of mustine with a naturally occurring substance would increase its activity. It is well absorbed from the intestinal tract. It differs from mustine in that after absorption it remains active for several hours.

Therapeutic use. Melphalan is largely used in treating multiple myelomatosis. It has also been used with some success in seminomas and ovarian carcinomas and in treating melanomas by local perfusion, about half the patients showing some response. The usual dose is 5–8 mg daily for 10 days. When the bone marrow has recovered this may be followed by a maintenance dose of 1–2 mg daily.

Contraindications and side effects. Melphalan is a powerful depressive of the bone marrow, producing leucopenia, and in particular, platelet depression. It may also cause nausea and with large courses some degree of alopecia.

THE ALKYL SULPHONATES

Busulphan

Pharmacological action. Busulphan is well absorbed from the intestine. It appears to react particularly with thiol groups and the major portion is excreted as sulphur-containing metabolites.

It depresses the myeloid series of cells and has much less effect on the lymphocytes.

Therapeutic use. Busulphan is used in chronic myeloid leukaemia where it nearly always produces remission. It is also occasionally used in polycythaemia rubra vera. It is the drug of choice for treating thrombocythaemia.

The initial dose is 3.0–6.0 mg daily. This is continued until the total white cell count reaches 20 000/mm³. The drug is then stopped and the white cell count usually continues to fall for 2–3 weeks.

If the white cell count then rises rapidly a continuous maintenance dose of busulphan is required, usually 2.0 mg daily, with the object of keeping the white cell count at about 10 000/mm³. If the white cell count only rises slowly further treatment is delayed until the white count rises to about 50 000/mm³ or troublesome symptoms develop. Intermittent courses are used in such cases. Blood counts are done at 2–4-week intervals.

Contraindications and side effects. Depression of the myeloid of cells has already been discussed, and it is important to remember that it is occasionally irreversible and may also affect the platelets. Pigmentation of the skin is quite common with prolonged treatment and is thought to be due to a disturbance of tyrosine metabolism.

A few patients complain of weakness, nausea and hypotension, reminiscent of adrenal failure—but adrenal function is normal.

Diffuse interstitial pulmonary fibrosis has been reported; its cause is unknown.

Mannitol myleran

Mannitol myleran is given orally but nausea is common. Its uses are similar to those of mustine and it has no particular advantages.

THE ETHYLENAMINES

Triethylene melamine

Triethylene melamine has been used in lymphomas. However its absorption is variable, and therefore the therapeutic dose varies between patients. Sometimes severe toxic effects may be produced. It is rarely used at the present time.

ThioTEPA

ThioTEPA is given by intramuscular or intravenous injection as it is rapidly hydrolysed in the stomach when given orally.

It appears most effective in carcinomas of the ovary and breast, and it has been suggested that this is due to depression of endocrine function rather than a direct action on the tumour.

ThioTEPA can be given:

1st week:	10 mg daily for 5 days
2nd week:	10 mg daily for 4 days
3rd week:	10 mg daily for 3 days
Thereafter:	2 mg weekly.

ThioTEPA produces bone marrow depression in a very arbitrary manner and as it has little advantage over other alkylating agents it is now rarely used.

ANTIMETABOLITES

These drugs resemble substances used by cells for metabolism and growth.

They compete with the normal substrates of cell metabolism and thus may prevent cell growth and ultimately cause cell death.

The action of antimetabolites is not confined to malignant cells but they are useful in certain types of malignant disease, probably because they have their greatest effect on rapidly dividing cells. Ultimately their usefulness is limited by their toxicity to normal cells, particularly those of the bone marrow, or to the development of resistance.

FOLIC ACID ANTAGONISTS

Methotrexate

Pharmacological action. Methotrexate competes with folic acid for the enzyme dihydrofolic reductase. It has a very much greater affinity for the enzyme than folic acid and thus effectively blocks the synthesis of tetrahydrofolic acid, an important substance in the synthesis of purines.

This block can be circumvented by giving folinic acid, which is 5-formyl-tetrahydrofolic acid, a stage further on in purine synthesis.

About half a normal dose is absorbed and largely excreted unchanged in the urine within 48 hours. Only a small quantity penetrates the blood-brain barrier (see later).

Therapeutic use. Methotrexate will produce a remission in about 50% of children with acute leukaemia. It is also used for maintenance treatment when a remission has been induced by other drugs. It is best used for maintenance rather than induction of a remission in acute lymphoblastic leukaemia.

To induce a remission the dose is 2.5–5.0 mg daily in children, and 2.5–10.0 mg daily in adults. Although methotrexate can be given by injection it is usually given orally as a single dose on an empty stomach. This is important, as multiple doses during the day may not produce the same effect. This regime is continued for 3–4 weeks, until a remission is induced or toxic effects appear.

There are a variety of schemes for maintenance treatment. One method is to give 20 mg/m² of body surface twice weekly.

Methotrexate can also be used in meningeal leukaemia. It is given intrathecally in doses of 0.2 mg/kg on alternate days for a total of four doses, and this should be combined with folinic acid 5.0 mg i.m. to reduce systemic effects.

Methotrexate is also used with considerable success in the treatment of chorionepithelioma. Higher doses are used and treatment requires special facilities.

Contraindications and side effects. In addition to bone marrow depression methotrexate causes oral ulceration which is preceded by patches of hyperaemia. It may also cause nausea, diarrhea and alopecia.

Methotrexate should be used with care in patients with impaired renal function, as a high proportion of the drug is excreted via the kidneys.

PYRAMIDINE ANTAGONISTS

5-Fluorouracil

Pharmacological action. This drug interferes with the synthesis of nucleic acid. It is poorly absorbed after oral administration, and is usually given intravenously. Most of the drug is metabolised, and about 20% is excreted in the urine.

Therapeutic use. 5-Fluorouracil is of some benefit in about 30% of patients with carcinoma of the ovary, stomach, intestinal tract and breast.

The usual dose is 15 mg/kg*/day for 5 days—the daily dose should not exceed 1.0 g. If there is no sign of toxicity a further four doses of 7.5 mg/kg can be given on alternate days.

Contraindications and side effects. Early signs of toxicity are nausea, anorexia and diarrhea. If mouth ulceration develops the drug should be stopped.

Bone marrow depression is common and usually starts within a few days of starting treatment. Reduced dosage should be used in those with bone marrow depression or jaundice.

5-Fluorouracil is contraindicated in patients who have had an adrenalectomy as they are particularly sensitive to the diarrhea and vomiting produced by this drug.

Cytarabin (Ara-C)

Pharmacological action. Cytarabin is a pyrimidine nucleoside which is incorporated in DNA and inhibits DNA synthesis. It is effective in acute leukaemias and also suppresses DNA viruses.

Therapeutic use. Cytarabin is most effective in producing remission in acute leukaemia. It is usually combined with one or several other cytotoxic agents, most commonly 6-mercaptopurine, cyclophosphamide, daunarubicin or thioquinine. In combination it produces a remission in about 25–50% of patients with acute myeloblastic leuk-

*This is ideal body weight.

aemia, but the remission is usually brief. Dosage is variable, depending on other cytotoxic drugs being given but is in the range of 3.0 mg/kg body weight.
Contraindications and side effects. Gastrointestinal upsets with nausea, vomiting and diarrhea are common. Bone marrow depression is usual.

PURINE ANALOGUES

6-Mercaptopurine

Pharmacological action. 6-Mercaptopurine interferes with the synthesis of DNA.

The essential stage is probably the conversion of 6-mercaptopurine to its ribose phosphate derivative which either prevents DNA synthesis or leads to the formation of abnormal DNA.

6-Mercaptopurine is well absorbed and widely distributed in the body. However, penetration into the CSF is poor. It is rapidly metabolised and the metabolites are excreted in the urine.
Therapeutic use. 6-Mercaptopurine is used in treating acute leukaemia, producing a remission in about 30% of children and a smaller proportion of adults. The dose is 2.5 mg/kg daily by mouth and is given as a single dose. The initial course should not exceed 6 weeks and is continued until a remission is produced or toxic effects appear. It is usually used in combination with other drugs in producing a remission. 6-Mercaptopurine can be used for maintenance therapy, the usual dose being 1.0 mg/kg daily.

6-Mercaptopurine in combination with other cytotoxic agents is used in treating chorionic carcinoma.
Contraindications and side effects. In addition to bone marrow depression 6-mercaptopurine occasionally causes nausea, vomiting and diarrhea. Jaundice, which can be either cholestatic or due to cellular damage, has been reported.

The concurrent use of allopurinol with 6-mercaptopurine increases the toxicity of 6-mercaptopurine and the dose should then be halved.

PLANT PRODUCTS

Vinca alkaloids—vinblastine/vincristine

A number of alkaloids have been isolated from the periwinkle and two of them, *vinblastine* and *vincristine,* have been shown to have useful cytotoxic action.
Pharmacological action. Both of these alkaloids inhibit cell division at the metaphase but this does not appear to be their chief mode of anti-tumour action.

They are poorly absorbed from the intestine and are usually given intravenously.

They are rapidly excreted by the liver and therefore any biliary obstruction will increase the effect of the drug.

Vinblastine

Therapeutic use Vinblastine is used in treating Hodgkin's disease, and chorion-epithelioma.

The initial dose is 0.1 mg/kg intravenously; this is increased by 0.05 mg/kg, each dose being given at weekly intervals until a remission is produced or toxicity occurs. Weekly dosage should not exceed 0.3 mg/kg. Maintenance treatment can be given weekly at a dose level which is found by trial not to produce leucopenia. A blood count should be performed before each dose.
Contraindications and side effects. Vinblastine can cause depression of the bone marrow. It usually occurs within a week of the dose and is short lived.

Vincristine

Therapeutic use. Vincristine is used as the initial drug in treating acute leukaemia. It can also be used in Hodgkin's disease and related conditions; it is particularly useful when there is bone marrow infiltration as it has little depressing effect on leucocyte or platelet formation. The initial dose is 0.01 mg/kg intravenously; this is increased but should not exceed 2.0 mg weekly.
Contraindications and side effects. The toxic effects of vincristine are mainly on the nervous system. Muscle weakness effects, particularly the dorsiflexors of the feet, the hands and larynx. This is followed by loss of reflexes and paraesthesiae. The autonomic nervous system is also affected, causing constipation and signs suggesting intestinal obstruction. Nerve damage usually recovers if the drug is stopped, but may persist indefinitely.

Vincristine also produces some alopecia. Bone marrow depression can occur but is usually preceded by neurotoxicity.

ANTIBIOTICS

Several antibiotics have been found to have anti-tumour activity.

Actinomycins probably produce their effect by interference with DNA and protein synthesis.

Actinomycin D is used in the treatment of Wilms' tumour in association with surgery and radiotherapy. It is given intravenously in doses of 15 μg/kg body weight daily for 5 days.

Toxic effects include dryness of skin, nausea, vomiting and bone marrow depression.

Actinomycin C can be used in Hodgkin's disease in doses of 200 μg daily until a total of 1.5 mg has been given.

Bleomycin is an antibiotic which is preferentially concentrated in epithelial tissues. It has some anti-cancer effect and has been used to treat cancers of the mouth and esophagus, and to some extent lymphomas. Its mode of action is not known, but it is almost unique among cytotoxic drugs in that it does not depress the bone marrow, unfortunately it is not very effective. It can be given by intravenous or intramuscular injection at weekly intervals in doses of 15–30 mg. Higher dosage is liable to cause ulceration of the mouth. Total dosage in excess of 200 mg may lead to widespread lung fibrosis. It is recommended that the drug is combined with steroids to minimise this complication and that the chest be X-rayed at regular intervals.

Daunarubicin

Pharmacological action and therapeutic use. Daunarubicin is believed to exert its cytotoxic effect by inhibiting DNA synthesis, forming a complex with preformed DNA. It is used in acute lymphoblastic and myeloblastic leukaemias. The dose is 30–60 mg/m² body surface/day for up to 5 days and it is usually used in combination with other cytotoxic agents.

Contraindications and side effects. include rapidly developing marrow depression (daily white cell counts are required), nausea, vomiting and ulceration of the mouth. Heart failure is produced by large doses.

MISCELLANEOUS COMPOUNDS

Procarbazine

Pharmacological action and therapeutic use. Procarbazine is most useful in Hodgkin's disease when it induces a remission in about 60% of patients. It may also produce some benefit in other lymphomas. Its mode of action is unknown. The initial dose is 50 mg daily orally, and this can be increased to 100 mg daily. A course usually lasts three weeks unless the white cell count or platelets become depressed.

Procarbazine can be used for maintenance treatment in smaller doses.

It can also be given intravenously but this is rarely necessary.

Contraindications and side effects. Procarbazine depresses the bone marrow. In addition it may produce nausea and vomiting. It is an amine oxidase inhibitor and potentiates phenothiazine which should therefore be used in half the normal dose if given concurrently. Combination with alcohol may produce general malaise.

Crasniton (L-asparaginase)

Pharmacological action. Crasniton splits the amino acid asparagine. Normal cells can manufacture this essential amino acid for themselves but certain types of leukaemic cells are unable to do so. They then become deficient in asparagine and die. Crasniton is usually obtained from *E.coli* but can also be obtained from *Erivinia carotorora.* It is worth noting that there may not be cross hypersensitivity between crasniton from these two sources (see later).

Therapeutic use. Crasniton is given intravenously in doses of 17 000 u/m² body area in 10 ml of saline twice daily. Preliminary testing with a small dose for hypersensitivity is advisable. The course may be continued for up to 4 weeks but will depend on the response of the patient. Crasniton is most effective in acute lymphatic leukaemia and is frequently combined with other cytotoxic agents.

Contraindications and side effects. Crasniton is often antigenic and hypersensitivity reactions of various types are common. Bronchospasm is an absolute indication to stop the drug.

Hormones

Estrogens and steroids are used in various neoplastic conditions.

IMMUNOSUPPRESSION

Certain diseases are thought to be due to malfunction of the immune system. In these diseases it is believed that the immune system fails to recognise certain cells as being part of the 'self' and regards them as 'foreign' invaders. These cells are then attacked by the immune system with subsequent development of disease.

Among the disorders which are sometimes treated by immunosuppressive drugs are some types of the nephrotic syndrome, rheumatoid arthritis, systemic lupus erythematosus, polyarteritis nodosa and Crohn's disease. The evidence for an autoimmune cause for some of these diseases is very tenuous and it may be that the effectiveness of these drugs is due to some other action. They are also used to prevent rejection of transplanted organs.

In general immunosuppressive drugs produce their effect by inhibiting the cells which are especially concerned in the immune response, particularly the lymphocytes and their precursors. Unfortunately they all suppress other rapidly dividing cells in the body, namely, the cells of the bone marrow (particularly the neutrophils and platelets) and the cells lining the gastrointestinal tract.

Azathioprine is a purine antimetabolite related to 6-mercaptopurine (see page 242). It is given orally and the dose usually lies between 50 mg and 150 mg daily. In addition to bone marrow depression azathioprine can cause diarrhea.

Cyclophosphamide is an alkylating agent and is widely used for treating neoplastic diseases (see page 237). It is given orally in doses between 50 mg and 100 mg daily. Bone marrow depression can occur and hair loss may be troublesome. Although the hair will grow again, the patient (particularly if female) may temporarily require a wig.

Corticosteroids are immunosuppressive as well as anti-inflammatory. They often have to be used for this purpose in large doses with all the attendant risks of high steroid dosage (see page 255).

General complications of immunosuppression. Infection of any type may occur but fungal or viral infection is particularly common. Patients who have had prolonged immunosuppression have an increased incidence of neoplastic disease, especially lymphomas.

Category 12

DRUGS USED IN THE TREATMENT OF HORMONAL DISORDERS

M. N. MAISEY and J. R. WALL

PITUITARY HORMONES

Growth hormone
This is only available in small amounts for the treatment of children with hypopituitary dwarfism.

Gonadotrophins

Preparations	Source
Human chorionic gonadotrophin injection.	Extract of pregnancy urine.
Human follicle stimulating hormone.	Extract of post-menopausal urine.

1. Female infertility. *Therapeutic use*: An accurate diagnosis is essential before treatment is begun, because primary ovarian failure and mechanical causes are not amenable to treatment with gonadotrophins. The essence of treatment is the initial treatment with FSH injection to induce maturation of the follicle, followed by the administration of HCG to induce ovulation. There are many different treatment regimes, but the treatment must always be monitored carefully with one or more of the following serial measurements: urinary estrogens, vaginal smears, basal body temperatures and pregnanediol.

2. Male infertility. This is less well established than female infertility, but successful results have been reported in patients with hypopituitarism and some types of testicular abnormalities.

3. Undescended testes and delayed puberty. HCG in doses of 4000–5000 units, twice weekly in 3-monthly courses is commonly used, but the exact indications and optimum ages are controversial.

Contraindications and side effects. Allergic reactions may occur.

Hyperstimulation syndrome during the treatment of female infertility with ovarian enlargement, abdominal pain and even ascites and pleural effusion.

Clomiphene
Preparation. Clomiphene citrate tablets, 50 mg.

Pharmacological action. Clomiphene is a non-steroid compound related to the estrogen chlorotrianisene. It has weak estrogenic properties but its principal property is the ability to cause increased secretion of gonadotrophins by the pituitary. Clomiphene may exert this effect by blocking the inhibitory effect of other estrogens on the hypothalamus.

Therapeutic use. Clomiphene citrate is used for the treatment of infertility due to disorders of ovulation. It is ineffective, however, in cases of complete pituitary or ovarian failure. The usual dose is 50 mg daily for 5 days; if this induces ovulation then the course is repeated until a pregnancy occurs. If not, then the dose is increased to 100 mg daily for 5–10 days.

Contraindications and side effects. Hot flushes due to the increased level of gonadotrophins are frequent; ovarian enlargement occurs, but with careful supervision the incidence can be reduced. Headache, diplopia, dizziness, transient scotomata, constipation, allergic skin reactions, and reversible alopecia have been reported and there is a higher incidence of multiple pregnancy.

Thyroid-stimulating hormone
Preparation. Thyrotrophin injection.

Therapeutic use. TSH, in conjunction with radio-iodine uptake measurements, is used diagnostically to differentiate between primary and secondary hypothyroidism, to diagnose myxedema in patients already receiving thyroid medication, and also to confirm hypothyroidism when the results of radioiodine investigations are borderline. It is sometimes used to increase the uptake of a therapeutic dose of radioiodine in the treatment of functioning thyroid carcinomas.

The dose is 2.5. to 10 units i.m. daily.

Contraindications and side effects. Local allergic reactions. In adrenal insufficiency TSH should not be given before appropriate steroid replacement therapy.

Vasopressin

Preparation	Main use	Dose
Vasopressin injection	Diagnosis of diabetes insipidus	0.1 unit i.v.
	Treatment of bleeding esophageal varices	20 units in i.v. infusion in 10 min.
Vasopressin tannate injection	Diagnosis and treatment of diabetes insipidus	2.5–5 units i.m
Lypressin injection*	Diagnosis of pituitary adrenal insufficiency	10 units i.m.
Lypressin nasal spray*	Treatment of diabetes insipidus	10 units 3–6 times daily
Pituitary (posterior lobe) insufflation	Treatment of diabetes insipidus	5–20 mg t.d.s.

*Synthetic preparations.

Vasopressin

Pharmacological action. Apart from its effect on smooth muscle causing a rise in arterial blood pressure and other manifestations of smooth muscle contraction, vasopressin is also the antidiuretic hormone increasing the permeability of the collecting ducts of the kidneys to water and thereby producing a hypertonic urine.

Contraindications and side effects. Vasoconstriction leads to skin pallor and a rise in arterial blood pressure.

Smooth muscle contraction may cause nausea, intestinal cramp and uterine contractions.

Constriction of the coronary vessels may occur and therefore should not be given if there is evidence of coronary artery disease.

Posterior pituitary snuff may cause local allergic reactions with nasal congestion, and allergic pulmonary infiltration has been described.

More recently chlorpropamide (250–500 mg daily) and also thiazide diuretics (e.g. chlorothiazide 500–1500 mg daily) have been used in the treatment of diabetes insipidus. These drugs are dealt with in more detail elsewhere.

THYROID HORMONES

Preparations	Equivalent doses
Thyroid extract tablets	30 mg
Thyroxine sodium BP	0.05 mg
Sodium liothyronine	10 μg

Pharmacological action. The main action of the thyroid hormones is to uncouple oxidative phosphorylation in mitochondria, but they undoubtedly also stimulate a large number of other enzyme activities.

The principal difference between thyroxine and liothyronine is in the duration of action; thyroxine has a peak action occurring at 9 days and lasting for about 18 days, whereas liothyronine has a peak action at 2–3 days and lasts for only 8 days.

Therapeutic use. Thyroxine is used in the treatment of primary or secondary hypothyroidism. The starting dose should be low (0.025–0.05 mg daily) and gradually increased at fortnightly intervals to a full replacement dose of 0.2–0.4 mg daily. Thyroxine is also used in the treatment of simple goitres, acute and chronic thyroiditis, and has been used in suppressive doses in the treatment of functioning thyroid carcinomas.

Liothyronine is used in the treatment of myxedema coma; the dose is 25 μg every 6 hours.

Contraindications and side effects. Excessive dosage is characterised by many of the features of thyrotoxicosis, in particular tachycardia, nervousness, tremor and sweating. During the initial stages of the treatment of myxedema, there may be precipitation of coronary insufficiency, cerebrovascular disease or failure of the pituitary adrenal axis.

ANTI-THYROID DRUGS

Thiocarbamides

Pharmacological action. The thiocarbamides act by inhibiting the oxidation of iodide to iodine, and interfere with the coupling of iodotyrosines in the production of tri-iodothyronine and thyroxine. They are rapidly absorbed by the gastrointestinal tract and excreted in the urine. They also cross the placenta and are excreted in breast milk.

Therapeutic use. They are used to treat thyrotoxicosis, either as the primary treatment or in

Thiocarbamides

Preparations	Initial dose	Maintenance dose
Methimazole	10 mg (5–20) 8 hourly	5–10 mg daily
Carbimazole	15 mg (5–20) 8 hourly	5–20 mg daily
Methylthiouracil	150 mg (100–200) b.d.	50–150 mg daily
Propylthiouracil	200 mg (100–300) b.d.	50–200 mg daily

preparation for thyroidectomy. The initial dose is high until the patient is euthyroid (3–6 weeks). Thereafter a smaller maintenance dose is required.
Contraindications and side effects. Skin rashes which may be associated with arthralgia and lymphadenopathy. Mild gastrointestinal upsets, leucopenia, agranulocytosis (which is usually reversible) have been reported.

The incidence of side effects is lowest with methimazole and propylthiouracil.

These drugs should be used with caution if there is tracheal compression, and thyrotoxicosis associated with pregnancy.

Other anti-thyroid drugs

Pharmacological action. Potassium perchlorate acts by competitive inhibition of the thyroidal iodine concentrating mechanism, and also releases any unbound intrathyroid iodine.
Therapeutic use. In view of the unacceptable toxicity in therapeutic doses, it is only used for diagnostic purposes; 600 mg of perchlorate will discharge radioiodine from the thyroid affected by some forms of dyshormonogenesis.
Contraindications and side effects. These include nephrotic syndrome, aplastic anaemia, neutropenia, skin rashes, pancytopenia and gastrointestinal upsets.

Iodine

Preparation. Aqueous iodine solution (Lugols) 5% iodine, 10% potassium iodide.
Pharmacological action. Iodine in thyrotoxicosis arrests the cellular hyperplasia, increases the storage of colloid and decreases the release of thyroxine. The vascularity of the gland is diminished. The maximum effect of iodine occurs at about ten days, but is only maintained for 2–3 weeks, in spite of continued administration.
Therapeutic use. After preparation for surgery with one of the thiocarbamide group of drugs, iodine may be used for 10–14 days preoperatively to diminish the vascularity of the gland. The dose is 0.3–1 ml of aqueous iodine solution daily in

milk. Larger doses are used in the treatment of thyrotoxic crises (2–3 ml daily).
Contraindications and side effects. Gastric irritation and rarely there is hypersensitivity to iodine with fever and skin rashes.

DRUGS AFFECTING CALCIUM METABOLISM

Parathyroid hormone

Preparation. Parathyroid injection (containing 100 units/ml).
Pharmacological action. Parathyroid hormone increases calcium absorption from the gut, increases calcium resorption from bone, and decreases renal excretion of calcium. It also increases the renal excretion of phosphate. The peak effect of one injection occurs at about 18 hours and lasts for up to 36 hours.
Therapeutic use. The only use is in the acute treatment of hypoparathyroid tetany. The initial dose is 100–300 units i.m. or s.c., followed by 20–100 units hourly, depending on the serum calcium level. Prolonged treatment is associated with the development of tolerance.
Contraindications and side effects. Hypercalcaemia and allergic reactions.

Vitamin D

Preparations
Calciferol injection   300 000 units/ml
Calciferol solution   3 000 units/ml
Calciferol tablets   50 000 units/1.25 mg tablets
Cholecalciferol   40 000 units/1 mg tablet
Dihydrotachysterol   0.25 mg/ml

Pharmacological action. Vitamin D is absorbed orally or by intramuscular injections. It is fat soluble and requires bile acids for absorption from the gut. The principal action is to increase the absorption of calcium from the gut and the resorption of calcium from bone; effects which are mediated through changes in protein metabolism and closely linked to the action of parathyroid hormone.

J

Therapeutic use

Main use	Dosage of Calciferol
Prevention of rickets	400 units/day
Treatment of rickets	3 000–4 000 units/day
Treatment of osteomalacia	5 000–50 000 units/day
Treatment of vitamin resistant rickets	up to 500 000 units/day
Hypoparathyroidism	50 000–500 000 units/day

Dihydrotachysterol has only 25% of the antirachitic activity of calciferol, but the same serum calcium raising ability, and is therefore the treatment of choice in hypoparathyroidism. The dose is 3 ml daily until the serum calcium is normal, thereafter reducing to a maintenance dose of about 1 ml daily.

Contraindications and side effects. Overdosage with vitamin D will produce metastatic calcification and renal failure, early symptoms are lassitude, thirst, nausea and vomiting. Convulsions and coma are also complications of acute hypercalcaemia.

Calcium

Preparations

Oral:	Parenteral:
Calcium gluconate tablets	Calcium gluconate injection i.m. or i.v.
Effervescent calcium gluconate	Calcium chloride i.v. only
Calcium lactate tablets	Calcium lactate s.c., i.m. or i.v.

Therapeutic use. Tetany (associated with hypoparathyroidism, rickets, chronic renal disease and celiac disease). Hypoparathyroidism. Acute colic associated with lead poisoning. Hypocalcaemic convulsions. Asystolic cardiac arrest. Osteoporosis. The dose is 5–20 ml of a 10% solution parenterally for emergency use, or 3–15 g orally.

Contraindications and side effects. Intravenous calcium should be given with caution to a patient on digitalis.

Symptoms of hypercalcaemia, metastatic calcification which may progress to renal failure.

HYPOGLYCAEMIC DRUGS

Insulin preparations

Pharmacological action. Insulin causes a fall in blood glucose concentration by increasing the entry of glucose into cells, and by reducing the output of glucose by the liver. In addition, insulin stimulates fat and glycogen synthesis, and decreases protein synthesis. It is not absorbed orally, being broken down by the gastric secretions.

Therapeutic use. Insulin sensitive diabetes mellitus. Diabetic hyperglycaemic coma. In the insulin tolerance test to assess the integrity of the pituitary gland. In the emergency treatment of hyperkalaemia.

Insulin has been used in the treatment of myocardial infarction, but its place is not established.

Insulin preparations

Preparations	Animal Source	Onset	Peak (Hours, approx.)*	Duration
Short acting				
Insulin injection (soluble)	Beef/pork or mixture	½	3–6	6–8
Neutral insulin injection (Actrapid)	Pork			
Insulin zinc suspension (Amorphous) (semi lente)	Beef	1	3–5	12–16
Medium acting				
Globin zinc insulin injection	Beef	1–2	6–12	18–24
Isophane insulin injection (BP) } NPH	Beef/pork or mixture	1–2	10–20	up to 28
Insulin zinc suspension (lente)	Beef/pork or mixture	2	4–4	24–28
Long acting				
Protamine zinc insulin injection (BP) } PZI	Beef/pork or mixture	4–6	8–20	24–36
Insulin zinc suspension, crystalline (ultra lente)	Beef	several hours	7–10	30+
Biphasic				
Biphasic insulin injection (Rapitard)	Mixture	½–1	4–6 8–24	12–24

*N.B.—An increasing dose increases the duration of action, but the figures given are representative. Individual patient variation may be over a wide range.

The dose in diabetes mellitus will vary from person to person, depending on the amount of endogenous insulin production, the diet and the amount of exercise taken. The requirements will increase in pregnancy, fever, thyrotoxicosis, infections and diabetic acidosis.

Contraindications and side effects. Hypoglycaemia. Local allergic reactions, including skin rashes, urticaria and angioneurotic edema. Local lipoatrophy or lipohypertrophy.

Sulphonylureas

Preparations	Relative potency	Average daily dose
Tolbutamide tablets	1 g	0.5–3 g in divided doses
Chlorpropamide	100 mg	100–250 mg daily
Tolazamide	100 mg	250–750 mg daily
Acetohexamide	200 mg	250–1500 mg daily
Glibenclamide	5 mg	2.5–20 mg daily

Sulphonylureas

Pharmacological action. These preparations are absorbed by the gut, partially bound to protein and excreted via the kidney. Their main action is to release insulin from the pancreatic islet cells although in addition they may potentiate the peripheral action of insulin.

Therapeutic use. The sulphonylureas are used in the treatment of mild uncomplicated diabetes mellitus without ketonuria. They are particularly suitable for the adult type maturity onset diabetics, but should not be used to replace adequate dietary therapy. Tolbutamide given intravenously is also used as a diagnostic acid in the differential diagnosis of hypoglycaemia.

Contraindications and side effects. They are unsuitable in diabetes following total pancreatectomy, diabetes with ketosis or ketonuria, and are best avoided in children with diabetes and patients with coexistent hepatic or renal disease.

Side effects include: Hypoglycaemia, particularly in the elderly and patients with hepatic or renal disease. Leucopenia and agranulocytosis. Skin rashes, including exfoliative dermatitis. Cholestatic jaundice. Gastrointestinal upsets. Transient ataxia and muscle weakness. Vasomotor disturbances with flushing, giddiness, tachycardia and breathlessness which may be precipitated by alcohol. Eosinophilic pulmonary infiltrations. Microgranulosis of the heart, liver and kidney have been described.

There may be biochemical evidence of hypothyroidism, but clinical myxedema is rare.

Biguanides

Pharmacological action. The exact mode of action is not established but probably the increased peripheral utilisation of both insulin and glucose is the major one.

The action of phenformin lasts 6–8 hours and that of metformin 8–12 hours, they are both excreted largely unchanged in the urine.

Therapeutic use. As for sulphonylureas. In addition, the biguanides have been used as an adjuvant to insulin therapy, where smooth control has proved particularly difficult, and in the treatment of obesity in diabetics. The starting dose should always be low and gradually increased to control the blood sugar.

Contraindications and side effects. As for sulphonylureas.

Side effects include: Gastrointestinal upsets, a metallic taste in the mouth, general malaise and weight loss, ketonuria without hyperglycaemia, skin rashes, lactic acidosis with phenformin.

CORTICOSTEROIDS

Pharmacological action. The steroids produced by the adrenal cortex and the synthetic products can be classified into three groups on the basis of their predominant physiological effects. These are the glucocorticoids (i.e. principally affecting carbohydrate metabolism), mineralocorticoids (i.e. mainly affecting sodium and potassium metabolism), and the sex hormones which will be dealt with in a later section.

The glucocorticoids increase gluconeogenesis, inhibit peripheral utilisation of glucose and increase glycogen deposition in the liver. In addition to these effects on carbohydrate metabolism, they

Biguanides

Preparations	Average daily dose
Phenformin hydrochloride tablets	25–150 mg in divided doses
Phenformin hydrochloride SA tablets	50–150 mg
Metformin hydrochloride	1–3 g in divided doses
Buformin hydrochloride tablets	50–300 mg in divided doses
Buformin hydrochloride SA tablets	100–300mg

Corticosteroids

Preparations	Equivalent oral dose	Route	Salt-retaining activity
Hydrocortisone	20 mg	Oral/i.m./i.v.	++
Cortisone	25 mg	Oral/i.m./i.v.	++
Prednisolone	5 mg	Oral/i.m./i.v.	+
Prednisone	5 mg	Oral	+
Methyl prednisolone	4 mg	Oral/i.v./i.m.	
Paramethasone	2 mg	Oral	
Dexamethasone	0.75 mg	Oral/i.v./i.m.	
Betamethasone	0.75 mg	Oral/i.v./i.m.	
Fludrocortisone		Oral	++++
Aldosterone		i.m./i.v.	++++

help to maintain normal renal function and raise the arterial blood pressure. In normal pharmacological doses they reduce the inflammatory responses, decrease antibody production, and stimulate production of gastric and peptic secretion.

Corticosteroids with predominant mineralocorticoid activity increase the transport of sodium into cells in exchange for potassium. The principal effect of this is an increased urinary loss of potassium, with sodium retention within the body.

Therapeutic uses. The corticosteroids are used therapeutically in three main categories.

1. *As substitution therapy.* In adrenocortical failure, in hypopituitarism and in congenital adrenal hyperplasia. The doses required are those which maintain normal health, electrolyte balance and arterial blood pressure. In primary adrenocortical failure, a powerful mineralocorticoid such as fludrocortisone (0.05–0.2 mg daily) is normally required in addition to cortisone (25–75 mg daily), whereas in hypopituitarism and congenital adrenal hyperplasia, cortisone alone is sufficient.

2. *In the treatment of some haematological disorders:* Such as autoimmune haemolytic anaemia, idiopathic thrombocytopenic purpura, and some forms of leukaemia, especially in children.

3. *To suppress unwanted inflammatory responses* in a wide variety of disease processes. These include systemic lupus erythematosus, asthma, dermatomyositis, polymyalgia rheumatica, cranial arteritis, polyarteritis nodosa, selected cases of rheumatoid arthritis and the nephrotic syndrome, and occasionally in tuberculosis.

The preparation chosen in the latter two categories is one having the minimal mineralocorticoid activity. The dose may be very high for a short period (e.g. prednisone 60–100 mg daily) in the early phase of the disease or during a relapse. But the correct dose at all times is the smallest dose necessary to produce a therapeutic response.

Contraindications and side effects. The contraindications are all relative, depending on the severity of the disease for which they are to be used. However, they should rarely be used when the following conditions are present:

Peptic ulcer, diabetes, osteoporosis, psychosis, active or possibly active tuberculosis, congestive cardiac failure, acute systemic viral or bacterial infections.

Side effects:

1. *Endocrine.* Production of iatrogenic Cushing's syndrome. Hyperglycaemia with accentuation or precipitation of diabetes. Retardation of growth rate in children. Salt and water retention with hypertension. Potassium loss. Mobilisation of calcium with osteoporosis. Aseptic necrosis of the femoral head. Suppression of the pituitary adrenal axis.

2. *Infections.* Reactivation or aggravation of tuberculosis. Increased susceptibility to viral, bacterial, fungal and parasitic infections.

3. *Eyes.* Exacerbation of infections which may lead to corneal perforation. Precipitation of glaucoma. Cataract formation.

4. *Skin.* Atrophy with the production of striae. Purpura. Hypertrichosis and acne.

5. *Gastrointestinal.* There is an increased incidence of peptic ulceration, and perforation. Acute pancreatitis. Increased incidence of toxic megacolon and perforation of ulcerative colitis.

6. *Nervous system.* Euphoria and psychosis. Precipitation of latent epilepsy. Raised intracranial pressure and papilledema in children. Pelvic girdle myopathy, especially with steroids having a F+ ion and the 9α position.

Corticotrophin

Preparations

Short acting:

Corticotrophin injection—i.v. or i.m. preparation.

Long acting:

Corticotrophin gelatin injection.

Corticotrophin zinc hydroxide injection.

Corticotrophin–carboxymethyl cellulose complex (ACTH/CMC).

Synthetic:

Tetracosactrin.

Tetracosactrin depot.

Pharmacological action. Corticotrophin stimulates the production and release of adrenal steroids. It also has some melanocyte-stimulating action by virtue of the structural similarity to MSH, and suppresses corticotrophin releasing factor both by the production of high levels of corticosteroids and by direct action on the hypothalamus.

Therapeutic use. Stimulation of the adrenals following long-term corticosteroid therapy.

Asthma in children during the growing period
Bell's palsy
Multiple sclerosis.

Corticotrophin is always given parenterally. A maximal response is obtained with 40 i.u. twice daily, but the dose should always be the minimal needed to control the disease. It is better to give a larger dose less frequently (e.g. twice weekly) than a small dose daily.

Corticotrophin is used to assess the function of the adrenal cortex by measuring either the plasma cortisol or the urinary 17-hydroxycorticoids response following stimulation with corticotrophin. The adrenal androgens are also increased following corticotrophin administration. An abnormal increase may be associated with hirsutism in women. More recently the synthetic preparations have been used with more consistent results.

Contraindications and side effects. As for corticosteroids with the addition of pigmentation, which may occur during treatment with both natural and synthetic corticotrophin, and the occasional allergic response.

ANABOLIC STEROIDS

Pharmacological actions. These compounds result from attempts to alter the chemical structure of the androgens, so as to reduce the androgenic effect and retain their protein anabolic function. At the present time all these drugs retain some virilising properties. Apart from causing nitrogen retention they also increase the retention of calcium, sodium, potassium, chloride and phosphate ions and increase bone growth and maturation.

Therapeutic use. There is no universal agreement regarding the indications for the anabolic steroids. Generally they are less effective in men than in women, they are rarely useful in acute catabolic diseases, and there is no indication for their use as a 'tonic'. They may contribute to nitrogen retention and protein anabolism in chronic debilitating diseases, post-menopausal and senile osteoporosis and chronic renal failure. They should be used with care in growth retardation, as epiphyseal closure may exceed increase in bone growth. Their place in the treatment of corticosteroid osteoporosis, burns and acute renal failure is not established.

Contraindications and side effects:

1. *Virilising.* This may occur in females with any preparation, and some patients appear to be excessively sensitive to this effect.

2. *Impotence.* An important side effect of long-term usage in males.

3. *Hepatic.* As with the androgens, those which have 17α alkyl substitution (the orally active preparations) cause liver impairment and may produce a reversible cholestatic jaundice.

Anabolic steroids

Preparations	Dose (mg/kg)	Route
Nandrolone phenylpropionate	0.75–1.0/week	i.m.
Nandrolone decanoate	1.0 –1.5/4 weeks	i.m.
Methenolone oenanthate	1.0 –2.0/10 days	i.m.
Norethandrolone	0.5 –1.0/day	Oral
Methandienone	0.2 –0.3/day	Oral
Methendone acetate	0.4 –0.6/day	Oral
Oxymetholone	0.25–0.5/day	Oral
Stanozolol	0.1 –0.15/day	Oral
Ethylestrenol	0.05–0.1/day	Oral

Progestogens

Preparations	Dose to produce a secretory endometrium
Progesterone injection	50–100 mg i.m. daily for five days
Progesterone derivatives	
Dydrogesterone tablets	10 mg daily orally for 10–15 days
Hydroprogesterone caproate	250 mg i.m.
Chlormadinone acetate	2 mg orally for two days
Medroxyprogesterone acetate	10 mg daily for 10 days orally
	50 mg i.m. once
19-Nortestosterone derivatives	
Norethisterone	10–30 mg daily orally for 10 days
Norethynodrel tablets	10–30 mg daily orally for 10 days
Dimethesterone tablets	15–40 mg daily orally for 10 days
Ethynodiol diacetate	1–2 mg daily orally for 10 days

4. *Others*. The oral preparations may also cause a rise in serum cholesterol and lipids, especially in conjunction with corticosteroids or in non-insulin requiring diabetics. Contraindications are the same as for androgens.

PROGESTOGENS

Pharmacological action. The progestogens produce the secretory changes in the endometrium, maturation of breast prior to lactation, and progesterone is responsible for the rise in basal temperature following ovulation, and the maintenance of normal pregnancy.

Therapeutic use. The treatment of functional uterine bleeding. Premenstrual tension. Contraception. Endometriosis. In the diagnosis of amenorrhea.

Progestogens have also been used in the treatment of habitual and threatened abortion, but their value is doubtful.

Contraindications and side effects. All progestogens may cause nausea, vomiting and weight gain. The nortestosterone derivatives are variably androgenic, and consequently can cause hirsutism, acne and deepening of the voice. If given during pregnancy, virilisation of the fetus can occur. The progestogens with an alkyl group in the 17α position (norethisterone, norethynodrel) may cause cholestatic jaundice, and should be avoided in patients with liver disease.

ESTROGENS

Pharmacological action. Estrogens stimulate the development and maintain the secondary sexual characteristics including stromal and duct growth in the breast. They are responsible for the proliferation of the endometrium, and for the cyclic changes of the cervix and vagina. The pubertal growth spurt and epiphyseal closure is also an estrogenic effect. There are a number of other general metabolic effects involving protein, fat, glucose and phosphate metabolism, and salt and water retention. Estrogens increase the proteins which bind corticosteroids and thyroxine, which may give rise to difficulty in interpreting plasma levels of cortisol and protein bound iodine. There are also effects on the blood clotting factors.

Therapeutic use. Replacement therapy in primary or secondary ovarian failure. Suppression of lactation. Suppression of ovulation in dysmenorrhea. With progestogens as a contraceptive. With progestogens in the treatment of endometriosis. Metropathic uterine bleeding. Delayed puberty. To encourage epiphyseal closure when there is excessive growth in girls. Control of menopausal symptoms. Treatment of carcinoma of the breast and prostate.

The dose will depend on the condition and will also vary with the patient. Examples of ethinyl estradiol are 0.01–0.05 mg daily for menopausal symptoms; 0.05–0.25 mg daily in replacement therapy and the treatment of primary amenorrhea; to control metropathic bleeding 0.5–2 mg daily should be given until the bleeding stops, or 20 mg of conjugated estrogens may be given intravenously in an emergency; 0.1 mg three times daily is given to terminate lactation. The highest doses are given in the treatment of carcinoma of the prostate, when doses up to 10 mg or more are given daily.

Contraindications and side effects. Nausea, headache, breast tenderness and weight gain due to sodium and water retention are frequent, usually transient, effects. More serious is the occurrence of thromboembolic phenomena. Estrogens should be avoided in patients particularly liable to thromboembolism, in renal disease, congestive cardiac failure and neoplasms of the female genital tract.

Serious side effects with estrogens containing oral contraceptives are uncommon when the dose of estrogen is not more than 50 μg per day.

Androgens

Pharmacological action. Testosterone and other androgenic steroids are responsible for the normal development of secondary sexual characteristics in

Estrogens

Preparations	Usual dose	Route
Ethinylestradiol	0.05–0.2 mg daily	Oral
Estradiol	0.25–10 mg daily	
	50–300 mg 4–6 monthly	By implantation
Estradiol benzoate	1–5 mg 1–3 times weekly	i.m.
Estradiol cypionate	1–5 mg every 3–4 weeks	i.m.
Estradiol dipropionate	1–5 mg weekly	i.m.
Estradiol valerate	5–20 mg every 2–4 weeks	i.m.
Piperazine esterone sulphate	0.75–4.5 mg daily	Oral
Estrogenic substances, conjugated	} 0.125–2.5 mg daily } 20 mg	Oral i.v.
Non-steroidal estrogens Stilbestrol	0.5–10 mg daily	Oral or i.m.
Stilbestrol diphosphate	250 mg–1g (Treatment of prostate carcinoma)	i.v.
Dienestrol	0.1–5 mg daily	Oral
Chlorotrianisene	12–48 mg daily	Oral
Methallenestril	3–9 mg daily	Oral

Androgens

Preparations	Dose, route and frequency
Testosterone implants	{ 200–1000 mg by subcutaneous { implantation every 4–8 months
Testosterone propionate	{ 5–25 mg intramuscularly one to { two times each week
Testosterone phenylpropionate	10–100 mg weekly intramuscularly
Testosterone enanthate	{ 100–200 mg intramuscularly every { 2–4 weeks
Testosterone cypionate	{ 10–100 mg intramuscularly every { 1–2 weeks
Methyl testosterone tablets	25–50 mg sublingually daily
Fluoxymesterone	5–20 mg sublingually daily
Mesterolone	50–200 mg orally daily

the male and for maturation of the spermatozoa. They also produce marked nitrogen retention and protein anabolism, which results in the growth spurt at puberty. They also cause maturation of bones, with fusion of the epiphyses.

Therapeutic use. The only clear cut indication of the use of androgens is in the treatment of primary or secondary male hypogonadism. Either a long acting preparation such as testosterone enanthate or testosterone implants are the most suitable preparations. Good sexual development is obtained in most cases. A new synthetic androgen, mesterolone, has been found useful in the treatment of idiopathic oligospermia.

Androgens have also been used in the treatment of carcinoma of the breast in females, aplastic anaemia, osteoporosis and growth disorders, but the value and indications are not well established.

Contraindications and side effects. A reversible cholestatic type of jaundice may occur with the androgens which are substituted in the 17α position (methyl testosterone and fluoxymesterone). This is a dose related not a sensitivity effect.

Other side effects include sodium and water retention, hypercalcaemia and virilisation if administered to females.

Androgens are absolutely contraindicated in pregnancy and carcinoma of the prostate. They should be used with special care in children, and when there is hepatic or renal disease.

Category 13

MISCELLANEOUS DRUGS

J. R. TROUNCE

THE CHELATING AGENTS

Desferrioxamine

Pharmacological action. This drug is an iron-free compound obtained from ferrioxamine, a meta-bolite of *Streptomyces pilosus*. It is an iron-complexing agent capable of eliminating iron from the body. It does not remove iron from haemoglobin or iron-containing enzymes. The iron complex formed with such substances as ferritin, haemosiderin and transferrin is rapidly excreted by the kidneys. The serum iron con-centration quickly decreases. The drug has almost exclusive affinity for iron.

Therapeutic use. The drug is of value in second-ary haemochromatosis, e.g. in aplastic anaemia, transfusion haemosiderosis, sickle cell anaemia and severe chronic acquired haemolytic anaemia. The dose is 1 g daily in one or two intramuscular injections; for maintenance purposes 500 mg is given daily.

Desferrioxamine is of great value in the treat-ment of children who have taken an overdose of iron tablets. After gastric lavage with bicarbonate solution desferrioxamine should be instilled into the stomach, suggested doses being 3–7 g in 50–200 ml of water or saline. This will prevent absorption of any iron still present in the gastro-intestinal tract. At the same time an intravenous drip should be set up and desferrioxamine infused in a maximum dose of 15 mg/kg of bodyweight/hour to a total of 80 mg/kg bodyweight. Des-ferrioxamine is rapidly absorbed from muscle and it may be wise to give 2 g i.m. before start-ing the time-consuming gastric lavage and intra-venous infusion.

Contraindications and side effects. Pain occurs at the site of intramuscular injection. The volume of urine may be temporarily decreased. The serum calcium is sometimes decreased.

Dimercaprol (British Anti-Lewisite)

Pharmacological action. The drug rapidly enters the circulation within five minutes after intra-muscular injection; it is rapidly distributed and eliminated within a few hours. The greater part of the drug is quickly metabolised and excreted in the urine. The dithiol forms relatively stable chelated complexes with arsenic, mercury, gold, and certain other metals. It is also highly effective locally.

Therapeutic use. The drug has been shown to be of value in arsenical intoxication, mercuric chloride poisoning and in toxic reactions due to gold.

In hepatolenticular degeneration it increases the already high copper output in the urine, causing some improvement in the disease.

The drug is given as a 5% solution of dimer-caprol in arachis oil with benzylbenzoate as solu-biliser. Administration is by intramuscular in-jection 8–16 ml in divided doses on the first day; 4–8 ml in divided doses on the second and third days; and 2–4 ml in divided doses on subsequent days.

Contraindications and side effects. Reactions are of minor importance, reversible, and of short duration; they usually occur with doses exceeding 3 mg/kg of bodyweight. They may be prevented by giving an antihistaminic drug or ephedrine beforehand. Paraesthesiae, pains or burning of the mouth, eyes, feet, sweating, lacrimation, sali-vation, vomiting, weakness, rise in systolic and diastolic blood pressure; these features last 30–60 minutes.

Care is required in patients with impaired liver function. Renal damage may be produced due to excretion of the drug with chelated metal. The intramuscular injection may cause severe local necrosis. Intravenous injection may cause cardiac collapse.

Sodium calcium edetate

Pharmacological action. The drug forms strong un-ionised complexes with cations. The calcium compound is used to avoid producing low calcium tetany.

Therapeutic use. The drug is effective in acute and chronic lead poisoning; it produces a marked in-crease in the urinary excretion of lead. In hepatolenticular degeneration it has been given with dimercaprol to increase the copper output in the urine. In digitalis intoxication and certain other arrhythmias sodium edetate has been used to bind calcium ions.

It is given by intravenous infusion, a maximum of 40 mg/kg bodyweight being given daily usually in two doses given over a period of one hour. A course of treatment usually lasts 3 days.

Penicillamine

Pharmacological action. This chelating agent consists of a portion of the penicillin molecule, which is an analogue of the amino acid cysteine. In copper, lead and iron poisoning it appears to increase the excretion of these metals.

Therapeutic use. The drug is effective in hepato-lenticular degeneration in promoting cupruresis. It has been used in copper, lead and iron poisoning.

Penicillamine hydrochloride is given in capsule form, 0.9-1.5 g daily, in divided doses, before meals.

Contraindications and side effects. It may produce morbilliform skin rashes, and renal damage has been reported. Agranulocytosis may occur.

Cholestyramine

Pharmacological action. Cholestyramine is an exchange resin which binds bile acids. Normally bile acids are excreted with the bile into the intestine and a high proportion is reabsorbed from the intestine and re-excreted by the liver. Bile acids are synthesised in the liver from cholesterol.

Therapeutic use. Cholestyramine is helpful for patients with chronic liver disease in whom retention of bile acids is causing intense itching. By binding bile acids in the intestine it prevents their reabsorption and thus lowers the blood levels.

It is also used to lower blood cholesterol. This is achieved partly by reducing cholesterol absorption from the gut, and partly by depleting the body of bile acids so that more cholesterol is switched to bile production.

The drug is available in sachets containing 9.0 g and these are given in a liquid vehicle 3 times a day.

Contraindications and side effects. The absorption of fat soluble vitamins (A & D) may be decreased by cholestyramine. It may also interfere with the absorption of other drugs which should not be given within two hours of taking cholestyramine.

DRUG USED TO LOWER BLOOD URIC ACID

Allopurinol

Pharmacological action. Allupurinol inhibits the enzyme xanthine oxidase, which converts hypoxanthine and xanthine to uric acid. This results in a lowering of plasma uric acid levels and uric acid excretion. Hypoxanthine and xanthine, which accumulate, are rapidly cleared from the blood by the kidney and being more soluble do not form stones except occasionally in the rare Lesch–Nyhan syndrome.

Allopurinol is rapidly absorbed from the gut and is converted into alloxanthine and excreted via the kidney.

Therapeutic use. Allopurinol is used in the treatment of chronic gout and also in hyperuricaemia complicating polycythaemia and leukaemias. The usual dose is 100 mg two or three times daily.

Contraindications and side effects. The most important side effects are hypersensitivity reactions causing rashes and drug fever. Leucopenia has been reported and patients may complain of headaches and nausea. An acute attack of gout may occur soon after starting treatment due to the initial mobilisation of uric acid.

URICOSURIC AGENTS

These drugs lower the plasma uric acid level by increasing excretion by the kidney. Uric acid is filtered by the glomerulus and a large proportion is then reabsorbed in the proximal tubule. At the same time a certain amount of secretion of uric acid into the urine also occurs at this level. Uricosuric drugs produce their effect of blocking reabsorption at the proximal tubule.

The main drugs are:

Probenecid

Pharmacological action and therapeutic use. Probenecid inhibits the transport of organic acids both into and out of the tubular fluid. It prevents the reabsorption of uric acid from the tubule and thus increases loss in the urine. Penicillin is partially secreted by the tubular cells into the urine; by blocking this process probenecid reduces penicillin loss in the urine and thus raises penicillin blood levels.

In treating gout it is usual to start with 250 mg in a single dose daily and increase weekly to 250–500 mg four times daily. To prevent penicillin excretion the dose is 500 mg four times daily.

Contraindications and side effects. Hypersensitivity reactions may occur and occasionally gastrointestinal upsets.

Sulphinpyrazone

Pharmacological action and therapeutic use. Sulphinpyrazone blocks tubular reabsorption of uric acid. Its uricosuric action lasts about 10 hours, the initial dose being 100 mg daily and increased slowly to 100–200 mg twice daily.

Contraindications and side effects. Sulphinpyrazone should not be combined with salicylates as this will reduce its uricosuric action. Gastrointestinal upsets can be troublesome and the drug should be taken with a meal. Finally, hypersensitivity reactions occur.

The sudden rise in urine uric acid levels following the use of the foregoing drugs in treating gout may cause stone formation or the precipitation of gravel in the urinary tract. In the early weeks of treatment their use should be combined with a large fluid intake and alkalinisation of the urine will make the uric acid more soluble.

ANALEPTICS

This group of drugs are central stimulants with a marked effect on the medulla. They were formerly used to reverse the effect of medullary depressive drugs, in particular with barbiturates, but it is now realised that their use is of doubtful value in treating barbiturate overdosage.

They are also occasionally used in increasing ventilation in those with respiratory failure.

APPETITE SUPPRESSORS

Phenmetrazine/diethylpropion

Pharmacological action and therapeutic use. These drugs are powerful suppressors of appetite with minimal adrenergic effect. They are used in the treatment of obesity. The dose is

Phenmetrazine 12.5–25 mg b.d.
Diethylpropion 25 mg t.d.s.

Contraindications and side effects. Dependence can occur with both these drugs. They should not be used in the early part of pregnancy, for there is some circumstantial evidence that one of them (phenmetrazine) may affect the fetus.

Fenfluramine

Pharmacological action and therapeutic use. Fenfluramine depresses appetite without apparently any stimulating effect on the central nervous system. In fact it sometimes has a mild sedative action. It is fairly long-acting and the recommended dose in obesity is 1 tablet (20 mg) 2 hours before the evening meal and 1 tablet mid-morning, but up to 6 tablets can be given daily. The main side effect is diarrhea, with occasional nausea. Overdosage, however, can produce agitation, confusion, convulsions and death.

THE ANTIHISTAMINES

Histamine has a wide range of pharmacological actions. In human disease histamine is usually released as the result of tissue injury due to some form of antigen–antibody combination when it produces the clinical syndrome of an allergic reaction.

Analeptics

Preparation	Dose	Uses
Picrotoxin	In barbiturate poisoning 6.0 mg at a rate of 1 mg/minute i.v.	Powerful central stimulant can produce convulsions, very short-acting.
Leptazol	In barbiturate poisoning up to 1.0 ml of a 10% solution i.v.	Powerful central stimulant can produce convulsions, very short-acting.
Nikethamide	2–8 ml of 25% solution i.v.	Less powerful central effect. Also sensitises carotid body. Very short-acting.
Amiphenazole	100–200 mg t.d.s., oral or 100 mg i.m.	Milder and longer-acting.
Bemegride	In barbiturate poisoning 50 mg i.v. repeated if necessary at intervals of 10 minutes to a total of 1.0 g.	Longer-acting.

Two forms of histamine receptor have now been described. H_1 receptors, when stimulated by histamine produce allergic manifestations. H_2 receptors stimulate gastric secretion.

The antihistamines described below are all H_1 blockers although they all have other actions.

The antihistamines are a large group of drugs, which in general are very similar in their actions, although they differ as to which particular action predominates.

Pharmacological action. The antihistamines are well absorbed from the gut and largely metabolised in the liver.

Their main pharmacological actions are:

1. They are competitive blockers of all the actions of histamine except they do not prevent histamine induced gastric secretion.

2. They are usually CNS depressors, producing some drowsiness and also are anti-emetics.

3. They have some mild peripheral anticholinergic action.

4. They have a weak effect on the heart, similar to that of quinidine.

Therapeutic use. Antihistamines are used in various allergic conditions, including urticaria and hay fever. They are rarely effective in bronchial asthma. Their effect on the CNS is used to prevent vomiting and they also may reduce the symptoms of Parkinson's disease.

Individual preparations

(a) Useful as antihistamines:

Promethazine: long-acting 25–50 mg at night often sufficient. Sedation marked.

Diphenhydramine: 25–50 mg four times daily. Sedation marked.

Mepyramine: 100–200 mg three times daily.

Chlorpheniramine: 4 mg three times daily or 10 mg i.m. Good antihistamine effect, some sedation.

Phenindamine: 25–50 mg three times daily. Little if any sedation.

(b) Useful as anti–emetics:

Dimenhydrinate: 50 mg four times daily. Sedation marked.

Cyclizine: 50 mg three times daily. Mild sedation.

Meclozine: 50 mg daily. Mild sedation.

Promethazine chlorotheophyllinate: 25 mg three times daily. Quite marked sedation.

Vomiting in pregnancy. All drugs should be avoided in early pregnancy, if possible. However, it is fair to say that the anti-emetics listed above have not been shown to produce fetal abnormalities.

Contraindications and side effects. Troublesome sedation is the commonest side effect. The anti-

cholinergic action of these drugs may produce dry mouth and gastrointestinal upsets. Rarely they produce bone marrow depression. It is interesting that both systemic and local use can produce sensitisation rashes.

Disodium cromoglycate

Pharmacological action. Disodium cromoglycate is thought to relieve bronchospasm in asthma by inhibiting the release of bronchoconstrictor substances which follows an antigen–antibody union on the surface of mast cells. It is not an antispasmodic. It is poorly absorbed from the gut and is given by inhalation.

Therapeutic use. Disodium cromoglycate is used to prevent attacks of asthma. It is given by inhalation and there are two formulations: either 20 mg disodium cromoglycate per Spincap capsule or 20 mg of disodium cromoglycate and 0.1 mg of isoprenaline per Spincap capsule. Initial treatment is one capsule night and morning and at 4–6-hourly intervals – this can be reduced when a satisfactory response is obtained. Disodium cromoglycate can be given concurrently with steroid or anti-spasmodics and may enable the dose of steroids to be reduced. If disodium cromoglycate is suddenly withdrawn in those whose steroid dose has been reduced the dose of steroids must be returned to their previous level or a severe relapse of asthma can occur.

Disodium cromoglycate has also been used in hay fever. The balance of evidence is that it may be effective. It is administered by nasal inhalation from a special inhaler, the usual dose being 10 mg given four times daily.

H_2 BLOCKERS

It has been known for many years that histamine was concerned in the secretion of acid by the stomach and may indeed be the final common pathway of a number of stimuli.

The receptors which are concerned are known as H_2 receptors and recently a number of drugs have been introduced which block the action of histamine on these receptors.

Cimetidine in doses of 0.8–1.0 g daily has been shown to reduce gastric acid secretion by some 50%. **Metiamide** will also reduce gastric acid but depression of the bone marrow has occasionally been reported.

Therapeutic use. H_2 blockers have been used in the treatment of duodenal ulcers and are effective in reducing the incidence of symptoms and increasing the rate of healing of the ulcer. Their place in the treatment of peptic ulcer remains however to be determined.

ANTACIDS

Antacids are used to relieve the pain of peptic ulcers. There is no evidence that they alter the rate of healing of an ulcer. They act by raising the pH of the gastric contents and thereby reducing the irritant effect of the gastic acid on the ulcer and decreasing the activity of pepsin. This is achieved if the pH of the gastric content is raised to around 4.0. The most widely used antacids are:

Sodium bicarbonate

Sodium bicarbonate is a rapidly acting antacid, but passes quickly through the stomach so its action is transient. It is absorbed and can thus produce alkalosis, although this does not occur with usual doses if renal function is normal. It is usually given in a dose of 1.0 g mixed with a little water.

Magnesium oxide

This salt is rather longer acting than sodium bicarbonate. There is no danger of alkalosis but all magnesium salts cause diarrhea due to the poor absorption of the magnesium ion. The dose of magnesium oxide is 0.3–0.6 g.

Magnesium trisilicate

A white powder given orally in a dose of 1.0 g mixed with milk or water. Much slower in action and longer activity than the previous magnesium salts. In order to spread the action of magnesium salts they are often combined in a single tablet.

Calcium carbonate

This is an efficient antacid in doses of 1–2 g. It is important to remember that calcium carbonate combined with excessive milk intake can cause hypercalcaemia in some individuals leading to thirst, polyurea and renal damage.

Aluminium hydroxide

Aluminium hydroxide is a useful antacid and can be given either as a gel or in tablet form. It is said to have some inhibiting effect on pepsin.

Bismuth salts

Pharmacological action and therapeutic use. Bismuth salts, in particular bismuth oxycarbonate have been used in the treatment of peptic ulcers. Although bismuth salts inactivate pepsin they are weak antacids and not very effective. Trisodium dicitrato bismuthate (DeNol) has been claimed to be more effective in that it combines with protein breakdown products in the base of the ulcer and forms a protective coating. The dose is 5.0 ml diluted half an hour before meals on an empty stomach and before retiring. A complete assessment of its effectiveness awaits further study.

Gaviscon

Gaviscon is a preparation containing arginates and antacids. It is believed to float on the gastric contents and thus coat and protect the lower esophagus if reflux should occur. It is used in peptic esophagitis being given after meals.

Carbenoxolone

Pharmacological action and therapeutic use. Carbenoxolone is a terpene derived from liquorice. There is good evidence that it increases the rate of healing of gastric ulcers in ambulant patients. Its usefulness in duodenal ulcers is not as yet proven. Its mode of action is not known but it provides increased secretion of mucus by the stomach and this may protect the ulcer. The usual dose is 50–100 mg t.d.s. It can cause sodium and water retention and should not be used in those in or near cardiac failure, and care should be taken in the elderly. It can also rarely cause potassium depletion and muscle weakness particularly if combined with a diuretic and it should be used with great care in patients taking digitalis. Carbenoxolone should not be used for more than two months.

A formulation of carbenoxolone which is released in the duodenum is also available for the treatment of duodenal ulcers. Its effectiveness is still open to some doubt.

There are other liquorice extracts used in treating peptic ulcers. **Caved S** which also contains antacids has been shown to have some effect in accelerating the healing of ulcers and does not appear to cause water retention although diarrhea has been reported.

PURGATIVES

Liquid paraffin. Acts by its lubricating action. It is useful particularly in the elderly and in painful conditions of the lower bowel. The dose is 15 ml twice daily or 5.0 ml, hourly for a few hours. Prolonged administration can cause vitamin A and D deficiency and inhalation by the very young or very ill can cause a paraffinoma in the lung.

Bulk purges. These act by increasing the bowel contents. There are a number of preparations available containing agar (dose: 4–8 g) or methyl-cellulose (dose: 1–1.5 g).

Saline purges. Magnesium sulphate is widely used in a dose of 8.0 g in 150 ml of water before breakfast.

IRRITANT PURGES

Phenolphthalein

Pharmacological action. Phenolphthalein is absorbed from the intestine and stimulates the colon. It is re-excreted via the bile and so a certain amount of recirculation occurs.

Therapeutic use and side effect. Phenolphthalein in a dose of 120 mg at bedtime produces a purge the next morning. It is relatively free of side effects but can produce rashes.

Anthracene purges

Pharmacological action. This group of purges contains a number of substances including emodin, which stimulates the colon.

Therapeutic uses

Senna – best given as the Senokot containing the purified active principles. The adult dose is 2–4 tablets or 1–2 teaspoonfuls of granules.

Cascara – Tablets of cascara (BP) 125–250 mg.

OTHER PURGATIVES

Bisacodyl

This purgative stimulates the colon when it comes into contact with the bowel wall. The dose is 5–10 mg.

Dioctyl-sodium sulphosuccinate

This substance is a wetting agent and softens the bowel contents. It is useful in faecal impaction in doses of 40–60 mg three times daily.

Lactulose

This substance is a disaccharide and is given in the form of a syrup. It passes unchanged through the small bowel but is changed by bacterial action in the colon to lactic acid. This appears to promote a mild laxative action. It can be useful in those with chronic constipation, and its effect on the intestinal bacterial flora has led to its use in hepatic encephalopathy. The dose of a 50%

lactulose solution is 30 ml as a laxative, and in liver disease 30 ml three times a day.

MUCOLYTIC AGENTS

The removal of sputum from the bronchial tree is an important aspect in treating a variety of chest disorders. For many years expectorants which usually contain *ammonium chloride, potassium iodide* or *sodium bicarbonate* were used. Although in emetic doses these substance would be expected to increase bronchial secretion and thus loosen sticky sputum, in the usual therapeutic dose it seems unlikely that they have much pharmacological effect. Among the older remedies the inhalation of steam is probably the most effective.

More recently however agents have been introduced which are claimed to liquefy sputum.

Chymotrypsin may be given by inhalation but its use has not obtained wide acceptance.

Acetylcysteine and **methylcysteine** can be given by inhalation or orally. They are effective in liquefying sputum *in vivo*, but are less useful in a clinical context.

Bromhexine is believed to liquefy sputum by breaking down mucopolysaccharide fibres, probably within the mucus secreting cell.

Clinical use. In doses of 8.0 mg three times daily bromhexine has been shown to produce some changes in sputum in asthmatics and bronchitics, although the effect on the clinical state of the patient is variable. Side effects are low but occasionally it can cause epigastric discomfort and nausea.

Metoclopramide

Pharmacological action. Metoclopramide is an anti-emetic but not an antihistamine. Its mode of action is not clear, but it decreases gastric emptying time, probably by stimulation of autonomic ganglia, and relaxes the duodenum.

Therapeutic use. Metoclopramide has been used in many types of vomiting and success has been claimed, although most of these studies are not very satisfactory. The oral dose is 10 mg and can be given three times daily. It can also be given intramuscularly in doses of 10 mg.

Contraindications and side effects. Metoclopramide can produce drowsiness with large doses. Dystonia has been reported and it should not be combined therefore with the phenothiazines. It should not be given in the first three months of pregnancy.

Category 14

VITAMINS

P. I. FOLB

Vitamin A (retinol)

Pharmacological action. Vitamin A is required for the formation of visual purple which is essential for the eye to see in dim light. Vitamin A also directly affects the metabolism of all epithelial tissues; it appears to be necessary for the normal formation of mucopolysaccharides.

Therapeutic use. Vitamin A is used for the treatment of xerophthalmia and of night blindness when this is due to dietary failure. It should also be given to malnourished people who show evidence of follicular keratosis.

Cod liver and shark liver oils are good natural concentrated sources of the vitamin. The prophylactic dose for children is 3000 i.u. and for adults 5000 i.u. daily. A therapeutic dose totalling 250 000 i.u. of retinol given in capsules over a period of one week usually achieves maximum therapeutic benefit.

Side effects. High doses taken by early Arctic explorers caused drowsiness, headache with increased cerebrospinal fluid pressure, vomiting and extensive peeling of the skin. Sporadic cases in children in recent years have generally been due to over-enthusiastic administration of fish liver oils. Rapid recovery follows withdrawal of the vitamin.

Vitamin D (cholecalciferol)

Pharmacological action. The vitamin probably has a direct action on bone; it is necessary for formation of normal bone and for the calcification of rachitic bone. After absorption vitamin D is modified to 25-hydroxycholecalciferol by the liver and then to 1,25-dihydroxycholecalciferol by the kidney. This compound is particularly active in promoting absorption of calcium from the intestine, thus ensuring a sufficient supply of the minerals to the growing points of bones.

Therapeutic use. For prophylactic use adults require 500 i.u. daily; growing children and lactating mothers require rather more. The therapeutic dose is 400–100 000 units daily; the vitamin is used in the treatment and prevention of rickets and osteomalacia. It is also useful in correcting low levels of serum calcium such as occur in the malabsorption syndrome and in hypoparathyroidism.

Vitamin D and its related compounds are broken down by enzymic action in the liver. Certain drugs, particularly phenytoin, increase this enzyme activity and this leads to an increased rate of metabolism of the vitamin. Occasionally patients who have been on phenytoin for a long time may show evidence of vitamin D deficiency.

Side effects. As this vitamin is fat soluble it is not rapidly metabolised or excreted. If taken in excessive amounts it may accumulate in the body and produce toxic effects. The earliest toxic symptom in children is usually sudden loss of appetite. Nausea and vomiting are frequently associated. Thirst and polyuria soon follow. There may be severe constipation, alternating with bouts of diarrhea. Headache and other pains are frequent. The child may become thin, wan, irritable, depressed and gradually fall into a stuporose condition which may suggest meningitis. In fatal cases metastatic calcification has been found at autopsy in the arteries, renal tubules, heart, lungs and elsewhere. The serum calcium may be elevated.

Vitamin K (menaphthon)

Pharmacological action. The vitamin is necessary for the normal formation of prothrombin in the liver; the manner in which vitamin K participates in this process is not understood.

Therapeutic use. The vitamin is given to neonates in order to prevent bleeding in a newborn infant who has suffered from trauma at birth, or who shows signs of bleeding. In underdeveloped countries where haemorrhagic disease of the newborn is an important problem there is a strong case for prophylactic use of vitamin K_1 as a routine. The dose for a baby is 1 mg of vitamin K_1 (phytomenadione) i.m., repeated in 8 hours if necessary.

In cases of biliary obstruction and fistula, and in malabsorption, if surgery is contemplated, vitamin K_1 is essential pre-operatively for 3 days in a dose of 10–20 mg daily i.m. When there is severe liver damage little or no improvement in the prothrombin level in the blood can be expected unless a blood transfusion is given.

In anticoagulant therapy with the phenindione group of drugs the 'prothrombin time' may increase to the point when bleeding results. In severe cases 20 mg of phytomenadione can be injected intravenously and repeated in four hours if the 'prothrombin time' has not returned to a safe level. In less severe cases the drug can be given by mouth (10–20 mg every 8 hours).

Vitamin C (ascorbic acid)

Pharmacological action. Ascorbic acid maintains a healthy state of the capillary walls and the intercellular substance. It is a hydrogen transport agent in oxidation–reduction systems.

Therapeutic use. Ascorbic acid has specific effects in the treatment of scurvy. The aim should be to saturate the body with as little delay as possible; 250 mg by mouth four times daily should achieve this within a week.

Side effects. Synthetic ascorbic acid is harmless even in large doses.

Vitamin B_1 (thiamine)

Pharmacological action. The pyrophosphate of thiamine is the coenzyme of carboxylase, the enzyme concerned with the decarboxylation and oxidation of pyruvic acid. The normal function of nerve cells and the kidney is dependent on this vitamin.

Therapeutic use. Thiamine is life-saving in the treatment of cardiovascular and infantile beriberi, and Wernicke's encephalopathy. It may be given, though without expectation of dramatic results, in cases of nutritional neuropathy. 25–100 mg daily for several weeks is required in the treatment of thiamine deficiency. Intramuscular injection may be efficacious where oral therapy fails.

Riboflavine (vitamin B_2)

Pharmacological action. Riboflavine is present in the prosthetic groups of the flavo-proteins, essential for cellular oxidation.

Therapeutic use. There are no incontrovertible indications for the use of synthetic riboflavine; however there is probably an indication for its use in cases of malabsorption syndrome with angular stomatitis. The vitamin may be given orally or parenterally in doses of 5 mg three times daily.

Side effects. No side effects of treatment with riboflavine have been described.

Nicotinic acid (niacin)

Pharmacological action. Nicotinic acid amide is required for the action of NADH and NADPH (prosthetic groups in certain tissue oxidising enzymes).

Therapeutic use. Nicotinic acid and nicotinamide have specific and dramatic effects in pellagra and in secondary deficiency in malabsorption syndromes. The therapeutic dose is 50–250 mg daily (orally or by injection). Large doses produce a generalized and transient vasodilatation.

VACCINES AND SERA

R. L. PARSONS and P. I. FOLB

Smallpox vaccine

Pharmacological action. Live cowpox (vaccinia: calf lymph) harvested from the inoculated skin of animals produces active immunity against infection with the *Variola* virus for many years. If stored dried, potency is retained for six months at room temperature in temperate climates, and a month in tropical climates. The vaccine remains potent for six months if kept consistently below 0 °C, 14 days at less than 10 °C, and 7 days at room temperature.

Therapeutic use. Routine childhood vaccination has now been dropped, since there is no evidence that it has reduced the number of cases of smallpox, and there is a real risk of considerable morbidity and mortality, from complications occuring in those at risk who are vaccinated by ancillaries, unaware of the contraindications. Encephalitis is more likely after childhood vaccination.

To ensure complete protection, vaccination should be performed every 3 years in those at risk (doctors, nurses, infectious disease hospital personnel) and immediately for smallpox contacts. Travellers may require an international certificate countersigned by a community physician when visiting areas where evidence of smallpox vaccination is compulsory. In cases where vaccination is contraindicated, a written statement giving the reason that vaccination is contraindicated, countersigned by the patient's physician, should be submitted to the appropriate embassy for approval prior to embarkation.

Technique. The minimum amount of lymph should be applied to the posterior aspect of the mid-deltoid region, preferably by multiple pressure using a heat sterilised needle. Scarification is more likely to produce a 'take', but should not be used routinely, as there is a greater risk of severe local reactions. The skin should not be sterilised with surgical spirit immediately prior to applying the vaccine, as inactivation of the lymph will result in no local reaction. After vaccination has been done, the excess lymph should be removed, to reduce the risk of a local reaction. No other immunisation procedure should be performed until the vaccinial lesions have completely subsided (about 21 days).

Interpretation of results. The normal responses and their timing after vaccination are summarised below. The times given are a general guide, considerable variation being the normal, rather than the exception. After vaccinating a smallpox contact, the lesions should be read after 3 days, to enable revaccination to be performed. In other individuals, the lesions may be read at 7-10 days.

Five types of reactions may occur. Revaccination will need to be performed if no local reaction occurs. The *typical primary vaccinia* usually reaches a maximum at about 7 days, and is associated with marked vesicular formation. An *accelerated vaccinoid reaction* occuring at 3-7 days usually indicates that previous immunity has only been partial. *Vaccinia necrosum (chronic progressive vaccinia)* is unpredictable and follows failure of the vaccinial lesion to undergo normal resolution. This may require treatment with anti-vaccinial gammaglobulin.

Some parents may request vaccination of their daughters on the leg, to avoid unsightly scars on the exposed area of the arm. This request should be resisted, since extensive local and general reactions may follow.

Complications of vaccination. Generalised vaccinia and postvaccinial encephalitis are the most lethal, being responsible for 26 deaths in one series of 5 million. Encephalitis is particularly likely to occur if vaccination is performed under one year. Generalised *Vaccinia* is a risk in eczematous children, and patients receiving steroids. Hypogammaglobulinaemia and immune deficiencies associated with the reticuloses are contraindications. Vaccination of the pregnant woman may lead to abortion, or vaccinia of the fetus. Table 1 summarises the contraindications to smallpox vaccination.

Vaccination of a child with eczema is hazardous, and should only be performed if there has been exposure to smallpox. Cover with hyperimmune vaccinial gammaglobulin and N-methylizatin β-thiosemicarbazone is required. A past history of childhood eczema in adults is less hazardous, vaccination frequently being uneventful. Atopy is a relative but not absolute contraindication to vaccination.

Table 1.   Contraindications to smallpox vaccination

(a) Absolute
1. Infantile eczema.
2. Hypogammaglobulinaemia.
3. Local skin sepsis.
4. Treatment with steroids and immunosuppressive drugs.
5. Pregnancy.

(b) Relative
1. Family contacts with eczema. Extreme caution is necessary to avoid contact, in view of the risk of generalised vaccinia.
2. Recent immunisation procedures.
   a: *Yellow fever* Smallpox vaccination may be performed 4 days after yellow fever immunisation, unless the patient is under 9 months old, when 21 days should be allowed to elapse. If yellow fever immunisation is delayed until after smallpox vaccination, 21 days must elapse before the second procedure is performed.
   b: *Triple vaccine* 2 weeks interval before smallpox vaccination.
   c: *Oral polio vaccine* 3 weeks interval.
   d: *Any other procedure* 3 weeks interval
   e: *BCG and measles* Immunisation may be performed simultaneously without impairing the immune response to smallpox or either condition. BCG should of course be given in the opposite arm.

Rabies vaccine

Pharmacological action. Inactivated (Semple) vaccine has superseded the older live attenuated (Fermi) vaccine, the WHO having advised that production of the incompletely inactivated Fermi vaccine should cease. Inactivated duck embryo vaccine is safer than the older vaccines prepared from adult brain which may be responsible for paralytic reactions. Following vaccination, antibody production commences in 10–14 days. All the vaccines can produce allergic reactions.
Therapeutic use. Prophylactic rabies vaccination, particularly in veterinary surgeons and attendants at quarantine kennels, is now widely practised. This group should be repeatedly vaccinated until there is evidence of antibody production. About 1 million people every year receive vaccination after being bitten by rabid animals. Bites in the region of the head and neck are the most serious.

After preliminary sensitivity testing, a course of 14–21 daily injections should be commenced immediately after exposure. If given rapidly within the 3–8 day incubation period of the disease, vaccination should effectively prevent the disease. Part of each injection should be given at the site of the infection. The animal should not be destroyed until evidence of infection is apparent, treatment is not required if the animal survives more than 10 days. This is because the risk of a paralytic reaction is directly related to the total number of injections given, and this should be reduced to a minimum.

In large continents, where quarantine cannot be effectively implemented, widespread vaccination of animals has now considerably reduced the incidence of rabies. It does unfortunately prolong the incubation period of the disease in the infected animal.

Poliomyelitis vaccine

Pharmacological action. The older inactivated polio virus (IPV: Salk) vaccine produces high levels of IgM and IgG. Its introduction led to a dramatic fall in the number of cases of polio during the 10 years it was in use prior to the introduction of the newer live attenuated oral polio vaccine (OPV: Sabin). The latter contains all three strains of virus. The OPV is given via the normal route taken by pathogenic virus. The OPV occupies receptors which otherwise would be available to be filled by pathogenic virus. The neuropathic potential of the pathogenic virus is limited by the continuous production of circulating antibodies. Early strains of OPV were responsible for some cases of polio, due to contamination with pathogenic virus.
Therapeutic use. The dramatic fall in the incidence of poliomyelitis that has followed the introduction of immunisation has engendered a false sense of security. It is still mandatory to immunise infants during their first year. Three 0.1 ml doses are given at 4–6-week intervals. This may be done immediately after the completion of the primary course of triple vaccine, or preferably combined as concurrent treatment. This course is not only administratively more convenient, but is likely to result in a greater success rate in the completion of immunisation programmes. Booster doses of Sabin vaccine should be given at 18 months and again upon school entry. The use of OPV during an epidemic may reduce the number of subsequent cases of polio.
Contraindications. These include intercurrent infections, diarrheal illness, the first four months of pregnancy, and steroid therapy.

Measles vaccine

Pharmacological action. The killed virus vaccine produces a short-lived and rapidly declining antibody response. The Schwartz (Glaxo) attenuated live virus vaccine was derived from the Edmonston B strain of the original Enders vaccine. It gives a better antibody response than the killed vaccine, and therefore better protection against measles. Prevention is achieved after a single injection in about 85%. A combined course of an early injection of killed vaccine, followed by live attenuated vaccine will produce a lower incidence of febrile reactions, which are more likely following a single dose of live vaccine. This is offset by a higher incidence of subsequent reinfection upon re-exposure to measles.

Therapeutic use. Measles immunisation is undoubtedly effective. U.K. trials have reduced the attack rate from 82% in the unprotected group to 6% in those treated with mixed killed and attenuated vaccine, and 2% in those who had live vaccine. Measles vaccination is particularly indicated in children with chronic cardiac and respiratory disease, cystic fibrosis, malabsorption, malnutrition and those with chronic suppurative infections of the upper or lower respiratory tract.

If killed vaccine is administered before live attenuated vaccine, there is a considerable risk of severe local or general reactions after the second injection. Subacute sclerosing panencephalitis may follow measles many years later and is due to activation of dormant measles virus within the CNS.

There is little point in immunising children before the age of one because maternal antibodies persist. Immunisation is best performed between the ages of 3 and 5, but in any case before school entry. Children may be immunised up to the age of 15, but when the population of immunised children is sufficiently large, the procedure will be restricted to the second year of life. An epidemic of measles does not contraindicate immunisation.

The Schwartz (Glaxo) freeze dried vaccine is reconstituted into a single dose of 0.5 ml which must be used within an hour of preparation. The freeze dried form remains viable for one year at 2–10 °C.

Contraindications and side effects. In the UK trial, anorexia and vomiting occurred in 31%, sleep disturbance in 45%, rashes in 19%, pyrexia in 6%, and convulsions in 0.19%. The incidence of encephalitis following measles has been dramatically reduced following the introduction of immunisation. Febrile reactions are most likely to occur between the 5th and 10th days and may resemble a mild attack of the disease. Fortunately they only last 24–48 hours. Leucopenia and lymphadenopathy have also been recorded.

Contraindications include intercurrent acute infections, particularly viral infections, a past or family history of febrile convulsions, a past history of allergy, particularly to egg protein, malignant disease including leukaemia, and intercurrent therapy with steroids and immunosuppressive drugs. These groups and other susceptible individuals such as those with hypogammaglobulinaemia should receive gammaglobulin. Measles vaccination should not be performed during pregnancy.

Rubella vaccine

Pharmacological action. Killed rubella vaccine has a low potency and is of little value. HPV-77 grown on vervet monkey cells is the oldest vaccine, from which the HPV-77 DE-5 vaccine used in the USA since 1969 has been developed. With these vaccines the risk of reactions from extraneous antigens is high. The Wistar RA 27/3 (B. W. Almevax) and Plotkin RA/27 vaccines are prepared from human diploid fetal cultures. The Wistar vaccine is the only one that can be given intranasally, being more effective by this route than when given subcutaneously. Concurrent respiratory infections preclude vaccination, since they reduce the normal antibody response, which is 4–8 fold lower than that induced by natural infection. The virus continues to be excreted in the nasopharyngeal secretions for 2–5 weeks after vaccination, but there is no risk of rubella occurring in contacts. The Candehill vaccine, which was introduced in 1970, prepared from rabbit kidney is the safest and least harmful. Since the virus crosses the placenta, it must not be given if there is any possibility of pregnancy, in view of the considerable risk of teratogenesis.

Therapeutic use. After immunisation, the rate of seroconversion is high (90–100%). Rubella vaccination is available for schoolgirls between the ages of 11 and 14, without prior screening to ascertain previous rubella infection. 80% of women during the childbearing age group, are seropositive, whether or not they have a past history of the disease. Vaccination should now be performed between the 2nd and 4th day of the puerperium to women exposed to infection from their children, or place of work, since the risk of pregnancy in the subsequent 6 weeks is at its lowest. If a woman is accidently vaccinated when pregnant, termination should be recommended in view of the 25% risk of fetal damage, stillbirth, and abortion during the first 16 weeks. After vaccination of women in the childbearing age group, contraceptive precautions backed up by pregnancy testing should be continued for at least two months. An interval of 3–4 weeks should elapse before any other immunisation procedure is performed. 0.5 ml of the vaccine may be given subcutaneously, or alternatively 0.5 ml of the RA 27/3 Wistar vaccine (Almevax) may be given into each nostril. The vaccine which comes in 1, 3, and 10 dose ampoules retains potency from 12 months at 2–10 °C. Reconstituted vaccine must be used immediately.

Contraindications and side effects. Reactions are most likely following the HPV-77 vaccine. In children, reactions are mild and include pyrexia, rashes, lymphadenopathy and paraesthesiae. In adults transient arthralgia and arthritis are more likely, but these side effects are less likely if the Cendevelt vaccine is used.

Contraindications include pregnancy, malignant disease including Hodgkin's disease and leukaemia, hypogammaglobulinaemia and other immune deficient states, and those receiving steroids and immunosuppressive therapy.

Mumps vaccine

Pharmacological action. Live attenuated mumps vaccine prepared from chick embryo cells produces an antibody response in over 90% of susceptible individuals. This antibody response is not blocked by the simultaneous administration of measles vaccine and/or gammaglobulin. The attack rate of mumps has been reduced from 61 to 2% after vaccination, but since levels of antibody slowly deteriorate, immunity only lasts for 5 years. Killed vaccines have been used in the past, but the protection following vaccination has only been temporary.

Therapeutic use. A single 0.5 ml dose of the Jeryl Lynn (mumpsvax M.S.D.) strain of lyophilised vaccine is given. Care should be taken to avoid contact with alcohol and other disinfectants. The place of mumps vaccine remains to be established. At 0–4 °C it retains its potency for 12 months.

Contraindications. As for measles vaccine.

Influenza vaccine

Pharmacological action. Antigenic variation, particularly of the more virulent influenza A virus is the factor behind each new epidemic, and subsequently for the production of a new vaccine incorporating the latest strains of both A and B viruses. There is a multiplicity of inactivated vaccines prepared from chick embryo allantois.

Potency has been increased by emulsification with highly purified oils, which enable high antibody titres to persist for several years. Saline vaccines are more likely than oil adjuvant vaccines to produce general and local reactions, but sterile abscesses, edema and thickening of the arm has followed the use of older oil–adjuvant vaccines.

Influenza cannot be controlled, since vaccination would have to be performed at yearly intervals to produce a sufficiently high group immunity. Vaccines containing recent strains of influenza A and B virus, such as the A_1 A_2 and Asian strains are the only ones of any value, producing protection in 40–80% of individuals.

Therapeutic use. At present there are three available vaccines. Admune contains formalin inactivated virus. Influvac has had virus inactivated by β-propionolactone. Flenzavax is a split vaccine treated with sodium deoxycholate after prior formaldehyde treatment.

The vaccine should not come in contact with alcohol or other disinfectants. For this reason it is manufactured in single 0.5, 1, and 10 ml multi-dose vials, coming as an injection pack. At 2–8 °C, the vaccine remains viable for 12 months. It should not be frozen, and should be protected from the light. After opening, the entire contents must be used in an injection session. The normal adult dose is 1 ml by deep subcutaneous or intramuscular injection. Children over six require half this dose.

Influenza vaccination is particularly indicated in those with chronic cardiac, pulmonary, diabetes and renal disease. If given to mothers whose pregnancies progress through the winter months, it should be recalled that influenza virus has been incriminated in the aetiology of childhood malignancy.

Those sections of the community who man vital services (transport workers, telephone operators, hospital personnel, firemen, policemen and teachers) should be given priority for vaccination during an epidemic.

Contraindications and side effects. Local reactions and nodules may occur at injection sites. These may be associated with malaise and headache. Pyrexial reactions may follow both the aqueous and oil adjuvant vaccines, and is due to impurities in the material used. Those individuals sensitive to egg protein or penicillin may develop reactions. Encephalitis, transverse myelopathy, polyneuritis and macular haemorrhages have followed influenza vaccine.

Vaccination should not be performed in those with a history of atopy, or allergy to eggs. It is contraindicated in active systemic lupus erythematosus, and in children under six. During pregnancy, the use of influenza vaccine should be tempered with the knowledge that it may be carcinogenic to the fetus.

BCG (Bacillus Calmette Guerin) Tuberculosis vaccine

Pharmacological action. This is an attenuated bovine vaccine which is non-pathogenic to man, but still effective in preventing subsequent infection by *Myco. tuberculosis, Myco. leprae* and *Myco. ulcerans.* Despite arguments over the efficacy (14–80% protection) of BCG, it is undoubtedly an important measure by which host resistance is increased. The annual attack rate of tuberculosis has been reduced from 1.28 to 0.28 per thousand over 15 years. BCG is given by subcutaneous and intradermal injection. Tuberculin conversion is more likely to be achieved by subcutaneous injection, but this may lead to the formation of intractable ulcers at the injection site. Intradermal injection with the dermo-jet injector has superseded the other two, being economical in the use of vaccine, requiring little technical skill, and enabling large numbers of schoolchildren to be rapidly immunised. Scar formation is much less than after the technically more difficult intradermal injection. The rate of tuberculin conversion is identical to that following intradermal injection. The main obstacles to more widespread use of this method are that a more concentrated vaccine (60–180 million viable organisms per ml) than the standard (20 million) one is required.

Therapeutic use. 0.1 ml of BCG is given by intradermal injection at the junction of the upper and middle third of the deltoid. Jet injection is not yet generally available.

Direct BCG vaccination without preliminary tuberculin testing is safe and efficient, serious reactions in infected individuals being rare. The Heaf test tends to produce false positives, and grade I results should therefore be interpreted as being negative for the purposes of administering BCG. Tuberculin conversion occurs at about six weeks after successful immunisation, and other vaccinations should be postponed until this has occurred. Second injections should not be given into a limb with an incompletely healed BCG lesion. Smallpox, diph-tetanus toxoid aluminium adsorbed vaccine and oral polio vaccine (OPV) vaccines may be given simultaneously but the first two should be given in the opposite arm. 80% of BCG-immunized individuals develop protection lasting 10 years.

About 10% of unimmunised adolescents are tuberculin positive in this country where tuber-culosis is waning. For this reason, BCG is better given at school entry or even in the neonatal period, since a high conversion rate can be achieved before exposure to tuberculosis. High risk groups (immigrant children, technicians handling tubercular material) should be tuberculin tested and immunised. Revaccination at the age of 15 may be necessary if it was originally performed early in life.

Complications. The commonest is the occurence of a severe accelerated local (the classical Koch) reaction followed by an indolent ulcer which leaves a larger scar than that usually following BCG. Local abscesses, lymphadenopathy, and caseation may also occur. Rarely, lupus vulgaris and other cutaneous tuberculides, urticaria, erythema nodosum, and keloid formation may occur. Fatal generalised BCG infections have been described, but accidental overdosage is not usually serious.

Diphtheria vaccine

Pharmacological action. Three vaccines are available. Purified toxoid aluminium phosphate (PTAP): purified toxoid aluminium hydroxide (PTAH) and toxoid antitoxin floccules (TAF). The first two contain a mineral adjuvant which increases efficacy, and the last is a suspension of the precipitate of floccules formed by mixing neutralising amounts of diphtheria toxoid and antitoxin. Reactions are more likely with the first two. Diphtheria vaccine is usually combined with tetanus and pertussis, since the antibody response to all three diseases is unimpaired and the number of visits to complete an immunisation course can be minimised. A quadruple vaccine containing inactivated killed Salk polio vaccine is available for those individuals where oral polio immunisation is contraindicated.

Therapeutic use. Diphtheria, tetanus, and pertussis (DTP/Vac) contains 25 Lf units of diphtheria toxoid, 5 Lf units of tetanus toxoid, and 20 000 million *Bordetella pertussis* in 0.5 ml. In those individuals in whom pertussis immunisation is contraindicated, DT/Vac may be used. TAF contains horse serum and is used in adolescents who are negative to Schick testing.

In infancy, three 0.5 ml subcutaneous injections are given at 6–8 week intervals, the last injection being given between 12–16 months. Immunisation procedures should not be started before 6 months of age, to allow maternal antibodies to subside. Booster doses are required at 5 years of age or at the time of school entry, and again at 15–19 years in Schick negative individuals.

Contraindications and side effects. Pyrexia, swelling of the arm and granulomatous nodules may be due to the diphtheria component of triple vaccine. The last is caused by the aluminium adjuvant, and the former are produced by antigenic components of the vaccine. Provocation poliomyelitis is the only serious hazard, and usually affects only the limbs into which diphtheria antigen has been injected. Oral polio immunisation has considerably reduced the risk of this complication.

TAF should not be used in those sensitised to horse serum. Diphtheria vaccination should be avoided in older patients since they are more likely to react, particularly if they already possess immunity to the disease.

Tetanus toxoid

Pharmacological action. There are two main types of tetanus toxoid, fluid, and the more potent aluminium adsorbed toxoid. The latter contains a very good antigen, capable of stimulating both primary and booster responses. After a full course of tetanus immunisation, antibodies may persist for as long as 12 years.

Therapeutic use. Universal primary tetanus immunisation should be performed, in an attempt to protect the whole community from tetanus, a disease that does not confer subsequent immunity. Three 0.5 ml doses of Tet/Vac/PTAP are given by either subcutaneous or intramuscular injection. The second dose should be given 6–8 weeks after the first, and the third 6–12 months after the second. Booster injections are required every 5 years to maintain immunity, and are indicated in susceptible groups.

Tetanus prophylaxis in the wounded. If exposure has occurred, then provided a full course of tetanus toxoid has been given, all that is required is a booster dose of 0.5 ml of Tet/Vac/PTAP; adequate surgical toilet; and systemic penicillin. Problems arise when the previous immune status of the injured is either unknown or inadequate. A combination of tetanus toxoid, surgical toilet and systemic antibiotics is generally considered adequate, although very occasionally the disease may still develop. Antitetanus serum (ATS) is for treating the developed disease.

Anti-tetanus serum (ATS)

Pharmacological action and therapeutic use. Tetanus antitoxin (ATS) 1500 u prophylactically is given by subcutaneous injection 30 minutes after a 0.05–2 ml test dose. A history of allergy, or past history of allergy to horse serum contraindicates ATS. If a reaction follows the test dose, then it should be repeated 6–12 hours later when the rash produced by the first test has subsided. A loaded syringe containing 1:1000 adrenaline should be available. Another alternative in those allergic to ATS is to use human tetanus immunoglobulin (Humotet B.W.) isolated from the sera of healthy human donors known to have high circulating levels of tetanus antitoxin, following active immunisation with tetanus toxoid. Each 1 ml vial contains 250 i.u. of tetanus antitoxin and is given by intramuscular injection.

Contraindications and side effects. Tetanus toxoid is responsible for urticarial reactions, sometimes with angioneurotic edema in about 1–2% of adults. In children, reactions are rare. They are more common with Tet/Vac/PTAH than fluid toxoid (FT), and tend to follow subcutaneous rather than intramuscular injection. Reactions are directly proportional to the total number of injections, being least likely after gluteal injection. Thiomersal, the antibacterial preservative used in the ampoule may produce delayed hypersensitivity reactions, and the aluminium adjuvant can be responsible for granuloma formation at injection sites.

Anti-tetanus serum (ATS) is responsible for 5–12% of reactions. Its use carries a 1:200 000 mortality. Human anti-tetanus globulin (ATG) rarely causes a reaction.

It must be emphasised that the non- or partially immune wounded and those recovering from tetanus *must* receive a full course of tetanus toxoid, when the immediate problem has been managed. Each patient should be given a card, a reminder being sent automatically at the appropriate time, to ensure that courses are completed.

Pertussis vaccine

Pharmacological action. 20 000 million killed *Bordetella pertussis* bacteria are contained in single Per/Vac and combined DTP/Vac vaccines. All three antigens should be included in the vaccine, since some batches which have not contained all the antigens have been less effective. Theoretically, early immunisation is desirable, both to reduce the risk of whooping cough in the young child, and also to lower the number of reactions which are more common in older children. There is no point in performing immunisation after the age of five, since at that age the disease is mild, and not followed by complications. There is a place for a more potent non-toxic vaccine. Present vaccines may produce a pertussis-like illness, or modify the disease when it occurs, making diagnosis difficult.

Therapeutic use. Combined prophylaxis with diphtheria and tetanus is usually given, the dosage and timing being identical to that outlined under the section on diphtheria vaccine.

Contraindications and side effects. The most serious complication is encephalopathy, which may be followed by chronic brain damage, and even death. This is rare (1:1 000 000). A past history of febrile convulsions means that immunisation is usually complicated by further fits. Pertussis vaccine is one of the most toxic, commonly being the cause of severe local and general reactions following triple vaccine. Despite the fall in the incidence of whooping cough that followed its introduction, pertussis vaccine has fallen into disrepute because of the incidence of serious toxicity, and the poor efficacy of some vaccines. In view of the low mortality from whooping cough it is doubtful whether it should continue to be used.

A past history of convulsions, or fits following the first injection precludes the further use of this vaccine, in view of the risk of encephalopathy following subsequent injections. Other contraindications are a history of recent infection, and a past history of allergy.

Typhoid–paratyphoid vaccine

Pharmacological action. There are a number of killed vaccines containing *Salmonella typhi, paratyphi* B and C. These may be combined with cholera or tetanus. The Vi antigens of *S. typhi* and *S. paratyphi* C are combined with the H and O antigens of all the other salmonellae.

The efficacy of *S. typhi* is proven, although it does not confer complete protection. That of the paratyphoid components is doubtful. If a potent vaccine is used, immunity should last for about 3 years.

Therapeutic use. An initial subcutaneous dose of 0.5 ml should be followed by 1 ml 4–6 weeks later. Reinforcing doses of 0.5 ml annually may be given to holidaymakers, or alternatively 1 ml every 3 years. An intradermal dose of 0.2 ml is equally effective and less likely to provoke reactions. However if this dose is inadvertently given subcutaneously, there is a risk of inadequate protection arising from a dose that is too small. Potent vaccines containing 5000 killed organisms /ml are used for intradermal injection.

Contraindications and side effects. Side effects are common. Local reactions, fever, malaise, headache, nausea, vomiting, and diarrhea may occur within 24 hours, but usually last only 1 or 2 days. Nephritis, arthritis, encephalitis and hypotension are more serious toxic effects. Herpes, polio, tuberculosis, and multiple sclerosis have been reactivated by TAB.

Contraindications include acute infections, chronic nephritis, and diabetes mellitus.

Cholera vaccine

Pharmacological action. A saline suspension of inactivated *Vibrio cholerae* containing 8000 million organisms/ml may be given alone or in combination with TAB. The vaccine contains equal parts of material from the Inaba and Ogawa serotypes, which possess the type O, and heat stable O antigen common to both types. Significant protection of a limited duration follows cholera immunisation. International certificates are valid 6 days after a first vaccination, and immediately after revaccination, provided this is performed within 6 months of the previous injection. The certificate remains valid for 6 months. Both cholera vaccine and TAB/Cho Vac may be given by either intradermal or subcutaneous injection.

Therapeutic use. An initial subcutaneous or intramuscular dose of 0.5 ml is followed by 1.0 ml between 7 and 28 days later. Alternatively 0.2 and 0.4 ml may be given intradermally at the same interval. Children under 12 should receive half these doses. If immunisation is being performed during an epidemic the initial dose should be doubled. Booster doses of 1 ml are given every 6 months.

Contraindications and side effects. 10% of individuals develop reactions consisting of swelling and tenderness at the site of injection. Fever, malaise, and general reactions also occur. A reaction which is mild usually occurs in most people. This persists for 2–3 days.

A past history of a florid sensitivity to the vaccine, and pregnancy are the only contraindications to its use.

DRUG INTERACTIONS

R. L. PARSONS and W. G. REEVES

INTRODUCTION

The risk of drug interaction always exists when more than one drug is prescribed, and this is particularly liable to occur in diabetics, hypertensives, patients treated for depression, and those receiving chemotherapy. The prescriber should regularly review and rewrite the prescription card, asking himself if any drug used, might interact with others prescribed simultaneously. Patients on monoamine oxidase inhibitors should receive a card with a list of proscribed foods, alcoholic beverages, and drugs (Table 1). Hypertensives should be warned not to buy nasal decongestants or cough mixtures which might contain sympathomimetic amines.

Table 1. Foods, alcoholic beverages, and drugs contraindicated with MAOIs

(a) *Foods*

Raw and cooked cheese
Marmite
Broad bean pods
Yoghurt
Bovril
Oxo
Game
Rich soups and gravies
Over-ripe bananas
Canned fish
Rollmops (delicatessen)

(b) *Alcoholic beverages*

German beers
Worthington
Bass
Chianti
Ginger beer

(c) *Other drugs*

Tricyclic anti-depressants	Anti-hypertensives
Barbiturates	Atropine
Alcohol	Reserpine
Narcotic analgesics	Methyldopa
L-dopa	Cocaine
Phenothiazines	Procaine
Sympathomimetic amines	Tetrabenazine
Insulin	
Oral hypoglycaemics (sulphonylureas)	
Thiazides	
General anaesthetics	

Table 2. Drugs responsible for the displacement of other drugs from protein binding sites

Phenylbutazone
Oxyphenbutazone
Indomethacin
Sulphonamides
Sulphonylureas
Coumarin antagonists
Mepacrine
Chloral
Nalidixic acid
Mefenamic acid
Diazoxide
Ethacrynic acid
Clofibrate

MECHANISMS

Interactions may occur during the absorption, transport, metabolism, and finally during excretion by the liver into the bile; or by the kidney into the urine. Parenteral combinations, particularly antibiotics mixed with infusion fluids, may be inactivated by physical or chemical incompatibilities.

INCOMPATIBILITIES IN SOLUTIONS AND INFUSIONS

Examples of mixtures that may result in inactivation of one or other component are: – suxamethonium and thiopentone; carbenicillin and gentamicin. Infusion fluids may be responsible for the inactivation of a large number of antibiotics; either in their own right, or following the addition of heparin and/or hydrocortisone, in a misguided attempt to prevent or delay thrombophlebitis, and maintain the patency of the drip. Parenteral antibiotics are best given either by intramuscular injection, or as in intravenous bolus in an isotonic infusion of saline (with the exception of methicillin or cloxacillin) to achieve a peak plasma concentration greater than the M.I.C. of the infecting organism, and to reduce the likelihood of interaction with the infusion fluid to a minimum. It is bad practice to make up solutions of drugs to be given over several hours with intravenous infusions. Apart from the risk of interaction the added substance may lose a considerable proportion of its pharmacological activity as a result of being left at room temperature.

INTERACTIONS PRIOR TO AND DURING ABSORPTION

The absorption of *tetracycline* may be considerably reduced by the simultaneous administration of calcium, aluminium and iron salts. The mechanism is by the precipitation of an insoluble tetracycline complex.

Cholestyramine should always be taken with a meal to produce maximum secretion of bile. Patients should be warned to take concurrent therapy at least two hours before cholestyramine to avoid chelation of drugs such as aspirin, phenylbutazone, warfarin, thyroxine, barbiturates and some antibiotics. This effect may be of value in the management of poisoning with paracetamol.

Improved absorption of *L-dopa* has been recorded in patients taking alkalis, and may be due to the inactivation of gastric hydrochloric acid. *Metoclopramide* has been shown to profoundly alter the timing and level of peak plasma concentrations of *paracetamol, digoxin* and *L-dopa*. Anti-cholinergic drugs such as *propantheline* may delay gastric emptying, and have been shown to reduce the peak plasma levels of both *digoxin* and *paracetamol*.

Steatorrhea may follow the administration of a number of drugs including *cholestyramine, neomycin, PAS* and *colchicine*. This may produce vitamin deficiencies and requires replacement therapy with fat soluble vitamins (A, D and K).

Tyramine, a potent vasopressor agent, is normally metabolised by monoamine oxidase situated in the gut wall. As a result of inactivation of this enzyme, patients taking *monoamine oxidase inhibitors* run a risk of severe and sudden hypertension if foods or alcoholic beverages containing large amounts of either tyramine or dopamine are ingested (Table 1). Subarachnoid haemorrhage has been described as a specific complication of this interaction. Hypertension occurs as a result of the tyramine induced release of large amounts of noradrenaline.

INTERACTIONS OCCURRING DURING TRANSPORT WITHIN BLOOD

A large number of compounds and natural hormones are carried to their receptors by the albumin molecules. Most drugs exist simultaneously as pharmacologically inert (protein bound) and pharmacologically active (free) forms. The free (unbound) form is available for diffusion into the tissues. Highly protein bound drugs usually have long half lives, a long duration of action, and owe their pharmacological activity to a relatively small proportion of the total plasma concentration. If displacement occurs, as a result of another drug competing with the first to occupy the receptors on the albumin molecules, then a sudden rise in the plasma concentration of free (unbound) drug may follow. This may produce a marked increase in the pharmacological activity of the first drug. Haemorrhage may result from such interactions in patients receiving anticoagulants. Profound hypoglycaemia may occur in diabetics on sulphonylureas. The drugs that may produce displacement of other drugs from the protein binding sites are listed in Table 2.

INTERACTIONS OCCURRING AT THE RECEPTOR

Drugs altering autonomic activity

The post-ganglionic adrenergic blocking drugs used in hypertension (guanethidine, debrisoquine, bethanidine) all reduce the normal sympathetic drive, and catecholamine release at the receptors. Concurrent therapy with sympathomimetic amines or fenfluramine in the treatment of associated problems such as obesity, nasal congestion, and obstructive airway disease antagonises the effect of the hypotensive agent by increasing circulating catecholamines at the receptors. Difficulty in controlling the blood pressure will occur until the second agent is discontinued.

Tricyclic antidepressants should not be prescribed for iatrogenic depression induced by hypotensive agents (reserpine, methyldopa, clonidine and propranolol) since they increase local receptor concentrations of catecholamines by preventing the re-uptake of noradrenaline, and thus may produce hypertension.

Tricyclic antidepressants

The problems of iatrogenic depression, and its treatment with tricyclic antidepressants in hypertensives have already been considered. It is considered hazardous to prescribe tricyclics to patients receiving monoamine oxidase inhibitors, and many authorities advise an interval of at least a fortnight before starting tricyclics in a patient who has previously received a monoamine oxidase inhibitor. Some psychiatrists regularly use both tricyclics and MAOIs concurrently, advocating it as a valuable regime. However this combination should only be used by an experienced psychiatrist. Glaucoma may require concurrent *anticholinesterase* therapy, and may be aggravated by the *atropinic* effect of the *tricyclics* on accomodation.

Monoamine oxidase inhibitors (MAOIs)

The hazards of *tyramine* induced hypertension, combined therapy with *tricyclics* and concurrent drug therapy (Table 1) have already been briefly considered.

Monoamine oxidase is a non-specific enzyme which is also involved in the metabolism of *narcotic analgesics* (in particular pethidine), *barbiturates, phenothiazines,* and *alcohol.* Therefore it is not surprising that the MAOIs may potentiate the effects of these drugs by enzyme inhibition.

Concurrent therapy with *rauwolfia, methyldopa,* and *tetrabenazine* in patients on MAOIs may be responsible for cerebral excitation. Orthostatic hypotension, a well recognised hazard of MAOI therapy, may be precipitated by *pethidine, phenothiazines* and *propranolol.* Finally MAOIs potentiate *insulin.*

L-dopa

L-dopa is a catecholamine precursor of noradrenaline and adrenaline. It is therefore not surprising that cardiac arrhythmias occur in the elderly patients receiving this drug. *MAOIs* should never be prescribed to patients on L-dopa, since one minor metabolic pathway of inactivation is blocked. This increases the likelihood of arrhythmias from increased concentrations of catecholamines at the myocardial receptors. Another hazard of this combination is severe hypertension and subarachnoid haemorrhage. Since L-dopa is a catecholamine, it goes without saying that its use in hypertensives receiving adrenergic blocking drugs renders the control of the blood pressure difficult. *Pyridoxine* antagonises the action of L-dopa, and since this is sold by the chemist as a constituent of a variety of tonics, it may explain therapeutic failure. Hypotension is a hazard when L-dopa is combined with *phenothiazines*, and *tricyclics*. It is not surprising that drugs which produce parkinsonism (*phenothiazines* and *butyrophenones*) will antagonise L-dopa. Conversely, the simultaneous prescription of anti-cholinergic drugs in the treatment of parkinsonism is an example of beneficial drug interaction. L-dopa is of no value in the management of drug induced parkinsonism.

Table 3.   Drugs contraindicated in patients receiving L-dopa

Phenothiazines
Reserpine
Butyrophenones
Methyldopa
Pyridoxine
CNS stimulants
Antacids
Large protein containing meals
Tricyclic anti-depressants
Monoamine oxidase inhibitors
Hypotensive drugs

INTERACTIONS OCCURRING DURING METABOLISM WITHIN THE LIVER

There are a large number of agents which may stimulate (induce) or inhibit the microsomal enzymes in the liver, which control drug metabolism (Table 4). Enzyme induction will result in a shortening of the half life, and therefore the duration of the action of a drug, whilst inhibition of drug metabolising enzymes, will prolong the action of the drug, producing cumulation, and even toxicity. The main problem arises when there is a sudden change, for example the cessation of an enzyme inducing drug when the patient leaves hospital. Patients on potentially dangerous drugs (i.e. oral anticoagulants) will continue to take the same dose as they were receiving in hospital, but once the stimulus to enzyme induction has been withdrawn, metabolic inactivation will return to normal and the level of anticoagulant may rise to dangerous levels. For this reason, patients on anticoagulants would be better avoiding enzyme inducing agents such as the *barbiturates, dichlorphenazone* and *glutethimide.* If an hypnotic is required, nitrazepam and the benzodiazepine tranquillisers have been shown to leave the plasma warfarin levels unchanged. Enzyme induction appears to be an individual characteristic, one individual inducing to a greater or lesser degree than another.

Prolonged anticonvulsant therapy may result in osteomalacia, since *25-hydroxycholecalciferol,* the main circulating pharmacologically active metabolite of *vitamin D* is metabolised to the inactive *21,25-dihydroxycholecaliciferol* metabolite by the hepatic enzymes induced by anticonvulsant therapy. Supplements of *cholecalciferol* or *25-hydroxycholecalciferol* may be required to correct this iatrogenic disease.

Table 4. Drugs producing enzyme induction and shortening the action of other drugs

Barbiturates
Glutethimide
Chloral hydrate
Dichloralphenazone
Antipyrine
Griseofulvin
Phenylbutazone
Phenytoin
Primidone
Dicophane (DDT)
Pheneturide

Some examples of extra-hepatic enzyme inhibition have already been considered. Some drug combinations may be beneficial, i.e. *6-mercaptopurine* and *allopurinol*. Allopurinol, an inhibitor of the enzyme xanthine oxidase, prevents the synthesis of uric acid, and so may be utilized to prevent hyperuricaemia and gout in patients undergoing cytotoxic chemotherapy.

Disulfiram (antabuse) is an inhibitor of acetaldehyde dehydrogenase, and is used in the treatment of alcoholism. It is of interest that a number of sulphonylureas will produce flushing and an 'antabuse-like' syndrome in diabetics who ingest alcohol. Other interactions due to enzyme inhibition are given in Table 5.

Table 5. Examples of enzyme inhibition with prolongation of action of drugs

(a) **Extra-hepatic**
  1. *Allopurinol* inhibits *xanthine oxidase*
  2. *Carbidopa* (alphamethyldopa *hydrazine*) inhibits *Dopa decarboxylase*
  3. *Monoamine oxidase inhibitors* (MAOIs)
     a: *Hydrazine* derivatives
         Iproniazid (Marsilid)
         Nialamide (Niamid)
         Phenelzine (Nardil)
         Pheniprazine (Catron: cavodil)
         Isocarboxazid (Marplan)
         Mebanazine (Actomol)
     b: *Non-Hydrazines*
         Tranylcypromine (Parnate)
         Pargyline (Eutonyl)
  4. *Anticholinesterases*
         Neostigmine
         Physostigmine
         Edrophonium
         Pyridostigmine

(b) **Hepatic**
  1. *Drugs inhibiting warfarin metabolism*
         Alcohol
         Chloramphenicol
         Disulfiram
         Allopurinol
         Methylphenidate
         Nortriptyline
         MAOIs
  2. *Drugs inhibiting phenytoin metabolism*
         Dicoumarol
         Disulfiram
         Isoniazid
         PAS
         Warfarin
         Methylphenidate
         Sulthiam
  3. *Drugs inhibiting sulphonylurea metabolism*
         Sulphaphenazole
         Phenylbutazone
         Dicoumarol (bishydroxycoumarin)
         Phenpyramidol
         Aspirin
  4. *Drugs inhibiting barbiturate metabolism*
         MAOIs
         Methylphenidate
         Dextropropoxyphene

INTERACTIONS OCCURRING DURING EXCRETION

A number of drugs compete for active transport within the renal tubules. *Probenecid* may successfully reduce the tubular secretion of *penicillin* and *indomethacin*. *Salicylates* and *sulfinpyrazone* both compete for the tubular transport systems involved in the transport of uric acid. Combined therapy may result in uric acid retention. This may lead to gout.

Phenylbutazone may inhibit the tubular secretion of *hydroxyhexamide*, the pharmacologically active metabolite of *acetohexamide* and thus cause hypoglycaemia.

Table 6. Drug interactions occurring as a result of competition for tubular transport mechanisms

Drug combination	Pharmacological effect
1. Probenecid and penicillins	Delayed penicillin excretion
2. Probenecid and indomethacin	Reduced tubular secretion and excretion of indomethacin
3. Salicylates and sulphinpyrazone	Retention of uric acid
4. Hydroxyhexamide* and phenylbutazone	Hypoglycaemia
5. Chlorpropamide and dicoumarol	Hypoglycaemia

*The pharmacologically active metabolite of acetohexamide

CONCLUSION

The number and complexity of drug interactions is increasing rapidly. Particular care is needed when prescribing for patients receiving treatment for depression, hypertension, diabetes and those receiving chemotherapy. Patients receiving a large number of drugs should have their prescriptions reviewed at regular intervals, and should carry a card with details of the drugs used, so that they can show this to all the doctors involved in their care.

Supplement B

DRUGS IN RENAL DISEASE

R. L. PARSONS

INTRODUCTION

Before prescribing any drug to a patient with renal failure, there are a number of important questions that must be answered. Firstly, how does renal failure affect the absorption, metabolism, and pharmacological activity of the compound in question? Secondly, are there any side or toxic effects which are particularly likely to occur as a result of retention of the drug? Thirdly whether the drug is removed by dialysis may be important in planning the detailed therapeutic regime.

The dose may be determined by measurement of the glomerular filtration rate, calculation of the rate of excretion or by checking the plasma concentration of the drug. Unfortunately plasma levels and glomerular filtration rates are unreliable guides to accurate dose requirements, and may not prevent serious toxicity (i.e. ototoxicity from aminoglycosides). In centres where sophisticated techniques are not available, a GFR of 30 ml/min or more is adequate when normal doses are used. The dose should be reduced to $\frac{2}{3}$ if the GFR is between 15 and 30 ml/min, and $\frac{1}{3}$ of the normal dose is required if below 15 ml/min. These rules however only apply to those drugs predominantly excreted by glomerular filtration.

Antibiotics

These may be subdivided into those that should never be used; those where a major dose adjustment is required; those where some minor dose adjustment is required; those where no dose adjustment is required (Table 1).

There is a considerable risk of an irreversible motor peripheral neuropathy following nitrofurantoin. Cephaloridine prescribed alone, or with frusemide has been shown to be nephrotoxic. Tetracyclines, except doxycycline, may produce an elevated blood urea in those with pre-existing renal disease. Prolonged storage of tetracyclines may lead to the formation of nephrotoxic anhydro and epianhydro tetracycline derivatives. The administration of chloramphenicol in renal failure does not alter the normal plasma concen-

Table 1. Antibiotics in renal failure

(1) *To be avoided altogether*
  Chloramphenicol
  Nitrofurantoin
  Tetracyclines (except doxycycline)
  Cephaloridine and frusemide (given together)
  Cephalothin and gentamicin (given together)

(2) *Potentially very toxic: therefore major dose adjustment + monitoring of blood levels required*
  Aminoglycosides
    Streptomycin
    Kanamycin
    Gentamicin
  Anti-fungal antibiotics
    Amphotericin B
  Cotrimoxazole
    (the sulphamethoxazole component)
  Anti-tuberculous drugs
    Sodium aminosalicylate
    Ethionamide
    Pyrazinamide
    Viomycin
    Ethambutol
  Other drugs
    Nalidixic acid
    Vancomycin
    Polymyxin B

(3) *Minor dose adjustments required*
  Penicillins
  Sulphonamides
  Isoniazid
  Rifampicin

(4) *Normal dose may be administered*
  Macrolide antibiotics
    Erythromycin
    Oleandomycin
    Spiramycin
  Novobiocin
  Fucidin

trations of the parent compound, but will lead to accumulation of toxic metabolites, increasing the likelihood of marrow aplasia.

The aminoglycosides and other anti-tuberculous drugs, with the exception of isoniazid and rifampicin, accumulate in renal failure. In this situation ototoxicity is a real hazard. After the first dose has been given, the plasma levels should be repeatedly estimated, to ensure adequate and optimum subsequent dosage.

Renal failure does not significantly alter the half life of trimethoprim. However, the total and acetyl sulphamethoxazole levels rise and may remain unchanged after a single dose of cotrimoxazole. Dosage adjustments may be required in those with severely reduced glomerular filtration rates. Patients with renal transplants should not be given cotrimoxazole even if their GFR is normal, since anuria and tubular necrosis have been reported.

Sedatives, hypnotics and anti-convulsants

Long acting barbiturates (barbitone, phenobarbitone, primidone) are excreted unchanged by the kidney. The medium, short and ultrashort acting barbiturates (chloral hydrate, methaqualone, dichloralphenazone, nitrazepam) are all metabolised by the liver, and so can be used at normal doses in renal failure. Phenytoin too is metabolised in the liver, and so can be used at normal doses.

Tranquillisers

Both phenothiazines and benzodiazepines are metabolised and excreted by the liver, and do not accumulate in uraemia. Oculogyric crises may occur in those treated with phenothiazines, and these may be erroneously diagnosed as uraemic fits.

Narcotic analgesics

Like the majority of the barbiturates, phenytoin and the tranquillisers, these are metabolised by the liver, and are therefore more hazardous in liver disease. If vomiting is troublesome phenoperidine (operidine—a narcotic analgesic) combined with droperidol (a neuroleptic) is a preferable alternative to morphine and pethidine.

Cardiovascular drugs

Digoxin. Cardiac glycosides should if possible be avoided in renal failure. They may produce nausea and vomiting and exacerbate renal failure. Rapid changes in the serum and myocardial potassium concentrations may produce an unpredictable pharmacological response and are potentially cardiotoxic, with arrhythmias and sudden death. The half life of digoxin is prolonged from 33 to 83 hours in advanced renal failure. A blood urea of 100 mg/ml requires halving the maintenance dose of digoxin. Several studies have shown a poor correlation between the blood urea, creatinine clearance, and the plasma digoxin levels. A more accurate way of determining dose is to use a computer predicted dose or alternatively radioimmunoassay of plasma digoxin, a procedure that is rapidly becoming standard in most laboratories.

Procainamide is partly metabolised, about 50% being excreted in the urine. It is contraindicated in those with digitalis intoxication and also those with renal failure.

Lignocaine is metabolised by the liver, about 5% being excreted unchanged in the urine. The pharmacokinetics of lignocaine in anephric patients is identical to that in normal individuals.

β-blocking drugs. Propranolol, oxprenolol and alprenolol are all extensively metabolised by the liver. There is evidence that the total amount of propranolol and its metabolites remains static in patients with renal failure. Practolol and acebutolol are excreted almost entirely by the kidneys and are not metabolised by the liver. Renal failure prolongs the half life of practolol to 78.2 hours.

Adrenergic blocking drugs are retained in renal failure. Their efficacy is reduced and they tend to aggravate pre-existing salt and water retention. Diazoxide and minoxidil are to be preferred, since these vasodilator drugs maintain renal blood flow.

Diuretics. Thiazides lose their diuretic effect if the GFR is reduced below 20 ml/min but they may still possess a useful extra-renal hypotensive effect. Frusemide and ethacrynic acid in high doses may produce a diuresis, even when the GFR is reduced below 5 ml/min. Large doses (500–4000 mg/day) of frusemide may be required. There is a risk of deafness with both of these potent diuretics. The serum potassium may also fall precipitately, and be a further cause of digitalis intoxication in uraemia.

Miscellaneous drugs used in renal failure

A list of these, together with side effects and alternatives are shown in Table 2.

Table 2. Miscellaneous drugs used in renal failure

Drug	Daily dose	Problem	Alternative
Antibiotics			
Carbenicillin	20–30 g	Sodium retention 1 g contains 5 mEq (Na$^+$) Daily intake = 100–150 mEq	
Cation exchange resins (sodium phase — SO$_3$$^-$)			
Katonium	15–60 g	Sodium retention	Calcium resonium
(potassium polystyrene sulphonate 25 %)			or
(ammonium polystyrene sulphonate 75 %)			Aluminium resin
Resonium A	15–60 g p.o.		
(sodium polystyrene sulphonate)	25–200 g p.r. (as an enema) Sodium retention		
Calcium resonium		Hypercalcaemia	
(calcium polystyrene sulphonate)			
Aluminium resin		Hyperaluminaemia	
Indigestion mixtures			
Magnesium trisilicate mixture BPC	15–180 ml	Sodium retention Hypermagnesaemia Diarrhea 10 ml contain 6 mEq (Na$^+$)	Aluminium hydroxide
Magnesium carbonate mixture BPC	15–180 ml	Sodium retention Hypermagnesaemia Diarrhea 10 ml contain 10 mEq (Na$^+$)	Aluminium hydroxide
Aluminium hydroxide	10–30 ml 50–100 ml	Hyperaluminaemia Hypophosphataemia nausea	Also used at high doses to treat hyper-phosphataemia

DRUGS IN LIVER DISEASE

R. L. PARSONS

The liver is the main site of drug metabolism. It is here that many lipid soluble drugs are converted to their water soluble metabolites which are excreted in the urine. This may result in inactivation. There are a number of changes occurring in patients with impaired liver function which may alter the plasma levels and duration of drug action. These effects can produce unpredictable pharmacological actions, for example as a result of the accumulation of toxic metabolites. There is always the possibility that injudicious therapy may precipitate hepatic coma. The main problem confronting the practitioner when treating a patient with liver disease is to decide which compounds he can safely use without the risk of cumulative or undesirable toxic effects.

Overenthusiastic use of diuretics is an important factor producing falls in the serum potassium, a well recognized precipitant of *hepatic encephalopathy*. In patients with ascites or peripheral edema, when a *diuretic* is indicated, a thiazide with adequate potassium supplements is usually satisfactory. If this is insufficient, spironolactone (an aldosterone antagonist) may be added. When more powerful diuretics are required, 40–80 mg of frusemide may be used, provided the serum potassium is monitored daily during the initial days of treatment.

The daily intake of sodium in the diet should be restricted to not more than 20–25 mEq Na^+. This is done to reduce water retention in the cirrhotic patient.

If possible the *narcotic analgesics* should be avoided, since they are metabolised by the liver, and their use may be followed by profound respiratory depression and coma. Small doses (25 mg) of pethidine are preferable. Normal doses of paracetamol may be safely used for conditions requiring minor analgesics. Aspirin is best avoided, since there is a risk of acute peptic ulceration and haematemesis. This may be severe if the patient already has hypoprothrombinaemia. If anti-inflammatory analgesics are required, the normal dose of indomethacin (25–50 mg t.d.s.) can be used. It should be remembered that both indomethacin and phenylbutazone produce peptic ulceration, and a severe haematemesis in the cirrhotic with a peptic ulcer is a life threatening hazard.

If a *hypnotic* is required the benzodiazepines and promethazine (25–50 mg) are preferable to the short and medium acting barbiturates, since there is less risk as a result of accumulation of these drugs. Phenobarbitone is mainly excreted by the kidneys and normal doses may be given.

When an *antidepressant* is indicated, small doses (25 mg) of amitriptyline should be given. Monoamine oxidase inhibitors are contraindicated in cirrhosis since they are almost entirely metabolised by the liver, and their use may cause hepatic coma.

There is a wide choice of *antibiotics* available for patients with liver disease. Although a proportion of all the penicillins and the cephalosporins is excreted in the bile, these drugs may be safely administered without fear of increased toxicity. All the aminoglycosides are excreted by the kidneys, so provided the patient has normal renal function, no modification of dose is required. Rifampicin, the tetracyclines and erythromycin (particularly the estolate) are best avoided since there is an increased likelihood of jaundice. Although Fucidin, lincomycin and clindamycin are mainly excreted in the bile, they may be given in half the usual dose. A short course of neomycin (4 g daily) may be required to sterilise the gut flora. This antibiotic is usually given to prevent the onset of hepatic encephalopathy which results from the absorption of the large protein load that follows a haematemesis from esophageal varices. The use of neomycin may be followed by deafness in cirrhotics. This is due to systemic absorption.

Since chloramphenicol is not metabolised in cirrhosis, its half life is prolonged, and there is a much greater risk of aplastic anaemia from the parent compound. Its use therefore should be restricted to those cirrhotics with septicaemia, whose infection is only sensitive to this antibiotic.

For *diabetics*, tolbutamide in small doses (0.5–1 g daily) is a safer sulphonylurea than the long acting chlorpropamide. The latter drug may produce prolonged hypoglycaemia and jaundice. Both these sulphonylureas are normally metabolised to inactive metabolites by the liver.

Impaired metabolism of *prednisolone* is particularly likely to be responsible for the rapid appearance of the features of Cushing's syndrome, even when small doses are used. Estrogens and the oral contraceptives are best avoided since they may be responsible for further fluid retention, and jaundice.

Drugs that may be prescribed

Drug	Dose
Sedatives Antihistamines/Tranquillizers	
Chlordiazepoxide	5–10 mg t.d.s. orally
Diazepam	2–5 mg t.d.s. orally
	5–10 mg i.m.
Nitrazepam	5–10 mg orally nocte.
Promethazine	25–50 mg orally
Chlorpromazine	25 mg orally
Sodium phenobarbitone	30 mg t.d.s. orally
	180 mg i.m.
Analgesics	
Codeine phosphate	30 mg t.d.s. orally
Dihydrocodeine	30 mg t.d.s. orally
Pethidine	25 mg b.d./t.d.s. orally
Paracetamol	0.5 g q.d.s. orally
Antibiotics	
Penicillins	
Cephalosporins	Normal doses
Aminoglycosides	

Drug	Dose
Fucidin	0.5 g t.d.s. orally
Lincomycin	0.5 g b.d.
Clindamycin	150 mg b.d.
Neomycin	1 g. q.d.s.
Diuretics	
First line	
Bendrofluazide	5–10 mg daily
Spironolactone	25–50 mg q.d.s.
Triamterene	100–250 mg daily
Second line	
Frusemide	40 mg b.d.
Ethacrynic acid	25 mg daily
Potassium Supplements	
Slow K	600–1200 mg t.d.s. sachets (24–48 mEq K$^+$ daily)
Effervescent Kloref	1–2 tablets t.d.s. (20–40 mEq K$^+$ daily)
Sando K	2–4 tablets daily (24–48 mEq K$^+$ daily)

The table is intended as a guide to those drugs that may safely be given to patients with liver disease, although the counsel of perfection is to avoid prescribing any drugs unless they are absolutely necessary. It is wise to realise that the effect of many drugs is unpredictable in these patients. Profound changes in normal physiological parameters may alter the absorption protein binding, and detoxication of drugs which may not exert their normal pharmacological effect.

USE OF DRUGS IN PREGNANCY

F. M. SULLIVAN

Although it had been known since the beginning of this century that the administration of drugs during pregnancy could affect the offspring, it was only following the thalidomide disaster that physicians became aware that the teratogenic properties of drugs could be a real hazard to their patients. From experiments conducted in animals it is quite clear that most drugs can produce embryotoxic effects if given in adequate doses and at appropriate stages of pregnancy, so one must regard embryotoxicity as only one aspect of general toxicity. The important question is therefore; which drugs are likely to produce toxic effects on the embryo or fetus at dose levels which are non-toxic for the mother? The true answer is, unfortunately, that we do not know. Thalidomide was such a drug although the increasing awareness of its neurotoxicity was raising doubts about its value as a hypnotic. Some other drugs are known to affect the development of the fetus but before considering these, we should look at the types of toxic effect which drugs can produce. It is simplest to consider these in relation to the stage of pregnancy at which they are administered.

Effects of drugs at different stages of pregnancy

1. *Implantation stage.* During the first two weeks or so following conception the blastocyst develops and implants. At this time drugs tend to exert all-or-none effects – they may have an antifertility action by preventing implantation or may cause abortion, but they are unlikely to produce any malformations at this time.

2. *Embryogenic stage.* This is generally accepted to cover the period between the second or third and twelfth week of pregnancy during which time the embryo develops from a simple ball of cells to a clearly recognisable fetus. It is during this period that drugs may produce gross structural defects such as missing organs or limbs, anencephaly, exomphalos, cardiac defects, etc. Large doses of drugs may produce widespread effects which are incompatible with further development

and so result in abortion, whereas lower doses may result in live but deformed babies.

3. *Fetogenic stage.* This covers the period from the twelfth week to term. It is mistakenly believed by many physicians that it is quite safe to use drugs in pregnant women during these last two trimesters since major congenital abnormalities will not be produced. While it is true that the major structures are already present by the twelfth week, a great deal of histological development continues through to term. In particular, cerebral cortical development occurs during this period and the time of maximum brain growth in man is in the last month before birth. Drugs acting during the last two trimesters may result in functional defects, e.g. mental deficiency, which are not incompatible with life and are therefore in many respects more important.

It is clear from the above, that the possible dangers of drug therapy must be considered at *all* stages of pregnancy, and that due care must be taken before using drugs at any time in pregnant women.

Difficulty of recognising teratogenic drugs

The simplest drug to detect would be one which produced an easily recognised and unusual type of deformity in a high percentage of women exposed to risk. These requirements were met with thalidomide which affected about 20% of women at risk, and yet it took 6 years and several thousand malformed babies before the association was recognised. With drugs producing more common types of abnormality the problem of recognition is even greater. For example in order to have a 95% chance of detecting a drug which doubled the normal incidence of anencephaly, studies on 23 000 treated pregnant women may be required. It is obvious therefore that many more drugs than are at present known, may be embryotoxic.

Even greater difficulties arise when one considers possible delayed manifestations of embryotoxic activity. It has been known for some time that in animals, administration of a single dose of a carcinogen which was non-toxic for the mother, could result in death of all the progeny from CNS tumours. These did not develop until 1–2 years after birth which was the middle of their expected life span. The possible relationship between the administration of drugs to pregnant women and the development of cancer subsequently in the offspring cannot be ignored. Vaginal adenocarcinoma which is very rare and then usually occurs in women over 50 years of age, has been reported recently in young women, aged 15–22 years. The most highly significant difference between these women and matched controls was that the mothers of the affected girls had been treated during pregnancy with stilbestrol. It is possible that this altered the vaginal epithelium *in utero* in such a way as to predispose it to develop adenosis leading to adenocarcinoma when subjected to endogenous estrogen at menarche. These observations have been confirmed by other workers, and it has also been suggested that diseases like chicken pox and influenza during pregnancy may also predispose to a higher than expected incidence of cancer in the offspring.

Specific recommendations

From all of this it is quite clear that since this is a relatively new and expanding field of study it is impossible to be dogmatic that any specific drugs are absolutely safe for use in pregnancy. On the other hand one should not be over pessimistic either and a nihilistic approach can be just as harmful if the pregnant patient is suffering from a condition which itself may lead to harm of the fetus.

It is impossible in a brief review to discuss all the evidence concerning individual drugs but the following summary gives an idea of the present state of knowledge in some of the fields which concern the general physician.

Analgesics

Narcotic analgesics. Morphine and pethidine like all centrally acting drugs cross the placenta easily and can produce dependence *in utero* so that both the fetus and newborn infant may have a withdrawal syndrome which in the latter can be fatal. There is of course also a risk of respiratory depression in the newborn if these drugs are given within a few hours of delivery. There is no evidence concerning their effects in early pregnancy. Provided one is aware of these risks the drugs seem to be safe to use.

Minor analgesics. There is some evidence in man that salicylates may be teratogenic in early pregnancy. In the later stages they can cause fetal hypoprothrombinaemia and neonatal bleeding as well as other toxic effects. It might therefore be advisable to use paracetamol instead of aspirin where possible.

Antibiotics

It is known that infections – rubella, cytomegalic inclusion disease, syphilis, toxoplasmosis and possibly influenza and mumps as well as febrile and toxic states of the mother — can all lead to fetal damage. Therefore it is never justified to withhold antibiotics or chemotherapeutics in situations where the mother really requires them. On the other hand practically all of the antibiotics have been suspected of causing fetal damage and they should definitely not be used for trivial indications.

Penicillins including ampicillin seem to be the least toxic and where appropriate should be the first choice. In the early stages of pregnancy, short acting sulphonamides like sulphadimidine also appear to be safe though towards the end of pregnancy it may be better to use alternatives since sulphonamides can cause jaundice and kernicterus in the newborn. Although there is no direct evidence of risk with cotrimoxazole, it does contain a folic acid antagonist (trimethoprim) and it would be advisable to avoid its use during pregnancy. Tetracyclines are definitely known to be teratogenic. They cause dark staining of the teeth with hypoplasia of the enamel and increased susceptibility to caries. They may also cause some retardation of skeletal growth. Since the period of risk is from about the 18th week it is advisable to avoid the use of tetracycline after that time. If it is necessary to use a tetracycline then oxytetracycline should be used since this only causes a creamy coloured staining of the teeth which is barely detectable.

Streptomycin is known occasionally to cause 8th nerve damage in the fetus and this drug together with gentamicin, viomycin and kanamycin should be used only if absolutely necessary. Isoniazid appears to be safe in pregnancy. Chloramphenicol should be avoided in late pregnancy since the fetus and neonate are unable to metabolise it and its use can lead to circulatory collapse and the 'grey syndrome'.

Like the highly protein bound sulphonamides, novobiocin should be avoided in late pregnancy due to a risk of neonatal jaundice or kernicterus, and nitrofurantoin has been reported to cause neonatal haemolysis after maternal administration.

Anti-diabetics

Because of the higher than normal incidence of fetal abnormalities in diabetic women it is difficult to assess the effects of individual drugs. There is however a very clear general opinion that insulin is the hypoglycaemic of choice in the treatment of pregnant diabetics. The sulphonylureas, especially chlorpropamide and tolbutamide have been associated with multiple fetal malformations, fetal death and severe prolonged neonatal hypoglycaemia and are best avoided during pregnancy.

Anti-emetics

The usual 'morning sickness' can often be helped by reassurance and without the use of drugs. However severe nausea or vomiting or hyperemesis gravidarum may themselves lead to fetal damage and should be treated. A rather strange situation exists in this field since suspicion of teratogenesis was levelled at two of the most commonly used anti-emetics — meclozine and cyclizine. A detailed review of the evidence failed to give a clear answer. However since more information on the use of these drugs in pregnancy exists than on any other anti-emetic, and since the risk with either is certainly low, it would appear that meclozine or cyclizine should be the drugs of choice for anti-emetic treatment. For very severe cases a phenothiazine, e.g. chlorpromazine should be used.

Hormones

Sex hormones. The sex hormones (estrogens, androgens and progestogens) have been demonstrated to be teratogenic in man, resulting usually in masculinisation of female fetuses. There is in any case little evidence that these drugs are of value in treating threatened abortion and their use should be avoided. If however, it is necessary to use an estrogen then for the reasons mentioned above concerning its possible carcinogenic action, stilbestrol should be avoided. Ethinyl estradiol appears to be the safest estrogen to use. The androgenic steroids and the synthetic progestogens ethisterone and norethisterone are most likely to cause masculinisation of females and should definitely be avoided. If a progestogen is required then progesterone itself or a 17α-OH progesterone derivative (e.g. Delalutin or Provera) may be safer than the 19-nor progestogens.

Adrenocortical hormones. Although ACTH and cortisone will regularly produce a high incidence of cleft palate in certain species and strains of animals, humans seem to be much less susceptible to this effect. Similarly, although there have been reported cases of infants with adrenocortical failure due to steroid withdrawal after large doses of prednisolone to the mother, this is relatively rare and many women have been treated with large doses of cortisone or prednisone for Hodgkin's disease during pregnancy, and with a completely normal outcome. If therefore, it is necessary to use steroids during pregnancy for treatment of any serious condition, this can be done with reasonable safety.

Thyroid hormones. Anti-thyroid drugs and iodides may cause goitres in the fetus to such an extent as to prevent adequate respiration after birth. They may also result in hypo- or hyperthyroid states though cretinism is extremely rare. It is recommended that minimum doses of anti-thyroid drugs should be used and that these should be tailed off with a view to ending treatment a month before the expected date of delivery. Radio-iodine should not be used since this may accumulate in and destroy the fetal thyroid.

Centrally-acting drugs

Anti-epileptic drugs have been shown in several studies to cause approximately a doubling of the expected incidence of heart defects and cleft palate in the offspring of epileptic mothers. Because multiple drug therapy is common in this situation, it is not possible to state which drugs are the most likely offenders. From a fairly large number of clinical and animal studies carried out, it seems possible that any or all of the commonly used anti-epileptic drugs (phenobarbitone, phenytoin, primidone, ethosuximide and trimethadione) may be involved. There is insufficient evidence available at present to recommend the use or avoidance of any specific drug or combination. Coagulation defects resulting in neonatal haemorrhages have also been clearly demonstrated following phenytoin and phenobarbitone therapy. This can be treated by administration of vitamin K_1 to the mother during the last month of pregnancy. As there is little alternative but to use drugs in epileptic patients, it would seem advisable to continue with the lowest doses of the most effective drugs. This whole question is however at present under active review and these recommendations may change within the next year or so.

Hypnotics. The rational choice of a hypnotic for pregnant women is not at present possible because of the lack of adequate information. Because of the suspicions mentioned above about phenobarbitone, it may be advisable to use a non-barbiturate. Chloral hydrate, dichloralphenazone and triclofos, seem to be harmless in early pregnancy as are the phenothiazines, e.g. promethazine (Phenergan), and these may seem a wiser choice than the newer and less well tested hypnotics.

Conclusions

All drugs must be considered as having a potential for fetal toxicity in the same way as they do for adult toxicity. This toxicity will not be seen in all women treated, nor even in all fetuses in one woman – it is known for only one of a pair of twins to be affected. Furthermore, whether the drug crosses the placenta or not is irrelevant since there are many ways in which teratogenic effects can be produced by an action on the mother or placenta. Thus it is probable that drugs represent one factor in a multifactorial system leading to congenital defects.

No drug should be used in pregnant women (nor in anyone else) unless there is a real need for its use, and likewise no woman should be deprived of a drug who really needs it. The present evidence suggests that humans are relatively resistant to the teratogenic effects of drugs, since, despite wide differences in drug usage throughout the world, the incidence of congenital abnormalities is remarkably similar in different populations. However, with the increasing awareness of the possible long term effects that drug administration during pregnancy can have on the subsequent growth and physical and mental development of the offspring, it is as well not to feel too complacent.

Section B

Selected Aspects
of Therapy

Selected
Aspects
of Therapy

Edited by H. W. PROCTOR and P. S. BYRNE

Contents

1

COMMON EMERGENCIES

JOHN FRY

INTRODUCTION

It is a truism that 'common diseases commonly occur and rare diseases rarely happen'.

In approaching the management of the so-called 'common emergencies' it is appropriate first to consider the meaning and significance of all these terms, – common, emergency and management.

This part is designed to assist the physician to deal with emergency situations that he may expect to encounter on a number of occasions in any one year. The management is considered from the viewpoint of the young physician in hospital or in general medical practice.

Each section sets out to present a profile of the condition, its presentation and diagnostic procedures and its management in an emergency situation.

ACUTE BACK

The 'acute back' is a frequent cause of sudden disability seen in general medical practice.

The annual prevalence is 25 per 1000, so that the general practitioner or primary physician who cares for a population of 2500 may expect to treat at least one such case each week.

More frequent in males than in females, the age-prevalence shows that it is a condition of active adult life with a peak in the sixth decade (50–59). This type of age-prevalence curve suggests a mixture of degeneration and physical overactivity. Below middle-age the lumbosacral region is still supple enough to tolerate the stresses to which it is subject and after the age of 60 there occurs a natural rigidity and less activity. It is important, nevertheless, to appreciate the natural tendency to spontaneous decline in prevalence, since it will influence our management of a condition that is likely to improve naturally with age.

The causes of the 'acute back' syndrome are many and various. Most frequently it results from sudden damage to either intervertebral joints, discs or ligaments in the region of the lumbar 4th and 5th and 1st sacral vertebrae. Rarely is it secondary to some more serious conditions such as secondary malignant neoplastic deposits from a primary in the breast, bronchus, prostate, thyroid or kidney, or myelomatosis; to osteoporosis which may be idiopathic or associated with hyperparathyroidism; to ankylosing spondylitis; to spondylolisthesis or following a missed vertebral fracture; or from osteomyelitis caused by tubercle, staphylococci or other organisms.

Presentation and diagnosis

The common history is that of a sudden incapacitating pain in the lower lumbar and sacral region following a trivial movement such as stooping to tie a shoelace, making a bed or on lifting heavy weights. The pain is disabling and all movements tend to be restricted. The back is held in an erect position with considerable spasm of the sacrospinalis muscles.

Examination may help to localise the site of the causal lesion. Pain may occur on stretching the sacro-iliac joints and there may be limitation of the straight-leg-raise indicating a probable lesion at the level of the 5th lumbar and 1st sacral vertebrae. Referred pain down the legs (sciatica) occurs in approximately 20% of acute backs but signs of nerve root pressure, such as loss of ankle jerk, weakness of calf or thigh muscles or anaesthesia over the appropriate nerve segments of the skin, are found in less than 5% of episodes.

No examination is really complete without a palpation of the rectum to exclude a possible carcinoma of the prostate or other pelvic lesions.

Special investigations are not indicated initially in most cases but where there is no improvement within one or two weeks then a radiograph of the lumbo-sacral region, haemoglobin level, white blood cell count and erythrocyte sedimentation rate and serum phosphatase (alkaline and acid) are indicated.

The course in most cases is a rapid improvement. Two-thirds will recover within 3 weeks irrespective of the treatment given and only 5% will still be disabled after 2 months.

Management

The simplest therapy is the most successful. Rest, heat and analgesics should be tried first and persevered with for at least 2–3 weeks. Rest should be in the most comfortable position. This most often is lying flat and supine in bed with a board, to avoid sagging, between the mattress and bedstead.

Heat may be with hot water bottles, electric blankets or hot baths at home, or with infrared lamps.

Analgesics such as aspirin or paracetamol are usually adequate, but rarely opiates such as morphine injection or its derivatives, such as pethidine, may be necessary to control severe pain.

If no improvement has begun to occur within 2–3 weeks, then various physical therapies may be considered such as support to the lumbar spine through a spinal corset or plaster of paris cast; traction to distract lumbar vertebrae and in theory allow replacement of a prolapsed intervertebral disc; or manipulation by those who believe in intervertebral joint displacements and who are experienced in the techniques. Alternatively, injections of local anaesthetics, such as $\frac{1}{2}$ to 1 per cent lignocaine, can be given either into areas of local tenderness or into muscle 'nodules' if they can be demonstrated or into the epidural space by those experienced in the technique.

Surgery such as removal of prolapsed intervertebral discs or bone grafts to stiffen the lumbosacral region are required in very few cases. The indications for surgery are persistent nerve root pressure and particularly if there is pressure on the cauda equina with interference of micturition, or, repeated severe attacks, when a bone graft may occasionally be considered.

In my own experience some 90% of 'acute backs' will settle with simple measures, 10% will require physical therapy and less than 0.1% will be operated upon.

THE ACUTE NECK

The syndrome of acute pain in the neck with radiation down the arms and up the neck and head has a similar age prevalence to that of the acute back but in contrast the acute neck syndrome affects more women than men.

The cause is that of a degenerative spondylosis affecting intervertebral joints and a narrowing and collapse of the intervertebral discs. These changes lead to nerve root pressure and referred pain.

Presentation and diagnosis

Pain and stiffness of the neck may occur suddenly and spontaneously, often on awakening or following an incident such as a jolt or 'whiplash' injury in a motor car accident.

Radiation of pain depends on the nerve roots affected and there is often wasting of the muscles supplied by the affected nerves.

The diagnosis is confirmed by radiographic signs of cervical spondylosis with narrowing of disc spaces and osteophyte formation around the intervertebral joints.

Management

Rest and analgesics are the sheet anchors of management.

Rest with restrictions of movements is supplemented by local immobilisation with a felt or plastic collar, which should be worn until pain ceases, which may be a month or longer.

Analgesics are as for management of the acute back.

Physical measures involving cervical traction and manipulation have never been proved conclusively to be more effective than less active therapy.

Surgery, involving the removal of prolapsed intervertebral discs and bone grafting to fix segments of the cervical spine, should never be undertaken without a great deal of consideration, because of the general tendency for the acute conditions to settle with less drastic measures.

ACUTE ABDOMEN

A section on the 'acute abdomen' in a medical textbook is not misplaced. The diagnosis and management of this condition faces all physicians who practise in the medical front line.

Although not required to undertake definitive technical surgical procedures the primary physician, whether in hospital or in the community, has the responsibility of early diagnosis and making the vital decision on when to refer the patient for surgery.

In making the diagnosis the physician should not be too concerned to fit the exact aetiological and pathological label but rather to answer the question, is there an acute intra-abdominal crisis present that requires urgent surgical care or is it a condition that can continue to be managed by the physician?

Table 1. Surgical and non-surgical causes of the acute abdomen syndromes (in order of frequency)

Surgical	'Medical' (non-surgical)
1. Acute appendicitis	1. Acute tonsillitis (in young children)
2. The colics—renal and biliary	2. 'Spastic colon', 'The periodic syndrome' and other psychosomatic conditions
3. Acute intestinal obstruction	3. Pneumonia
4. Diverticulitis of colon	4. Cardiac and vascular—myocardial infarction, pericarditis, dissecting aneurysm and mesenteric thrombosis
5. Perforation of peptic ulcer	5. Herpes zoster (T.8–12)
6. Haemorrhage (intra-abdominal)	6. Bornholm disease (epidemic myalgia)
	7. Intestinal worms
	8. Acute haemolytic crises in malaria, sickle cell trait and other haemolytic anaemias
	9. Diabetic pre-coma
	10. Acute porphyria
	11. Tabes dorsalis

There are numerous non-surgical conditions with similar clinical manifestations which have to be excluded.

Aetiological types

The annual prevalence of the acute abdomen is approximately 3–4/1000. This means that the primary physician with 2500–3000 patients to care for will encounter some 7–12 cases each year or less than one each month, and the large district general hospital may expect to admit around 500–700 'acute abdomens' each year, or two a day.

There are many possible types of 'acute abdomen' and some of these may be non-surgical. Table 1 gives a list of these in the order of frequency as seen by the primary physician.

Clinical presentation and diagnosis

The prominent symptoms of an acute abdomen are abdominal pain and vomiting. Any abdominal pain that persists for more than 6 hours is increasingly likely to be a surgical case.

Abnormal signs may consist of abdominal tenderness, rigidity and distension. General features of collapse and shock may be present.

A systematic diagnostic approach is essential for correct management.

The history, possibly, is of greater importance than the examination or even the investigations and as much time should be allowed for talking with the patient and relatives as for examination and investigation.

Since pain is the most striking symptom, attention must be paid to its analysis.

The exact time and mode of onset are helpful. The most sudden and dramatic onset is with perforation of a gastric or a duodenal ulcer or with conditions such as a rupture of the ab-

dominal aorta with dissection and tracking of the blood. Equally dramatic is the collapse and faint that may accompany an acute pancreatitis or rupture of a pregnant uterine tube.

A more gradual build up of pain occurs in appendicitis, the colics and intestinal obstruction, but where there is strangulation of bowel or torsion of a cyst then the onset usually is quite sudden. With medical conditions the onset tends to be gradual except in rupture of the abdominal aorta; and in some cases of myocardial infarction, pneumonia and porphyria.

Information on the nature of the pain depends on the ability of an acutely sick person to tell his story. In intestinal obstruction and the colics the pain is intermittent and in women is likened to labour pains; in appendicitis it is constant, dull and aching; in a perforated gastric or duodenal ulcer it is diffuse, burning and immobilising; in dissecting abdominal aneurysm it is tearing; in acute pancreatitis it is agonising and unremitting.

The site may be fixed or the pain may shift or radiate. In a perforation it is usually 'all over the abdomen' from the start. Small intestine and appendicular pain is felt first in the epigastric and umbilical regions. Pain from the large bowel is generally in the lower abdomen. Biliary colic is referred to the epigastric or to the right subcolics and appendicitis than with obstructions of groins.

Pains referred to the abdomen from non-surgical conditions are generally mid-abdominal. Thus pain from a myocardial infarction, diabetic pre-coma or hiatus hernia tend to be epigastric, whereas in the 'periodic syndrome' of children and in tonsillitis, porphyria and haemolytic crises the pain is central or lower abdominal.

Vomiting may occur as a result of obstruction of the bowels, ureters or biliary ducts or from reflex nervous irritation. Pain tends to precede vomiting in most acute abdominal conditions and it occurs earlier with reflex causes as in the colics and appendicitis than with obstructions of the small and large bowel.

Any significant change in bowel habits is important. Constipation with no flatus may be indicative of a large bowel obstruction but this may occur over a few days. Diarrhea is a confusing symptom. It is dangerous to assume that it is suggestive of a common enteritis; in association with lower abdominal pain and tenderness it may well be a feature of a much more serious pelvic peritonitis. The presence of blood is always highly significant and may occur in intussusception or with a neoplasm of the large bowel or rectum.

Special attention should be paid to the menstrual pattern and any changes or characteristics suggestive of ovulatory pain, and irregular losses together with a late onset of a period may occur in a tubal pregnancy or in an abortion.

The examination of a patient with an acute abdomen must always include a rectal and vaginal examination, as well as a routine examination of the chest, cardiovascular and central nervous systems.

Investigations are by no means always necessary to establish the diagnosis but should always be carried out in assessing patients for possible surgery.

Radiographs of the chest and abdomen may be required. The former to exclude an intrathoracic lesion or to assess the state of the lungs and the size of the heart in surgical cases, and the latter in possible cases of intestinal obstruction to observe distension of coils of intestines and fluid levels, in cases of an intussusception following a barium enema and in biliary or renal colic to detect calculi.

Blood examination should check the level of haemoglobin and the various indices, a blood smear should be examined for leucocytosis, abnormal red blood cells (sickling and spherocytosis), white blood cells (leukaemia) and malarial parasites. Serum electrolytes should be measured in order that any correction by intravenous therapy may be made.

The urine must always be examined not only for albumin and sugar but also on a slide for pus and red blood cells. In difficult and uncertain situations the urine should also be tested for porphyrins.

Management

The physician has a number of decisions to make and to make them fairly quickly.

1. Is the condition an 'acute abdomen' or is it secondary to some other disorder?
2. Is it surgical and therefore to be referred to a surgeon?
3. If uncertain can one wait and observe and investigate or proceed to more active measures?

These decisions must be taken alone or in consultation on the clinical diagnostic bases enumerated. It is best always, and it should be possible, to seek the advice of a surgeon when in doubt over diagnosis or management.

In general terms the management comprises the following components. During the first 24–48 hours it is advisable to withhold solid food but to allow fluids if there is no vomiting.

Vomiting, if it is repeated, will require tubesuction in association with intravenous fluids.

Control of pain will generally require potent analgesics such as morphine or pethidine, but it is dangerous and unsafe to rely on these before a diagnosis has been made and a plan of management decided upon. Specific therapy must depend on the causal condition.

ACUTE VOMITING AND/OR DIARRHEA

There are two main portals of entry into the human body – through the respiratory and the alimentary tracts. It is not surprising therefore that both tracts are liable to suffer from infections and irritants that are inhaled and ingested, and that respiratory and gastrointestinal infections are the two most common disorders in the community.

Not only is the alimentary tract affected directly by infection or irritation but it can be affected also indirectly through metabolic disturbances as in diabetes, pregnancy, thyroid and renal disorders and through the central nervous system by involvement of the vomiting centre in the brain.

The most frequent causes of vomiting and diarrhea are acute infections. It is possible that most of these are viral when no pathogenic bacteria can be found on investigation. The condition is more or less endemic in all places with bouts of extra cases that may add up to local epidemics on occasions. Local inhabitants appear to become resistant to these local organisms but visitors, especially to the tropics, soon succumb but even here often no specific bacterial organisms can be isolated from the stools.

Of course there are specific bacterial infections such as dysentery, typhoid fever and cholera but these are much more rare, particularly typhoid and cholera, than the non-specific and possibly viral gastroenteritis.

In infants certain strains of *E. coli* are pathogenic and may in institutions assume epidemic proportions, whilst in certain situations such as after prolonged antibiotic therapy in debilitated patients *Staphylococcus pyogenes* may cause severe and dangerous entero-colitis.

Food poisoning

Food poisoning may occur from bacterial toxins, bacterial infection, chemical contaminants or allergy.

Staphylococcal food poisoning is caused by the ingestion of preformed toxins which have accumulated in foods such as artificial cream, custards, trifles and cream cakes. The foods are contaminated by handlers with staphylococcal lesions and the organisms and their toxins are not destroyed by cooking.

The onset with vomiting occurs a short while after ingestion (1–3 hours) and is followed by diarrhea and a variable degree of malaise and collapse.

Cl. welchii is another organism that causes a toxin type of food poisoning. It is transmitted by stored or recooked meat products such as meat pies.

Bacterial food infections are caused by the salmonellae, especially *Salmonella typhimurium,* dysentery, staphylococci or occasionally streptococci.

The onset usually is delayed until the ingested bacteria have grown sufficient in numbers to cause symptoms, that is 24–36 hours after infection. Profuse diarrhea is the main symptom and in a salmonella infection is likely to persist for many days unless treated with antibiotics.

Chemical, plant or allergic food poisoning from cooking vessels, cooking ingredients, fungi and berries or shellfish results in vomiting followed by diarrhea within 2 hours of ingestion.

Vomiting

Apart from accompanying the common acute gastro-enteritis this vomiting may occur without diarrhea. Epidemics of vomiting do occur and are probably also caused by a variety of undefined viruses. The so-called 'epidemic winter vomiting' disease is one such syndrome.

Repeated and sudden vomiting may occur in cases of duodenal ulcer when obstruction as a result of spasm, edema or scar stenosis develops.

As part of the 'acute abdomen syndrome' vomiting usually follows pain.

Acute vomiting may occur in myocardial infarction in association with chest pain and collapse; in renal conditions such as renal colic,

acute nephritis and anaemia; in diabetic precoma and glaucoma.

Vomiting may be the first feature of pregnancy and when a young woman, previously fit, comes with recent nausea and vomiting as symptoms the first question that should be asked is the date of her last menstrual period.

In migraine, vomiting follows headache and in other central nervous system conditions such as meningitis and space occupying lesions the vomiting is but one feature, the others being headache and disturbance of consciousness.

Acute diarrhea

Infections, already referred to, are the most frequent causes of acute diarrhea but on rare occasions ulcerative colitis with slime, pus and blood in the faeces, and cancer of the colon and rectum may present acutely.

Clinical presentation and diagnosis

Nine out of ten cases of acute vomiting and diarrhea are caused by an infection.

Vomiting followed a few hours later by watery diarrhea and accompanied by abdominal pain, fever and various degrees of malaise and collapse are the clinical features of a gastrointestinal infection.

The course in most instances is towards a natural and spontaneous resolution within 2–3 days.

In the majority of cases special investigations are unnecessary and unhelpful. It is only when some unusual cause or epidemic is suspected such as food poisoning, a metabolic disease, an intracranial lesion or an acute abdomen, or if the condition is not beginning to settle within 48 hours, that special investigations are indicated.

If food poisoning is suspected then specimens of or the whole remnant of the possible causal food should be sent for bacteriological examination, and faeces should be examined for salmonella and dysentery organisms.

If the person has collapsed then blood examination for electrolyte and haematocrit levels is necessary as a preliminary to possible intravenous fluid therapy.

Management

On the assumption that most cases will resolve spontaneously within 48 hours and provided that no other serious condition is suspected and that the general condition is good then 'expectant measures' are all that is required.

These measures consist of avoiding solid food, taking fluids by mouth if they are retained, and rest. If it is felt that the patient expects some medication then a mixture of kaolin, 10 ml 2-hourly, is reasonable.

It is quite wrong to give antibiotics or sulphonamides or some other chemical antiseptics blindly on the assumption that the cause is a bacterial infection. In the great majority of the common infections no pathogenic bacteria can be detected and the condition settles rapidly and well without these potent drugs.

It is also wrong to take prophylactic antibiotics (these themselves can cause diarrhea) or chemical antiseptics on travelling to foreign lands. There is no proof that they are helpful.

Naturally specific conditions once diagnosed will require specific remedies and in severe cases dehydration will require intravenous fluids, particularly in infants and in the aged.

GASTROINTESTINAL HAEMORRHAGE

Bleeding from the gastrointestinal tract may occur from any part but in practice it is the esophagus, stomach, duodenum and the large bowel that contain the lesions which account for most of the incidents.

Bleeding from the esophagus, stomach and duodenum is manifest by vomiting of blood (haematemesis) but if some of the blood passes through the stomach and intestines it will pass through and be excreted as black altered blood (melaena). Bleeding from the small and large intestines tends to be unaltered and bright red.

Serious gastro-duodenal haemorrhage is not all that frequent in practice. A primary physician caring for a population of 2500–3000 may expect no more than 1–2 cases a year, whereas a large district hospital may admit annually between 100–200 cases.

Profuse bleeding from the lower bowel is less frequent, although minor bleeds are common and present as diagnostic rather than therapeutic problems.

Causes

Haematemesis and melaena

Acute and chronic gastric and duodenal ulcers account for 85% of all cases. The acute erosive ulcers occur chiefly in the stomach and are a separate condition from the chronic penetrating varieties. In many acute ulcers there is a history of ingestion of aspirin or similar drugs immediately before the bleeding occurs and it is likely that these substances are responsible.

Bleeding from esophageal varices which develop from cirrhosis of the liver or some other obstruction of the portal circulation accounts for between 2.5 and 5% of all cases, depending on the prevalence of chronic alcoholic cirrhosis.

Hiatus hernia and gastro-esophageal reflux (2.5%) cause an esophagitis with occasional ulceration of the lower esophagus. This tends to cause chronic bleeding but on occasions this may be acute and profuse.

Other possible causes are gastric or esophageal neoplasms (2.5%), rupture of the lower esophagus (Mallory–Weiss syndrome) (2.5%), and a variety of conditions such as rupture of an aortic aneurysm, gastric polyps and acute gastritis.

A condition of uncertain origin causing diffuse bleeding from the stomach is gastrostaxis. This is rare but extremely difficult to treat.

When considering haematemesis it is always necessary to differentiate between a true bleeding from the gastro-duodenal region and vomiting of swallowed blood after dental or nasal haemorrhage.

Bleeding through the rectum

Blood per rectum may originate anywhere along the intestinal tract from the duodenum downwards. Blood that has passed through the stomach by regurgitation will be altered and black (melaena) but blood from the small and large bowels may pass through quickly and be bright red in colour.

Causes of sudden and profuse bleeding per rectum are in order of frequency, melaena from bleeding gastric or duodenal ulcers; haemorrhoids, although usually the bleeding is slight and recurrent; rectal or colonic neoplasms that have eroded largish vessels; polyps of the small and large intestines; ulcerative colitis (although rarely is bleeding profuse, more often it is of small amounts and mixed with slime and pus); an ectopic gastric ulcer in a Meckel's diverticulum; lesions in the terminal ileum such as ileitis; and sometimes in spite of repeated investigations no cause for a single sudden and profuse bleed can be found.

Gastrointestinal haemorrhage may occur in a haemorrhagic disorder such as thrombocytopenia or telangiectasia, or in someone on anticoagulants, and this possibly should be borne in mind when no clear explanation is evident.

Clinical presentation

The case may present clearly with a history of vomiting blood or bleeding per rectum, but it is not unusual for it to present as some feature of a sudden and hidden internal haemorrhage.

Vomited blood may be either fresh, but darker than normal, or it may appear as 'coffee grounds' as a result of some retention and digestion in the stomach.

Blood per rectum may be black and tar-like if its passage has been through the stomach and intestines or bright red from lesions in the large intestine.

Sometimes the first feature is not an obvious bleed associated with vomiting or passage of blood per rectum but an effect of the sudden and severe hidden internal haemorrhage. An unexpected faint in a previously fit man; collapse with malaise, headache, pallor, thirst, cold sweat and dyspnea; and sudden onset of angina of effort and even myocardial infarction, all these may delay the early diagnosis unless specific questions are asked about the colour of the stools and nature of any vomit.

General investigations are designed to determine the presence of any coincident diseases and a chest radiograph, electrocardiograph, urinalysis and estimation of blood urea, serum electrolytes and blood cells may be indicated.

Diagnosis

Cause of the bleeding

Remembering that more than four out of five gastro-duodenal bleeds are caused by acute or chronic ulcers, it is possible from the history, physical examination, endoscopy and radiography to establish an accurate diagnosis in the majority.

A history of intermittent dyspepsia supported by a positive finding after a barium meal makes a chronic ulcer likely.

Acute gastric ulcers or erosions have no previous history of dyspepsia but often are associated with taking aspirin, alcohol, phenylbutazone and similar drugs, or corticosteroids.

Esophageal varices should be considered where there is a palpable spleen, spider naevi, 'liver palms' and of course a history of alcoholism.

Alteration of bowel habits, symptoms of intermittent intestinal obstruction, colicky abdominal pain and distension, are suggestive of neoplasms of lower bowel and all cases must have a rectal examination performed.

The extent and detail of investigations must depend on the state of the patient, on the available facilities and expertise and on the confidence in the clinical assessment. In most specialist units esophagoscopy, gastroscopy and sigmoidoscopy with the less traumatic fibrescopes, and radiology with barium or gastrografin contrast media are possible within a few hours after resuscitation.

Assessment of blood loss

It is dangerous and inaccurate to rely solely on the history and the general state of the patient to assess the amount of blood loss. A persistent pulse rate of over 100 per minute and a systolic blood pressure below 100 mmHg make blood transfusion urgently necessary. An initial level of haemoglobin may be fallacious as it may be falsely high before haemodilution has taken place.

Haematocrit levels and indices such as MCV and MCHC are more useful.

Management

Although the bleeding ceases spontaneously in many instances it is safer to transfer to hospital all cases with anything more than apparently small bleeds. However, no cases should be transported if in a state of severe shock. It should be possible to resuscitate the patient at home or wherever the incident has occurred with intravenous fluids and other measures before the ambulance ride which may itself be traumatic and disturbing.

In general the following steps should be taken in hospital after the preliminary case history has been taken and examination carried out:

Arrangements for possible blood transfusion

A blood sample should be taken for haemoglobin and other blood examination and for blood grouping and cross matching with at least 2–3 litres of blood, which must then be kept available constantly. Blood transfusion is indicated in patients who appear clinically shocked with a pulse rate of over 100 and systolic blood pressure below 100 mmHg. It is indicated particularly in the elderly but here the dangers of circulatory overloading are very real.

Constant observation and assessment

Pulse rate and blood pressure levels should be recorded every half-hour and close attention paid to any clinical deterioration.

Rest and sedation

Bed rest is essential until it becomes clear that bleeding has ceased and the general condition is improving.

In spite of theoretical objections, morphine in 15 mg subcutaneous injections every 4–6 hours still is, in my opinion, the best sedative in these cases.

Gastric aspiration is indicated only with repeated vomiting and where it is thought that there is residual blood in the stomach.

Diet

A light diet with adequate fluids should be allowed from the very onset. Starvation does not prevent re-bleeding and leads rapidly to dehydration.

Surgery

Gastrointestinal bleeding is a situation for joint action by physician and surgeon. Emergency surgery is now relatively safe, even in the elderly, and it will be indicated when bleeding continues or recurs over 2–3 days, in the elderly more than in the young and middle-aged, and where there are causal lesions that may require definitive surgical treatment.

The results of management of gastrointestinal bleeding severe enough to require hospitalisation should aim at a mortality of less than 1% in those under the age of 60, and less than 10% in those over 60.

ACUTE POISONING BY OVERDOSAGE OF DRUGS

In the United Kingdom there are 24 000 attempted suicides admitted to hospital each year and 6000 suicides. This means that there will be 1–2 cases annually per general practitioner and more than one case admitted each week to a large district hospital.

More than two-thirds of these suicides and attempted suicides are the results of overdosage with drugs.

Acute poisoning by drugs comprises two other smaller groups – accidental poisoning, most often in young children who discover some attractive looking pills and eat them, and criminal poisoning in an attempt at murder.

The whole question may be associated with emotional drama, legal and police involvement.

The following are the most usual drugs that are responsible for acute poisoning:

1. Barbiturates   60% } 2/3 of total cases
   Tranquillizers   5% }
2. Salicylates   15%
3. Coal gas   10%
4. Others   10%

The high frequency of poisoning by barbiturates and similar preparations is a result of the prevalent use of these drugs for persons suffering from depression and other emotional disorders. It is not surprising therefore that access to an accumulating quantity of sleeping pills offers ready opportunities for overdosage.

The specific effects of the common poisons depend on the individual drug but in large doses they affect the central nervous system, respiration and circulation, and when death occurs it is due to the depression and ultimate failure of these systems.

Presentation and diagnosis

The presentation is dramatic. The victim usually is discovered by friends or relatives in a drowsy or unconscious condition. The situation is full of emotion and upset.

As much information as possible should be obtained from all available sources on the recent mental state of the victim and on previous physical and mental illnesses. Suicide notes are useful guides. The approximate time of the ingestion of the drugs is important in assessing the duration of its action. Identification of the drug should be established as soon as possible. Some may remain and the name of the drug may have been written on the container.

The case may present as one of 'coma' and in the elderly and the middle-aged, overdosage of drugs must be considered in the differential diagnosis of a cerebrovascular accident.

If the victim is not found for some hours, and particularly if he decides to perform the act of suicide out of doors, there will be the added dangers of exposure and hypothermia.

General management

The aim of treatment of acute poisoning must be to save life and restore the victim to health. Under modern conditions in a well-equipped and staffed unit it should be possible to reduce the mortality, in patients admitted alive, to below 1%.

The general management comprises a mixture of supportive measures and active therapy and skill lies in arriving at the best mix of the two.

It is safer to admit to a hospital with necessary services all patients who have taken an overdose of drugs, either intentionally or accidentally. The primary physician has the role of making the probable diagnosis of overdosage, of collecting information on the drugs ingested and in applying emergency aid and arranging for the transfer of the patient to hospital. It may be necessary to carry out resuscitation and intubation and mechanical ventilation prior to moving the patient in severe cases.

The definitive management consists of the following steps:

1. Keeping the patient alive.
2. Removing the poison.
3. Increasing the elimination of the drug.
4. Managing any underlying psychiatric condition that led to the self-poisoning and arranging for after-care of the individual.

5. Deciding on the steps, if any, to be taken to inform the police or other authorities.

6. Applying, if in difficulty, to an information service (e.g. 'Poisons Bureau' – or the drug manufacturer) on the nature and content of preparations ingested and on the correct management.

Keeping the patient alive

During the journey to hospital it is essential that the airway be kept clear in the unconscious patient who should be transported in the semi-prone position with an airway in place.

Admission should be to a ward or unit equipped for intensive care and blood-gas analysis.

If the patient is deeply unconscious then the airway must be maintained by means of a cuffed endotracheal tube which can be left in place for up to 72 hours.

Oxygen should be given in high concentration. Bronchial and tracheal secretions should be aspirated and assisted mechanical ventilation started if the patient is cyanosed with feeble spontaneous circulation or if the blood gases are seriously disturbed.

Shock and hypotension should be treated by elevating the foot of the bed and injecting intra-muscularly metaraminol 5 mg and repeated once only after ½–1 hour if necessary. If there is no response and blood pressure remains low then blood transfusion or the infusion of plasma or dextran should be started and the amounts given controlled by frequent recording of the pulse rate and blood pressure and by monitoring the central venous pressure.

For dehydration and electrolyte balance in the patient who is unconscious for more than 24 hours, one litre of 5% dextrose and half a litre of normal saline in alternation should be administered (in 24 hours).

Cardiac failure requires rapid but careful digitalisation and cardiac arrhythmias, which are likely with overdose of the tricyclic anti-depressants should be controlled with lignocaine or propranolol.

Convulsions may occur in unconscious patients in poisoning with tricylic antidepressants and phenothiazines, and curarisation with controlled ventilation may be necessary.

Prophylatic antibiotics are rarely necessary and should be used only when there is evidence of respiratory infection. Bladder catheterisation is not required and analeptics have no virtue.

Successful outcome will depend to a large extent on a high standard of nursing team care.

Removal of the poison

If the poison has been swallowed then removal can be helped by vomiting and washing out the stomach.

If the poison has been inhaled then the patient should be moved into the fresh air and oxygen administered.

If the poison has been absorbed from the skin then the clothes should be removed and the skin washed.

Most poisons are ingested. It is dangerous to induce vomiting in the drowsy or unconscious patient. Ipecacuanha and apomorphine should not be used. Vomiting should not be induced in the very old and the very young, in petroleum or corrosive poisoning, in those with previous gastric operations and in alcoholics, and it is useless to wash out the stomach more than four hours after ingestion.

In the conscious patient vomiting can be induced by drinking salt water or by inserting fingers down the back of the mouth.

In the unconscious patient the stomach can be washed out through an adequately sized tube (Jacques 30 English gauge) but only with a cuffed endotracheal tube in place.

Elimination of poison

There are no general antidotes. Most cases of poisoning through overdosage will recover without active measures designed to increase elimination provided that supportive measures are adequate.

If increased elimination is required then forced diuresis (by frusemide or intravenous mannitol), peritoneal dialysis, haemodialysis, passage of blood over ion-exchange resins or even exchange transfusions may be considered.

Barbiturate overdosage

Poisoning with barbiturates accounts for 60% of all cases of poisoning and most of these occur in patients already being treated for depression or other psychiatric illnesses. The risks should be appreciated whenever these drugs are prescribed and when they are all containers should be labelled with the name of the contents.

The effects of excessive barbiturates are depression of the central nervous system leading to drowsiness and coma, to depression of respiration and respiratory failure, to depression of the vasomotor centre with shock and hypotension, and to interference with temperature control and thus leave a liability to hypothermia.

Diagnosis depends on a good history, the

identification of the ingested preparation and on the level of blood barbiturates.

The prognosis depends on the degree of severity which is measured by the depth of unconsciousness:

Mild cases (60% of all barbiturate poisoning) are those who are drowsy but conscious.

Moderate cases (30%) are stuporose but responsive to painful stimuli.

Severe cases (10%) are comatose and non-responsive. Assessment of these grades is often more accurate clinically than biochemically.

The levels of serum barbiturates are useful. With moderately quick-acting barbiturates levels of more than 2–3 mg/100 ml are indicative of a severe overdose and the rapid absorption of the drug and with slow-acting barbiturates a level of more than 8–10 mg/100 ml of barbiturate suggests severe overdose.

Management

The mild cases do not require any specific therapy but should be seen and assessed by a psychiatrist prior to discharge. He should arrange after-care and support.

The moderate cases who are stuporose but rousable require the application of standard methods.

The respiration must be maintained through a clear airway (intubation if necessary) with oxygen and assisted mechanical ventilation if necessary.

The stomach may be washed out (with endotracheal tube in place) up to four hours after ingestion.

Shock and hypotension may require raising foot of bed, metaraminol and transfusion.

The severe cases in order to maintain life may require increased elimination of drugs by forced diuresis with intravenous dextrose and saline, mannitol or frusemide, or by peritoneal or haemodialysis.

Salicylates

Ingestion of large numbers of aspirin tablets is the second most common form of drug overdosage (15% of all poisoning).

The effects are to cause salicylism with ketosis, respiratory alkalosis and metabolic acidosis. Accompanying this there is dehydration and acid–base upsets.

Clinically there is vomiting, tinnitus, deafness, dizziness and excitability. There is sweating, over-breathing, fever and dehydration. Eventually, in severe cases, coma, collapse and death ensue.

Blood salicylate levels offer a guide to severity. In adults cases are considered to be severe when the blood salicylate level is more than 70 mg/100 ml, and moderate when it is over 50 mg/100 ml. In children a level of 30 mg/100 ml and over, is dangerous.

Management

Up to twelve hours after ingestion a stomach wash out with sodium bicarbonate under suitable precautions is advisable.

Mild cases can be treated with copious oral fluids.

Moderate cases showing a blood salicylate level of over 50 mg per 100 ml should have forced diuresis encouraged with intravenous saline, dextrose and sodium lactate.

Severe cases in coma and with a salicylate level of more than 70 mg per 100 ml may require haemodialysis in a special unit.

Iron

Ingestion of brightly coloured iron tablets is a hazard in young children and causes a haemorrhagic gastritis and acidosis.

Many cases settle spontaneously under observation.

In severe cases the chelating agent desferrioxamine should be used to inactivate the iron as soon as possible. It can be used intravenously, instilling 80 mg/kg over 24 hours, or by intramuscular injection 2 g 12-hourly until the condition improves. It is also useful to wash out the stomach and leave a 5 g solution in 50 ml of fluid in the stomach.

ACUTE CORONARY ARTERY DISEASE

The clinical spectrum of acute coronary artery disease is a wide one.

Sudden and unexpected deaths account for 20% of all forms. There is usually a preceding history of 'indigestion' that may be worse on effort, for a few hours or even days before the victim is found dead or collapses and dies within minutes.

Angina is the first sign of acute coronary artery disease in another 20% of cases. The presternal pain that radiates down the left or both arms is brought on by effort, cold or emotional upsets.

In myocardial infarction the chief clinical feature is a heavy and constant presternal pain that persists for hours.

The category of acute coronary artery insufficiency is unnecessarily confusing and represents a mild form of infarction rather than a specific category.

Clinically three grades of severity can be recognised:

The 'mild' myocardial infarction (12% of all presenting types) is that type where the patient often walks into the consulting room with a history of classical coronary chest pain for variable periods during the preceding days associated with 'indigestion'. Electrocardiography confirms the diagnosis of myocardial infarction.

In the 'moderate' variety (35%) the patient is often seen at home, or is brought to hospital, with a history of severe anterior chest pain for an hour or longer. The patient is distressed but there are no signs of shock or cardiac failure. The pain and general condition improve and then clear within a few hours after an injection of morphine, or similar analgesic.

In the 'severe' type (13%) there is shock, hypotension, collapse and heart failure often from the very onset.

Coronary artery disease is a condition of ageing and degeneration and is not one affecting only middle-aged men, although it is this group that tends to present most suddenly and dramatically.

The place and time of the sudden deaths are of relevance. In a study in my own practice I found, for example, that 65% of all deaths from coronary heart disease occurred on the first day.

Of these 'first-day deaths' 70% occurred in the victim's own home, 13% in hospital and 17% elsewhere.

50% were 'instant' within 15 minutes of onset, 30% within 15–60 minutes of onset and 20% between 1–24 hours.

In theory, after excluding instant deaths and those with associated conditions that would have made resuscitation impossible, it was found in 36% of these sudden first-day-deaths resuscitation would have been possible and feasible – but 72% of these 'possibles' died at home and 80% within the first hour, so that speedy resuscitation outside hospital would have to have been available.

Presentation

The presenting clinical features of an acute myocardial infarction may be pain, collapse, dyspnea or arrhythmia.

The pain is most often presternal. It is a heavy pain as 'though someone is sitting on me' or 'crushing' or 'constricting'. It may radiate down the arms (left more often than right), up to the chin or through to the back. It may occur only at the referral sites namely arm, chin or back. The severity varies and the mild types may be regarded by the patient as unimportant 'indigestion'.

Diagnosis

The electrocardiogram (ECG) is the most useful investigation. Characteristically positive findings of a transmural infarction are deep Q waves, elevation of the S–T segments in leads facing the damaged area with reciprocal S–T depression in remote leads and symmetrical T wave inversion (further reference to a standard book on this subject should be made).

When present these changes are confirmatory but they may take a few days to develop and in some instances may never appear even in otherwise definite cases of myocardial infarction. In my opinion more reliance should be placed on the clinical assessment than on an ECG and other tests, and if it is considered clinically that the patient has sustained a myocardial infarction then, and if there is no evidence of other conditions, he should be managed as such in spite of repeated negative ECG changes.

A chest radiograph should be taken when diagnosis is uncertain to exclude other conditions such as pericardial effusion and lung lesions.

An elevation of the temperature often develops and persists for several days and, like an elevated erythrocyte sedimentation rate (ESR) and polymorph leucocytosis, is evidence of muscle damage.

Serum enzyme levels may be helpful with equivocal ECG tracings.

The serum glutamic oxaloacetic transaminase (SGOT) reaches its peak level 24–48 hours after infarction and should be tested for only at this time.

The serum lactic dehydrogenase (SLDH) is maximal later at 48–72 hours.

Management

The objectives of management are to save life during the immediate acute stage, prevent complications and rehabilitate to normal life whenever possible.

The most dangerous period is the first day and in particular the first hour after infarction. If care is to be optimal then the feasibility of special emergency ambulances staffed by physicians able to use resuscitative equipment should be considered. These ambulances are being used successfully in the large cities such as Moscow, Leningrad and Kiev in USSR, and in Belfast in Northern Ireland.

Whilst it is not possible to predict the course of any myocardial infarction and complications may occur even in 'mild' cases, in the first few days after onset the course and outcome are related closely to the clinical severity. The primary physician therefore is in a dilemma when faced with the management of the 'mild' and 'moderate' cases. Complications may occur but the course is benign in the majority of these cases. In an ideal situation the patient with a proven (or probable) myocardial infarction should be admitted to a hospital coronary care unit, equipped to deal with all possible complications, for 2–3 days. It is of doubtful value for the patient to be admitted to a hospital without such facilities, and he might as well be nursed at home.

The steps in management are:

1. Diagnosis and resuscitation at home or wherever the victim is found.

2. Transport to hospital if admission is considered necessary.

3. Intensive care and supervision for 2–3 days.

4. Progressive care in hospital for up to 2 weeks.

5. Rehabilitation at home.

The possibility of resuscitation at home by an emergency team has been referred to and facilities for resuscitation should be available also in the ambulance taking the patient to hospital. A sizeable proportion die in transit and if intensive care is to be given then it should commence as soon as skilled assistance reaches the patient.

Intensive care implies constant supervision by trained nursing staff, ECG monitoring and appropriate treatment for any complications that may arise.

Since the danger period is chiefly in the first two or three days after the infarction the patient's stay in the unit need not be any longer, unless he is on active treatment for a complication.

From the intensive care unit the patient is transferred to the general hospital wards where progressive ambulation can be carried out over the following weeks. Complete bed rest is not necessary and the aim should be for the patient to be ambulant in the ward within two weeks in an uncomplicated case.

Immediate care

Pain must be controlled and morphine is still the analgesic most widely used, 15 mg intramuscularly, or 5–10 mg intravenously for severe pain, should be given at once and repeated within an hour if there is no relief. Vomiting occurs in a proportion of patients after morphine, and diamorphine (heroin) is recommended by some as a better preparation in similar dosage. Those who do not wish to use opiates because of respiratory depression give pethidine 100 mg intramuscularly.

Oxygen is given when available at a rate of 4 1/min.

Anticoagulants are effective in reducing the likelihood of thromboembolic complications. They have no effect on the infarction. They are safe and should be given to younger patients, up to 65, and for all severe attacks unless there is a history of active peptic ulcer, presence of a pericardial friction rub, suggesting a transmural infarct, or a history of haemorrhagic disorders.

To effect immediate anticoagulation heparin in an initial intravenous dose of 10 000 units should be followed by an intravenous infusion for 48 hours. This should contain 40 000 units of heparin in 1 litre of 5% dextrose per 24 hours and will keep the whole blood-clotting time at twice the normal. Oral phenindione should be started on admission at 100 mg daily and the dose controlled by estimation of prothrombin time.

Complications

The death rate of patients admitted to hospital with acute myocardial infarctions is still between 15 and 30%.

The causes of death are:

Arrhythmias – 50%

Shock and heart failure – 43%

Thromboembolism – 5%

Ruptured myocardium – 2%

Arrhythmias should be detected by the continuous ECG monitor. Digoxin 0.5 mg followed by 0.25 mg 6-hourly is indicated for persistent atrial tachycardia and fibrillation (providing there is no history of previous digitalisation, when the dose must be modified).

Frequent ventricular ectopic beats predispose to ventricular fibrillation and are best prevented by adding lignocaine into the intravenous drip. The dose will depend on what is needed to achieve control of the arrhythmia but up to 6–8 g can be given in 24 hours. Alternatively oral propranolol up to 40 mg 6-hourly can be used.

Ventricular fibrillation is an emergency that is best treated by immediate electrical version with a synchronous DC defibrillator. If this is not available up to 50 mg of lignocaine should be injected slowly.

Cardiac arrest is due either to asystole or ventricular fibrillation. Mouth to mouth resuscitation and external cardiac massage should be started immediately and assistance summoned. Endotracheal intubation should be carried out and mechanical ventilation with oxygen commenced.

For ventricular fibrillation correction should

be attempted with the defibrillator and for asystole, pacing with an intracardiac pacemaker is indicated.

Metabolic acidosis should be anticipated and once the heart beat has been restored intravenous infusion with some bicarbonate (100 mEq initially) should be started.

Complete heart block is an early complication if it occurs and should be treated by pacing with an intracardiac pacemaker until rhythm is restored and the pacemaker should be left in situ for 5 days more. If not available then a long acting isoprenaline (such as Saventrine) may restore normal rhythm and prevent recurrence. Atropine by injection may also be tried.

Hypotension in association with shock is difficult to manage and when persistent carries a bad prognosis.

Raising the foot of the bed, oxygen and intravenous therapy are all that can be done.

Cardiac failure is treated with digitalisation, and diuretics.

CARDIAC ARRHYTHMIAS

Cardiac arrhythmias are not infrequent as medical emergencies. Some are benign and may occur in normal and healthy persons and others are the results of various disorders of the heart itself or conditions affecting the heart.

There are two groups. The ectopic tachycardias, including atrial, nodal and ventricular tachycardias and various forms of heart block.

Extrasystoles

Extrasystoles may occur in young persons with no cardiovascular abnormalities. There is no reliable treatment that controls them and reassurance with, perhaps, a sedative or minor tranquillizer, are all that is required.

In the middle-aged and elderly the appearance of extrasystoles may be the result of ischaemic heart disease and when they occur after an acute myocardial infarction they often are danger signals that herald paroxysms of ventricular tachycardia or fibrillation.

Extrasystoles may result from excessive dosage with digitalis and coupled rhythm is almost always due to this cause.

Control of extrasystoles that may be associated with ischaemic heart disease may be treated with digitalis (provided that it has not been given in the past few weeks), or with quinidine.

Paroxysmal supraventricular tachycardia

This usually occurs in young persons who often give a history of repeated attacks which start and stop suddenly. The function of the heart is usually not disturbed and the rhythm is regular. However, some cases may be associated with various underlying conditions such as thyrotoxicosis, rheumatic fever and ischaemic heart disease. Digitalis overdosage may cause a dangerous form of paroxysmal tachycardia in persons with heart failure and potassium depletion.

The attacks may last a few seconds or up to some hours. The rate is around 170–200 and the diagnosis is confirmed by ECG.

The management should be non-specific unless serious functional disturbance occurs.

Reassurance and sedation are necessary. Simple manoeuvres such as holding a deep breath, massage of the carotid sinus, eyeball pressure or an ice-cold drink may all cut short an attack.

Specific measures are rapid digitalisation, provided it has not been used in the past few weeks, quinidine, propranolol or electroversion.

Atrial flutter and fibrillation

These conditions are almost always portents of serious underlying disorders such as ischaemic heart disease, hypertension, rheumatic heart disease and thyrotoxicosis.

Paroxysmal bouts may occur for some years before a persistent arrhythmia is established.

Functionally, atrial fibrillation and flutter interfere with the work of the heart and may lead to left or right cardiac failure, and because there is some stagnation of blood in the atria, thrombi may form, and produce emboli in the lungs or peripheral arteries.

In atrial flutter the jugular vein pulsation is often more than twice the ventricular rate. The pulse is regular. Fibrillation produces a completely irregular pulse.

Diagnosis should be confirmed by ECG, which in flutter shows an inverted 'saw-tooth appearance' and in fibrillation a totally irregular ventricular rhythm with normal QRS complexes and fine coarse irregular 'f' waves.

Management of the acute case is by full digitalisation. An initial dose should be given of digoxin 1.0 mg followed by 0.5 mg 6-hourly for 48 hours and then 0.25 mg two, three or four times a day until control with minimal dosage is established.

In flutter the rhythm may be converted to fibrillation and then normality; fibrillation may persist; or the rhythm returns to normal. Recurrences are not uncommon.

In fibrillation the objective is primarily to control the heart failure and not simply the irregular rhythm.

In cases with a sudden and recent onset there

is a place for electroversion. This has now replaced quinidine for this purpose.

Paroxysmal ventricular tachycardia

This is associated with ischaemic heart disease and carries a serious prognosis and a high risk of death. There is always considerable functional disturbance with breathlessness, low blood pressure and raised venous pressure.

The ECG shows wide bizarre splintered complexes.

The most satisfactory treatment is electroversion. If this is not available then intravenous lignocaine should be given.

Heart block

Complete heart block is most frequent in old persons. It is most likely to be associated with ischaemic heart disease.

Heart block by itself causes little serious functional disturbance if it is stable. It is the Stokes–Adams attacks of syncope or near-syncope that occur with complete heart block and when there is a change from partial to complete block, that require emergency care.

The attacks occur when the heart rate suddenly drops to an unacceptable level of 10–15 beats/min or ceases altogether for a few seconds. There may be transient loss of consciousness with convulsions at times which may be confused with epilepsy. In other attacks consciousness is not lost but there is faintness, giddiness and a feeling of dying.

In most attacks the heart beat soon returns to its regular rhythm of around 30–40 beats/min, consciousness returns and circulation is restored. If this does not happen then a pacemaker (external or internal) is needed but this is not often readily available. Isoprenaline should be given intravenously or even intracardially.

The most satisfactory drug for prevention is the long-acting preparation of isoprenaline, Saventrine, which is given in 30 mg doses every 3–6 hours.

ACUTE DYSPNEA

In practice there are two important groups of sudden and severe breathlessness.

There are the various conditions that lead to acute left ventricular failure and those that lead to acute pulmonary insufficiency.

A result of better care and facilities for controlling the causes of both groups has meant that the numbers that present as emergencies has fallen – and since these were the reasons for

many 'night calls', so have the number of night calls.

ACUTE LEFT VENTRICULAR FAILURE

The condition occurs when the left half of the heart pump suddenly fails and the function of the right half remains unimpaired. The effects fall largely on the lungs and there is a build-up of back pressure in the small alveolar and pulmonary vessels with a slowing of blood flow and an outpouring of fluid into the alveoli, to produce pulmonary edema.

The pulmonary venous engorgement and edema fluid in the alveoli and connective tissues of the lungs, result in a decrease of lung compliance – leading to increased efforts to breathe, and a disturbance of ventilation and perfusion relationships. These abnormalities in function and the nerve reflexes from the distended tissues lead to the severe dyspnea of left ventricular failure.

The causes are:

1. Myocardial infarction. Acute myocardial infarction may present as acute left ventricular failure but more often it develops from the myocardial weakness some time after the acute episode.

2. Hypertension is found frequently in those who suffer from left ventricular failure. The reasons for its sudden appearance at night are uncertain but presumably it is as a result of strain on the left ventricle from attempting to circulate the blood against the high arterial resistance or as a result of the recumbent posture.

3. Less frequently the condition may complicate aortic valvular disease (aortic stenosis, regurgitation or mitral regurgitation).

4. Rarely paroxysmal tachycardias, intracardiac tumours and cardiomyopathies may also cause acute left ventricular failure.

5. Iatrogenically overloading the circulation in too rapid, or too profuse, intravenous transfusions may lead to pulmonary edema and breathlessness.

Clinical presentation

Although the severe attacks of breathlessness occur at night, often in the early hours between 11 p.m. and 1 a.m., there is usually a history of some dyspnea and cough on exertion for a few days before the acute episode.

The patient awakens with a 'heavy' 'tight' chest, severe breathlessness and a dry cough. Sitting up on the edge of his bed helps, but not very much. Clothes are then removed or loosened and finally the victim gets out of bed on to an open window to try and overcome the frightening suffocation. After a while the cough becomes bubbly and productive of a large amount of thin, frothy, pink, blood-stained sputum.

There is extreme distress and fear. The patient is ashen grey in colour with a cold and clammy skin. Auscultation reveals fine crepitations that are most marked at the lung bases. Triple rhythm of the heart is usual and often better felt than heard.

The rapid and alternating pulse may be felt or detected on measuring the blood pressure with a sphygmomanometer.

Management

No time should be lost in carrying out any further investigations such as chest radiography and electrocardiography.

The patient should be propped up in bed, if he is not already sitting up. Oxygen, if available, should be given at a rate of 6–8 1/min through a face mask until the breathing improves.

Morphine is the drug of choice and 15 mg should be given intramuscularly, or 10 mg intravenously in severe cases. The danger of morphine when there is uncertainty over the differentiation of this condition from chronic airway obstruction has been exaggerated and, as it is a life-saving measure, decision and action must be taken quickly.

The response is often dramatic and within 10–15 minutes breathing is easier and the patient relaxed and comfortable. If there is no satisfactory response then aminophylline 0.25 g should be given slowly intravenously. Intramuscular and rectal routes are unsatisfactory.

Diuretics should always be given. Frusemide 40 mg may be given by mouth, but there will be a delay of 30–60 minutes before diuresis commences. To obtain a more rapid response intravenous frusemide (20 mg) can be given.

The subsequent (within hours) treatment of the causes may include digitalisation, control of hypertension, management of the myocardial infarction and assessment of valvular lesions and possible surgical treatment.

Venesection used to be recommended as a heroic measure for acute left ventricular failure. It is a messy and unsatisfactory measure but it may have a place when the condition is the result of circulatory overloading by transfusions.

ACUTE PULMONARY INSUFFICIENCY

Acute dyspnea from pulmonary causes may be the result of the following:

1. Acute airways obstruction associated with wheezy bronchitis and bronchopneumonia or asthma. The obstructed airways may extend from the larger bronchi down to the smallest bronchioles and alveoli. The factors concerned in the obstruction may be contraction of the bronchial muscles, mucosal swelling from congestion and edema, plugging by viscid mucus and collapse of the smallest airways due to destruction and other damage.

2. Spontaneous pneumothorax is most often a disease of young healthy adults with no serious underlying disease. The cause is rupture of a small bulla or other lesion on the surface of a lung. This spontaneous rupture leads to a communication between the vacuum of the interpleural space and the air-containing lung. Air is rushed into the pleural cavity until the defect closes. The size of the pneumothorax depends on how much air escapes before self-closure of the defect. After closure the air is reabsorbed gradually and the lung expands. Recurrences are frequent.

Occasionally the defect may remain patent with a valve-like effect allowing air to escape into the pleural cavity but not to re-enter the lung. A gradual build up of positive intrapleural pressure results, this tension pneumothorax may compress vital mediastinal structures and lead to death. Occasionally spontaneous pneumothorax may complicate chronic airways disease and here it is always a most serious matter.

3. Massive lung collapse occurs most often after abdominal operations due to blockage of the large airways by sticky mucus and weak respiratory movements. This leads to an absorption collapse of the lung distal to the block.

Other causes of massive collapse are found in catarrhal children and chronic bronchitics whose thick, sticky and profuse sputum may cause similar blockage and distal collapse.

4. Laryngitis stridulosa. Although not strictly a pulmonary defect, inflammation and swelling of the larynx cause a 'croupy' cough and dyspnea.

Clinical presentation

In acute airways obstruction there is the shortness of breath accompanied by generalised expiratory wheezing in the chest and areas of collapse and crepitations. Severe obstruction results in carbon dioxide retention and hypoxaemia with cyanosis, confusion and restlessness, hot hands, rapid bounding pulse and signs of cor pulmonale (raised jugular venous pressure, triple rhythm and accentuation of pulmonary second sound).

There is almost always a history of previous attacks and 'chest troubles' with cough and sputum.

Spontaneous pneumothorax, when large enough, is detected clinically by reduced air entry, hyper-resonance, lack of movement and displacement of the mediastinum.

Diagnosis

Clinical findings are most helpful but in hospital a chest radiograph, sputum culture and measurement of arterial carbon dioxide and oxygen levels are useful.

Management

Acute airways obstruction is managed in the same way, whatever the cause.

1. Oxygen should be given with caution because with hypercapnia a vicious cycle may result with excessive oxygen, due to an unresponsive respiratory centre.

2. Bronchodilators. Aminophylline 0.25 g intravenously is safest for quick action. Corticosteroids should not be withheld for long in severe asthma and they may be beneficial also in chronic bronchitis and emphysema. If given by mouth a loading dose of up to 80 mg prednisone on the first day followed by a reduction of 5 mg daily is appropriate. In emergencies 100 mg of hydrocortisone hemisuccinate can be injected intravenously and then followed by oral prednisone.

3. Broad-spectrum antibiotics such as oxytetracycline or ampicillin 0.25 g 4-hourly should be started and continued until the results of sputum culture are available.

DIFFERENTIATION BETWEEN ACUTE CARDIAC AND PULMONARY DYSPNEA

Because management of these two types of dyspnea is different, differentiation is important.

It is usually not difficult and the following are useful clinical points.

1. A history of previous chest illnesses is always present with pulmonary causes, but it may well be that a respiratory cripple may suffer occasionally from an acute left ventricular failure.

2. Wheezing and rhonchi are features of pulmonary dyspnea, bubbling and crepitations are characteristics of left ventricular failure.

3. In acute cardiac dyspnea there are generally other features of heart trouble such as triple rhythm, alternating pulse, and features of causal disease such as myocardial infarction, hypertension or valvular heart disease.

SUDDEN COMA

The list of possible causes of coma is long and includes many unusual situations. For practical purposes the most frequent types of sudden coma

(prolonged unconsciousness) encountered in primary medical care are, in order of descending prevalence:

1. Cerebro-vascular accidents (strokes)
2. Head injuries
3. Drug overdosage (including alcoholism)
4. Epilepsy
5. Intracranial neoplasms
6. Meningitis and other intracranial infections
7. Metabolic disturbances such as uraemia, hypoglycaemia and diabetic coma.

The approach to any cause in coma must be orderly and systematic. It is necessary first to make as accurate a diagnosis as possible in order that suitable management may be carried out.

Although the initial situation is dramatic, once steps have been taken to ensure a free airway and satisfactory respiration, further diagnostic assessment need not be hurried.

Clinical presentation

The ways in which the case presents depend on the cause of coma and the form of onset, and the circumstances in which the patient is found will be helpful in diagnosis.

There may be a history of past disease as in diabetes and epilepsy, and the immediate history may suggest possible causes such as trauma, overdose with drugs, infections which may be related to a meningoencephalitis, or a history of progression to coma, as in some cerebro-vascular occlusions and haemorrhage.

Diagnosis

The clinical examination, whilst concentrating on the central nervous system must cover all systems.

Examination must be delayed until respiration is adequate and cerebral anoxia due to respiratory distress has been corrected.

The examination should be conducted towards answering questions that will influence management.

1. Is the cause intracranial?
2. Are there any specific and urgent therapeutic measures that ought to be taken?

In the central nervous system the pupils, fundi, muscle tone and reflexes must be examined and an assessment made of the level of consciousness. This is best tested by noting the response of the patient to certain stimuli such as shouting, shaking, pin pricks and pressure of the tendo-achilles. These tests should be repeated at regular intervals and a comparative record made.

Investigations should include urinalysis, radiograph or skull, blood count, ESR, and Wassermann and Kahn tests.

A lumbar puncture and examination of the cerebrospinal fluid should be made unless there is thought to be a raised intracranial pressure, with papilledema when it would be a dangerous act.

Management

The first essential is to ensure a free airway with adequate oxygenation. Routine care must include attention to posture, care of the skin, the state of hydration and control of urinary incontinence by an indwelling catheter.

Specific therapy will be necessary once a diagnosis has been made as in the management of drug overdosage, diabetes, hypoglycaemia, uraemia and meningitis.

Surgical intervention may be needed for head injuries and the possibilities of extradural or subdural haematomas should be borne in mind even after minor trauma.

ACUTE CHEST INFECTIONS

Acute chest infections are the most frequent group of major (life-threatening) disease in the community.

In the United Kingdom the annual prevalence rate of these conditions is 30 per 1000 and the general practitioner with a practice of 2500 may expect to treat 75 cases each year. Of these less than 10% require admission to hospital. The others respond satisfactorily to treatment at home.

Certain groups are particularly vulnerable and liable to chest infection. Males at all ages are more vulnerable than females; the young and the old are the age groups most likely to suffer and in children the peak prevalence is between 4 and 7 years of age, and in the elderly there is a gradual rise with age from 50 onwards. Sufferers from other chest conditions such as chronic bronchitis and emphysema, asthma, pneumoconiosis and other pulmonary fibroses and bronchiectasis are particularly liable to recurring infections. Tobacco smokers and those living in atmospherically polluted areas and the lower social groups all suffer from more than average amounts of chest infection.

The *classification* of acute chest infections may be on an *aetiological* basis where the condition is related to the specific causal organism or on a more practical *clinical or radiological* basis of presenting signs.

Aetiologically, chest infections may be caused by bacteria such as *Streptococcus pneumoniae, Staphylococcus pyogenes, Haemophilus influenzae, Klebsiella pneumoniae,* tubercle bacillus, or mycoplasma or viruses such as adenovirus, respiratory syncytial virus, the ornithosispsittacosis group, Q-fever, influenza and measles.

Unfortunately there is no clear and ready correlation between the causal organisms and the presenting clinical picture, and often there is a mixture of organisms responsible.

Clinically, diagnostic terms such as acute bronchitis, bronchopneumonia and various forms of pneumonias such as lobar, lobular, aspiration and segmental are described. However in practice it is better to rely on a combination of a number of co-ordinates such as the general condition of the patient, the clinical and radiological picture and the results of bacteriological and virological tests.

It should be recalled always that the acute chest infection may be secondary to a lesion such as a carcinoma of the bronchus or some other primary condition of the lungs.

Physio-pathological effects

The two major effects of acute chest infections are the infection and the results of interference with aeration because of airways obstruction with infiltration, and edema of the alveoli and pulmonary parenchyma. This results in anoxaemia, retention of carbon dioxide and acidosis. Interference to, and obstruction of, the pulmonary blood flow leads to pulmonary hypertension which may in turn lead to cor pulmonale or right heart failure.

Clinical presentation

Cough with sputum that is generally yellow or green in colour and which may be blood-stained, shortness of breath and pain in the chest are the local symptoms that suggest an acute chest infection. More generally, there is fever, with rigors on occasions and malaise; there may be cyanosis.

The signs in the chest fall into four main groups:

'Acute wheezy chests' with bilateral rhonchi and rales represent the diffuse type of acute bronchitis or bronchopneumonia. It is impossible to differentiate between the two clinically except on severity of illness and on radiographic signs of patchy consolidation. The acute wheezy chest is the most frequent clinical type of acute chest infection, accounting in the United Kingdom for more than one-half of all cases.

Segmental pneumonia denotes a specific clinical syndrome with irritating cough and some mucopurulent sputum and only a minor or moderate degree of illness. Chest signs are those of a local area of inspiratory moist rales or crepitations usually at one or other base of the lower lobes or over the lingula or middle lobe. This type of acute chest infection is also very frequent and accounts for up to 40% of all cases.

Amongst the remaining 10% of cases there are lobar pneumonias with a more severe illness and clinical signs of consolidation, the empyemata and other effusions which are now rather uncommon, acute pleurisy with a pleural rub as the only abnormal sign and others which may be variants of all the types or which may yield no abnormal physical signs although there is radiological evidence of infection.

Clinical evidence of a high carbon dioxide retention (more than PCO_2 of 49–50 mmHg) is hypercirculation with hot hands and a bounding pulse, congested retinal veins, papilledema on occasions, mental confusion, drowsiness and tremor of the hands.

Cor pulmonale (right heart failure) may be recognised by a raised jugular venous pressure, enlargement of the liver, edema of the legs and sacral pad and an accentuation of the second pulmonary heart sound.

Investigations must include a chest radiograph, bacteriological and possibly virological examination of the sputum, haemoglobin, ESR, white blood cell count and possibly levels of PCO_2 and PO_2. An electrocardiograph may also be useful.

Management

There are four parts to the management of acute chest infections:

Infection

Treatment should be started at once in most cases without waiting for the result of the bacteriological identification of the causal organism, which is only possible in less than one-half of all cases.

The antibiotics most suitable are either intramuscular penicillin 1 megaunit 8–12 hourly, oral ampicillin 0.25–0.5 g 6-hourly or oxytetracycline 0.25–0.5 g 6-hourly. One of these preparations should be started and the progress reviewed. If there is no improvement within 36–48 hours, or if the report on the sputum suggests resistant organisms then other antibiotics should be considered.

Airways obstruction

It is the 'acute wheezy chest' that presents the greatest problem with a mixture of bronchospasm, edema and mucus obstruction. Aminophylline by intravenous injection (0.25 g) or by suppository; corticosteroids by intravenous injection of hydrocortisone (100 mg) or by oral prednisone, up to 60–80 mg daily to start with; or various antispasmodics such as salbutamol (4 mg) or orciprenaline (20 mg) – 4-hourly – all these may be tried, but often without much success.

Respiratory failure

In respiratory failure carbon dioxide retention occurs and the respiratory centre becomes less sensitive to the stimulus of the circulating levels of oxygen and carbon dioxide.

Whilst oxygen is essential for respiratory failure it must not be given continuously or in too high a concentration too quickly, because this may lead to even greater hypercapnia.

When the respirations are weak and there is difficulty in expectoration then aspiration and sucking out of bronchial secretions through a bronchoscope may be necessary and in more severe cases a temporary tracheostomy or intubation and mechanical ventilation may be indicated.

Cor pulmonale

When present treatment should be by digitalisation and diuretics.

ASTHMA

It is difficult to separate 'asthma' from the other types of 'acute wheezy chests'. It is true, as Chevalier Jackson remarked many years ago, that 'not all that wheezes is asthma'.

In looking at 'acute wheezy chests', we find that age-prevalence is a U-shaped curve with greatest involvement of the young and elderly.

The syndrome of the acute wheezy chest includes three definable and separable types – wheezy children, acute episodes in chronic bronchitis and emphysema, and asthma.

Acute wheezing in the chest affects no less than one child in every four in their first decade (Fry, J. 'The Catarrhal Child', 1961, London).

The great majority (95%) cease these attacks, which are a response of a sensitive and immature respiratory tract to infection, as they grow older and fewer than 5% become true asthmatics.

Acute exacerbations of chronic bronchitis are characterised by wheezing in the chest and dyspnea and have to be distinguished from asthma.

Excluding these two large groups of chest wheezers there is asthma which may be defined as 'paroxysmal attacks of acute airways obstruction unassociated with any underlying pulmonary disease'.

The annual incidence of asthma in my own practice over 20 years has been 2/1000, which means that in a country such as the United Kingdom there are 1 million asthmatics.

The annual mortality from 'asthma' in the United Kingdom is 2000 but this may include a number of non-asthmatic chronic bronchitics. In 10 years there was a sudden and an unexpected increase in deaths of young asthmatics and it is believed that these were iatrogenic as the result of over-treatment with the newer aerosol sprays of isoprenaline and similar antispasmodics.

It is customary to divide asthma into extrinsic (allergic) and intrinsic (non-allergic) types. The allergic type tends to start in early childhood and the non-allergic in adult life. Asthma is a genetic condition and in one-quarter of the cases there is a near relative with asthma.

The natural history of asthma shows a strong tendency to spontaneous improvement, particularly in those whose attacks begin in childhood. In a long-term follow-up of asthmatics in my own practice I found that only 15% were disabled after 20 years.

Effects of asthma

An attack of asthma is produced by an acute airways obstruction due to a combination of spasm of the bronchiolar muscles, edema of the bronchial and bronchiolar mucosa and excessive production of sticky mucus which causes plugging of the smaller bronchioles with some alveolar collapse.

This results in difficulty in breathing with consequent anoxaemia and hypercapnia and acidosis and respiratory failure – if the condition continues in a severe form.

Clinical presentation

There is almost always a history of previous attacks.

The patient is breathless sitting up, with the accessory muscles of respiration being used and there is expiratory wheezing to be heard in the chest. The severity of attack varies from a minor inconvenience on effort or associated with some other trigger-factor to very severe distress, breathlessness, cyanosis, shock and even sudden death.

Signs of danger that indicate the need for urgent and intensive care are:

1. Increasing restlessness and confusion indicating cerebral anoxia.
2. Increasing breathlessness with decreasing wheeze suggesting more complete obstruction of the airways.

3. Decreasing expectoration with retention of bronchial secretions and further increase of obstruction and collapse of alveoli.
4. Increasing pulse rate and evidence of right heart failure with cyanosis, gallop rhythm, raised jugular venous pressure and ECG features of cor pulmonale.
5. Exhaustion and peripheral circulatory failure.

Diagnosis

Conditions to be considered in differential diagnosis are acute left ventricular failure, acute wheezy chests associated with an exacerbation of chronic bronchitis and spontaneous pneumothorax. In relation to the latter it should be remembered that pneumothorax may sometimes complicate an acute attack of asthma and may be the reason for a sudden and serious deterioration of the patient's condition. Likewise, acute left ventricular failure may occur in patients with a previous history of asthma.

Investigations

In an acute asthmatic attack there is no need to await investigations before commencing treatment. A chest radiograph is useful to exclude any local lesions and in particular pneumothorax. Radiological features in asthma are over-inflation of the lungs, and patchy collapse.

If the attack follows an acute respiratory infection and the sputum is purulent then bacteriological examination for antibiotic sensitivity is useful, but should not delay antibiotic therapy.

In prolonged attacks knowledge of the blood levels of PO_2 and PCO_2 is necessary to control therapy.

Management

Many chronic asthmatics have become able to abort and control their acute attacks with a variety of preparations such as adrenaline and isoprenaline inhalers and antispasmodics such as ephedrine.

The physician is only called in to help these chronic asthmatics when the attack is particularly severe or when there is no response to their usual measures.

The physician on seeing the patient in an acute attack has to make an assessment of severity, based on duration of the attack, the general state of the patient, including the pulse rate, degree of dyspnea and cyanosis and the nature of previous attacks.

On this assessment a decision has to be made whether the patient is to be treated at home or admitted to hospital. Whatever the decision, and each situation has to be managed individually, the following are the most useful measures.

Reassurance and confidence

Although the role of emotions in an acute asthmatic attack are secondary to the physical effects, a vicious circle is created if the victim is tense, anxious, unsure and afraid. A part of successful management is the instillation of confidence and assurance by the physician.

Bronchodilators

Bronchospasm is only one reason for the acute airways obstruction and hence oral and inhalant bronchodilators are not always successful once the attack has persisted for more than an hour or so. They are helpful however in aborting some attacks and in long term management.

A dangerous situation arises when there is no response and the patient is tempted to increase the number of ephedrine and similar tablets taken and to use more frequently his aerosol inhalers of isoprenaline. The over-use of such preparations may lead to dangerous levels in the body and cause death from acute heart failure.

If there has been no response to the patient's usual preparations after an hour then intravenous aminophylline (0.25–0.5 g) should be given slowly, or alternatively a subcutaneous injection of adrenaline (0.5–1.0 ml of 1 in 1000 solution) may be used.

Oxygen

Oxygen is essential in all severe attacks and can be given in high concentration, providing there is no history of chronic airways obstruction with a raised arterial PCO_2 when a lower oxygen concentration should be given.

Steroids

Corticosteroids should be given early in a severe attack of asthma. They are safe preparations given intermittently and in large doses for short periods.

They are best used in high dosage for a few days followed by a gradual reduction over 2–3 weeks.

In a severe attack an initial injection of 100 mg of hydrocortisone hemisuccinate should be given followed by 80 mg of oral prednisone daily for 2–3 days and then reduction by 5–10 mg daily providing that satisfactory improvement occurs.

Antibiotics

Respiratory infection is a frequent precipitating cause of an attack and broad-spectrum antibiotics such as oxytetracycline (0.25–0.5 g 6-hourly or ampicillin 0.25–0.5 g 6-hourly) should be given whenever infection is suspected or the sputum is purulent.

Sedation

In the past asthmatics were over-sedated. Asthmatics are anxious because they cannot breathe. Once they have responded to treatment they become less anxious. Sedatives are not an important part of treatment. If one is considered necessary, then chlorpromazine 50 mg intramuscularly can be given, and repeated, or administered orally every 6–8 hours.

Expectorants

There are no reliable expectorants or mucolytics. Dehydration is one cause of increasing viscosity and intravenous therapy should not be delayed, if clinical dehydration is present.

Mechanical ventilation and bronchial lavage

When the attack fails to respond to the above regime and there is danger to life because of respiratory and circulatory failure then the possibility of assisted mechanical ventilation, aspiration of the bronchi and even bronchial lavage must be considered urgently, but provided at a special centre.

After care

Successful management of an acute attack must be followed by long term supervision of the patient in order to try and prevent further attacks.

SPONTANEOUS PNEUMOTHORAX

Spontaneous pneumothorax is not uncommon, with an annual incidence of approximately 1 per 5000, implying that a primary physician may see a new case every 2 years.

It is a condition of young adults, apparently in good health and in the great majority it is not associated with any underlying primary disease. It is often recurrent and this suggests some local structural defect of lung or pleura.

The condition is believed to be due to small sub-pleural bullae which rupture, and when this happens air is sucked into the vacuum in the pleural space causing a collapse of the lung. The pleural defect generally seals itself off and lung re-expands within a short time, depending on the size of the pneumothorax. Occasionally the pleural opening acts as a one-way valve allowing air out of the lung but not back again. This leads to a build-up of air under pressure in the pleural cavity with displacement of vital mediastinal structures producing circulatory and respiratory embarassment and failure.

Rarely the pneumothorax may be secondary to pulmonary diseases such as tuberculosis, primary or secondary neoplasms, asthma, or chronic bronchitis.

Clinical presentation

The presentation generally is undramatic with a vague pain in the chest followed by some breathlessness. The pain may be sharp and pleuritic at first but soon becomes an ache. The degree of breathlessness depends on the extent of the pneumothorax and on the state of respiratory function.

Examination of the chest reveals hyperresonance, diminished air-entry and, perhaps, shift of mediastinal contents away from the side of the chest that has a sustained pneumothorax.

The course in the majority of cases is towards gradual absorption of air within 2–4 weeks, but recurrence on the same side or on the opposite side is not uncommon.

Tension pneumothorax results in considerable breathlessness, distress and shock and urgent treatment is required.

The diagnosis is confirmed by chest radiography.

Management

In most cases no special intervention is necessary and unless there is appreciable dyspnea the patient should be managed by close supervision with radiographic control until the lung re-expands. Tension pneumothorax, when it occurs, does so from the start and is not a later complication.

There is no need to admit these patients to hospital unless there is some complication or primary disease that requires special investigation.

If there is increasing breathlessness or other evidence of tension pneumothorax then it is necessary to release air from the pleural cavity. This is carried out by inserting a wide bore needle or intra-pleural catheter through the second or third anterior intercostal spaces or the fourth intercostal space in the axilla.

Recurrent attacks may require pleurectomy or other surgical measures to seal the pleural defect and to obliterate the inter-pleural space.

ACUTE THROAT INFECTIONS

Acute throat infections are common in any community. The annual prevalence is between 30–40 per 1000. They are chiefly conditions of children and young adults.

Aetiologically, in approximately one-half of cases a pathogenic organism will be isolated from a throat swab. Thus in 46% *Str. pyogenes* will be grown and in 3% a variety of organisms such as Vincent's organisms (*B. fusiformis* and *S. vincenti*) and *Candida albicans* but in 50% no bacteria are isolated and it is assumed that the cause is a virus. Diphtheria is now an extremely rare cause of an acute throat infection but must always be borne in mind as a possibility, particularly in patients in developing countries.

Acute throat infections may also be the presenting feature of blood disorders such as glandular fever (infectious mononucleosis), leukaemia or agranulocytosis.

Clinical presentation

Sore throat, fever and malaise are the presenting features.

There is tonsillar swelling, if the tonsils are present, with a follicular, gelatinous or membranous exudate. It is quite impossible to make an accurate aetiological diagnosis from the appearance of the fauces because the appearance is similar, irrespective of the cause. The condition is not usually confined to the tonsils and the adjacent pharynx and soft palate are generally red and swollen. A punctate erythema of the soft palate sometimes occurs in glandular fever. A solitary dirty ulcer in one tonsil with foul breath is suggestive of an infection with Vincent's organisms.

The degree of general disturbance is variable, ranging from sudden onset of high fever and prostration to a sore throat that is only an inconvenience in one's daily routine.

Cervical glands are usually tender and palpable. With streptococcal infections, glandular fever and some viral infections, skin rashes may occur. These are a diffuse scarlatiniform erythema with streptococci, blotchy pink macules over the neck and trunk in glandular fever and a more generalised confluent rash in viral infections.

Diagnosis

A throat swab should be examined for causal organisms in all cases that do not resolve quickly and a differential white blood cell count and Paul–Bunnell or Monospot tests to exclude glandular fever or other blood conditions.

Course

The natural course is for the condition to clear over 4–7 days. Complications are unusual and consist of peritonsillar infection (quinsy). Acute nephritis and rheumatic fever are, nowadays, rare complications of streptococcal infections. Recurrences are frequent.

Management

One-half of all acute throat infections are caused by viruses which do not respond to antibiotics. The results of a bacteriological examination take 1–2 days. Antibiotics may be prescribed for all but the mildest cases in the knowledge that in many they will be ineffective, or they can be withheld for 48 hours to see if natural resolution will occur.

Penicillin is the most effective antibiotic and in my opinion, should be given intramuscularly, 1 megaunit twice daily for 48 hours followed by oral penicillin 0.25 g 6-hourly for a further 4–5 days. Improvement should occur within 2–3 days. If this has not occurred then bacteriological investigations and blood tests (white cell differential count and Paul-Bunnell or Monospot tests) should be carried out.

Glandular fever

Glandular fever is a condition of adolescents and young adults with the main age-prevalence in the teens (13–20). It presents as a sore throat, enlarged cervical glands and fever. These persist in spite of treatment with penicillin. The acute phase lasts 1–3 weeks often followed by weakness and malaise for some months.

It is diagnosed by a mononucleosis and a positive Paul-Bunnell or Monospot tests.

The cause is uncertain and the condition does not respond to antibiotics. In severe cases with considerable local and systemic disturbance corticosteroids (prednisone 50 mg each day for 3 days and then a daily reduction by 5 mg) may have dramatic beneficial effects.

ACUTE LARYNGEAL DYSPNEA

The causes of acute laryngeal obstruction are:
1. Acute laryngo-tracheo-bronchitis (croup)
2. Acute epiglottitis
3. Laryngeal diphtheria
4. Angioneurotic edema
5. Foreign body or other laryngeal irritants
6. Acute retropharyngeal abscess
7. Papillomata of the larynx.

Acute laryngo-tracheo-bronchitis (croup)

This is a frequent condition in young children (6 months–3 years). Most cases are associated with a viral upper respiratory infection but the same syndrome may be caused by such bacteria as *Haemophilus influenzae*, streptococci and pneumococci.

The onset often is sudden and in the middle of the night. The child awakens with a dry, irritating, barking and seal-like cough with hoarseness and an inspiratory crowing and breathlessness.

The child is frightened and is usually sitting up in bed or on the parent's lap with the accessory muscles of respiration being used. In severe cases cyanosis is present and sudden death may occur.

Fortunately most cases are not severe and will settle with simple measures such as warm moist air – a steam kettle is an excellent improvisation at home – and oxygen, if available.

Severe cases with considerable respiratory distress, restlessness and cyanosis should be admitted to hospital speedily with oxygen and medical supervision during transport.

Tracheostomy may be a life-saving measure and should not be over-delayed. Alternatively endotracheal intubation may be carried out.

The question of antibiotics is a difficult one because many cases are caused by viruses. To start with, until bacteriological investigations are available, a mixture of intramuscular penicillin and streptomycin is reasonable.

Acute epiglottitis

A condition of young children caused by viruses or *Haemophilus influenzae*. Since the inflammation is above the larynx there is no hoarseness or stridor. The main feature is an obstructive dyspnea.

The appearance of the fauces is characteristic – on depressing the tongue the epiglottis is seen as a red cherry-like swelling behind the tongue.

The condition is a serious one with an appreciable mortality and the child must be admitted to a hospital able to deal with the management of this form of respiratory obstruction quickly by intubation or tracheostomy, supported by antibiotics.

Laryngeal diphtheria

This is now a rare condition but should be considered in all cases of laryngeal dyspnea. A membrane may not be seen and the child may have a history of immunisation.

If there is any suspicion of diphtheria an immediate intramuscular injection of 24 000–48 000 u of diphtheria antitoxin should be given pending the results of throat swabs.

Angioneurotic edema

Laryngeal obstruction in angioneurotic edema is accompanied usually by other features such as swelling of the face and generalised urticaria.

Treatment is with subcutaneous injections of adrenaline (0.5 ml of 1/1000 solution) repeated in 5 minutes if no improvement has occurred.

INFLUENZA EPIDEMICS

The impact of an influenza epidemic is considerable on all local medical services and emergency actions are required to cope with the rush of patients who require treatment for the primary infection and its complications.

Influenza is massive and unpredictable. The 2- or 3-yearly epidemics are unexpected and disorganising, but the pandemics that seem to occur once every 10–20 years are disastrous, not only in toll of life but in their economic effect on the community as well.

The influenza viruses belong to the myxovirus group. There are three types, A, B and C. Each type is antigenically distinct and there is no cross immunity.

Influenza A causes the most serious epidemics and pandemics.

Influenza B is responsible for milder but local epidemics.

Influenza C has been blamed for only minor epidemics in closed communities.

The extent and severity of an epidemic of influenza depend on the virulence of the organisms and the prevailing state of mass immunity. The most severe epidemics occur when a new mutant strain of influenza virus develops and gains a foothold on an unprotected population.

The effects of the influenza viruses are on the respiratory tract causing damage to the mucosa and making a secondary bacterial infection likely. The clinical features are those of an acute respiratory infection and complications tend to be limited to the lungs.

An epidemic lasts some 6–8 weeks starting insidiously with a few sporadic cases. By the end of the second week, with a build-up of cases, it becomes obvious that an epidemic is on. As a rule school children tend to be the first to be affected, then their families and the elderly are affected only in the later stages or may escape altogether.

The peak of the epidemic is reached after 3–4 weeks and is followed by a gradual decline in the number of cases over the following month.

Clinical features

The onset is sudden, often the victim is able to record it to the minute. Intense malaise with aching limbs, back, head and eyes predominates.

Coughing, sore throat and nasal discharge denote involvement of the respiratory tract. Additional symptoms may be present, such as vomiting, diarrhea and abdominal pain, but these are not necessarily evidence of viral involvement of the gastrointestinal tract but more likely to be general non-specific reactions to an acute infection.

The course of an uncomplicated attack is for a slow improvement over 4–5 days followed by a period of weakness and depression.

Complications

The case fatality of influenza overall is less than 1 per 1000. Complications are almost confined to the respiratory tract and consist of pneumonia, acute bronchitis, otitis media or sinusitis.

Over 10 influenza epidemics during the past 25 years (1950–1975) the rate of chest complications in my own practice has been 11%. These complications principally affected young children and old persons and the chronic bronchitic and cardiac cripples.

Management

There is no specific treatment of the acute attack. It is best treated with bed rest, fluids, analgesics and a linctus that relieves the irritating cough.

Vulnerable groups such as those with a history of chronic bronchitis or other chronic chest conditions or those with cardiac failure should be given broad-spectrum antibiotics such as ampicillin or oxytetracycline prophylactically (0.25 g 6-hourly) during an attack.

Chest complications should be treated with these broad-spectrum antibiotics and if there is no improvement within 48 hours then the sputum should be tested for possible resistant bacteria.

Prevention. Influenza vaccines are available but it is difficult quickly to prepare the vaccine appropriate to the strain and type of influenza virus causing the epidemic. There are no influenza vaccines that will protect against all types of infection because of the changing antigenic strains of the viruses. The beneficial effects of any vaccine will last for only 2–3 years.

The best approach is to prepare as quickly as possible a vaccine suitable against the type of virus causing the epidemic, and once available, use it selectively for certain vulnerable individuals such as chronic chest and cardiac cases and for key workers such as physicians, nurses, hospital and ambulance workers and others particularly exposed to the infection.

L

ACUTE OTITIS MEDIA

Pain in the ear due to an acute otitis media is a common emergency in practice.

Acute otitis media is now quite a different condition from that of twenty years ago. With the availability of antibiotics and because of the lower virulence of causal organisms it has now lost the earlier terrors of mastoiditis and even death. Yet, in spite of the success of antibiotics in controlling the acute infection, many problems remain. Slow resolution and persistent and sometimes permanent deafness are dangers which have to be controlled and avoided.

Prevalence

Acute otitis media is now chiefly a condition of children although attacks do occur in adults, particularly recurrent attacks in already damaged ears. No fewer than one-third of all children in the United Kingdom suffer one or more attacks of acute otitis media during their first ten years. In any year a physician with a population of 2500 to care for may expect to treat 50–60 children with attacks of acute otitis media.

The age distribution is characteristic of all forms of respiratory infection in childhood, namely, a rising prevalence from the age of 2, a peak between 4 and 8, and then a rapid decline which continues in adult life. The pattern is explained by the time at which children are most exposed to cross infection, that is when they start to mix with other children and begin to attend school. It seems that after 2 or 3 years the child builds up a natural resistance to infections which then become less severe and less frequent.

Clinical pathology

Acute otitis media is part of the catarrhal child syndrome, namely, recurrent coughs, colds, sore throats, wheezy chests and ear infections.

Infection of the middle ear is secondary to an upper respiratory infection, which is often viral. The ear infection, however, is caused usually by pneumococci, streptococci, *Haemophilus influenzae* and staphylococci bacteria. This secondary infection reaches the middle ear along the eustachian tubes which become obstructed by inflammatory swelling or pressure by enlarged adenoids. Infection with an obstructed eustachian tube leads to accumulation of muco-pus in the closed middle ear space with interference with movement of the ossicles and swelling and inflammation of the drum.

The symptoms related to these changes are pain due to inflammation, deafness from accumulation of fluid, and some discharge from a perforation of the drum.

Complications such as mastoiditis, brain abscess and chronic otitis media are rare now but deafness may occur due to the persistence of thick mucus in the middle ear (catarrhal deafness or 'glue ear').

Clinical presentation

The painful red drum is the most usual type. Nine out of ten cases present in this way. The child is unhappy and feverish. The older child is able to localise the trouble and complain of earache but in younger children and infants the presentation may be that of high fever and malaise. Examination of the ears, imperative in all sick children, reveals a red drum, sometimes bilaterally.

The discharging ear may on occasions be the first symptom in a disturbed child (in 5% of cases), but more often any discharge, when present, follows earache.

Deafness to some degree occurs in all attacks.

Course

In the typical case the acute phase with pain and fever persists for 3–4 days and then proceeds to a natural resolution. This tendency to natural resolution should be recalled since it is likely that even without antibiotics most ears would resolve. Although the pain and fever soon settle the appearance of the drum may not return to normal for 1–4 weeks and with redness and swelling of the drum deafness is present. Discharge generally settles within 2–3 weeks, but there are a few cases in which it continues in spite of antibiotics.

Recurrent attacks are frequent and two-thirds of children with otitis media suffer more than one attack.

The final outcome is related to social factors as well as clinical severity. Thus, the outlook is worse in lower social groups, in larger families (of any class) – the more children making cross infection more likely – and where there is a family history of ear disease or deafness.

Management
Antibiotics

Although it is so easy and cheap now to prescribe oral antibiotics it is salutary that I can use them in less than one-half of all attacks with good results. My indications for antibiotics are the severity of pain and fever, presence of discharge, recurrences and where there has been no improvement within 2–3 days of onset.

Penicillin is still the most satisfactory antibiotic, either by intramuscular injection or by mouth.

Myringotomy (or aspiration)
Myringotomy (or aspiration) of mucus from the middle ear is now reserved for those cases in which there is persistent deafness after some weeks and where the cause is considered to be a 'glue ear'.

Adenoidectomy
This is a useful procedure with recurrent attacks where it is considered that the enlarged adenoids obstruct the eustachian tube.

Follow up
An essential part of management must be careful and continuing follow up of all cases until the drum and hearing have returned to normal. Ideally all children old enough to cooperate should have a pure-tone audiogram carried out 3–6 months after the attack.

COMMON EMERGENCIES IN CHILDREN

The three most frequent emergencies in children are acute chest infections, gastro-enteritis and dehydration, and convulsions.

The approach to these must be systematic and the first step is an accurate diagnosis followed by appropriate therapeutic measures. Not only has the child to be treated but the parents have to be managed and it is important to develop good rapport and communication with them and explain in understandable terms the situation and the steps being taken.

Acute chest infections
These have been referred to already in general terms.

Acute chest infections are frequent in early childhood with the peak prevalence between 4 and 8 years of age.

The 'acute wheezy chest' is the most common type and it is an acute diffuse bronchitis with airway obstruction. It is not the forerunner of asthma in later life.

Segmental pneumonia, presenting a cough, and variable malaise and fever with a local area of inspiratory rales at one or other base, is the next most frequent type.

A less common but important type is acute bronchiolitis of infants. Most cases are caused by the respiratory syncytial virus but other viruses and bacteria can produce the same conditions. The infection affects the smaller bronchioles which become obstructed with secretions and inflammatory edema.

Following an upper respiratory infection there is a fairly sudden onset of breathlessness with a frequent spasmodic cough. There is difficulty in both inspiration and expiration with indrawing of the lower chest wall. The child becomes restless and agitated and grey.

There are many scattered rales and rhonchi in the chest and the radiograph shows hypertranslucency and depression of the diaphragm with no consolidation and little collapse.

The management of these cases is based on antibiotics, treatment of respiratory distress and failure, and general care.

Although many of the infections are caused by viruses and are insensitive to antibiotics, it is impossible to differentiate these cases and it is safer to prescribe one of the broad-spectrum antibiotics such as ampicillin or co-trimoxazole.

Humidified oxygen is necessary when there is respiratory distress and if the condition continues to deteriorate then bronchoscopic suction or even tracheostomy with mechanical respiration or bronchial aspiration must be considered as life saving procedures.

Although less of an influence than in the past, good skilled nursing makes a great contribution to the care of the really sick child.

Gastro-enteritis and dehydration
Gastro-enteritis is second only to acute respiratory infections as the most frequent condition in children.

Caused by a variety of organisms and irritants most cases will settle quickly by withholding food, but not fluids, for 12–24 hours. It is not necessary to give antibiotics because only a small number are caused by sensitive bacteria.

In management, care has to be taken to distinguish in these children the presenting symptoms from a possible 'acute abdomen' or secondary to infection elsewhere, such as acute throat or chest infections.

Dehydration is suggested by anxiety, restlessness, throat and dry tongue, weight loss and oliguria requires hospitalisation and fluid replacement under biochemical control.

Convulsions
There are many causes of convulsions in childhood but the commonest are the 'febrile convulsion' and epilepsy.

The febrile convulsion occurs in an apparently normal child at the height of some acute infection with high fever. Rare before 6 months and after 3 years, it often recurs in the same child in subsequent fevers and there is frequently a family history of similar episodes.

The convulsions are usually generalised tonic and clonic seizures. Usually the fit is solitary and of short duration. Attacks which continue to recur or last for more than ½–1 hour raise more serious possibilities, such as meningo-encephalitis.

In most cases no special treatment is necessary because the convulsion does not last very long. More important than treating the convulsion is the establishment of an accurate causal diagnosis.

Continuing convulsions require attention to maintaining a free airway and administration of anticonvulsants such as paraldehyde (1 ml/7 kg of body weight) or sodium phenobarbitone (60 mg at 6–12 months and 120 mg at 2–3 years), or diazepam (5–10 mg) intramuscularly.

Repeated bouts require further investigations to consider the possibilities of epilepsy, intracranial lesions or metabolic disturbances.

ANAPHYLACTIC SHOCK
ANGIONEUROTIC EDEMA AND URTICARIA

Three forms of allergic reactions are anaphylactic shock, angioneurotic edema and urticaria.

Anaphylactic shock is a violent systemic reaction to foreign proteins and other substances to which the patient has become previously sensitised. Injections of serum, vaccines, especially those grown in chick embryos, and penicillin are the most frequent causes.

The reaction may be immediate or delayed depending on the dose of allergen and the route of administration.

The patient complains of feeling unwell with pallor, vomiting, tightness in the chest, abdominal pain and a feeling of impending doom. The blood pressure falls, the pulse becomes rapid and thready with a shock-like state. Cardiac arrest may occur or the patient may become comatose. Death may occur.

Obviously before potentially dangerous drugs which may cause anaphylactic shock are given the patient must be questioned as to any previous reactions.

Once the reaction occurs the patient should be laid down. Adrenaline 0.5 ml of 1/1000 solution should be injected intramuscularly at once and repeated in 5–10 minutes if no response. Oxygen should be administered. If there is no response in 5–10 minutes an intravenous injection of hydrocortisone hemisuccinate 100 mg should be given. When bronchospasm is marked and persistent in spite of adrenaline and hydrocortisone administration, then aminophylline (0.25 g) should be given intravenously.

With cardiac arrest, mouth to mouth breathing and external cardiac massage should be applied.

Angioneurotic edema occurs in sensitive individuals as a result of ingesting a food to which the victim has been sensitised. There is swelling of the lips, tongue, eyelids and face and there may be generalised urticaria as well.

The swelling may involve the perilaryngeal tissues and cause an acute respiratory obstruction.

Adrenaline should be injected immediately (0.5 ml intramuscularly) and repeated in 5–10 minutes if no response. Hydrocortisone hemisuccinate (100 mg) may be given intravenously and if successful prednisone should be continued by mouth in reducing dose from 50 mg/day.

If there is severe laryngeal obstruction then intubation or tracheostomy may be required urgently.

Urticaria of the skin is a common condition, but its cause is often undetermined. Most frequent in children it tends to recur.

As it does not usually last for more than a few days, symptomatic measures are all that are required. Where there is considerable distress antihistamines or corticosteroids may be given. Chronic urticaria is a very troublesome condition which may persist for years and which in the main responds poorly to most of the standard forms of treatment.

2

THE TREATMENT OF NEOPLASIA

J. M. A. WHITEHOUSE

INTRODUCTION

The word cancer is for many people an emotive one, conjuring up visions of chronically ill relatives, friends or of others who have died prematurely. Since those who are cured of their malignancy are rarely recognised it is not surprising that the general attitude to this condition is one of pessimism. It is frequently said that any attempt to put cancer into perspective must depend upon an accurate evaluation of the incidence and prognosis of the disease. This is indeed true, but more important still is the emphasis that must be placed on the fact that cancer is not one disease but many. The collective use of this word to describe a group of widely differing conditions with enormously different prognoses is, to say the least, unfortunate and at best profoundly misleading.

Malignant tumours share in common the uncontrolled proliferation of cells and propensity for dissemination which is their hallmark. But there the similarity ends. Tumours derive from different tissues and even among those of the same histological type, comparison between each tumour shows that there is a wide variation in the degree of differentiation of the tumour cells. Thus the rate of growth of tumours differs just as does their tendency to metastasise for, while some tend to remain localised, metastasising only rarely, others disseminate widely.

That there is great variation between tumour types becomes even more apparent when their sensitivity to treatment is compared. Some are highly sensitive to radiotherapy and chemotherapy and others very resistant; yet others are sensitive to one modality of therapy but resistant to another. Unfortunately, such sensitivity to therapy does not necessarily equate with curability. The size of the therapeutic problem becomes apparent when it is realised that in 1970, 154 351 new cases of malignant disease were reported in England and Wales in a population of 48 987 700. The number of cases presenting with various malignancies may be compared in Table 1.

Table 1. Some of the commoner new cancers 1970 in England and Wales (Total population 48,987,700—Males 23,830,900—Females 25,156,800).
(With acknowledgement to the Office of Population Censuses and Surveys).

Tumour	Males	Females	Total
Carcinoma of trachea, bronchus and lung	23 797	5187	28 984
Carcinoma of the breast	168	18 156	18 324
Carcinoma of the stomach	6538	4556	11 094
Carcinoma of the large intestine	4729	6350	11 079
Carcinoma of the bladder			10 058
Carcinoma of the rectum	4134	3413	7547
Carcinoma of the pancreas	2412	2002	4414
Carcinoma of the prostate	5247	—	5247
Carcinoma of the cervix	—	4099	4099

Changes in the incidence of certain malignancies have become apparent in recent studies and may be due to a variety of factors, for example an increased awareness of the need for early diagnosis so that the patient with mild symptoms presents early; increased screening, such as has been carried for lesions of the cervix and previously for the lung; improvements in diagnosis; and lastly, a real increase in the incidence of the disease. Real increases in the incidence of leukaemia, cancers of the ovary, pancreas and prostate, appear to have occurred, while that of carcinoma of the stomach is declining. Carcinoma of the cervix also appears to be less common, despite intensive screening methods which might have been anticipated initially to increase the number of cases identified with this condition.

Little is understood about the factors which may predispose to neoplasia, variations which may, in part, be responsible for the changes in the incidence of individual tumours. However, ionising radiation and chemical carcinogens are well recognised to predispose to neoplasia. The increased incidence of leukaemia in survivors of the atomic bombs at Hiroshima and Nagasaki, and in patients who received radiation for ankylosing spondylitis is well known. Among the carcinogens, those in tobacco have received most publicity and the rising incidence of carcinoma of the bronchus is attributed to them. The identification of other carcinogens such as beta naphthylamine (carcinoma of the bladder), asbestos (mesothelioma), benzypyrine (carcinoma of the skin) to mention but a few, has led to their strict control and thus diminished their significance as causes of these tumours. Such restrictive measures obviously play an important part in the prophylactic precautions which must be taken against cancer. Recently, exposure to vinyl chloride has been associated with the increased incidence of a rare tumour, the hepatic angioblastoma, in those who work closely with the chemical. Other aetiological agents may soon be identified. As yet there is only one malignancy where an infective aetiology has any support, namely Burkitt's lymphoma. This derives from the limited geographical localisation of patients with this lymphooma and the identification of an associated virus in the tumour, the Epstein Barr (EB) virus. The same virus has also been incriminated as the infective agent of infectious mononucleosis.

Some attempt has been made to incriminate an infective agent in acute leukaemia and the lymphomas by demonstrating time–space clustering of cases, but the evidence is as yet unconvincing. While a careful study of the characteristics of a particular malignancy is an essential prerequisite to any approach to therapy, the elimination of any predisposing factors is an obvious preliminary to its control. The logical approach to the management of neoplasia is thus to attempt to identify such causative factors and, where possible, to identify high risk groups of individuals. Since early diagnosis of any neoplasm facilitates its management and increases the possibility of complete cure, screening procedures are theoretically attractive. However, the frequency with which these need to be carried out to identify certain neoplasms and the variation in sensitivity of the methods available, restricts their usefulness considerably. At the present time their greatest use would appear to be when applied to high risk groups.

The intention of treatment of a cancer must ultimately be to reduce the tumour cell population to zero. Where the tumour is well localised this end may be achieved by simple excision or radiotherapy alone. Commonly, however, microscopic deposits of cells have extended to more distant sites and such therapy is insufficient to achieve cure. How then may these potentially lethal deposits be eradicated? If this question were simply answerable then malignant disease would no longer present a therapeutic problem. At the present time the only way to determine whether all neoplastic cells have been eradicated is by awaiting macroscopic evidence of recurrence. Such a crude assessment is of little assistance to the clinician attempting cure. Indeed, individual variations in the behaviour of tumours means that these isolated recurrences may not, in some tumours, such as carcinoma of the breast and malignant melanoma, become apparent for many years.

Prior to planning any treatment, a crucial decision has to be taken; that is whether the clinical situation justifies an attempt at cure, or whether the aim should be control of the disease or palliation alone. The morbidity associated with the therapeutic extremes of the major treatment modalities increases as the likelihood of cure becomes more certain. Each patient's disease must be assessed in the light of available therapies and the morbidity associated with each weighed against the possible therapeutic advantage. Temporary severe morbidity is acceptable in the treatment of a potentially lethal disease if the outcome offers either a possibility of complete cure or a significant prolongation of useful life. The complications of therapy may be considerable involving for example permanent disability such as lymphedema of a limb, loss of a limb or other organ, the formation of an alternative structure such as a colostomy or ileal bladder. Less permanent complications include loss of hair and damage to other rapidly proliferating normal tissues resulting in diarrhea and other gastrointestinal upsets (gastrointestinal mucosa); anaemia, thrombocytopenia and granulocytopenia (bone marrow) leading to risks of haemorrhage and infection; infertility (testes and ovaries); cutaneous reaction to radiotherapy and the more permanent late complications which may result from fibrosis in irradiated tissues.

The therapy of a neoplasm depends on its histology, its site and whether it is localised or disseminated. There are three major approaches to treatment – radiotherapy, surgery, and chemotherapy. Immunotherapy has as yet earned no permanent place among this group, but is under extensive study. Preliminary results using immunotherapy with injected irradiated leukaemia cells and BCG to maintain complete remission in acute myeloblastic leukaemia, suggest that this concept has minor therapeutic potential.

Radiotherapy

The majority of malignant tumours are treated by some form of X-ray or gamma ray. The super voltage X-ray machines have the advantage that they are able to deliver large doses of radiation to depths of the body with a lesser effect on the intervening structures than is possible by other means, so avoiding the unpleasant skin reactions seen in the past. The commonly used source of gamma rays is Cobalt 60, an artificially produced isotope, which provides beams of gamma rays which are used in essentially the same way as the super voltage X-ray machine. Other sources of radiation are the isotopes which can be used in diagnosis or therapy, and radioactive implants.

For radiotherapy to be of any value a tumour must be radio-sensitive, that is susceptible to alteration of its growth by ionising radiation. Many tumours are more susceptible to ionising radiation than their tissue of origin but newer techniques make this less important. As with other therapeutic measures, radiotherapy has its place in the cure as well as the palliation of malignancy, and the combination of this with other therapeutic modalities is proving of increasing value in the management of many different tumours.

Surgery

The biopsy or excision of a neoplasm is an essential preliminary to diagnosis. The role of surgery in effecting a cure then depends on the individual tumour. Certainly radical surgery which once was regarded as the prerequisite of cure is losing favour. It is increasingly realised that the addition of irradiation or chemotherapy to more moderate surgical procedures may subordinate the need for radical operations and offer the optimum chance of cure. The place of surgery in the diagnosis of malignancy, in the removal of bulk disease and in reconstructive procedures, remains unchallenged.

Chemotherapy

Since 1948 when Farber described folic acid antagonists which were capable of producing remissions in acute leukaemia, a plethora of various chemical agents have been described for treating cancer. The effectiveness of some newer agents in causing regression of neoplastic disease, particularly in the leukaemias and lymphomas, is now well established.

With a greater understanding of the mode of action of these drugs, certain principles of therapy have become accepted. Combining two drugs with different toxicities and different modes of action permits an anti-tumour effect which could only be achieved by using toxic doses of the drug alone. In some cases drug combinations may even be synergistic. Continuous therapy with one drug has the disadvantage that it suppresses normal tissue recovery and that in theory the tumour escapes in a way analagous to the development of antibiotic resistant strains of bacteria. High dose intermittent therapy produces tumour destruction; normal tissues recover more readily than those of the tumour, on each occasion that chemotherapy is given to a sensitive tumour a progressive reduction in tumour mass occurs. The value of effective drug combinations used alone or in conjunction with surgery or radiotherapy in the management of certain solid tumours is becoming increasingly apparent. This applies particularly to childhood tumours such as neuroblastoma, Wilm's tumour, rhabdomyosarcoma and osteogenic sarcoma.

Immunotherapy

Provided that the immunological system of the host is capable of recognising a tumour as foreign tissue, it is likely that some kind of immunological reaction to the tumour cell is possible. The form that this may take is the subject of much study and debate, but if immunity to a tumour could be stimulated it might, in theory, be possible to eradicate all remaining tumour cells after the bulk of the tumour has been excised or destroyed by chemotherapy or radiotherapy, thus achieving a complete cure. The fact that cures are not universal, despite attempts to use a whole variety of techniques, testifies to the weakness of such an hypothesis. Nonetheless, there is encouraging evidence that some benefit may be obtained from immunotherapy. Whether this results from a nonspecific stimulus of immunity as may be obtained by injecting BCG, or from a specific stimulus as when irradiated tumour cells are injected, is not yet clear.

THE SOLID TUMOURS

Unlike the leukaemias which are disseminated at presentation and the lymphomas which arise in a widely distributed system, most solid tumours develop in tissues confined to a limited anatomical site. It follows that the management of these tumours is influenced by this fact. Many tumours remain contained within the tissue of origin long before metastatic disease becomes apparent. The treatment of choice for localised disease is surgical resection of the tumour or whole organ of origin. Unfortunately, it is only possible to make a relatively crude assessment to exclude extension of the tumour beyond the operation site. Since tumour cells may be presumed to break away from the tumour mass prior to and during the operation, additional 'blanket' therapy has been given following the excision of many tumours. Chemotherapy may possibly have a place pre-operatively, although there is a strong argument for giving chemotherapy effective for a particular tumour post-operatively since stray cells released at operation should theoretically be destroyed even at distant sites.

Customarily localised disease, for example carcinoma of the breast, is followed by a therapeutic course of irradiation to the operation field in the hope of achieving cure. Where the mode of spread is predictable and predominantly local, such an approach may influence the course of disease and favourably influence survival. However, in many cases, by the time the primary has become apparent, sufficient numbers of cells will have separated from the primary becoming lodged at sites remote from the prospective treatment area, thus surviving local adjuvant therapy and establishing the risk of metastases.

Why some tumours metastasise and others do not, why some do so via the lymphatics and others via the blood stream, why some tend to metastasise to specific organs, and why some remain dormant for long periods of time, are questions which remain to be explained. However, a knowledge of the behaviour of a particular tumour is an essential adjunct to its treatment.

The management of disseminated disease is much more problematic. Surgical intervention has little direct relevance, except for those tumours which have been found to be hormone dependent where the removal of organs secreting these hormones may profoundly change the course of the disease. In some tumours, however, hormone antagonists may be equally effective. Radiotherapy has a useful place in the treatment of localised metastatic disease of bony deposits and in the palliation of locally invasive disease. The role of chemotherapy has yet to be fully assessed but appears to have a growing place in the management of many malignancies, both therapeutically and palliatively. The combined approach of resection of bulk disease with chemotherapy and radiotherapy may open new avenues of approach to malignant diseases which have previously been regarded as untreatable. These principles are best examined in relation to the management of individual solid tumours.

Carcinoma of the breast

This is the second most common malignancy in England and Wales after carcinoma of the bron-chus. In 1970 there were 18 156 new cases in females, while in males only 168 cases were reported. Forty per cent of the patients who develop this condition survive for 5 years and approximately 10 000 deaths per year are caused by it. It is disturbing to find that this figure has remained the same over a period of years despite advances in diagnostic and therapeutic techniques. The clinical diagnosis of carcinoma of the breast tends to occur after the tumour has been present for some considerable time. In theory this prejudices the chance of cure and thus any aids to early diagnosis may improve the prognosis in this condition. Several such aids are available; these include thermography which utilises the changes in temperature resulting from the altered vascular supply to a tumour, mammography, and best of all xeroradiography which shows more detail than can be seen on a mammogram. These techniques complement clinical examination but do not replace it. A variety of surgical methods have been used to treat carcinoma of the breast, ranging from simple removal of the lump to more radical and mutilating operations which were thought originally to offer a greater chance of cure.

The morbidity associated with supra-radical operations is high and many surgeons have chosen a middle course of a simple mastectomy with or without axillary clearance as the optimal treatment available today. This can then be followed by radiotherapy if indicated. The morbidity of this procedure is relatively low and the results in terms of survival have been shown to be better than simple removal of the lump and no worse than radical mastectomy. While it is customary to follow a mastectomy with regional radiotherapy, it has been shown that the survival of these patients can be equalled if no radiotherapy is given routinely post-operatively, but is held in reserve for those with recurrent disease. This avoids over-treating one third of the patients without detrimentally affecting the survival of those who do relapse. Pre-operative radiotherapy is no longer contemplated because of the delay in skin healing which may result post-operatively. However, there is some encouragement from early studies for the idea that adjuvant chemotherapy for carcinoma of the breast can materially alter survival, and it may be that a judicious combination of all three modalities—surgery, radiotherapy, chemotherapy—will offer the opportunity of improving the outlook of this condition.

For the patient with disseminated disease at presentation or in those who relapse, there are several therapeutic options open. Localised recurrence may best be treated with radiotherapy. Surgical removal of the ovaries, adrenals or pituitary have become standard procedures in the management of advanced carcinoma of the breast. In general terms, oophorectomy alone may be sufficient to achieve dramatic regression in 30–40% of pre-menopausal women. Post-menopausally, a trial of stilbestrol by mouth should be tried, followed by an adrenalectomy should this fail. Endocrine manipulations do not prejudice the response to chemotherapy, and since such a response using existing regimes may be of short duration, chemotherapy should remain a sequel to endocrine ablation. Various ways of predicting the endocrine responsiveness of the patient's tumour have been under study for some time, but their value in general use has not yet been established.

Carcinoma of the lung

Malignancies of the trachea, bronchus and lung accounted for 28 984 of the new malignancies reported in England and Wales in 1970. That there is a relationship between smoking and the epidermoid and undifferentiated neoplasms of the lung is now undisputed and since most tumours are relatively advanced by the time the patient becomes symptomatic, only palliative therapy is possible. In the chance radiographic demonstration of a bronchial neoplasm where disease is localised so that it may be totally removed by resection of a lobe or of the whole lung, surgery offers the greatest chance of cure. Where the disease is more extensive, radiotherapy may halt progress for a few months. Similarly, in those painful lesions resulting from local invasion, such as may be seen in a Pancoast tumour, radiotherapy to the area may prove far more effective than powerful analgesics in relieving pain. At the present time chemotherapy has made little impact on survival in this disease, but it may, in selected cases, particularly in undifferentiated neoplasms such as oat cell carcinoma, produce a marked regression in tumour volume. It may also prove useful in the palliation of disseminated disease.

Carcinoma of the gastrointestinal tract

Carcinoma of the stomach and of the colon and rectum account for the bulk of tumours of the gastrointestinal tract. Surgical resection in the case of localised disease with lymph node dissection is the treatment of choice. If the lesion is incurable because of local fixation or the presence of distant metastases, palliative procedures may be necessary, but wherever possible the tumour is resected since this offers the best chance of palliation. At the present time radiotherapy and chemotherapy are principally reserved for palliation and the control of recurrent or metastatic disease, but gastrointestinal tract tumours haves proved in the main fairly resistant to long term control with chemotherapy. Some newer regimes do suggest, however, an increasingly important role for chemotherapy in conjunction with surgery.

The identification of a tumour-associated antigen in the blood of patients with carcinomas of the gastrointestinal tract (carcinoembryonic antigen—CEA) suggested a promising role for this substance as a marker of malignant disease. Extensive surveys have however shown that the levels of this antigen are raised in many patients with non-gastrointestinal tract malignancies and indeed in non-malignant disorders such as alcoholic liver disease, pancreatitis and even in the presence of inflammation alone. The usefulness of CEA as an indicator of malignancy is thus severely restricted but it may have a place in the monitoring of disease in individual patients whose levels return to normal following therapy.

Carcinoma of the uterus (cervix)

This tumour is slightly more common in those sexually active before the age of twenty and has a peak age incidence at 45 years. In screening surveys it has been possible to identify carcinoma in situ which may be satisfactorily treated by excisional cone biopsy alone. A survey carried out in British Columbia suggests that by using such screening it is possible to reduce the incidence but not to eliminate this tumour. In Britain the bulk of the screening is carried out by the general practitioner, family planning clinics and hospital obstetricians. Intra-cavity irradiation in association with external radiotherapy offers the best chance of control. Surgery has a declining role in the management of this tumour.

Carcinoma of the ovary

This tumour is more common in single and nulliparous women than in those who are married and parous. Unfortunately, because of the site of these organs, it is unusual to find localised disease at operation. Indeed more than 50% of patients have disseminated disease at presentation. However, those infrequent cases found to have well localised disease have a relatively good prognosis. The conventional treatment for carcinoma of the ovary is a hysterectomy and bilateral salpingo-oophorectomy in conjunction with local clearative surgery. The hysterectomy is carried out because of the recognised association between carcinoma of the endometrium and carcinoma of the ovary. The contralateral ovary may not be removed in the younger female, but is generally excised because of the small risk of bilateral tumours. Radiotherapy has a minor role as an adjunct to surgery in locally advanced cases, but continuous single agent chemotherapy with alkylating agents has proved very effective in the temporary, and in some cases prolonged control of advanced disease.

Carcinoma of the bladder

The role of carcinogens, particularly the aniline dyes in the aetiology of this neoplasm is well documented and strict controls within the chemical industry have eliminated this risk. For the purposes of treatment, all papillomata of the bladder are regarded as potentially malignant and only small, apparently benign papillomata are treated with local diathermy. Neoplasms of this organ tend to metastasise late and being readily visualised by cystoscopy are thus readily followed up to exclude recurrence. Sequential levels of carcino-embryonic antigen (CEA) in the urine may provide a useful monitor of disease state, rising when recurrence occurs. It is possible that once substantiated as an indicator of relapse in a particular patient, regular monitoring of CEA levels may override the need for frequent cystoscopy. With larger localised tumours, partial cystectomy may be required. Large fulminating lesions require total cystectomy with the construction of an ileal or rectal bladder. Radiotherapy is useful in palliatory procedures and in the management of inoperable lesions, particularly in controlling haemorrhage.

Carcinoma of the prostate

This tumour is usually a well differentiated adenocarcinoma, but anaplastic forms do occur. Since part of the posterior lobe of the prostate remains following prostatectomy for benign hypertrophy, carcinoma of prostatic tissue may occur despite prior prostatectomy. Local lymphatic invasion is common, although involvement of lymph nodes is unusual. The tumour may be slow growing, usually metastasising to bone, but ultimately to lung, liver, and brain. The most useful therapeutic feature of the well differentiated adenocarcinoma is the fact that the tumour and its metastases are nearly always responsive to estrogens. Commonly, stilbestrol 1 mg t.d.s is used. Radical prostatectomy for localised disease is no longer the treatment of choice in this country, but remains popular in the United States of America. Although stilbestrol has become the hormonal treatment of choice for carcinoma of

the prostate, there is some evidence that its use is associated with an increase in cardiovascular disease. Orchidectomy alone can decrease the pain from bone metastases and reduce prostatic size relieving partial urinary retention. Using palliative treatment alone, a 50% five year survival has been achieved.

Tumours of the testis

Eighty per cent of testicular tumours occur below the age of forty. Malignant change occurs in 10–15% of undescended testes and orchidopexy does not protect against this. Several histological types of tumour occur in the testis; about 40% are seminomas, these spread predominantly via the lymphatics and are highly radiosensitive; a further 40% or so are teratomatous tumours which tend to be highly malignant, metastasising early via the blood stream; other tumours are much less common. Delay in presentation of patients with testicular swelling means that many will have metastases at the time of presentation. Some of the embryonal tumours and teratomas secrete human chorionic gonadotrophin which may prove useful as a marker of tumour recurrence. The treatment of choice where the disease is clinically localised is immediate orchidectomy and high ligation of the testicular vessels and of the spermatic chord. In the case of localised seminomas, operation followed by radiotherapy to the iliac and para-aortic lymph nodes offers a 95% 5-year survival rate. The other histological types of tumour are more radioresistant, but some chemotherapeutic regimes using vincristine, actinomycin and methotrexate have proved useful in controlling the disease for a period of time.

Miscellaneous solid tumours

The difficulty is assessing different forms of treatment in the management of various less common tumours has made the identification of the optimum treatment for each one a matter of the individual clinician's preference, although group studies are now overcoming this problem. The general principle of wide excision of local disease followed in some cases by local radiotherapy, has been applied to many tumours, and as more experience accumulates in dealing with each of these conditions, so customary therapies are being called into question. Indeed, the addition of various chemotherapeutic regimes to surgical and radiotherapeutic procedures has opened up new horizons of treatment.

THE LEUKAEMIAS

Acute myelogenous leukaemia

This disease affects all ages equally, apart from a very slightly increased incidence in middle age. The presenting symptoms and signs are unremarkable and usually those associated with an anaemia with thrombocytopenia or granulocytopenia, and the diagnosis is entirely dependent on bone marrow examination. Frequently the patient is well until as little as 2 to 3 weeks prior to presentation. Untreated, such a patient might not be anticipated to survive much over 2 months; some less, others more, and until about 10 years ago even with treatment survivals in excess of 6 months were rare.

The introduction of chemotherapy has radically changed the attitude of the physician to the management of this disease. Experience in Hodgkin's disease has shown that it is no longer unrealistic to anticipate cure in some malignancies, but that to do so requires not only intensive study into the character of each disease, but specialist management in centres familiar with the problems of the disease and its therapy. Applying such principles to the acute myelogenous leukaemias has raised the median survival from 2 months to well in excess of a year, with some patients surviving for 5 years or more

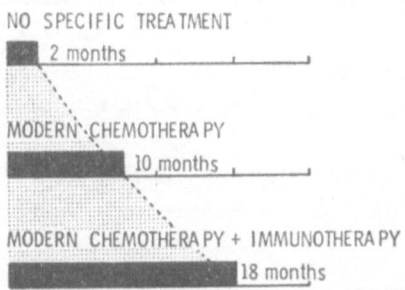

NO SPECIFIC TREATMENT

2 months

MODERN CHEMOTHERAPY

10 months

MODERN CHEMOTHERAPY + IMMUNOTHERAPY

18 months

Figure 1. The improvement in median survival of adult patients with acute myeloblastic leukaemia as therapy has improved.

(Figure 1). Perhaps most hopeful of all is the fact that these patients are not invalids, but are able to follow their occupations and lead normal lives. Such a situation is not achieved easily. Of those patients (all age groups) referred to special centres, in some the disease is so advanced that they die before treatment can hope to be effective, and others die within the first 6 weeks of referral from the complications of their disease and the

prolonged bone marrow depression that may occur from treatment.

The aim of therapy is to eradicate from the bone marrow all the leukaemic blast cells, thus allowing repopulation of the normal marrow elements. The best drugs so far described to do this include daunorubicin, cytosine arabinoside and 6-thioguanine, but their effect on the bone marrow is not only to kill the leukaemic cells but also to damage normal bone marrow. Normal marrow repopulates more readily than the leukaemic element, but following treatment all the bone marrow elements are depressed even further. At this time the patient is at an increased risk from haemorrhage or infection and supportive care is vital if death in a patient whose disease is being progressively eradicated is to be prevented. Anaemia is readily corrected by blood transfusion, but any sign of infection requires rapid and efficient management with intravenous antibiotics and possibly of granulocyte transfusions in a patient who is virtually agranulocytic. The role of such granulocyte transfusions, using granulocytes leucophoresed from close relatives or other donors, is not established as beneficial in agranulocytic patients with life threatening infections, but is theoretically attractive. The facilities required for this technique are extensive, as are those for managing the patient in a sterile environment which offers the alternative situation of prophylaxis. The latter facility is not available in every centre and is in the process of being evaluated.

The thrombocytopenic patient with occult (retinal haemorrhages or haematuria) or overt signs of haemorrhage, requires platelet transfusions to prevent catastrophic haemorrhage, and theoretically HL–A matched platelets collected from a relative survive longest in the patient. Such transfusions require to be given daily while bleeding persists.

The process of eliminating visible evidence of leukaemic infiltration by chemotherapy to achieve bone marrow and peripheral blood normality is known as the 'induction' of complete remission. The number of patients achieving complete remission varies depending on the centre, from as low as 30% to as high as 65%, although the criteria for complete remission vary somewhat from centre to centre so that these figures are not entirely comparable. A patient with acute leukaemia who achieves complete remission (that is a normal bone marrow, a normal peripheral blood picture and no clinical evidence of disease) is still assumed to have occult disease and for this reason it is customary to give 'consolidation' chemotherapy in the hope of eradicating this.

The greatest problem is only posed once the patient has achieved complete remission, as it is obviously to no advantage to achieve this position only to be faced with relapse shortly afterwards. Thus 'maintenance' of complete remission is the vital prelude to complete cure of acute leukaemia. Since most patients eventually relapse it is obvious that no ideal form of maintenance exists. Repeated courses of chemotherapy at intervals may adequately suppress recurrence for a period of time but it is unlikely, if minimal residual disease remains, to eradicate it. Further intensive chemotherapy at 1 year after complete remission has been reported to prolong survival significantly in patients who have remained in complete remission thus far, but it is too early as yet to know whether any of these patients represent cures.

An alternative means of achieving a complete cure would be to so boost the patient's own immunological resistance to the disease that every leukaemic cell would be eliminated. There is some experimental evidence to suggest that the patient in complete remission is capable of identifying his own leukaemic cells as foreign tissue. Various centres have attempted to accentuate this recognition so that the leukaemic cells are rejected by the host as would be a foreign tissue graft. Using allogeneic leukaemic cells to stimulate active immunity specifically and BCG to stimulate nonspecifically, one group has improved the complete remission length to a median of 374 days compared with a control group who had identical maintenance chemotherapy but no immunotherapy (median 180 days). The median survivals were also improved, the immunotherapy patients having a median survival of 530 days whereas the control group had a median survival of 295 days. The improvement in chemotherapeutic techniques and the advent of more sophisticated methods of supportive care, coupled with research advances, make the outlook for the future in this disease steadily more promising.

Acute lymphoblastic leukaemia

This variety of acute leukaemia has a peak incidence at 4–5 years, but occurs sporadically in all other age groups. It differs little in its presenting features from the acute myelogenous leukaemias, although lymphadenopathy and splenomegaly are found more frequently. In the older age groups the features of the disease may more resemble a lymphoma than a leukaemia. The complications of the disease and its treatment are similar to those of AML. However, acute lymphoblastic leukaemia of childhood is more readily treated. The combination of vincristine and prednisolone is much more specifically toxic for the lymphoblastic cells than for the normal bone marrow components. Indeed complete remissions in this disease have followed blood transfusion alone. Excellent clinical trials by Professor Pinkel and his group at Memphis, Tennessee, have shown that it is possible to achieve complete remission rates in excess of 90% and 5 year survivals in excess of 50%, the latter using maintenance chemotherapy with daily 6-mercaptopurine and weekly methotrexate plus cyclophosphamide.

More recent studies have shown that identical results can be obtained without the cyclophosphamide. Maintenance chemotherapy is continued for 3 years following complete remission with regular follow-up checks which include full blood counts and bone marrows when indicated. The incidence of central nervous system disease in this condition is much higher than in acute myeloblastic leukaemia and since Pinkel has shown that cranial prophylaxis (cranial irradiation plus a course of intrathecal methotrexate) can radically reduce the risk of CNS disease, this procedure has now become routine for all patients achieving complete remission. The progress achieved in the management of this condition in patients up to the age of 15 can be measured in the difference between the median survival in 1940 (2 months) and the median survival in 1973 (>5 years) (Figure 2). Adults with this disease pose a

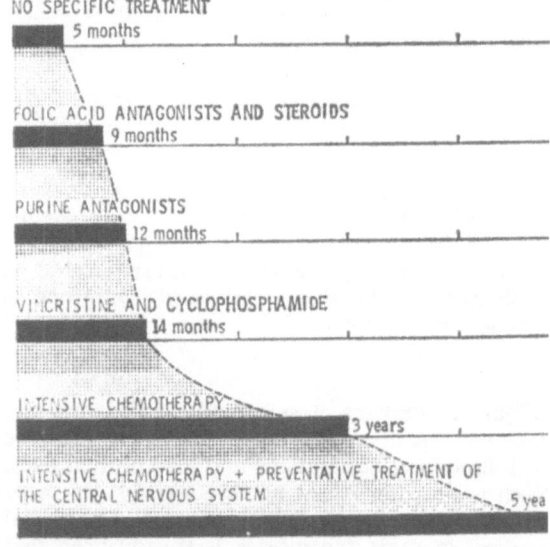

NO SPECIFIC TREATMENT
5 months

FOLIC ACID ANTAGONISTS AND STEROIDS
9 months

PURINE ANTAGONISTS
12 months

VINCRISTINE AND CYCLOPHOSPHAMIDE
14 months

INTENSIVE CHEMOTHERAPY
3 years

INTENSIVE CHEMOTHERAPY + PREVENTATIVE TREATMENT OF THE CENTRAL NERVOUS SYSTEM
5 yea

Figure 2. The improving median survival of patients with acute lymphoblastic leukaemia as new treatments have become available.

greater problem since, although the eradication of visible disease is usually fairly readily achieved, recurrence is frequent and survival in no way equals that of the childhood group.

Chronic myeloid leukaemia

This disease, predominantly presenting in middle age, is characterised by moderate splenomegaly and anaemia. Thrombocytopenia may occur and very much less commonly, localised deposits of leukaemic tissue may be seen. The diagnosis is unequivocal in the presence of the Philadelphia chromosome. The median survival for this condition, either following treatment with busulphan or radiotherapy to the spleen, is $2\frac{1}{2}$ years, but fewer problems are associated with the use of busulphan and this remains the treatment of choice. Despite progress in other fields, the median survival for this disease has remained the same. The terminal phase of the illness is associated with a change in character of progression, resulting in a clinical and bone marrow picture which in many cases is indistinguishable from acute myeloblastic leukaemia. This is relatively refractory to treatment, although some long survivors are reported. In an attempt to reduce the number of patients whose disease undergoes this transformation, various centres are examining the role of splenectomy in the chronic phase of the disease. So far there is little evidence that this has reduced the tendency to blastic transformation, but since the terminal phase is often associated with massive splenomegaly, the complications associated with this have been reduced. The place of early intensive chemotherapy is also under study.

Chronic lymphocytic leukaemia

This, the most frequently identified of the leukaemias, occurs most commonly in the older age groups. It is associated with long survival and its chronicity is well demonstrated by the fact that some cases are identified on a chance blood count. Some patients develop Coombs positive haemolytic anaemia, but in general this is steroid responsive. Both this, the raised lymphocyte count, the lymph node enlargement and mild splenomegaly respond well to chlorambucil which remains the drug of choice for treating symptomatic disease, but radiotherapy can usefully reduce bulky lymphadenopathy. There is no evidence to suggest that patients with moderate lymphadenopathy derive any benefit other than cosmetic from treatment. In comparison with chronic myeloid leukaemia, the tendency for a terminal blastic phase of the illness to occur is less common, but the

possibility of a change in character of the patient's disease merits continued surveillance.

THE LYMPHOMAS

Hodgkin's disease

This disease, above all others, illustrates the value of cooperative studies between physicians, surgeons and radiotherapists. It commonly presents as regional lymphadenopathy, with or without symptoms of weight loss, fever, pruritus and occasionally alcohol pain in lymph nodes. The marked improvement in prognosis of this condition reflects a careful study of the disease and the rational application of therapeutic techniques. Four histological varieties of Hodgkin's disease have been identified; lymphocytic predominance, nodular sclerosing, mixed cellularity and lymphocytic depletion. The first two have a better prognosis than the third, and the last is significantly poorer than all others. Localised disease can be cured by adequate radiotherapy alone, but since it is essential to know the extent of the disease and thus avoid undertreating (and possibly failing to cure) a patient with occult but more extensive disease than is clinically apparent, a widely accepted staging procedure is now used. This includes assessment of liver function, bone marrow, lymphangiogram and laparotomy and splenectomy. During the last procedure the liver is biopsied and selected lymph nodes are removed for histology. These include lymph nodes from standard sites plus any which appear involved on lymphangiogram. Once these procedures are complete the extent of the disease is summarised by a simple staging procedure (Table 2). When the patient is symptom free this is sub-classified

Table 2. The currently used staging procedure for Hodgkin's disease.

Stage I	Involvement of a single lymph node region (I) or of a single extra-lymphatic organ or site (I_E).
Stage II	Involvement of two or more lymph node regions on the same side of the diaphragm (II) or localised involvement of extra-lymphatic organ or site and one or more lymph node regions on the same side of the diaphragm (II_E).
Stage III	Involvement of lymph node regions on both sides of the diaphragm (III) $\pm$ involvement of the spleen (III_S) or localised extra-lymphatic organ or site (III_E).
Stage IV	Diffuse or disseminated involvement of one or more extra-lymphatic organs or tissues, e.g. liver, marrow, pleura, lung, bone and skin.

Systemic symptoms — Weight loss, fever, sweating. If absent = 'A'.   If present = 'B'.

as A disease. Weight loss or fever are regarded as B disease. The latter is a less favourable prognostic sign.

It has been customary in many centres to treat disease above the diaphragm, stages IA to IB, with 'mantle' radiotherapy either down to or just below the diaphragm, and with disease above and below the diaphragm (IIIA) to treat with radiotherapy to all lymph node groups (a mantle followed by an inverted Y). The remaining stages are treated with chemotherapy alone, either MOPP (mustine, vincristine, prednisolone and procarbazine) or MVPP (mustine, vinblastine, prednisolone and procarbazine). These are given as two weekly courses at either monthly or 6-weekly intervals. The total number of courses given varies from centre to centre, ranging from six to as many as sixteen given over 3 years with decreasing frequency. The morbidity associated with this treatment is low but a minority of patients find the nausea following mustine intolerable so that oral cyclophosphamide has to be given in its place.

The dosage of radiotherapy above and below the diaphragm varies from centre to centre and some clinicians follow radiotherapy with six courses of quadruple chemotherapy in those patients with a poor histological type of Hodgkin's disease. Using these intensive investigational and therapeutic measures, the overall survival in patients with Hodgkin's disease regardless of stage of histology, is 77.6% alive at 5 years (Figure 3). With localised disease and good histology the percentage of adequately treated patients alive and free of disease at 5 years exceeds this last figure.

Other lymphomas (non-Hodgkin)

While the classification of Hodgkin's disease is well accepted and the prognostic implications of the sub groups recognised, that of other lymphomas is less clear. However, a workable classification has evolved and has formed the basis of many clinical studies. This is compared with the older classification in Table 3. The histology of

Table 3. **A widely accepted histological classification for non-Hodgkin lymphomas.** *Compared with the international classification*

Classification 1
(Gall and Mallory, 1942)

Lymphocytic lymphoma
Lymphoblastic lymphoma
Stem cell lymphoma
Clasmatocytic lymphoma
Follicular lymphoma

Classification 2
(Rappaport, 1966)

Nodular   Diffuse

Undifferentiated
Histiocytic
Mixed histiocytic-lymphocytic
Lymphocytic well differentiated
Lymphocytic poorly differentiated

these lymphomas may show either a nodular or a diffuse pattern and it is apparent clinically that those with the nodular pattern have a better prognosis than those in which the lymph node architecture is lost. The clinical presentation may resemble Hodgkin's disease, but unlike the latter, non-Hodgkin lymphomas do not follow a predictable pattern of behaviour and preliminary studies have not yet shown that aggressive extended field radiotherapy holds the same advantage for these diseases as it does for Hodgkin's disease. Indeed, the clinical spectrum of these lymphomas is greater than that associated with the different histological varieties of Hodgkin's disease, for patients with a well differentiated diffuse lymphoma may live for many years with mild or non-existent lymphadenopathy requiring no treatment, whereas a localised histiocytic lymphoma, proven at laparotomy to be localised

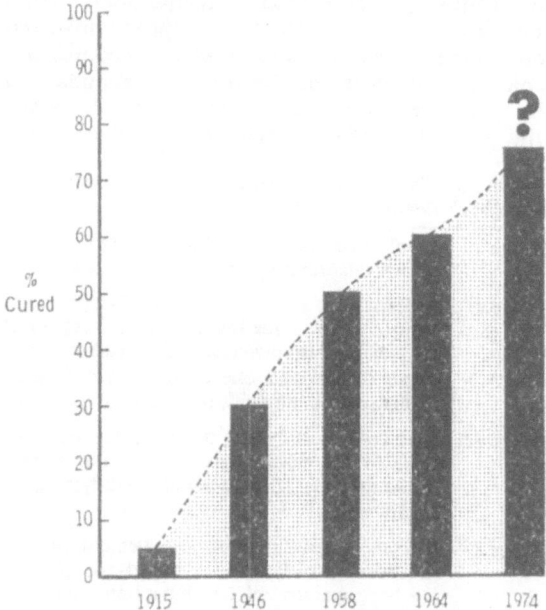

Figure 3. How the estimated chance of being cured of Hodgkin's disease has changed from 1915-1974.

may, despite adequate treatment by radiotherapy, recur and extend rapidly from another site.

In this last condition particularly, extra nodal disease is not uncommon. An undifferentiated lymphoma may more resemble a leukaemia than a lymphoma. Various chemotherapeutic regimens used alone or with radiotherapy are in the process of evaluation. Of these, CVP (cyclophosphamide, vincristine and prednisolone) has been reported to give good results in the better differentiated tumours, although the superiority of this over chlorambucil alone has not yet been established. In the less well differentiated tumours, including the histiocytic lymphomas, it has been shown to be more effective than single drug therapy.

Improved classification methods based on the immunological characteristics of the lymphomatous cells may offer the best chance of assessing prognosis and susceptibility to the therapeutic measures so far available. As yet the discipline developed for Hodgkin's disease can not be applied to this other group of lymphomas.

Choriocarcinoma

Although rare—only 37 new cases were reported in 1970—choriocarcinoma merits discussion since it is a malignancy which can be cured by chemotherapy alone. Slightly more than 50% of cases follow a hydatidiform mole and a high titre of HCG (human chorionic gonadotrophin) following evacuation of such a mole is very suggestive of the presence of a choriocarcinoma. Distinction between an invasive mole and a choriocarcinoma may prove more difficult but where possible curetings should be examined histologically to distinguish the two. There is no indication for hysterectomy unless to control unmanageable uterine haemorrhage.

It is customary to nurse patients admitted for treatment in sterile isolation units since therapy may produce profound bone marrow suppression. Anti-folate drugs alone can produce complete remission in up to 75% of patients, but in refractory cases drug combinations are indicated. The HCG levels are monitored at regular intervals following treatment as a means of detecting early recurrence. About 50% of patients presenting with this condition can be completely cured.

The major centre in the United Kingdom specialising in the management of this tumour is the Department of Medical Oncology, Charing Cross Hospital, London.

Conclusions

As the management of individual neoplasms becomes more and more specialised, so the available resources for managing cancers tend to become aggregated within special centres. The results of the treatment of particular malignancies within such centres, and the contribution they have to offer not only to the standard of specialist care available for the patient, in the training of those associated with managing a cancer patient, but also in developing a greater understanding of malignant disease, more than justify their existence. Unfortunately at the present time these specialist centres are often geographically far removed from the home of the patient and his family and the difficulties likely to be encountered by them as a result of such a referral must obviously be weighed carefully against the possible benefit which may result. Much greater guidance will ultimately have to be offered to the family physician to assist him in recognising those of his patients who would previously have been regarded as unrescuable, but for whom recent advances offer considerable opportunities of recovery.

This text would not be complete without some brief comment on the management of the terminal cancer patient. This problem, all too familiar to the clinician, is no less demanding than one where anti-cancer therapy is required. The decision that a patient is beyond beneficial therapy for his malignancy is often not an easy one, and indeed it is tempting to go further than is really justifiable in the hope of achieving some regression of disease, if only temporary. Rapidly advancing disease in the face of therapy or the risk of toxicity or of side effects worse than the disease itself are indications that therapy should be changed or abandoned. Once the decision to abandon an attempt to reduce the disease has been taken, the therapeutic endeavour should be directed towards making the patient's life tolerable. In this day of powerful analgesics, pain should no longer be a necessary suffering. Pleural effusion and ascites may be relieved temporarily by drainage and their recurrence delayed in some cases by an intra-cavity injection of a cytotoxic agent. Both local radiotherapy and chemotherapy used judiciously may play a useful palliative role.

The intelligent use of the resources available, both pharmacological and otherwise can diminish the intolerable burden to the terminal cancer patient and to those who surround him, and in many cases reduce the period of the patient's dependence on others to an absolute minimum.

Progress in the management and treatment of many different malignancies has made the promise of complete cure much less remote, and the next decade will hopefully offer a better prospect to those with advanced and disseminated disease.

3

PAIN AND TERMINAL CARE

E. WILKES

PSYCHOLOGICAL FACTORS

Because of the advances in medical care most patients now die at the end of a chronic and tedious illness rather than as a consequence of pneumonia or other short-term disease. This gives rise to many psychological, social and physical problems so that the essential factor in attaining good terminal care is a knowledge of the whole situation of the patient and his family.

The patient will often complain of pain – this is indeed by far the commonest complaint and it occurs in between half and three-quarters of cases dying from malignant disease. It does seem however that pain is sometimes used by the patient as a complaint when their real problem may be more of emotional desolation and spiritual loneliness consequent on their general predicament. It is not respectable to complain of desolation or loneliness so the patient will complain of pain. Depression, for example, may magnify discomfort to a genuinely severe or even intractable pain. It is extremely important, therefore that the doctor in charge should not restrict his therapeutic intervention to the control of pain impulses along the lateral spino-thalamic tracts. He must be dealing with the patient and not just the pain. Personal relationships may be more vital here than any drug.

The knowledge of the diagnosis can have an important influence on the degree of suffering felt by the patient. Many patients do not wish to know that they are dying and they will take the problems of each day without long-term worries, and without too much curiosity. Such patients tend to be popular with doctors and nurses as they are easier to handle and, indeed, they often include people of poor education who accept old-fashioned attitudes from those in charge of their case. There is little doubt, however, that such patients are gradually becoming less typical in our society and that more and more patients are requiring to know the truth about their situation than was the case 10 or 20 years ago. These patients are sometimes kept in a state of acute anxiety and uncertainty because of the unwillingness of doctors to face the truth about their own therapeutic impotence and to take their patients more fully into their confidence. Many patients experience a strange sense of relief when they are told that their illness is not curable. They no longer feel that they have to fight, they no longer feel surrounded by a wall of lying and deception. Although general practitioners still tell the truth to only a minority of their dying patients, the proportion told seems to be increasing steadily: and more doctors now hesitate to be caught out in a flagrant and damaging lie.

The major support of the patient must come from the family. But the family in turn need educating and supporting, and this integral part of terminal care has an important influence on the control of what the patient will call pain. The family must have their lives organised for them in a kindly and perhaps slightly authoritarian way so that, for example, never more than one member of the family is on duty at night and some kind of shift system is devised to help ride out an illness of 6 or 12 months, or even longer. The members of the family sharing the care must be taught as much as they can deal with, depending on their physical state and their nursing capacity. Most relatives, if given calm instruction from the home nurse, or indeed from the hospital nurse, will be able to keep the patient's pressure areas in reasonable repair. They will be able to change urine bags if the patient is catheterised. They will be able to give drugs appropriate in dosage and in the timing of that dosage and they will maintain a suitable fluid intake and prepare a sensible diet.

In many of these facets of care the standard of a well-briefed family may indeed be shamefully superior to the standards attainable in a busy and under-staffed hospital ward. This will only be so, however, if the family is really well briefed and this necessitates the doctor, his home nurse, and his health visitor carving time out of a hard-pressed day to talk about the symptoms which may be worrying the relatives, the purposes for which drugs are prescribed, the way they should be used for maximum help, and the action to be taken in certain emergencies. This necessitates no less than a simple, often repeated training programme which will give the family not only trust in their professional advisers but also confidence in their own ability to cope.

They must be given clearly to understand that for the great majority of those cases who die fairly slowly pain is severe in only a tiny minority. In the conditions of general practice 50% of the cancer cases dying at home have no pain at all and only some 10% to 15% of cases stretch the nursing and medical resources in controlling the situation. These facts alone should be given early on in the illness to the relatives, and if the nurse or the doctor can promise always to be available, either personally or through a well-briefed colleague, and that the pain will always be tolerable and well controlled, this simple message can transform the whole atmosphere of the sick room for the whole duration of the illness – no matter how tedious and harrassing this may be. The doctor, on his side, needs candour from the family about the patient's reactions, worries and quality of life. Without this his care must be uncertain and based on inadequate data.

All this does not mean that everything is going to be easy and that the patient will become a more noble animal than ever he was in health. Patients will become bored, demoralised and demanding, despite all than can be done for them. They will complain bitterly that the tablets or medicine do not suit them and are upsetting them. This should be accepted by the doctor and slight modifications tried. This sort of patient will be helped by blaming the doctor rather than the basic disease process and by these changes and manipulations of drugs time is used up; and time is an important weapon for the doctor.

Patients may also become somewhat unreasonable in their requirements. They may want to go into the garden, or drive the car, or they may exaggerate minor complaints while trivialising more central and vital disabilities. A small proportion of them become disturbed and feel that their doctors are poisoning them or they become frankly aggressive towards their wives. The hypercalcaemia of disseminated malignant disease, or renal or hepatic failure will alter personalities as well as drug metabolism, and yet another factor may be the presence of cerebral metastases. In all these syndromes confidence in the doctor and the nurses and effective management of the situation in a familiar environment is more important than drug therapy, tremendously helpful though the drugs can be. Other non-pharmacological factors of great importance in this situation are the religious background of the patient, the accommodation of the patient, and

the preservation of the self-respect of the patient. These three factors merit a brief discussion.

Even in an increasingly pagan society, many people who are losing ground in a long illness tend to revert, naturally enough, to the religious practices of their childhood and they clearly derive comfort and consolation from a routine which carries with it a backward-looking connotation of youth and vigour. It is important to remember from Hinton's study (Hinton, 1963) that the more religious patient may well be the more depressed. Clearly, however, deeply religious people are tremendously helped by the discipline and support of their familiar religious practices, and facilities for these must be immediately and informally available without any unnecessary conforming pressures.

The accommodation of the patient is ideally in their own home: but dying at home is getting rarer and now only a third in an ageing society succeed in ending their days there. Simple extras—a hand-rail or a wheel-chair, a home-help or a night-nursing service—may allow terminal cases to stay at home without too much improvisation or loneliness. The family usually accept their responsibilities well: but if there is only a small or aged family or no family at all, then an institutionalised dying may be imperative. That there are only a few units especially geared to the needs of the dying patient is inevitable and wholly excusable. What is not so easily tolerated in our hospitals is the poor catering, the rushed and haphazard nursing, the general lack of amenity and privacy and dignity, and the insensitive or inadequate attitudes of the staff that may find expression in visiting regulations more suited to the open prison than to the last few weeks of life.

Simple and easy occupational therapy lightens the tedium of the illness and if it can create something which is genuinely useful and demands an effort that is still practicable, this can alter the whole attitude of the patient towards his own body image and greatly reduce the tendency for self-rejection and disgust. This latter tendency is especially distressing for the younger man or the woman who can gain enormous help—and sometimes a diminished need for analgesics—from a visit by the beautician or the skilled administrations of a hairdresser. Domiciliary occupational therapy or a hairdressing and beauty-care service would be no sentimental fantasy but a helpful expansion of medical care.

PAIN CONTROL

If the patient is well cared for, calm, resigned

and able to adjust to the disability either through a great and conscious effort or through the stoicism of advancing years, then mild analgesics such as paracetamol or dextropropoxyphene tablets are all that may be needed. Such patients may complain more bitterly of their weakness, their anorexia and cachexia, rather than of pain.

Unhappily, however, it is common for the patients of even the most conscientious and involved practitioners to suffer severe and unnecessary pain. Cartwright (1973) discovered that while some 85% of practitioners were thought by relatives to be friendly and approachable people, no less than 30% of the dying patient's symptoms were not communicated to or discussed with the doctor. This must be a major cause for the frequent and excessive delay in the use of potent analgesics, such as the opiates and their synthetic analogues.

These drugs are used for some three-quarters of terminal cases in hospitals but in only about half of cases dying at home. Even when they are used, they are not always used effectively. Junior doctors may be over cautious or timid in their dosage, while their nursing colleagues are prone to accept for too long a regime that is clearly inadequate. Pain should be prevented by a regular routine of medication with extra drugs available as and when required. Even the routine 3-hourly schedule may not be enough for the most difficult case: and the 4-hourly schedule may be more a convenience to a busy staff than to the patient in pain. Relatives must be instructed to give relief in a responsible way but without improper delay. This seems easier to organise at home than in many big hospitals.

There are many ways of using the opiates but one of the varieties of mixture known as the Brompton cocktail is a reliable stand-by. Gin is used often as a vehicle here but its use is best restricted to those who like it. A perfectly adequate alternative is to use 10 mg of cocaine and 10 mg of diamorphine in 10 ml of chloroform water. The dosage can vary from 5 to 20 ml but if the higher dosage is often needed the mixture can be altered to 10 mg of cocaine but with 30 mg of diamorphine in 10 ml of chloroform water. Here again from 5 to 20 ml may be given every 3 or 4 hours and other drugs can be added to the mixture if needed. Diazepam, prochlorperazine or chlorpromazine are probably most often used in this way. If it is desired to use morphine, 2.5 ml of nepenthe—a liquid opium with added morphine—can be used similarly with phenothiazines. This is a good preparation, but since diamorphine (heroin) may cause less nausea and vomiting and seems to give better mood-control

and euphoria it is marginally preferred to morphine, for all that it has a shorter duration of action.

If the patient has been in pain for some time he will often benefit from the speedy imposition of really effective control even if this makes him drowsy. The dosage can be reduced with caution after a few days, when he is rested, refreshed and more confident.

In very ill patients injections of diamorphine (6–20 mg) or of morphine (10–20 mg) are more effective by subcutaneous or intramuscular injection than orally. Morphine works after 15 minutes for some 4 hours, diamorphine perhaps only for 2 or 3 hours. Intravenous injections help after 2–5 minutes.

Patients in great distress or who have been on such drugs for a long time form a small minority but they may well need greater than routine dosage. 30 mg of diamorphine or 60 mg of morphine are quite often needed for such patients. Tolerance combined with an increasing need for these drugs is atypical however and in most terminal cases the appropriate analgesic dosage may well need little alteration for weeks or months. Conversely, when the patient says he is in more pain and needs more help he is usually right. Individual needs vary more than is usually described.

The common side effects of morphine and to a lesser degree diamorphine are nausea, vomiting, anorexia, dizziness, constipation, impairment of bladder control, restlessness, mood changes, and respiratory depression. Nausea is more frequent than vomiting and is usually controlled by antiemetics. Dizziness is met with in the ambulant patient. Constipation is always a problem. In the usual doses the other side effects are, like the allergic reactions (urticaria, pruritus), rare enough to be only occasionally a nuisance in general practice.

Paracetamol and dextropropoxyphene have been mentioned as effective for the control of discomfort or milder pain. Paracetamol is more free from side effects and is as effective as compound codeine tablets. Dextropropoxyphene more resembles morphine in its toxic effects, and can lead to dependence. It is therefore to be used with care alone or in combination with tranquillisers but is a useful drug although less potent slightly in its analgesic effects than codeine. The usual dosage is 65 mg 3 or 4 times in the day.

Codeine produces the same side effects as morphine but more rarely and less severely. It only rarely produces dependence, and is, of course, a much less powerful analgesic. If pain is not controlled by 60 mg of codeine, it will be ineffective in higher doses. It produces no euphoria, and rather less constipation than morphine. It is valuable as an anti-tussive in doses of 45 to 120 mg daily in divided doses.

There are comparatively few drugs of real value in the control of intermediate grades of terminal pain. Most cases will do well on paracetamol or dextropropoxyphene. If not, then they will need the opiates. Many more intermediate drugs exist, of course, and some are very often prescribed. The most popular are dihydrocodeine tartrate and dextromoramide. Dihydrocodeine tartrate may produce nausea, vomiting or vertigo in the therapeutic dosage of 30 mg, but by mouth or injection it is effective for mild to moderate pain. Dextromoramide by mouth or intramuscular injection (in a dose of 5 mg usually but this can be doubled or even quadrupled) or as a 10 mg suppository is also a popular drug. Pentazocine (intramuscularly 30 mg or orally 50 mg every 3–4 hours are average doses) and phenazocine (by mouth 5–10 mg or by injection 2 mg) are preparations that lack the euphoriant and sedative effects of diamorphine but are not greatly inferior to morphine or diamorphine in their purely analgesic properties. Their use in general practice is likely to increase. Another useful drug is dipipanone, of which 25 mg by injection is said to be equivalent in effectiveness and duration to 10 mg of morphine. In tablets 10 mg of dipipanone are combined with 30 mg of the anti-emetic cyclizine. When morphine or diamorphine do not suit the patient one or two tablets of this preparation every 4 hours may often prove both acceptable and efficient, more closely resembling the effectiveness of the opiates.

The short duration of action of pethidine and the lack of sedative action of methadone make these drugs only occasionally useful in terminal pain control.

OTHER SYMPTOMS

Confusion and anxiety are common. Diazepam (2–10 mg) or chlordiazepoxide (5–10 mg) combine well with routinely used analgesics and in certain cases the muscle-relaxant and anticonvulsant action of diazepam can be an added advantage, as can its association with amnesia in high or intravenous dosage.

Haloperidol (1–2 ml of the liquid or tablets of 1.5 or 5 mg given two or three times daily) is valuable in disorientated or anxious patients and is not used as often as it merits. It has a less anti-emetic and less sedative effect than chlorpromazine but its clinical effects resemble closely those of the phenothiazines.

Chlorpromazine is the most frequently prescribed member of the phenothiazine group. It can be used orally or by injection in dosages of 10–100 mg. It has an anti-emetic effect, potentiates the analgesic action of the opiates (the syrup can be added to the Brompton cocktail), is valuable in the treatment of hiccoughs and calms the agitated or confused patient. Serious blood dyscrasias, cardiomyopathies, or jaundice can occur but only the latter is fairly common; and if it is indicated the drug can be administered safely to cases of terminal malignant disease in the presence of obstructive jaundice.

Such a valuable drug tends to be frequently prescribed: but if it is given in high dosage to patients in pain it impairs their inability to communicate without necessarily keeping them comfortable. Sometimes the high dosage of chlorpromazine so sedates a patient that confusion is exacerbated and bedsores occur prematurely. The parkinsonism syndrome associated with a daily dosage of 800 mg or more may contribute to this last problem.

Of other phenothiazines trifluoperazine (1–5 mg) is equally effective as an anti-emetic but is more stimulating than sedative. Perphenazine and promazine are generally similar to chlorpromazine but are slightly less sedative and therefore are often used for older patients.

Insomnia often afflicts the terminal patient unless they are kept really comfortable. Triclorofos tablets or syrup (1–2 g) or nitrazepam tablets (5–10 mg) are adequate for most cases but patients habituated to a barbiturate or other hypnotic are best kept with their accustomed routine to the end.

Care must be taken to ensure that the sleeplessness is not caused by inadequate analgesia. The insertion of a 60 mg morphine suppository at bedtime will deal with this. Another less frequent cause is a depressive illness not out of place in their state. The tricyclic anti-depressants should be given a thorough therapeutic trial in such cases but despite the occasional success the results are disappointing. The monoamine oxidase inhibitors are only rarely indicated since their interaction with other drugs makes the general management of the case more complicated. A drug combination hardly ever indicated nowadays save for terminal mood-control is the amphetamine–barbiturate combination and this can prove most helpful in the short term.

Cachexia is usually progressive but occasionally the symptom is mitigated by cytotoxic drugs and when anorexia is associated to a marked degree small doses of steroids such as prednisolone 5 mg twice daily are a genuine help.

Nausea and vomiting are also common problems. The usual anti-emetics are prochlorperazine by mouth, injection or suppository (5–25 mg), cyclizine tablets, injections or suppositories (25–50 mg) which are less sedative, and metoclopramide (10 mg in tablets or syrup) which induces gastric peristalsis and emptying. It must be remembered that intractable vomiting may deserve palliative surgery even if life is short. Milder cases respond often to the antihistamine tablet promethazine theoclate 25 mg twice daily.

If the vomiting is due to cerebral deposits, injections of dexamethasone 8 mg two or three times daily can reduce cerebral edema and cause a great, if temporary, amelioration of symptoms. This is a costly treatment but can give weeks of sane life in primary cerebral tumours.

Dyspnea is associated with anxiety even more often than pain, and can prove difficult to control. The aspiration of pleural effusions can be at times enormously helpful and yet on other occasions makes disappointingly little difference. When associated with widespread pulmonary metastases relatives should be warned that an unexpectedly rapid turn for the worse can take place without warning. On the other hand chronic bronchitics can adjust well for months to a greatly restricted exercise tolerance.

Spasmolytics (orciprenaline, salbutamol, steroids) and oxygen are of some help but refractory cases are best helped by cautiously graduated doses of diamorphine (2.5 mg is a reasonable starting dose) combined with diazepam (2–5 mg). This is the most helpful combination of drugs for the dyspnea due to disseminated malignant disease and is also helpful in terminal cardiovascular disease in which β-blockers, intensive diuretic therapy and digoxin may all be indicated. Mucolytic agents such as bromhexine hydrochloride (24–32 mg in three or four divided doses) certainly reduce sputum viscosity *in vitro*. Bromhexine has been reported as increasing the tetracycline content of bronchitic sputum while producing a subjective feeling of improvement. It is doubtful however whether this comparatively expensive preparation has been associated with any large-scale improvement in pulmonary function and it is best left to trial in difficult cases clinically troubled by tenacious sputum. It is probably being over-prescribed and is contraindicated in cases with a history of gastric ulcer.

Cough can be a most distressing symptom in cases of pharyngeal or lung neoplasm. Codeine has already been mentioned as effective in milder cases, but in those exhausted by their paroxysms routine doses of diamorphine (5–10 mg) can be supplemented regularly, or at need, by linctus

methadone, containing 4 mg in 10 ml of syrup. The combination of diamorphine and methadone will give good control in almost all cases.

Patients on opiates are often anorexic and inactive too. This combination leads to a formidable degree of constipation both worrying and uncomfortable to the patient. Some cases prove stubborn and are best dealt with by twice-weekly enemata or regular manual removals. Bran in the diet, bulk laxatives like methyl cellulose granules (1–4 g in divided doses), daily sub-laxative doses of routine preparations such as liquid paraffin and magnesium hydroxide emulsion (10–20 ml) or a standardised senna preparation may obviate the need for these measures or render them more acceptable to the patient. It should be emphasised that constipation is of major interest since it menaces the patient's comfort although not his health.

Urinary or faecal incontinence tremendously increase the difficulties of domiciliary care. Indwelling catheters usually solve the urinary problem and faecal incontinence is usually due to impaction with spurious diarrhea that needs energetic treatment to produce rapid relief. When the incontinence is due to malignant fistula(e) this tends to make transfer to a suitable institution, if it exists, appropriate. Tenesmus can also be troublesome and cryosurgery, cytotoxic therapy or palliative radiotherapy may be indicated.

When haematuria is a problem, surprisingly effective control can be given by the energetic treatment of urinary infections, a high fluid intake, and by the exhibition of the haemostatic substance aminocaproic acid. This is an antifibrinolytic agent which inhibits plasminogen activity and is largely excreted in the urine. It is contraindicated in severe renal failure and can give rise to nausea, diarrhea, hypotension and the usual allergic reactions, such as rash, pruritus or nasal stuffiness. A dosage usually safe and effective is in 6 g sachets three times daily.

Relatives must be taught that as the end draws near they are likely to be suffering a good deal more than their patient. They must be discreet at the bedside since the patient's comprehension may long outlast their ability to communicate. Relatives as well as the doctors and nurses, need to remember that as sensory perception is dimmed so touch becomes more important, the pressed shoulder or the clasped hand is more comforting than any words.

Fluid intake must be maintained as long as possible in very small, frequent sips yet relatives must not harrass a patient unduly to eat or drink.

Oral moniliasis is common at this stage and needs simple treatment by a fungicidal suspension such as nystatin suspension 1 ml four or five times daily.

As chest secretions accumulate the noisy breathing is best treated by an injection of hyoscine hydrobromide (4 mg). This dries up the secretions well and its sedative effect makes hyoscine more suitable than atropine which can excite the patient. The purpose of this, as of all other measures, must be made clear to the whole team involved in conveying their patient on the last journey. Such involvement is a major help in the future management of bereavement.

4

SOME USES OF LOCAL ANALGESICS, PHENOL AND ALCOHOL IN INTRACTABLE PAIN

FRANK WILSON

Persistent pain is the dominant symptom in a wide variety of conditions which embraces all branches of medicine. The purpose of this chapter is to discuss a few of the conditions where patients may sometimes respond dramatically to the disruption of the transmission of pain impulses by local analgesics such as lignocaine hydrochloride or bupivacaine or by the injection of phenol or alcohol. However, it is important to appreciate that specific treatment of this type should be used in conjunction with other available treatment such as the administration of analgesics, sedatives, anti-depressants or cytotoxic drugs. Equally important is a close liaison between the social worker and district nurse who should be made fully conversant with the problems involved. Procedures such as posterior rhizotomy, surgical cordotomy or percutaneous electrical cordotomy may also need to be considered, all of which necessitate admission to special units.

In the simplest classification, with respect to their regional sites of origin, there are several main types of pain which may confront the practitioner. These include peripheral pain, as for example cutaneous and deep somatic pain, visceral, peritoneal and pleural pain and also referred pain which is felt at a site different from its place of origin. Various combinations and overlappings of these types of pain may occur. Decision regarding the origin of the pain and the route it takes may be difficult, but choice of agent and site of injection depend on correct interpretation of the site of stimulation and route of the affected pain fibres.

TYPES OF PAIN

The reception, transmission, perception and response to pain constitute a very complex subject which is not completely understood but a wide variety of views has been formulated.

Because a lesion sometimes involves more than one type of sensory nerve pathway, successful interruption of one particular group of sensory fibres may only reduce the intensity of the pain or diminish the area in which it is felt. Complete abolition of the pain will only occur after interruption of the remaining affected pathways (see Case history 9.

PERIPHERAL PAIN

Pain pathways

Excessive stimulation of sensory receptors produces pain impulses which pass along the peripheral nerves to the region of the spinal cord which they enter by way of the dorsal nerve roots. Entry into the spinal cord itself separates the pain and temperature fibres from other sensory fibres such as some of the touch fibres and those conducting position, joint and vibration sense. The pain fibres in the cord either proceed upwards on the same side or decussate to form the spino-thalamic tracts, all of which proceed to the thalamus which is intimately connected with the cerebral cortex.

Types and characteristics

1. *Superficial (cutaneous) pain.* The site of origin of the pain often determines the type of sensation. Cutaneous pain is familiar to all people and can usually be perceived as two different sensations. Sudden penetration of the skin by a needle, for example, gives rise to an initial sharp pain which is followed by a longer lasting burning sensation even if the original stimulus is immediately removed. The initial pain is referred to as the 'incident pain' and the more persistent pain is regarded as 'continuous pain.' The time lag between reception and perception of the two pains is due to different rates of conduction through the different types of pain conducting fibres. Incident pain is transmitted through the larger myelinated A fibres whereas

the longer acting continuous pain passes along the smaller non-myelinated C fibres. Appreciation of the fact that two types of pain can exist is of clinical importance in some patients because incident pain is usually relieved by immobilisation or rest whereas continuous pain is not. A patient who develops a pathological fracture may experience a sudden incident pain which is aggravated by movement. Fixation of the appropriate site by plaster, corset, sling, sand-bag, pin, nail or plate can give considerable relief.

2. *Deep somatic (non-visceral) pain.* Pain arising from bone, tendon, ligament, fascia, joints and muscle travels up the same nervous pathways as cutaneous pain but their segmental innervation does not always correspond with those of the overlying skin (see Referred Pain). Deep somatic pain tends to present as a dull ache and is not as well defined as cutaneous pain. It is often associated with muscle spasm or rigidity.

VISCERAL PAIN

Pain pathways

The nerve pathways which transmit the pain fibres, although separate from the autonomic nervous system, accompany either the sympathetic or parasympathetic nerve fibres on their way to the dorsal nerve roots and ganglia, thalamus and cortex. In the upper abdomen the pain fibres pass with the sympathetic nerves through the lumbar and thoracic sympathetic ganglia and into the dorsal nerve root ganglia via the white rami communicantes. The pelvic pain fibres, however, accompany the parasympathetic nerve fibres in the pelvic nerves, the nervi erigentes, on the front of the sacrum to reach the dorsal nerve root ganglia and spinal cord at the level of S_2 and S_3.

Types and characteristics

Interference to the outflow of any viscus by an obstructing carcinoma gives rise to the pain and other symptoms typical of acute or chronic obstruction. Reduction of visceral blood supply can cause gangrene. However, intractable cancer pain is due to infiltration of the sensory nervous pathways causing a characteristic dull ache which often becomes severe and continuous.

PERITONEAL AND PLEURAL PAIN

The parietal layers of the peritoneum and pleura are sensitive to pain.

Characteristics

Parietal sensations are conducted directly from the parietal peritoneum and pleura and are localised directly over the painful area. They can also be referred to other regions well away from the initial site of stimulation.

REFERRED PAIN

Pain from deep structures such as muscle, bone and deep joints is not referred to beneath the overlying dermatome, except when the two embryologically coincide in position such as in the intercostal region. It is referred to another deep structure area known as a sclerotome which may be some distance away from the diseased area but which is innervated by the same nerve. For example, pain in the pectoral region, although underlying the T_4 dermatome, may be caused by disc involvement of the C_7 nerve root because this nerve supplies the lower pectoral muscle. Similarly, involvement of the hip muscles may cause referred pain to the knee and diaphragmatic pain to the shoulder because the shoulder and diaphragm are both supplied by C_4.

SPECIFIC CONDITIONS

The following section describes a few conditions where local injection may be beneficial. The case histories included are brief and only state a few of the relevant points pertinent to the particular treatment described.

HERPES ZOSTER

Post-herpetic neuralgia is a common cause of intractable pain. The pain may persist for years after the acute phase and may cause considerable misery. The affected site of the nervous system is thought to be the dorsal nerve root ganglia and naturally it would be supposed that any treatment directed towards the nervous pathways, to alleviate pain, should be directed towards these ganglia. In actual fact many people respond remarkably well to the injection of 2–10 ml 0.5% bupivacaine or 0.5% lignocaine into the region of the painful area of the skin. It is the practice of the author to inject the local analgesic subcutaneously beneath the old skin lesions, and also to form a barrier of analgesia proximal to the cutaneous scarring, in the hope that any sensory impulses originating from the scarred region may be interrupted on their way to the spinal cord.

In spite of the fact that local analgesics theoretically act for only 3 or 4 hours it is sometimes found that pain is relieved for 24–48 hours. After further injections the periods of analgesia often begin to increase in duration so that after 3 or 4 injections the analgesia may last a week. Following 6 or 12 injections of local analgesic the pain may permanently disappear or become faint enough to need only 2 or 4 aspirins per day.

Not all patients respond to this treatment and it should be pointed out to them that it is the intention to reduce the pain to a tolerable or acceptable level and that only in a few people will there be complete and permanent abolition of pain. Where the peripheral nerves are easily located, as for example the intercostals, they may be infiltrated by means of a paravertebral block but the author prefers the more generalised infiltration of the region in and around the actual painful area.

Case history 1
Past history. Male. Aged 74 years.

August 1974. Referred to pain relief clinic by general practitioner with 4½ years history of post-herpetic pain around left side of chest, which prevented him from moving his left arm sufficiently to cope with the gear change in his car.
Treatment: He was injected with 2% lignocaine hydrochloride beneath the old herpetic scars and also around the 6th intercostal nerve proximal to the old lesion. The pain was abolished and he was pain free for 1 week during which full arm movements were restored. 10 injections at weekly and then fortnightly intervals resulted in him being pain free and able to drive his car in comfort.

Trigeminal neuralgia
A prior injection of local analgesic, such as bupivacaine or lignocaine hydrochloride, into the trigeminal ganglion allows the patient to experience the abolition of pain and also the associated loss of other sensory sensations before embarking on a phenol or alcohol block which is of much longer or permanent duration.

Many patients develop trigeminal neuralgia following an attack of herpes and it is always worth while injecting bupivacaine beneath the lesions or around the accessible sensory nerves such as the supratrochlear, supraorbital and lachrymal division of the ophthalmic nerve.

The author recently, in a patient with post-herpetic trigeminal neuralgia, successfully reduced the intensity of the pain which was distributed over the ophthalmic division of the trigeminal nerve by a series of bupivacaine injections, similar to those described in Case history 1, so that analgesics were no longer necessary.

Amputation stumps
Pain in amputation stumps can be very distressing and is often very difficult to treat. The author has had no success in treating the pain and tenderness in amputated thumbs. Occasionally, however, in amputated limbs there may be found areas which are localised and excruciatingly painful to the touch. Local analgesics, injected around and then into these areas, often cause freedom from pain from anything up to 1 or 2 days. Repeated injections prolong the duration of time that he is pain free and after 6 or 12 injections there may be no need for further treatment.

Case history 2
Past history. Male. Aged 69 years.

1962. Right arm was caught in the rollers of a conveyor and was literally pulled off. Amputation performed at junction of middle and lower third of humerus.
1968. Fell and bruised stump. Complained of severe pain in stump. Painful neuroma excised which relieved his pain.
July 1972. Pain returned. Two large and two small neuromas removed with sections of the nerves from which they were arising.
August 1972. Was taking 10–12 dihydrocodeine tartrate (DF118) 30 mg tablets daily. Referred to pain relief clinic by orthopaedic surgeon. Very tender areas in tissues deep to operation scar and at end of stump. Slight pressure caused excruciating pain over these areas.
Treatment: 1st local infiltration with 1% lignocaine hydrochloride around and into painful areas caused relief of pain for 3 hours.
2nd injection lasted 4 days.
3rd injection lasted 6 days.
4th injection lasted 14 days.
5th and subsequent injections lasted 14 days and pain was then controlled with 2 DF118 tablets a day.
November 1973. Was still free from pain and injections were stopped.
May 1974. Still free from pain.

Trigger points
The painful back or neck can be notoriously difficult to cure, but it is always worth while looking carefully for a local trigger point. This can sometimes be found only on deep pressure by the palpating fingers and often it responds to local infiltration of 0.5% bupivacaine or 0.5% lignocaine followed by gentle massage, manipulation and exercise. Such treatment can have dramatic results and a search for trigger areas in the muscles or ligaments should not be omitted just because the patient has obvious radiological evidence of arthritis which could give pain in that

particular area. Likewise, the presence of a neo-plasm should not always be blamed for causing pain. An associated spinal arthritis may be the main culprit and phenylbutazone may alleviate the pain thus obviating the need to give an intra-thecal injection of phenol.

Case history 3
Past history. Male. Aged 53 years.

May 1973. 1 year history of pain in neck radiating to occiput, shoulder and arms. X-ray showed severe cervical spondylosis at many levels, most marked between C_3 and C_4, C_6 and C_7. Pain in the shoulders and arms disappeared after traction, physio-therapy, collar and phenylbutazone (Buta-zolidin).

June 1973. Pain in neck and back of head returned and made his life miserable.

2nd October 1973. Referred to neuro-surgeon who referred him to pain relief clinic requesting to see the effect of local analgesic infiltration of affected occipital nerve.

25th October 1973. Seen at pain relief clinic. Acute deep tenderness was discovered just below occipital protuberance, to left of mid line.

Treatment: 0.5% bupivacaine was injected into tender area with instantaneous abolition of pain which did not return for 2 days. Repeated injections of bupivacaine resulted in longer periods of analgesia until eventually, after 12 injections, weekly infiltrations of local analgesic kept him pain free.

7th June 1974. Neurosurgeon exposed and avulsed the left greater occipital nerve.

Postoperatively he developed an area of anaesthesia over the appropriate area and he was pain free.

INTRATHECAL PHENOL INJECTION IN CANCER PATIENTS

Intrathecal injection of phenol can completely abolish the intractable pain due to cancer. In about one third of patients the results are dra-matic. A miserable looking patient who has been confined to bed, and who has not slept continu-ously for more than 2 hours for months due to constant pain, suddenly undergoes a complete transformation. His countenance changes, the age-ing years flow away from his face, his eyes fill with disbelief and a cautious smile creeps across his face as he begins to realise that the pain has gone.

Unfortunately, approximately a further one third of these patients show only moderate or slight improvement and the remaining one third show none at all. Nevertheless the fact remains that improvement can be dramatic and phenol injection should always be considered.

Technique

All the details of techniques are not included in this chapter but it is important that the prac-titioner knows the principle, the difficulties in-volved and the complications of intrathecal injections. The principle underlying intrathecal injections of phenol is to place it in contact with the dorsal nerve roots and thereby destroy the pain fibres. Originally it was thought that the small non-myelinated pain fibres were selectively destroyed but recent opinion indicates that the phenol is non-selective and can damage all types of nerve fibres. However, if the phenol is cor-rectly placed it can abolish pain and have re-markably little effect on other sensations so that the perception of touch in the affected segments may remain or be only slightly reduced.

Control of the phenol is assisted by making a solution of 5% phenol in glycerine[1] which more or less has the flow characteristics of pure glycerine. It is therefore much heavier than cerebrospinal fluid and when introduced within the theca it runs down to more dependent levels.[2] In the case of cutaneous pain the operator decides which dorsal nerve root he wishes to treat, if necessary with the help of dermatome charts (Figure 1). Pain from viscera, bone and muscle is more diffuse and it is not so accurately represented in these charts. It may involve treatment of a greater number of nerve roots, some of them being some distance from those which serve the overlying skin of the painful area (see Referred Pain).

---

[1] Phenol B.P. 5% w/v in glycerine BP.

[2] Some doctors use intrathecal alcohol which is less dense than cerebrospinal fluid. Because of this hypobaric property, and the fact that the alcohol should be placed where the twiglets of the dorsal nerve roots enter the spinal cord, a different tech-nique is needed.

The patient is positioned so that he lies painful side up. At this stage it must be remembered that the spinal nerves join the spinal cord at a higher level than the correspondingly numbered vertebral bodies. For example the 6th thoracic nerve emerges from the cord at the level of the body of the 4th thoracic vertebra and the 1st lumbar nerve joins the cord at the level of the 10th thoracic vertebra. Fail-ure to appreciate these points may result in nerve blocks lower down the cord than are desired.

The spread of alcohol is more difficult to control than phenol and consequently is not as popular as 5% phenol in glycerine.

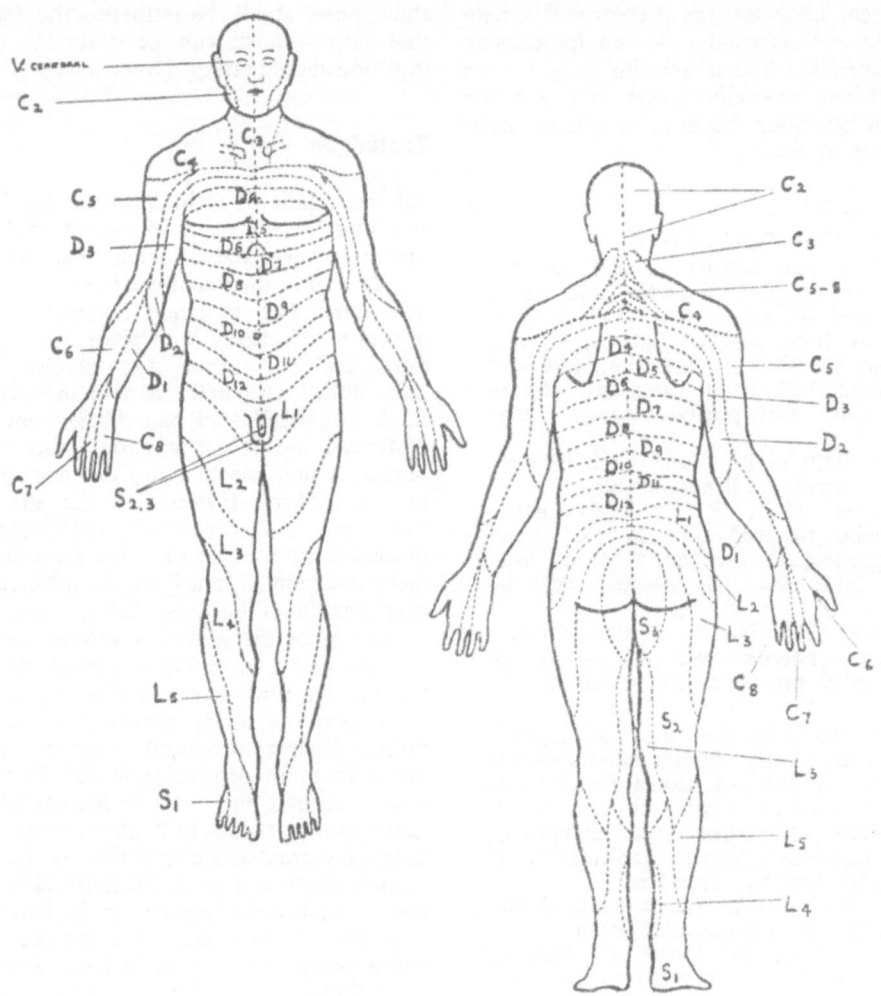

Figure 1A. Dermatome charts

It is recognised that it is easiest and safest to apply the phenol to the dorsal nerve roots where they enter the intervertebral foramina. Consequently, once it has been decided which dorsal nerve roots are to be treated, their position of exit through the side of the dura into the intervertebral foramina must be decided either by palpation of vertebral spines, combined with the well known anatomical landmarks[3] or by means of an X-ray using a well placed marker such as a paper-clip. The dura is penetrated by the lumbar puncture needle over or adjacent to either the top one or the bottom one of the selected dorsal nerve roots. The patient is then turned onto his side and rolled 30°–40° backwards so that the dorsal nerve roots of the painful side become dependent. He is then tilted head up or head down and maintained in such position so that when the phenol is injected it will gravitate and 'fix' onto those dorsal nerve roots which need the block.

The needle is then withdrawn gradually until a position is reached in which cerebrospinal fluid just flows out so that the needle point is as far away from the cord as is possible. At this stage the dura will be coned, and with the needle bevel directed towards the affected spinal nerves the drops of phenol are injected which slide down

---

[3] (i) The 12th rib, leading medially to the body of T_{12} helps to locate the body of L_1. (ii) The highest level of the iliac crest is at the level between spines (or bodies) of L_3 and L_4. (iii) The dimples over the posterior superior iliac spines lie at the level of the spine of S_2.

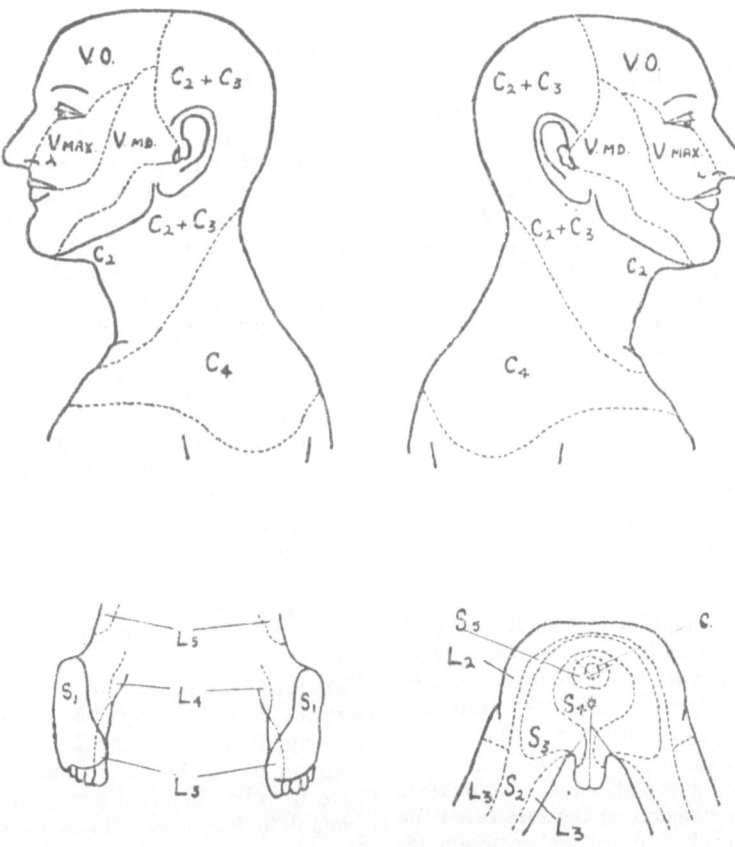

Figure 1B. Dermatome charts

the coned dura onto the dorsal nerve roots as they leave the dura to enter the intervertebral foramina. The quantity of 5% phenol in glycerine injected varies from 0.2 ml to 3.0 ml in the lumbar region and up to 2.0 ml to 3.0 ml in the thoracic region. In these quantities the phenol affects 2 or 3 segments. The patient is then kept in the selected position for half an hour after which there is no danger of further spread.

Attempts to cone the dura prior to injection of the phenol in glycerine sometimes results in accidental withdrawal of the needle from the intrathecal space. Re-entry into the intrathecal space may require re-posturing the patient to the sitting position or other more convenient position.

Prolonged or frequent attempts to cone the dura upset the patient, mostly due to the fact that rolling him 'into a ball' to help the operator causes considerable distress, especially if he is elderly, obese or dyspneic. It is essential, therefore, that the patient is not subjected to any unnecessary pain which may result from the intrathecal injection. Consequently, the author always

infiltrates the structures liberally with local anaesthetic as the lumbar puncture needle is advanced towards the theca. As a result some local analgesic may enter the epidural space and abolish any pain which is transmitted along the nerve roots in contact with the local analgesic. This causes further problems because according to most authors the introduction of phenol in glycerine into the theca results in certain well defined symptoms, indicating that it is being introduced onto the correct nerve roots. Typically the patient is said to feel immediate loss of pain over the affected nerve roots followed by creeping paraesthesiae or warmth according to the direction of the flow of the phenol in glycerine. These symptoms are followed by diminished sensation to pin prick but no reduction in sensation to light touch. The author has only occasionally been able to elicit these symptoms, probably due to the fact, already mentioned, that he infiltrates the tissues generously with local analgesic in advance of the lumbar puncture needle. However, even if a local analgesic is not used prior to puncture of the dura, too much reliance cannot be placed on this abolition of pain followed by para-aesthesia because frequently the mere introduction of a needle into the skin, at the site of proposed entry of the lumbar puncture needle, results in temporary abolition of a pain which the patient has had for months. Furthermore, in elderly patients, paraesthesiae frequently appear due to the position in which they are being held. They also find paraesthesia difficult to assess, describe and localise and the operator may be misled. Consequently too much reliance cannot be placed on either the abolition of pain or the production of paraesthesiae as regards the correct approximation of an intrathecal needle to the selected nerve roots.

Some anaesthetists use phenol in radio-opaque iophendylate so that the path taken by the phenol may be observed on the X-ray screen. Others think that iophendylate interfers with the effects of the phenol.

The significance of the need to posture the 'phenol patient' and maintain him in that chosen position during and after the injection is obvious because it does limit where the injection can be performed. Some anaesthetists carry out the treatment in the patient's home but the author feels that only rarely is this warranted.

Furthermore, finding the theca can sometimes be difficult and time consuming because often the patient is old, his back is deformed, osteophytes are present and ossification of the spinous ligaments has taken place. Collapse of the vertebral bodies may cause further deformities and add to the difficulties.

Complications

Complications are similar to those of an ordinary lumbar puncture, but phenol can affect all types of nerve fibre and it is because of this that more immediate and serious complications can arise.

5% phenol in glycerine, run onto the spinal cord or onto the ventral nerve roots, can cause motor weakness so that the patient has difficulty in walking. Usually this improves after 2 or 3 days.

Contact with the nerve supply to the bladder causes urinary retention which usually lasts for 2 or 3 days and therefore careful watch must be kept on the urinary output and catheterisation performed if necessary. This can of course be a further problem in the home. In isolated cases the retention may persist for 10 days but it can be permanent. Absence or difficulty of urinary control before the injection should be carefully noted so that the injection is not blamed for causing an already disfunctioning bladder.

Discussion of complications with the patient

Decision as to whether intrathecal injection is justified warrants careful consideration. The patient should be told of the possible complications but if too much emphasis is placed on them then he will invariably refuse to have anything done even though he is in severe pain. He is then denied a technique which may remove his pain completely. It is advisable to mention the possible complications to the patient but also to tell him that they usually clear up in 2 to 3 days.

Treatment of extensive lesions

It is neither always possible nor wise to treat all the affected segments at once if more than three are involved. Further injections can be given for the other segments at 2 or 3 days interval. It is also probably safer to treat the dorsal nerve roots, one side at a time, at 2 or 3 days interval if the pain is bilateral. If complications occur, such as urinary retention, they should be given ample time to clear up before further segments are treated.

Extent of pain relief

Relief of pain may be permanent. In other patients it recurs after 2 to 3 weeks but may respond to further injection. Spread of the disease to other nerve segments necessitates further phenol to the newly affected area. Failure to relieve pain is due to faulty technique or possible involvement of the nerve roots with cancer tissue which prevents contact with the phenol.

Sites of injection

Intrathecal phenol can be given to treat nerve roots in the cervical, thoracic or lumbo-sacral region.

CERVICAL REGION

Cervical injections are not too difficult to perform but they have the reputation of not being so successful for cancer as are those made lower down the vertebral column. Nevertheless the author has seen one patient, who was on diamorphine hydrochloride (heroin) and cocaine due to pain in her arm as a result of secondaries from lung cancer, who received immediate relief and took no further heroin or cocaine until she died 2 months later (see Case history 4).

Great care must be taken to ensure that the phenol does not run upwards to the brain. Therefore, if the patient faints during, or shortly after, the introduction of phenol the operator must not follow his normal practice of lowering the head! The correct treatment is to raise the feet and at the same time keep the head elevated.

Case history 4

Past history. Female. Aged 48 years.
Smoked 20 cigarettes a day for past 30 years.
September 1971. Normal X-ray and broncho-scopy.
April 1972. Diagnosed as carcinoma bronchus. Treated with radiotherapy to right supra-clavicular node enlargement and to mediastinum for very advanced carcinoma of the lung.
21st October 1972. Referred from general practitioner to pain relief clinic because of intractable pain inside right arm near anterior border of axilla and in outer side of shoulder going towards inside of the arm, i.e. C_4, C_5 distribution. He stated 'for 5 months she has been on increasing doses of a diamorphine hydrochloride (heroin) mixture—now on heroin 30 mg, chlorpromazine 25 mg and cocaine 5 mg 3-hourly orally plus morphine 10 mg at night by injection. In addition she is on pentazocine hydrochloride 50 mg and dipipanone hydrochloride 10 mg with cyclizine 30 mg from time to time'. These failed to control her pain. She had a very edematous right arm with marked anaphylactic type swellings of both infra-orbital regions. These were probably gravitational due to the fact that for several months she had been unable to lie down with comfort and used to sleep sitting up leaning over 4 pillows.
22nd October 1972. **Treatment:** 18.00 hours. Needle inserted intrathecally between C_3 and C_4 with patient in sitting position. She was postured so that she was leaning backwards and also laterally to the right so that the 0.75 ml 5% phenol in glycerine injected intrathecally gravitated towards the dorsal nerve roots of C_4 and C_5. She was maintained in this position with pillows for a further half hour. She developed pins and needles down the arm but no loss of sensation.
20.00 hours. Fell asleep and slept all night without sedation. When she awoke the pain had gone. She had no further heroin or morphine until 2 months later when she died of pneumonia.

Comment. This patient illustrates that it is possible to cease taking narcotics voluntarily even after a regular substantial intake over 5 months once the intractable pain has been removed.

THORACIC REGION

Injections in the mid-thoracic region are the most difficult to perform because of the marked obliquity of the thoracic spinous processes. However, as regards complications, provided the needle is correctly sited, they are the least dangerous because the curve of the thoracic spine can usually be easily controlled and varied to control the deposition of the phenol onto the affected segments. Intractable pain due to infiltration of the thoracic spine and ribs with cancer often is completely relieved by this treatment.

Case history 5

Past history. Male. Aged 68 years.
April 1973. Haematuria. Biopsy of growth right lateral wall of bladder showed 'not too well differentiated transitional cell neoplasm.'
May 1973. Radical course of X-ray treatment to his bladder carcinoma.
September 1973. Developed right sided pain extending from middle of back, around chest, to just below nipple.
March 1974. 'At end of his tether' with pain in chest.
April 1974. Straight X-rays of thoraco-lumbar spine showed no abnormality. Bone scintiscan showed increased uptake in the lower thoracic and lumbar regions consistent with metastases.
24th June 1974. Referred by general practitioner to pain relief clinic with following complaints:—

1. Severe continuous pain in right side of chest along distribution of T_5, relief of which was obtained by 2-hourly dose of Brompton mixture, every dose containing diamorphine hydrochloride (heroin) 20 mg and cocaine 20 mg, plus heroin 30 mg intramuscularly at night.
2. Grossly distended abdomen with rock like faeces palpable per rectum. This was relieved by 3 enemas.

25th June 1974. **Treatment:** A marker was placed on T_2–T_3 space and 2 ml 5% phenol in glycerine were injected intrathecally between T_3 and T_4 with him positioned on his right side and in the semi-supine position in order to gravitate it onto the right dorsal nerve roots. At the same time the head was elevated to prevent upward spread towards the brain, and the pelvis was raised to prevent gravitation onto the nerve supply of the bladder.
Pain immediately disappeared. Slightly restless in night. Brompton mixture was neither asked for nor given.
27th June 1974. Completely free from pain. Had not requested his Brompton mixture since his intrathecal injection. Discharged home.
29th July 1974. Completely free from pain. Had had no Brompton mixture since leaving hospital. Takes sodium amytal 400 mg at night and an occasional Diconal tablet during day.
14th September 1974. Died from uraemia.

Comment. As in Case history 4 voluntary abstinence of the taking of high doses of heroin and cocaine was immediate once the pain was removed. Withdrawal symptoms can be slight or non-existent. The constipating effect of the opiate can cause considerable abdominal discomfort and distress. Ordinary plain X-ray films may show no evidence of metastases in the spine. In this patient there was useful evidence provided by scintiscan. When this is not available intrathecal injection of phenol should not be withheld in a patient who has a normal plain X-ray when he has obvious malignant disease.

LUMBO-SACRAL REGION

Lumbo-sacral injection is probably the easiest to perform but the most prone to produce complications. If the patient is continent the needle should always be kept away from the termination of the spinal cord, the conus medullaris, which is situated at the level of the body of the 1st lumbar vertebrae.[4] Here, at the origin of the cauda equina, there is a concentrated accumulation of spinal nerves so that many nerve roots can be affected by a small quantity of phenol.

Case history 6

Past history. Female. Aged 51 years.

October 1972. Diagnosed as stage II squamous carcinoma of cervix with induration of anterior vaginal wall.

Treated with radiotherapy.

October 1973. Developed node in right groin. Many nodules in vagina.

17th June 1974. Referred by gynaecologist to pain relief clinic because of pain in left leg. She was taking pentazocine hydrochloride 50 mg 4-hourly. She complained of an aching pain in the lumbar region spreading to the outside of the left buttock, shooting round to the groin and down to the inside of the thigh above the knee. On examination she was analgesic to pin prick over the distribution of L_2. The knee jerk (L_2 L_3 L_4) of the left leg was markedly brisker than that of the right side. Plain X-ray of the lumbo-sacral spine showed 'a destructive, probably metastatic, lesion affecting the left pedicle of L_4 and probably spreading onto the lower border of L_3'.

24th June 1974. **Treatment:** Admitted to hospital. Needle was introduced intrathecally between L_3 and L_4 with patient on her left side. She was rolled backwards to the semi-supine position to bring the left dorsal nerve

roots to the most dependent position. The pelvis was elevated so that the 0.6 ml 5% phenol in glycerine introduced between L_3 and L_4, gravitated upwards, towards and over the dorsal nerve roots of L_2.

27th June 1974. Pain had gone from L_2 distribution. Left knee jerk was absent. Had some weakness of left quadriceps but could walk with support.

29th June 1974. Walked well but left knee had let her down twice. Had had no pentazocine hydrochloride since her intrathecal injection. Pain completely disappeared. Discharged home with corset to support back.

9th July 1974. Could stand for 15 minutes before she became tired. Before intrathecal injection she could only stand for 2 minutes because of pain.

Left knee jerk definitely present but very diminished. Walked normally. Completely pain free over distribution of L_2.

Comment. The painful nerve root was L_2 and the phenol could have been introduced between L_1 and L_2 but any error of technique, such as having the needle too far through the theca, might have resulted in dropping the phenol over the concentrated accumulation of lumbar and sacral nerve roots, near the conus medullaris, with a very real danger of bladder paralysis. It is better, if in doubt, to keep away from L_1 (see Footnote 4). At the level of the body of L_4 the lumbar and sacral nerve roots are not so close together and the chance of an unwanted involvement of many nerve roots with 0.6 ml 5% phenol in glycerine is greatly reduced.

Case history 7

Past history. Female. Aged 46 years.

26th February 1972. 4 weeks' history of diarrhea—3–4 times a day. Had lost 7 kg in weight during last 12 months. P.R. anterior tumour of rectum.

8th March 1973. Abdomino-perineal excision of rectum. Pathological examination of the specimen showed well differentiated adenocarcinoma which had extended through the muscle coats but had not invaded the lymph nodes.

15th October 1973. Abdomen soft, no masses palpable.

16th March 1974. Large abdominal mass was diagnosed as local recurrence of the rectal tumour. Given a course of cytotoxic drug fluorouracil which appeared to make mass softer.

22nd August 1974. Referred to pain relief clinic with 6 weeks' history of localised pain in perineum which was treated by morphine injection 30 mg night and morning and flurazepam 30 mg orally at night. Very lethargic and weak.

---

[4] The anaesthetist usually says 'keep away from L_1,' meaning that the needle point should never, unless entry cannot be made elsewhere, be introduced between T_{12} and L_1 or L_1 and L_2. If L_1 nerve root requires treatment it should be approached from two segments higher up or lower down and the phenol allowed to flow towards L_1. Between T_{10} and T_{11} and between L_2 and L_3 the nerve roots are not so closely packed together.

23rd August 1974. 12.00 hours 0.5 ml 5% phenol in glycerine injected intrathecally between L_5 and S_1 with patient on right side leaning backwards with 20° caudal slope. Then turned gently onto her back with 20° caudal tilt for 10 minutes. She was allowed to sit up a little having her head on 4 pillows for a further 10 minutes when she was allowed to sit up almost upright. 19.00 hours passed 100 ml urine; 21.00 hours passed 180 ml urine; 22.00 hours passed 100 ml urine.
24th August 1974. No analgesic had been asked for nor given since her intrathecal injection. Completely free of perineal pain.
4th September 1974. Still completely free of pain—no analgesic necessary. Much more alert and happier due to withdrawal of morphine.
Comment. Sudden withdrawal of her morphine injections, when the perineal pain had disappeared, caused no withdrawal symptoms. Her abdominal masses were neither painful nor tender and it is interesting to compare her symptoms and the treatment of the tender abdominal masses in Case history 9.

INTRATHECAL PHENOL IN NON-MALIGNANT PATIENTS

Non-malignant causes of intractable pain which were not amenable to surgical treatment were, at one time, considered unsuitable for treatment by intrathecal phenol because of the possible complications. However, the present view, due to increased knowledge of the technique, is that some conditions such as osteoarthritis, spondylitis and vertebral collapse may respond better than malignant patients provided that the pain is localised to 1 or 2 segments on one side of the body.

MANAGEMENT OF UPPER ABDOMINAL CANCER PAIN

Pain fibres from the upper abdominal viscera on their way to the spinal cord, accompany the sympathetic nerve fibres. On their way they pass through the celiac plexus which lies on the front of the 1st lumbar vertebra. This plexus is the obvious place to block if it is considered necessary to disrupt pain transmission in these pain fibres. Such a block, known as a celiac plexus block, with 50% alcohol in water[5], has been used successfully for intractable pain due to cancer of the stomach, liver, gall bladder, pancreas, (see Case history 8, and retroperitoneal tumours. Some authors have also claimed its success in the treat-

[5] Dehydrated alcohol BP (absolute alcohol)

ment of uterine and rectal cancer. Case history 9 describes such a success in rectal cancer, after previous treatment with intrathecal phenol.

Relief of pain can be very dramatic and although it is believed that the block should be performed before addiction to analgesics has developed it is sometimes found that the patient already on large doses of narcotics (see Case histories 7, 8 and 9) may cease to require them and be content with an occasional dose of a mild analgesic.

Technique

The injection should be performed in hospital. The patient is placed face downwards and the needle is inserted through the skin, lateral to the spine of the 1st lumbar vertebra. It is then withdrawn slightly, re-directed and advanced until it penetrates the celiac plexus.

A trial run is performed with 0.5% lignocaine to see if it abolishes the pain after which 50% alcohol in water (see Footnote 5 this page) is injected the following day.

Complications

Apart from the danger of injecting the alcohol into the cerebrospinal fluid, major blood vessels or pleura, there is the complication of hypotension due to interruption of the vasoconstrictor fibres passing through the celiac plexus on their way to the lower part of the body. Hypotension can occur after injection and may result in the elderly patient fainting when he gets out of bed. For 48–72 hours after injection it is advisable to bind the limbs from the feet up to the upper thigh and preferably also to apply an abdominal binder until the time when the vessels apparently re-adapt themselves as regards the maintenance of the vascular tone. Frequent blood pressure readings are advisable for 2 or 3 days, especially in the elderly and note should be taken of the urinary output in case it is affected by the hypotension.

Case history 8

Past history. Female. Aged 63 years.
February 1974. Weight loss 14 kg in 2 months. Abdominal pain for 4 months—worse for last 2 months. Tenderness in left hypochondrium.
March 1974. Liver scan showed decreased uptake of isotope in region of porta hepatis. Pancreatic scan showed a region of decreased uptake in the body. Laparotomy showed inoperable carcinoma of body of pancreas fixed to aorta, invading stomach, with hepatic metastases.

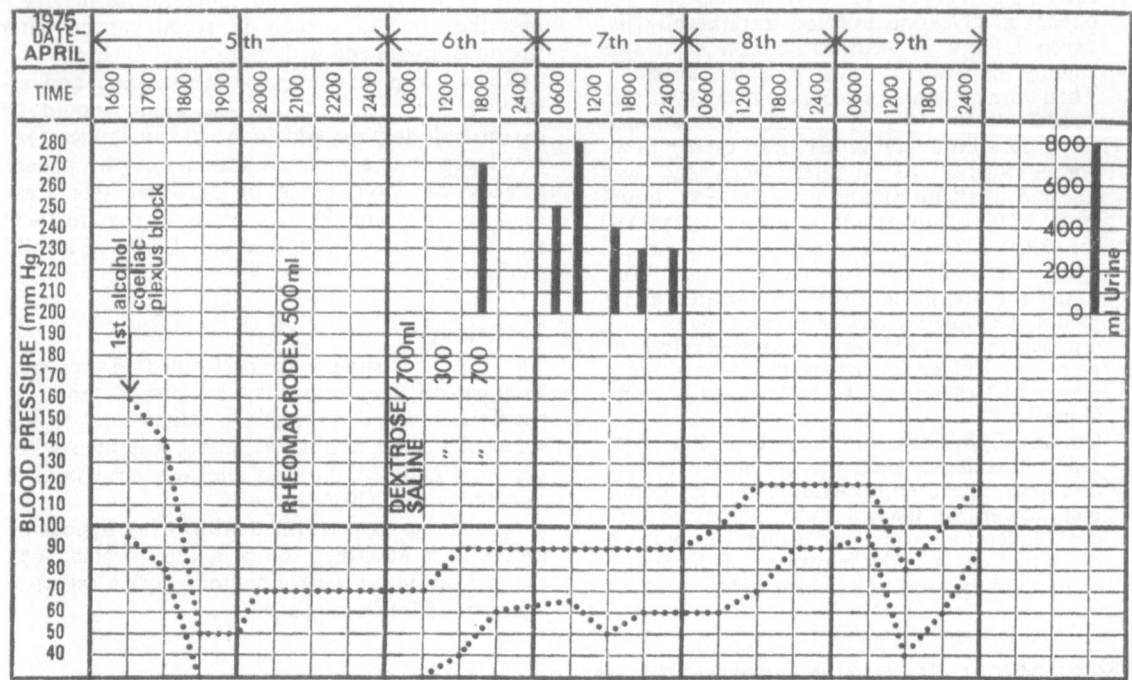

Figure 2. Case history 8. Blood pressure and 3 day urinary output chart after 1st celiac plexus block with 50% alcohol. Note prolonged and severe hypotension and absence of urinary output for 36 hours after block. Oral intake of fluids was normal before and after the block

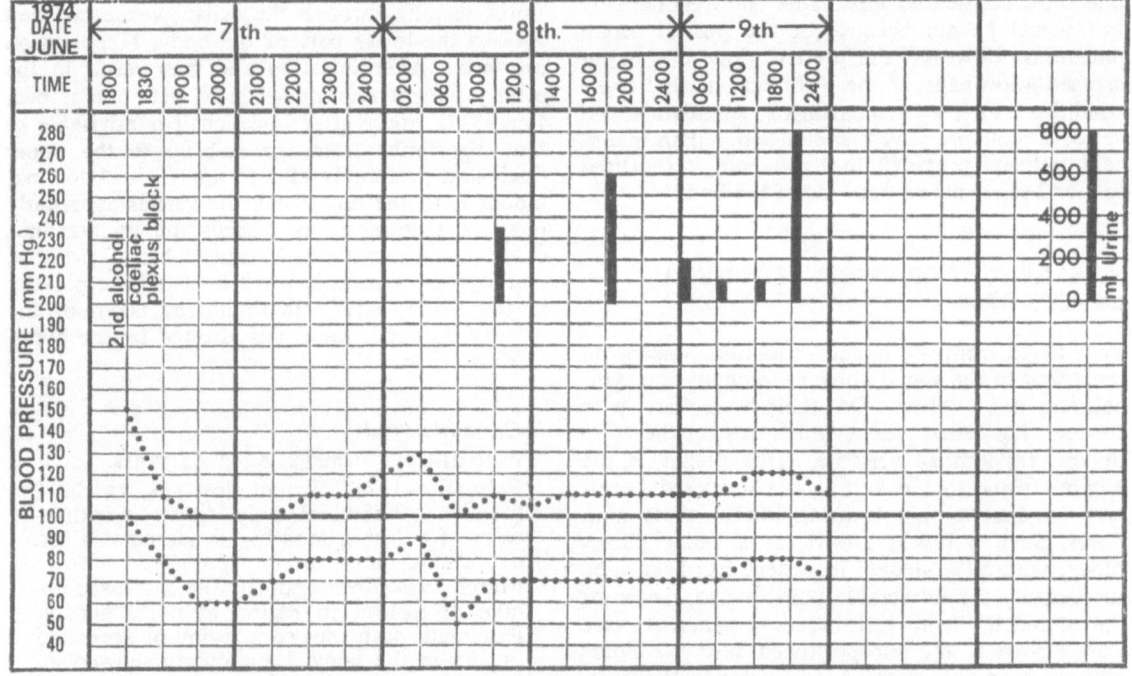

Figure 3. Case history 8. Blood pressure and 3 day urinary output chart after 2nd celiac plexus block with 50% alcohol. Note short duration of slight hypotension and satisfactory urinary output

3rd April 1974. Referred to pain relief clinic by general surgeon because of severe pain and acute tenderness in lower abdomen and lumbar regions. BP 140/90 mmHg. Pentazocine hydrochloride 50 mg 6-hourly, intramuscularly or pethidine hydrochloride 100 mg 4-hourly, intramuscularly. Nitrazepam 10 mg at night, orally.

Treatment: 10.00 hours. Temporary celiac plexus block with 20 ml 0.5% lignocaine gave complete relief of pain on left side and almost complete pain relief on right. BP fell to 70/50 mmHg for 4 hours.

5th April 1974. 16.00 hours. Celiac plexus block repeated with 40 ml 50% alcohol (20 ml to each side). BP fell to 70/40 mmHg for 12 hours and then rose to 90/50 mmHg, reaching her pre-operative value 72 hours later (Figure 2).

Passed no urine.

6th April 1974. Pain and tenderness completely gone in right side. Localised area of tenderness left lumbar region just below 12th rib.

15.00 hours. Passed 700 ml urine.

7th April 1974.

03.00 hours. Passed 500 ml urine.

06.00 hours. Passed 800 ml urine.

The pain in the left side was controlled by dextropropoxyphene hydrochloride and paracetamol but after a few weeks began to get worse.

7th June 1974. Celiac plexus block performed left side with 20 ml 50% alcohol with complete abolition of pain and tenderness. Hypotension occurred as before but was not so profound (Figure 3).

Passed no urine.

8th June. 10.00 hours. Passed 350 ml urine.

16.00 hours. Passed 600 ml urine.

Completely free from pain.

4th September 1974. Has to take 10 minutes to get out of bed in morning because she feels that she would faint if she stands up quickly. After this she is all right. Goes shopping. Completely free of pain and original tenderness.

Comment. Some workers believe that it is only necessary to perform a celiac block on one side because the alcohol is supposed to spread throughout the celiac plexus. In this patient abolition of pain in the right side with the first alcohol block (5th April 1974), leaving residual pain in the left side, suggests one of three alternatives. First that the author 'missed' the ganglia with the left injection. Second, if he did miss it, that 20 ml alcohol is insufficient to spread adequately to the other side (but see Case history 9) or third, that the spread of alcohol in the ganglia is not always unimpeded from one side to the other.

Another interesting point is that abolition of pain was complete after the second alcohol celiac plexus block (7th June 1974) but the hypotension was neither as profound nor as long lasting as after the first alcohol celiac plexus block (5th April 1974). This raises the question as to whether only a proportion of the vasoconstrictor fibres had remained functional after the first alcohol celiac plexus block (5th April 1974) and whether the blood pressure was therefore being well maintained from compensatory sources or pathways which did not involve passage through the celiac plexus.

In view of the successful pain relief, indicating that the alcohol had been put in the correct place at the second celiac plexus block (7th June 1974) it would have been very interesting to see if a third celiac plexus block would have caused any hypotension at all. Absence of hypotension might then have indicated a complete and satisfactory take over by compensatory mechanisms controlling the blood supply to the lower part of the body, uninfluenced by the fibres passing through the celiac plexus.

Case history 9

This patient is interesting because she needed to have a celiac plexus block to relieve her abdominal pain after her main complaint, severe anal pain, had been removed by an intrathecal injection of phenol.

Past history. Female. Aged 75 years.

February 1974. Diagnosed as having a large cauliflower growth of anterior wall of rectum. Considered inoperable.

X-ray of chest showed 'There are several small opacities of varying size in both lungs, presumably secondaries'. Was given a course of the cytotoxic drug fluorouracil.

27th June 1974. Referred to pain relief clinic because of severe pain:—

1. Around anus which was very tender after defaecation.

2. In R.I.F. which was very tender.

Current medication was: Dextropropoxyphene hydrochloride 65 mg and paracetamol 650 mg i.e. 2 tablets, 4-hourly. Pethidine hydrochloride 50 mg 6-hourly orally. Nitrazepam 10 mg at night orally.

The pain after defaecation 'sometimes needed 6 pain relieving tablets to take the pain away.'

Treatment: Very deaf lady—difficult to get her to co-operate. A needle was introduced between L_5 and S_1. She was placed onto her right side, rolled backwards to the semi-supine position and 0.6 ml 5% phenol in glycerine was injected intrathecally. Then she was turned onto her back with 10° foot down tilt for half an hour.

2nd July 1974. Complete absence of pain around anus. Very diminished sensation to pin prick in area 8 cm wide around anus.

5th July 1974. Complained of abdominal

M

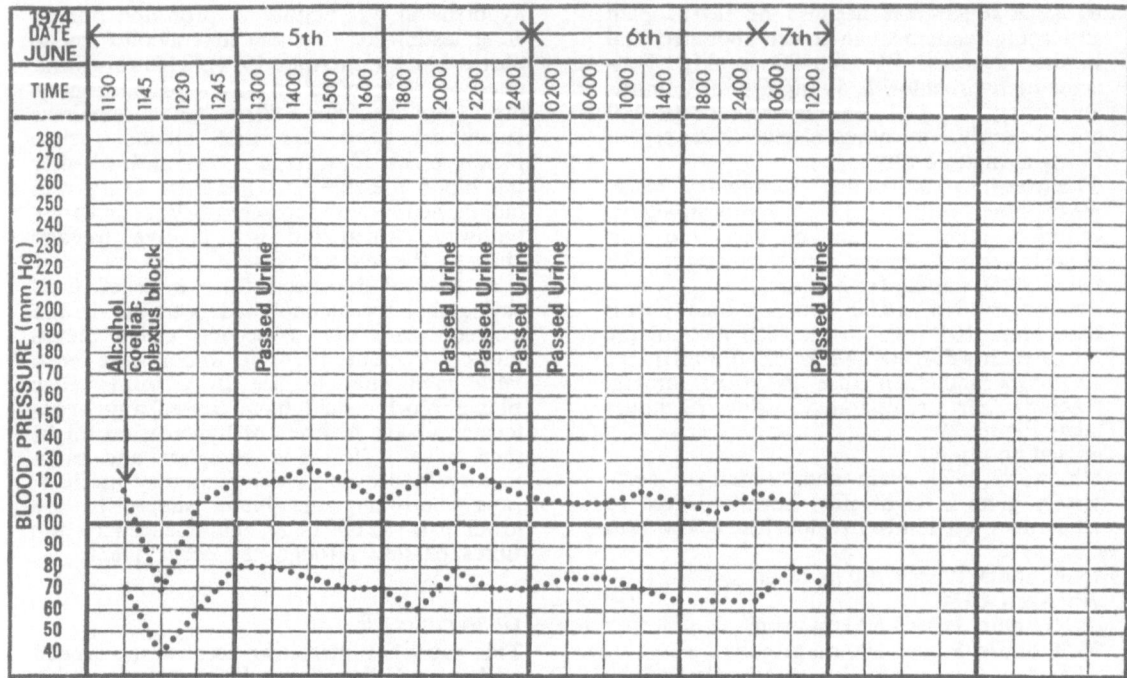

Figure 4. Case history 9. Blood pressure and urinary chart after celiac plexus block with 50% alcohol, the legs having been bound with crepe bandages prior to the block. Note only transient drop of blood pressure. Urinary output appeared to be normal but it was not possible to measure because micturition was accompanied by passage of liquid faecal material per rectum

pain. Very tender over palpable lower abdominal mass. BP 116/70 mmHg. Legs bound with crepe bandages from toes to thigh.

11.30 hours. Celiac plexus block 20 ml of 50% alcohol injected into celiac plexus right side (Figure 4).

Complained of severe pain in back. Felt faint —sweating. BP 70/60 mmHg. In view of the general condition left sided block was not done.

12.30 hours. Free from pain. Tenderness had gone.

6th July 1974. BP maintained itself at pre-operative level. Allowed to walk around bed. Felt faint—was put back to bed. BP 114/70 mmHg.

8th July 1974. Patient allowed to walk up and down ward. No feeling of faintness. Crepe bandages removed from thigh to knee —allowed to walk around ward. No feeling of faintness.

Crepe bandages removed from knee to ankle —no feeling of faintness.

Advised: Before getting out of bed—to sit up for 5 minutes and then hang legs over bed for 5 minutes keeping them moving.

5th September 1974. No pain in anus, abdomen or back. Slightly tender over left upper abdomen. Masses palpable in right iliac fossa, left iliac fossa and suprapubic region had increased in size. Mass also palpable in epigastrium.

Comment. If both methods, namely intrathecal phenol and celiac plexus block with alcohol, are used in one patient then a period of several days should be permitted to elapse between the two techniques. This allows the doctor to evaluate the urinary output so that confusion does not arise between a possible retention of urine due to sacral root involvement and a diminished renal outflow due to hypotension.

24 hours after a celiac plexus block it is customary to bind the legs and possibly the abdomen before the patient is allowed to stand up. This patient had her legs bound from toes to thigh with crepe bandages before the block was performed. Her abdominal pain and tenderness disappeared, showing that the alcohol had been injected at the correct site. Also, that some vasomotor instability did exist was indicated by her tendency to feel very faint when she stood up 48 hours after the block. However, during the 24 hours which she spent on the operating table or in bed after the block, apart from a few minutes at the time of injection, she had no hypotension and no obvious impairment of urinary output by the kidneys. It therefore seems reasonable to advise that patients who

are to have a celiac plexus block should have their legs bound **before** the alcohol is injected in the hope that support to the vessels of the legs will help to prevent hypotension and thus ensure an adequate urinary output.

20 ml alcohol was sufficient to alleviate pain. Either it spread throughout the entire celiac ganglion or the author was just fortunate in blocking the affected pain carrying fibres.

Celiac block is usually advocated for upper abdominal pain but infrequently for rectal cancer. Without laparotomy it cannot be accurately known which intra-abdominal tissues are involved but it appears that a celiac plexus block may be worth considering in intractable pain in the lower as well as the upper abdomen.

In contradistinction to the patient in Case history 8, who did not find the block unpleasant, this lady said that the pain was terrible whilst the alcohol was being injected.

SPASTIC PARAPLEGIA

Transection of the cord eventually leads to a spastic paraplegia. Often associated with this spasticity are violent, spontaneous and uncontrollable jerky movements of the legs. Some patients eventually progress to the scissor-like position of the legs where the thighs are adducted and the feet crossed over each other. The paraplegia confines the patient to bed because his legs will not bend and allow him to sit comfortably at a table or be transported by means of an ordinary car. To add to his misery he develops bed sores and is incontinent of urine and faeces.

The amount of pain varies but may be severe. Usually it is intermittent and is often associated with attacks of muscular spasms. Pain may be a secondary effect from the muscular spasms, in which case abolition of these spasms should be achieved by preventing the passage of motor impulses along the ventral nerve roots by depositing onto them a necrotising solution such as phenol. This has been successfully performed by some physicians, but it is important to realise that diminution of muscle spasms will naturally result in muscular weakness. If, therefore, a person is able to stand with support or transfer himself from one chair to another and the phenol causes him to lose the muscle tone he may no longer be able to stand with support and may be condemned to life in a wheel chair. In the opinion of the author this treatment must never be performed where the patient is able

to utilise his spasticity to some extent in order to perform some action which would be impossible if the affected muscles were rendered flaccid.

Other workers believe that the spasms can be stopped by interrupting the sensory pathways by depositing phenol in the vicinity of the dorsal nerve roots. Breaking the reflex arc at this point can abolish both the pain and the spasms. (See Case history 10.

After the initial injection of the phenol the spasms may temporarily become much worse and the pain most intense. The author is therefore always ready to give pethidine 100 mg intravenously. Analgesics must be prescribed for the next 24–48 hours.

Later the legs become more relaxed and can be moved thus enabling the patient to be taken from his bed and sat in a chair. Further injections of phenol may be required at 3 or 6 monthly intervals.

Complications

Intrathecal injection of this type invariably affects the nerve supply to the bladder and rectum. This may lead to no further problems if he is confined to bed and already has urinary incontinence or requires manual removal of faeces. However, the patient who goes out to work often manages to regulate the emptying of his bladder and bowels or is aware of the times at which such actions will take place. Alteration of these functions by intrathecal phenol can upset a patient's routine and causes him some embarrassment and distress. Sometimes the bladder and bowel may resort to the original habits which they had before the phenol injection but the patient may have to re-adapt his daily routine to fit in with the changes of his ablutions.

Case history 10

Past history. Male. Aged 56 years.
1964. Involved in a car crash. Suffered a severe whip-lash injury to the neck. Was left tetraplegic due to C_6 lesion. Treated in paraplegic and rehabilitation centres.
1st May 1973. Referred to pain relief clinic with following complaints:—
1. Severe spasms in legs which almost threw him out of a chair—eventually they confined him to bed.
2. Severe pain which:—
   a. made him scream.
   b. started in lumbo-sacral region shooting down back of legs around heel and instep.
   c. occurred every few seconds, often for several days at a stretch.

d. failed to respond to the following combination of drugs:—
Amitriptyline hydrochloride 100 mg 3 times daily orally. Chlorpromazine hydrochloride 100 mg 3 times daily. orally. Pentazocine hydrochloride 50 mg 3 times daily orally. Pentazocine hydrochloride 30 mg i.m. at night. Pethidine hydrochloride 100 mg 6-hourly i.m.

3. Adduction of lower limbs with absence of passive movement at hips and knees.
4. Bed sores over right greater trochanter.

2nd May 1974. **Treatment:** Because he had no control of his bladder, a larger quantity, **1.5 ml of 5% phenol in glycerine,** than is usual, was injected **intrathecally** between L_2 and L_3 with the patient on his side. Immediately after injection he was turned onto his back. He felt pins and needles in the legs. Sedated with pethidine 100 mg intravenously.
4th May 1974. Had 2 days of severe pains in legs in spite of sedation.
7th May 1974. Spasms and pain had almost gone. Was able to sit in chair again and lie comfortably on his back and on both sides.
25th February 1974. Spasms had begun to return.
5th March 1974. 1.2 ml of phenol in glycerine was injected intrathecally between L_2 and L_3. Positioned as on 2nd May 1973. Developed severe pain in both legs which became freely movable, passively, at knees.
6th March 1974. Spasms had disappeared. No pain in legs but complained of severe pain from lumbo-sacral region through to scrotum.
19th March 1974. All pains had gone.
16th July 1974. He said that sometimes he gets slight pains in legs but they do not distress him. Routinely he is out of bed and comfortable in a chair from 08.00 hours to 17.00 hours daily. Both legs could be moved passively through 30°–45° at knees and hips. Total sedation in 24 hours is amitriptyline hydrochloride 100 mg three times daily and pentazocine hydrochloride 50 mg nocte orally.

VASCULAR DISORDERS OF THE LOWER LIMBS

Pronounced reduction of the blood flow to the lower limbs causes pain in the feet or calves and often leads to gangrene. Interruption of the vasoconstrictor fibres to the vessels of the lower limbs can be achieved either by surgical lumbar sympathectomy or by chemical lumbar sympa-thectomy in which local analgesics or 5% phenol in water[6] are injected in the region of the lumbar sympathetic ganglia.

Performance of a lumbar sympathetic block with lignocaine often causes the foot to become warm with a reduction in the intensity or with complete removal of the pain. Sometimes the patient remains free of pain for 3 or 4 hours or perhaps for 1 or 2 days. There are, however, some who remain symptomless for 3 to 6 months. This is not easy to explain. It may be due to interruption of some well established reflex arc or it may be a sudden sufficient vasodilatation of the collaterals which never again resort to their original lesser calibre, thus ensuring a regular adequate flow of blood to the limb. If the ligno-caine is successful then 5% phenol in water may be injected but it is advisable to do this under X-ray control. Spillage of the phenol onto the spinal nerves can cause troublesome pain in the groin or upper part of the thigh.

CONCLUSIONS

Addiction to frequent doses of narcotics is generally thought to be easily acquired and diffi-cult to cure. However, the reaction of the patients in Case histories 5, 6, 7, 8 and 9 and others treated by the author strongly suggests that patients with intractable pain, whose increasing demand for larger and more frequent dosage are well known, appear to be able to do without drugs such as morphine, pethidine, cocaine and Fortral without distress, provided that the pain is removed.

Many of the patients who attend the pain relief clinic have been examined, diagnosed and treated by members of many specialities but unfortunately, by some doctors, the pain relief clinic is regarded as a last resort. Consequently, some of the cancer patients die within a few days of being referred. The doctor who runs such a clinic often realises that his efforts will be in vain. However, to those patients who have advanced malignancies, he appears as another interested person on whom they can pin their hope and trust. He can often do much to make the last few weeks or months of their lives bearable both to themselves and to their families.

---

[6] Phenol B.P. % w/v in water for injection BP

5

HYPERLIPOPROTEINAEMIAS AND THEIR TREATMENT

M. C. STONE

There is now a formidable body of evidence linking hyperlipidaemias (or hyperlipoproteinaemias) with the development of premature atherosclerosis and ischaemic heart disease. There is also some recent evidence that hyperlipoproteinaemias are common in countries like the UK and the USA. For example, about 17% of males and females aged 15 to 80 years in a UK general practice were found to have abnormal lipoprotein patterns.

The mechanism whereby raised lipoprotein concentrations influence the risk of ischaemic heart disease (IHD) is still uncertain, but they appear to act together with other 'coronary risk factors' such as raised blood pressure, glucose intolerance, cigarette smoking, etc., the greatest risk being found when several risk factors are present at the same time. Hyperlipoproteinaemias appear to be particularly important in younger males and it has been found that the majority of young males who develop acute myocardial infarction, or who die suddenly from ischaemic heart disease, have hyperlipoproteinaemia.

Interest in hyperlipoproteinaemias has been stimulated in the past two decades by a number of factors:

(1) Simpler methods of lipid and lipoprotein analysis have been described recently, some of which are well within the capacity of most hospital laboratories and some are even suitable for use in health centres.

(2) The classification of lipoprotein patterns described by Fredrickson and his colleagues has provided a simpler basis for investigating and treating hyperlipoproteinaemias.

(3) It is now possible to reduce lipoprotein levels by diet and drugs in the majority of patients.

Recent clinical trials have suggested that reduction of lipoprotein levels may reduce the risk of developing a myocardial infarction in some groups of subjects, and although the results are far from conclusive, this has stimulated much activity in this field.

In view of the changing situation, it is appropriate to review briefly the present position with regard to the diagnosis and management of hyperlipoproteinaemias, with special emphasis on the situation facing the general practitioner.

THE HYPERLIPOPROTEINAEMIAS

The blood plasma of even healthy young subjects contains substantial concentrations of the lipids cholesterol, triglycerides and phospholipids which are transported within macromolecular complexes named lipoproteins. These particles contain both the lipids and globular proteins called apoproteins, which have a special capacity for binding many times their own weight of lipid.

The plasma lipoprotein spectrum contains four main families of particles which differ in size and composition as well as in their sites of synthesis and in the functions which they perform within the body. These four families are represented diagrammatically in Figure 1. The figure also shows the terminology which is now recommended for general use, i.e. high density, low density and very low density lipoproteins, and chylomicrons (HDL, LDL, VLDL and chylomicrons).

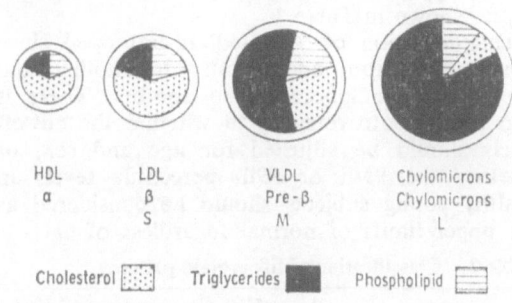

RECOGNITION OF HYPERLIPIDAEMIA AND HYPERLIPOPROTEINAEMIA

The presence of hyperlipoproteinaemia can be recognised if cholesterol and triglyceride estimations in serum or plasma are available. However, a more precise identification of the lipoprotein

Table 1.   Lipoprotein pattern analytical techniques

Lipoprotein fraction	Abbreviation	Alternative names and separation technique		
		Electro-phoresis	Membrane filtration and nephelometry	Analytical ultracentrifugation
High density lipoproteins	HDL	Alpha-lipoproteins	—	—
Low density lipoproteins	LDL	Beta-lipoproteins	Small (S) particles	S_f 0–20 lipoproteins
Very low density lipoproteins	VLDL	Pre-beta lipoproteins	Medium (M) particles	S_f 20–400 lipoproteins
Chylomicrons	—	Chylomicrons	Large (L) particles	$S_f > 400$ lipoproteins

pattern is obtained by the use of analytical techniques which separate (and especially if they also quantify) the major lipoprotein fractions.

A number of techniques are available by which this can be done and each has generated its own terminology. These terminologies are shown in Table 1, but for clinical purposes the terms used for each of the lipoprotein fractions can be regarded as interchangeable. Since electrophoresis and 'membrane filtration and nephelometry' are the simpler techniques they will be more commonly encountered in clinical practice.

CLASSIFICATION OF LIPOPROTEIN PATTERNS

It is possible to classify lipoprotein patterns on the basis of either lipid or lipoprotein analysis and at the present time the most popular of the classifications is that introduced by Fredrickson and his colleagues and modified by a WHO expert committee. The typing of the patterns is based on the concentrations of the LDL, VLDL and chylomicron fractions as shown in Table 2 and can be applied to the results of any of the techniques shown in Table 1.

The definition of 'elevated' is left open since it will vary from one country to another and even from one laboratory to another. There is also some controversy as to whether the cut-off levels should be adjusted for age and sex, or whether the 95th or 99th percentile levels in healthy young subjects should be considered as the upper limits of normal regardless of age.

Table 2.   Classification of lipoprotein patterns

Lipoprotein fraction	Type of lipoprotein pattern						
	Normal	I	IIa	IIb	III	IV	V
LDL	−	−	+	+	−	−	−
VLDL	−	−	−	+	+*	+	+
Chylomicrons	−	+	−	−	±	−	+

−, Normal; +, Elevated; *, Indicates abnormal concentration of a lipoprotein intermediate in size and composition between VLDL and LDL (floating β-lipoproteins)

CLASSIFICATION OF LIPID PROFILES

If only cholesterol and triglyceride estimations are available, the lipoprotein pattern can be estimated from Table 3, but it will be seen that there are a number of lipoprotein patterns which have the same lipid profile. Identification of the pattern is somewhat improved by allowing a sample of the serum to stand in a refrigerator for 24 hours at 4 °C. The sample should then be inspected for the presence of a creamy chylomicron layer and the infranatant serum should be examined for turbidity. It can be seen from Table 3 that this will separate types IIb and IV on the one hand from types III and V on the other.

The different types of lipoprotein pattern may be produced in a number of ways. For example, they may be primary, i.e. genetic, or may be secondary to one of a number of different influences, e.g. nutritional, endocrine diseases, drug or emotional stress. A simple classification of hyperlipoproteinaemias is given in Table 4.

It must be emphasised that each of the types of lipoprotein pattern shown in Tables 2 and 3 may be either genetic or secondary, and that any given type of lipoprotein pattern may be secondary to a number of different diseases. For example, hypothyroidism and nephrotic syndrome may both produce a type IIa pattern or, alternatively, type IIa may be due to a single mutant gene, i.e. familial hypercholesterolaemia (FH). Similarly, the type IV pattern may be familial, but it may also be secondary to obesity, diabetes mellitus, alcoholism or to the use of an oral contraceptive.

The picture is further complicated by the fact that the same primary disorder may be associated with a different type of lipoprotein pattern at different stages of the disease. For example, mild nephrotic syndrome often produces type IIa patterns, whereas in its most florid stage the type IIb or type IV patterns are common.

Table 3. Recognition of lipoprotein patterns from cholesterol and triglyceride concentrations

Serum lipids	Type of lipoprotein pattern						
	Normal	I	IIa	IIb	III	IV	V
Cholesterol	–	–	+	+	+	+ or –	+
Triglyceride	–	+	–	+	+	+	+
Appearance of chilled serum Chylomicron layer	Absent	Present	Absent	Absent	Present or Absent	Absent	Present
Appearance of infranatant	Clear	Clear	Clear	Turbid	Turbid	Turbid	Turbid

–, Normal; +, Elevated.

Table 4. Clinical classification of hyperlipoproteinaemias

(In the majority of subjects with hyperlipoproteinaemia the type and severity of the abnormality is determined by a combination of polygenic and nutritional factors).

Genetic
   Polygenic
   Monogenic

Nutritional
   Excess of total calories leading to obesity
   High intake of certain dietary constituents, e.g.
      saturated fats, sucrose or alcohol

Secondary to other diseases and conditions
   Pregnancy
   Endocrine—diabetes mellitus, hypothyroidism
   Metabolic—gout
   Renal—nephrotic syndrome, chronic renal failure,
      dialysis and renal transplantation
   Liver—obstructive disease, e.g. biliary cirrhosis
   Dysglobulinaemias, e.g. multiple myeloma,
      macroglobulinaemia, systemic lupus erythematosus

Secondary to drug-induced hormonal changes
   Oral contraceptives—estrogens
   Steroids

Induced by other factors
   Stress situations—driving in traffic, lecturing, etc.

VARIABILITY OF LIPOPROTEIN PATTERNS

A further important consideration is the variability of the lipoprotein pattern in an individual at different times. These changes may be produced by changes in diet, (there is a marked fall in lipoprotein concentrations with weight loss), seasonal variation, and particularly as a result of some major upset or illness, e.g. a surgical operation, a major fracture or a myocardial infarction, may each produce a marked fall in lipoprotein concentrations lasting for several weeks.

THE DIAGNOSIS OF HYPERLIPOPROTEINAEMIAS

It is clear from the previous sections that the diagnosis of hyperlipoproteinaemia cannot be made merely by knowing that the patient has, for example, a type IIa or a type IV lipoprotein pattern. In order to arrive at a diagnosis, one should have examined the blood under standardised conditions and have carried out a full physical examination.

One must ensure that:

1. The blood is drawn after an overnight fast of about 14 hours and with the minimum of venous stasis.

2. The patient has been taking his usual diet for at least 2 weeks and is not losing weight.

3. He is not taking any drugs likely to affect the lipoprotein pattern, e.g. clofibrate, thyroxine, or phenformin.

4. He is not within about 10 to 20 weeks of a major illness likely to have affected the lipoprotein pattern, e.g. acute myocardial infarction.

He should also be examined carefully to exclude the presence of any of the secondary causes of hyperlipoproteinaemia given in the clinical classification above, and should be questioned as to the possibility of a familial incidence of hyperlipoproteinaemia. His eyes should be examined for evidence of premature arcus corneae and his skin and tendons should be examined carefully for xanthomata. Laboratory tests should be carried out to exclude the presence of any underlying disorder which may account for the lipoprotein abnormality. If, as a result of these examinations, it seems likely that the patient is suffering from a familial type of hyperlipoproteinaemia, other members of the family should be examined to confirm this possibility.

HOW COMMON IS HYPERLIPOPROTEINAEMIA?

In the relatively small number of population studies published so far, types IIa and IV lipoprotein patterns have been found more commonly than the other types. In a UK general practice study* it was found that in males, type IV was the most common pattern (about 10%), with type IIa as the next most common (about 5%). In females, however, type IIa was the most common (11%) with type IV the next most common (4%). Type IIb patterns occurred in about 2% of males and 1% of females, whereas types III and V were much less common, and type I was not seen at all.

In some groups of subjects commonly encountered in general practice, hyperlipoproteinaemias are much more common than in the population as a whole, e.g. those with obesity, ischaemic heart disease, diabetes mellitus, and also those who regularly take a good deal of alcohol. The other secondary causes of hyperlipoproteinaemia shown in Table 4 are less commonly encountered in general practice although they form a substantial proportion of patients seen in hospital lipid clinics.

Primary or genetic hyperlipoproteinaemias are also found in general practice, for example, each practice has at least one or two families with familial type IIa hyperlipoproteinaemia (familial hypercholesterolaemia). These families may be detected initially when a young male member has an acute myocardial infarction or dies suddenly, or may be made manifest when xanthomata appear in the skin or tendons of one of the family members.

WHOM SHOULD WE TREAT?

Only a small proportion of subjects with hyperlipoproteinaemia develop symptoms and signs directly attributable to the abnormal concentration of lipoproteins. These include attacks of acute abdominal pain, acute pancreatitis, and skin and tendon xanthomas, all of which are manifestations of severe degrees of hyperlipoproteinaemia. It is clearly justifiable to treat this group of patients.

The majority of subjects, however, are not aware of their hyperlipoproteinaemia, yet the severity of atheroma in these subjects is greater than in those with lower lipoprotein concentrations and the risk of developing ischaemic heart disease is also greater. Atherogenesis is a chronic process, starting in childhood, and it has yet to be established conclusively that reduction of lipoprotein levels in middle aged subjects is capable of producing regression of these lesions or even

---

*Stone *et al.*, *Clin. Chim. Acta*, **31**, 333 (1971).

of halting their progress. In spite of this lack of conclusive proof, many workers in this field consider that correction of hyperlipoproteinaemia and also of other factors such as hypertension and cigarette smoking is justifiable at present, especially in subjects who have more than one of these coronary risk factors.

We should therefore, seek to treat those subjects with hyperlipoproteinaemia who are most vulnerable, e.g. those subjects with any of the following findings:

1. Severe degrees of hyperlipoproteinaemia, especially in young males with types IIa and IIb.

2. Angina pectoris, ischaemic changes in an ECG or signs of left ventricular hypertrophy.

3. Raised blood pressure or cigarette smoking. These two risk factors should also be treated at the same time as the hyperlipoproteinaemia.

4. Abnormal glucose tolerance.

5. A family history of premature ischaemic heart disease or other vascular disease.

Subjects with hyperlipoproteinaemia secondary to other diseases will probably not require treatment aimed specifically at the lipoprotein abnormality. In these subjects spontaneous remission or successful treatment of the primary disease will often correct the lipoprotein abnormality. However, if this does not occur, diet or drug therapy of the hyperlipoproteinaemia itself may have to be considered.

MONITORING THE RESULTS OF THERAPY

Two methods are in common use for the monitoring of therapy:

1. Changes in the plasma or serum cholesterol and triglyceride concentrations will give a good indication of the success or failure of therapy.

2. Changes in the concentrations of LDL, VLDL and chylomicrons can be estimated by membrane filtration and nephelometry. The results of this technique can be expressed in the form of a lipoprotein profile (the SML profile) whose changing shape and changing position on the reference frame gives a graphic representation of the alteration in lipoprotein pattern produced by treatment (see Figure 2).

TREATMENT OF HYPERLIPOPROTEINAEMIAS

We can now treat hyperlipoproteinaemia successfully in a great majority of subjects but in order to ensure maximum reduction of lipoprotein levels, both diet and drug therapy are usually necessary.

Time (months)	0	1	3	7	8
Cholesterol (mg/100 ml)	294	306	232	200	215
(mmol l^{-1})		8.0	6.3	5.25	5.5
Weight (kg)	72.7	67.3	64.1	64.6	63.6

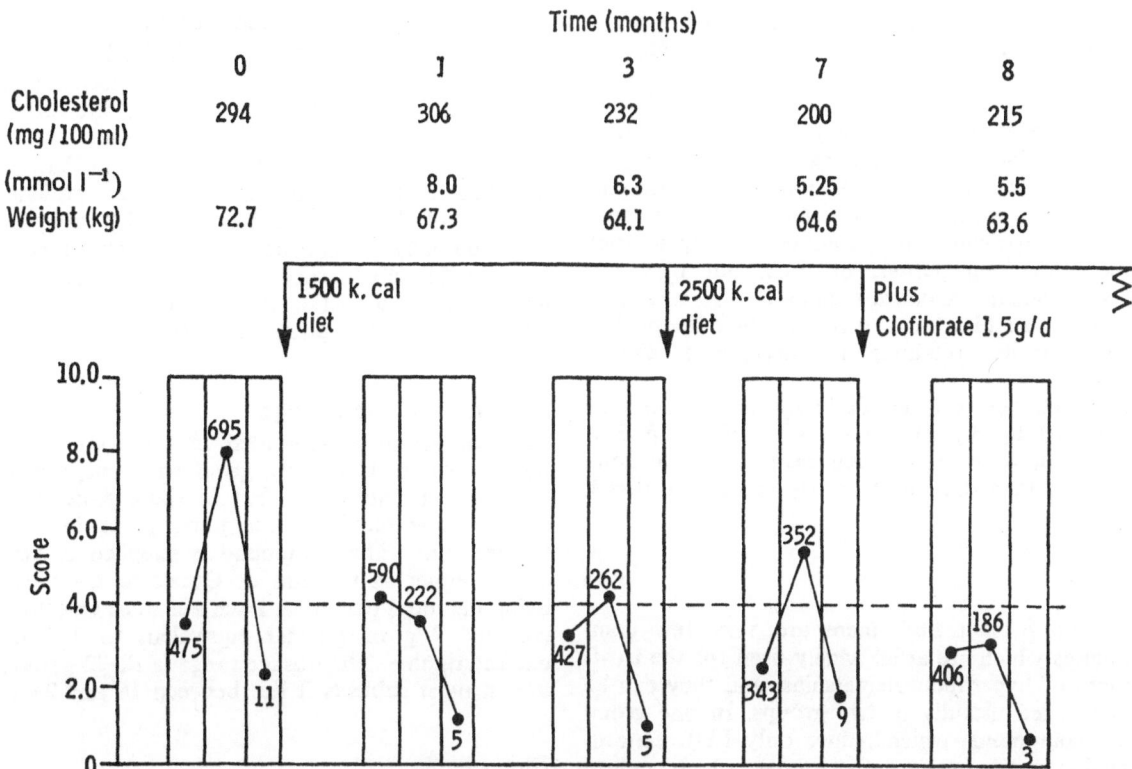

DIET

The role of diet is twofold, first to correct obesity, which is a common cause of the milder hyperlipoproteinaemias found in the community, and second (in all subjects) to keep the lipoprotein concentrations to the minimum levels consistent with adequate nutrition. In the obese subjects any low energy diet usually produces a fall in lipoproteins during the period of weight loss, but when the energy value of the diet is raised to maintain the new weight level, lipoprotein concentrations often rise again to some extent (Figure 2). In these subjects, and in those who are not obese, the composition of the diet should be altered to secure the minimum level of lipoproteins at any given level of total energy intake. This can be done by reducing the intake of those foods which exert a major influence on the plasma lipoproteins. For example:

1. *LDL and plasma cholesterol*—These are increased by the intake of saturated fats and cholesterol, and decreased by the intake of polyunsaturated fats and oils. On a weight for weight basis the saturated fats are twice as effective at increasing the levels of LDL

as the polyunsaturated fats are at decreasing them.

2. *VLDL and triglycerides*—These are increased by high levels of carbohydrates in the diet but particularly by the intake of simple sugars and alcohol.

3. *Chylomicrons*—In subjects with types I and V hyperlipoproteinaemia the concentration of chylomicrons is determined by the daily intake of fats with a chain length of C-12 or greater (i.e those which are incorporated into chylomicrons in the intestinal wall cells). These include the majority of animal fats and dairy products.

The average UK diet contains about 100–130 g of fat/day. About 79 to 80% of this is saturated and of animal origin, for example, meat fat, butter, milk, hard cheese and eggs. We also consume about 800 mg of cholesterol/day mostly in those same foods which are rich in saturated fats. However, certain foods are particularly rich in cholesterol, e.g. egg yolk, butter, fish roes and organ meats such as heart, brains, sweetbreads and liver.

Thus, by avoiding foods which induce hyperlipoproteinaemia the constituents of the diet can be chosen to produce the maximum fall in any abnormal lipoprotein fraction, though this will usually distort the patient's accustomed dietary pattern. Detailed diets suitable for the treatment of hyperlipoproteinaemias can now be found in standard textbooks of nutrition and can also be obtained from most hospital dietetic departments.

Many patients will not adhere strictly to such diets for long periods of time, but they will accept general guidance such as that given above, and this enables them to reduce their lipoprotein levels whilst retaining an acceptable dietary pattern.

If satisfactory levels of lipoproteins cannot be obtained by dietary measures, or if the patient is reluctant to suffer such restrictions for long periods, then drug therapy has to be considered.

DRUGS

At the present time there are very few compounds which are at all widely used for the treatment of hyperlipoproteinaemias, and they can be considered usefully in two groups. In one group are compounds which reduce only LDL concentrations and in the other those which reduce LDL and VLDL concentrations.

DRUGS REDUCING LDL CONCENTRATIONS

CHOLESTYRAMINE

Cholestyramine, the chloride form of an anionic exchange resin, is not absorbed from the intestinal lumen. It prevents the reabsorption of bile acids in the intestine by binding them to the resin in exchange for chloride. This interferes with the bile acid enterohepatic cycle and results in an increased rate of cholesterol oxidation in the liver to replace bile acids lost in the faeces. At high dosage of resin the normal absorption of cholesterol from mixed micelles, and its incorporation into chylomicrons may also be diminished.

Cholestyramine also produces an increased endogenous synthesis of cholesterol to compensate for the increased oxidation in the liver, but in most subjects this is not sufficient to counter the increased oxidation.

Indications

The treatment of hyperlipoproteinaemias in which LDL levels are substantially raised, e.g. types IIa and IIb.

Effect on lipoprotein concentrations

Cholestyramine produces a fall in LDL concentrations which therefore results in a decrease in plasma cholesterol. Falls of 20–35% are often observed.

There is sometimes an early rise in VLDL (and therefore triglyceride levels) in patients taking cholestyramine, and occasionally this persists and may be substantial. However, in contrast to this effect, very large doses of the resin may reduce the VLDL and triglyceride levels by producing malabsorption and weight loss.

Presentation and dosage

The compound is presented in the form of a powder which is usually given as a suspension in water or fruit juice, but in some patients it is only tolerable in a thin porridge made with fat-free milk. The compound is supplied in two forms, either as Cuemid or Questran, the latter being the more palatable. Each sachet of Questran contains 9 g of powder equivalent to 4 g of cholestyramine. The dosage range is 12–32 g/day, but in most subjects it lies between 16 and 24 g.

Side effects

A substantial proportion of subjects complain of one or more of the following symptoms.
1. A bloated feeling
2. Constipation
3. Epigastric discomfort or pain
4. Nausea and sometimes vomiting

Large doses (greater than 28 g/day) may produce some malabsorption, which can be detected by measurement of faecal fat excretion. Theoretically, there may also be malabsorption of the fat soluble vitamins A, D and K, though this does not seem to occur in practice if the vitamin content of the diet is adequate.

Cholestyramine also binds a number of drugs including digoxin, thyroxine, phenylbutazone, thiazide diuretics and warfarin, and thus prevents their complete absorption from the intestinal tract. Spacing the drugs so that the resin is given 1 hour after each drug dose is usually satisfactory. However, in the case of warfarin, considerable difficulty may be encountered in stabilisation; therefore if the anticoagulant is considered essential, the cholestyramine may have to be discontinued.

NEOMYCIN

Neomycin is a virtually unabsorbable antibiotic which lowers plasma cholesterol in man. The mode of action is still uncertain but it increases the faecal excretion of neutral sterols and bile acids, possibly by preventing the formation of mixed micelles in the intestinal lumen by precipitating bile salts from aqueous solutions.

Presentation and dosage

The compound is available as neomycin sulphate tablets 500 mg. The recommended dose is 1 to 2 g daily given in two doses.

Effects on lipoproteins and indications

Neomycin reduces the concentration of LDL and is therefore indicated for types IIa and IIb hyperlipoproteinaemia.

Side effects and contraindications

1. Cramping abdominal pain and diarrhea have been reported, usually during the first 2–3 weeks of treatment and usually disappearing after that time.

2. It may cause steatorrhea and malabsorption syndrome.

3. The drug is very poorly absorbed but in subjects who have poor renal function there may be impaired excretion of even the small amount which is absorbed.

DEXTROTHYROXINE (D-THYROXINE)

Thyroid hormones lower the plasma cholesterol of hypothyroid patients and also that of hypercholesterolaemic subjects who have normal thyroid function. The dextro isomer is used because it is less calorogenic than the naturally occurring laevo isomer.

Mechanism of action

Thyroxine stimulates endogenous synthesis of cholesterol in man, but it also stimulates cholesterol degradation and removal. It is the latter effect which appears to predominate, and the excretion of bile acids is increased. Thus the mode of action of D-thyroxine is to increase the rate of removal of LDL and cholesterol.

Presentation and dosage

The compound is presented as tablets of sodium D-thyroxine 2 mg. The dosage is 1 mg daily for 7 days increasing by 1 mg/day every 7 days until an effective dose is reached, with a maximum of 8 mg/day.

Effect on lipoprotein levels and indications

D-thyroxine produces a fall in plasma cholesterol of about 20% by decreasing the level of circulating LDL, but has virtually no effect on VLDL. It can be used to treat hyperlipoproteinaemias of types IIa and IIb.

Side effects and contraindications

1. Signs of hypermetabolism occur in some patients, e.g. tachycardia and a feeling of heat.

2. In some subjects the drug may induce or aggravate an arrhythmia or anginal pain. These symptoms have been controlled by giving 40–80 mg of propranolol per day in two doses. However, some observers regard the presence of an arrhythmia or evidence of ischaemia in an ECG, as contraindicating the use of D-thyroxine. They base this advice on evidence that subjects who had extrasystoles before starting D-thyroxine were found to have an increased death rate whilst taking the drug.

3. It has been reported that D-thyroxine may potentiate the effects of anticoagulants by a so far unexplained mechanism. The dose of anticoagulants may therefore require some reduction in patients who are being given this compound.

DRUGS REDUCING BOTH VLDL AND LDL CONCENTRATIONS

In this group there are only two compounds in general use, clofibrate (Atromid-S) and nicotinic acid.

1. CLOFIBRATE

Clofibrate is an ester of oxyisobutyric acid. It is hydrolised rapidly in the body to clorophenoxyisobutyric acid (CPIB) which is carried in the plasma bound to albumin.

Mode of action

There is still some doubt as to the precise mode of action, but it is believed to exert its effects at a number of different sites including the liver, intestinal wall cells, and adipose tissue cells. The following actions have been suggested:

1. Displacement of thyroxine from its binding sites on albumin, with subsequent increase in the liver thyroxine concentration, leading to increased catabolism of cholesterol.

2. Decreased cholesterol biosynthesis.

3. Increased efflux of cholesterol from tissue pools via the plasma compartment to the liver, and increased excretion of neutral sterols through the biliary tract with subsequent faecal excretion.

4. Decreased mobilisation of free fatty acids (FFA) from adipose tissue cells, with reduced levels of plasma FFA.

5. Decreased synthesis and release of VLDL into the plasma from the liver and intestinal wall.

Effect on lipoprotein concentrations

Clofibrate is particularly effective in reducing VLDL concentrations, but it also reduces LDL concentrations to some extent. As a general rule the degree of reduction in VLDL and LDL is proportional to the initial level, i.e. the higher the initial levels of lipoproteins the greater the fall in concentration on clofibrate therapy. There are however, some differences in the way this affects the different types of lipoprotein pattern.

In type IV hyperlipoproteinaemia about 20% of subjects show no significant response, but in the remainder, a mean fall in VLDL of 40–50% can be expected. In subjects with types IV/V HLP in whom the LDL levels are low (i.e. below about 400 mg/100 ml) some rise in LDL may occur, but usually not into the abnormal range.

In type IIa and IIb subjects about 40% show no response to clofibrate, but, in those who have no tendon xanthomas, LDL fall by an average of about 17%. The maximum fall has usually occurred by about 3 months of therapy and changes little thereafter. In subjects with type IIa who have tendon xanthomas, the fall in lipoproteins on clofibrate therapy may be delayed, for example, in five subjects Stone and Dick (unpublished data), found that there was no significant fall in LDL after three months of therapy, but at the end of 1 year the mean fall was 30%.

In patients with type III hyperlipoproteinaemia there is usually a very marked fall in VLDL levels (about 70–80% reduction is common), and the VLDL concentrations are often reduced to normal within a few weeks.

Effect on xanthomata

Xanthomatosis associated with types III and IV hyperlipoproteinaemia will usually regress and eventually disappear if the lipoprotein levels fall with clofibrate therapy, but patients with types IIa and IIb who have skin and tendon xanthomas have usually failed to show any change in these lesions. However, there are a small number of reports which suggest that long-term clofibrate is capable of reducing these lesions, sometimes to a significant extent. It is interesting that the reduction in size of the xanthomas occurs even though the lipoprotein levels have not returned to the normal range. This supports the view that clofibrate is reducing the size of the tissue pools of cholesterol but that these changes are not fully reflected by falls in the plasma lipoprotein concentrations.

Indications

Since clofibrate is particularly effective in reducing VLDL concentrations, it is indicated for the treatment of types III and IV hyperlipoproteinaemia but it may also be effective in some patients with types IIb and IIa.

Presentation and dosage

The compound is supplied in red gelatine capsules each containing 500 mg of clofibrate. The recommended dose is 1.5–2.0 g per day given in two doses, but in practice 1.5 g per day is usually sufficient (see Side effects).

Side effects and contraindications

Over the past 12 years many thousands of subjects have been treated with clofibrate, but few have reported significant side effects. However, a small proportion suffer from one of the following:

(a) *Gastrointestinal symptoms.* Some subjects complain of loose bowel motions during the early weeks of therapy and may also have upper abdominal discomfort and occasional nausea. These symptoms can often be prevented by starting treatment with one 500 mg capsule daily for the first week, increasing this to 500 mg twice daily for the second week and then giving 1.5 g daily thereafter. It is rarely necessary to give more than this.

(b) *Liver.* Some patients have increased levels of the enzymes SGOT and SGPT during the early weeks of treatment. This rise is usually modest and transient and does not indicate the need to reduce or stop the medication. It is believed that increased enzyme levels reflect an adaptive change on the part of the liver rather than a true toxic effect on the liver parenchyma.

(c) *Muscle pains.* Muscle pains or myositis has been reported in a few cases and the muscle enzyme creatine–phosphokinase (CPK) may be elevated. This is more likely to occur if the drug is given to subjects with low plasma albumin levels, for example in nephrotic syndrome. It is recommended that in such cases the dose of clofibrate should not exceed 500 mg/day for each 1 g/100 ml of serum albumin concentration.

Care should be exercised when clofibrate is given to any subject with impaired renal function since almost all of the drug is excreted through the kidneys.

(d) *Potentiation of anticoagulant effect.* If anticoagulants are being given their effect will be potentiated when clofibrate is added. It is recommended that the dose of the anticoagulant be reduced to two-thirds or one half of the previous level and then adjusted on the basis of the laboratory results.

(e) *Pregnancy*. Clofibrate should not be administered during pregnancy since the fetus cannot conjugate the drug and excessive levels of the free compound may occur.

(f) *Arrhythmias*. Clofibrate-induced arrhythmias have so far been reported in two patients.

NICOTINIC ACID

It has been known for almost 20 years that nicotinic acid could reduce plasma cholesterol levels and more recently it has been shown that it has an even more pronounced effect on triglycerides.

Mode of action

The mode of action of nicotinic acid has not been fully resolved but a number of more or less well substantiated actions have been described:—

(1) It decreases free fatty acid (FFA) release from adipose tissue and produces a decreased uptake of FFA by the liver.

(2) There is a decreased synthesis of hepatic triglycerides and a decreased release of VLDL from the liver.

(3) The peripheral uptake of triglycerides from the blood may be increased.

(4) LDL synthesis is probably decreased. This may be secondary to the decrease in VLDL synthesis which is itself secondary to reduced FFA uptake by the liver.

The net result of these actions is reduction of VLDL and LDL levels in patients with hyperlipoproteinaemia.

Effect on plasma lipoproteins

Nicotinic acid administration decreases both VLDL and LDL levels and therefore reduces both triglyceride and cholesterol concentrations in the plasma. It is indicated in the treatment of all types of hyperlipoproteinaemia except type I.

Presentation and dosage

The compound is available as tablets of 50 and 100 mg. It is given initially at a dose of 100 mg orally three times per day. This is increased gradually to the maintenance dose of 1 g three times per day. The dose required will depend on the fall in lipoprotein concentrations and on the presence and severity of side effects. In some cases up to 6 g daily will be required to achieve

a satisfactory response, and in subjects with severe homozygous type II hyperlipoproteinaemia even higher doses have been used.

Side effects and contraindications

Nicotinic acid frequently causes side effects sometimes of such severity that the drug has to be discontinued.

(a) *Skin*. The major side effect is flushing and itching of the skin starting within 1–2 hours after each dose. After about 14 days of therapy this decreases or disappears but in approximately 15% of patients it persists. Brown hyperpigmentation has been described in the skin of some subjects and is sometimes severe.

(b) *Gastrointestinal tract*. Epigastric discomfort or pain, and aggravation of peptic ulcer symptoms occur in some patients.

(c) *Liver*. Liver toxicity has been described, with early changes in liver function tests, e.g. SGOT and alkaline phosphatase. Occasionally jaundice occurs, but the changes are reversible if the drug is stopped early. Liver fibrosis has been reported after prolonged usage.

(d) *Glucose tolerance*. Reduced glucose tolerance sometimes occurs and patients may exhibit glycosuria but this reverts to normal when the drug is withdrawn.

(e) *Hyperuricaemia*. It is common for the uric acid level to rise slightly during therapy but attacks of gout have occurred only rarely.

COMBINATIONS OF DIET AND DRUG THERAPY

The combination of diet and drug therapy is often more effective than either treatment alone, and similarly some subjects with resistant hyperlipoproteinaemias will respond more satisfactorily to a combination of drugs than to any single member of the combination.

Types IIa and IIb are often somewhat resistant to therapy and it is in these types that diet and drug combinations may be successful. It is logical to use one drug which reduces the synthesis of cholesterol and lipoproteins (i.e. clofibrate or nicotinic acid) and another which increases the catabolism of cholesterol and LDL either indirectly, by interfering with the intestinal absorption of bile acids and cholesterol (e.g. cholestyramine, or neomycin), or directly by increasing the breakdown of cholesterol and LDL in the liver (e.g. D-thyroxine). A number of these combinations have been used successfully but the ones which are likely to be used most commonly in general practice are clofibrate with either cholestyramine or Secholex. However, other combinations such as cholestyramine with nicotinic acid and clofibrate with D-thyroxine have also proved effective in some subjects.

SUMMARY

The hyperlipoproteinaemias are common disorders which are associated with an increased risk of developing ischaemic heart disease.

They can be recognised by a number of relatively simple methods and can be classified morphologically on the basis of the lipoprotein pattern, and clinically according to the influences which contribute to their development.

Although there is at present no conclusive proof that treating hyperlipoproteinaemias reduces the risk of developing ischaemic heart disease, there are groups of subjects who are especially vulnerable, and in these subjects treating the hyperlipoproteinaemia seems amply justified.

Before such treatment can be carried out, a reliable lipoprotein or lipid analysis should be performed and a careful clinical appraisal carried out to identify the probable cause of the lipoprotein abnormality.

The majority of hyperlipoproteinaemias will respond to diet and drug therapy, but the choice of regime should be based on a rational assessment of the lipoprotein pattern and the clinical picture.

6

HOME RENAL DIALYSIS

A. J. RALSTON

INTRODUCTION

During a recent conversation with a colleague in general practice, he made the observation that home haemodialysis was the one situation in his professional life where he found the patient invariably knew more about his own treatment than himself, and it is the purpose of this chapter to attempt to remedy some of this potential deficiency.

There are approximately 1000 patients being treated by this method in the United Kingdom and the numbers are increasing steadily. The technique, originally developed both in this country and the United States in 1964, has been more widely applied in his country following a decision by the Department of Health and Social Security to develop facilities for home haemodialysis, so that well over half the patients being treated by this method in Europe live in the United Kingdom. The possibility of treating patients with end-stage chronic renal failure by intermittent haemodialysis developed from the description in 1960 by Scribner and his associates from Seattle in the United States of a plastic indwelling cannula made of Teflon which permitted ready and repeated access to the circulation eliminating the major problem which prevented the development of regular haemodialysis. Scribner allied his shunt to a low resistance dialyser of the parallel plate type and was able subsequently to demonstrate good results clinically using regular haemodialysis treatment of patients with end stage chronic renal failure.

The methods of access to the circulation as well as the techniques and equipment for haemodialysis, as one might expect, have been refined over the years and these will be dealt with later in this chapter.

SELECTION OF PATIENTS

The age range at which patients may be treated has tended to increase, and nowadays some children from the age of 5 upwards are treated. The upper limit of age is usually 55–60. Above that age the increasing incidence of vascular disease tends to preclude successful treatment.

'Single' patients can dialyse at home quite successfully though it is preferred that a relative such as a spouse, parent or sibling lives with the patient. It is essential that the patients are emotionally stable and have a reasonably satisfactory social situation to help enable them to withstand the stresses that the treatment imposes.

The treatment is contraindicated where the renal failure is part of a generalised disorder, such as a collagen disease or amyloidosis. Diabetes is usually considered to be a contraindication though if there are only minor vascular, neurological or ocular complications, haemodialysis may be attempted. Severe cerebrovascular or coronary artery disease is a contraindication to treatment.

The presence of active peptic ulceration and old tuberculosis are relative contraindications, the former because of the risk of bleeding and the latter for the possibility of re-activation.

The risk of hepatitis associated with regular haemodialysis treatment is well known and all patients are screened to make sure their blood does not contain Australia antigen, before they are accepted on a haemodialysis programme.

The level of glomerular filtration rate at which patients are admitted to home dialysis training programme varies from 5 ml/min down to less than 1 ml/min. In the latter case the patient will usually have been maintained on a low protein diet of the modified Giovanetti type and intermittent peritoneal dialyses, for some months prior to starting haemodialysis therapy.

PRINCIPLES

In any form of haemodialysis therapy the blood is brought into contact with a semi-permeable membrane, usually a variety of cellophane, which separates it from the dialysis fluid. The composition of the blood is altered by two physical processes, firstly diffusion along concentration gradients across the membrane and secondly the use of hydrostatic pressure across the membrane—so called ultrafiltration —(Figure 1). The composition of dialysis fluid varies and the ranges that are commonly used are given in Table 1.

single-pass type of dialysate system. Using the coil type of dialyser it is more common to use a fixed amount of dialysate and pump this round the coil in a recirculating type of system. In addition to

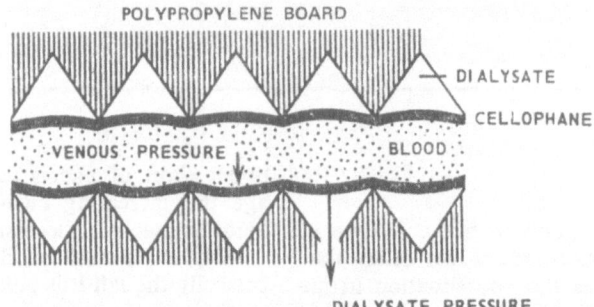

Figure 1. Diagram of Kiil dialyser. The venous pressure and dialysate pressure (the latter is often referred to as 'suction' or 'negative pressure') together make up the trans-membrane pressure. This governs the degree of ultrafiltration which will take place.

Table 1. Composition and ranges of dialysis fluid.

Composition	Range
Na$^+$	120–140 mEq/1
as (NaCl)	90–100 mEq/1
(Na acetate)	30– 40 mEq/1
K$^+$	1.0–2.0 mEq/1
(KCl)	
Ca^{++}	2.5–3.1 mEq/1
(CaCl$_2$)	
Mg^{++}	1.0–1.7 mEq/1
(MgCl)	
Dextrose	Nil–400 mg%

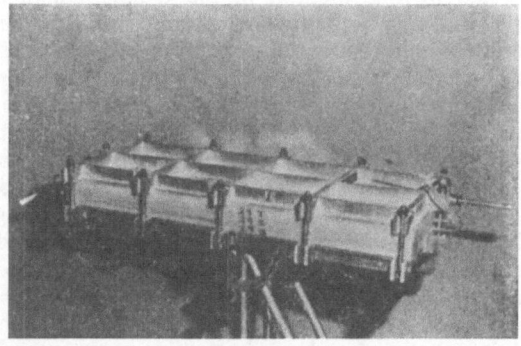

Figure 2. (A) A Kiil dialyser complete showing the metal clamping frame, and tilt trolley.

The dialysate is most commonly produced continuously by a preportioning machine which mixes tap water, softened or de-ionised if necessary, with a concentrated dialysate solution. Occasionally the concentrated dialysate solution is diluted prior to dialysis in a large tank.

The membrane which separates the blood from the dialysate is supported in the artificial kidney or dialyser. The most commonly used variety of this in this country is some form of modified parallel plate dialyser of the Kiil type (Figure 2). Also in quite common use is the coil type of dialyser in which the membrane is wound round a plastic mesh as a support (Figure 3).

The dialysate in the Kiil dialyser only passes along the membrane once before it goes out to waste down the drains, the blood flowing in the contra-lateral direction. This is referred to as a

this there are compromise varieties called mingle-pass systems in which, although recirculation is taking place, a small amount of the total volume is allowed to go to waste and the loss is made good by fresh dialysate.

The patient's blood is connected to the dialyser by means of lines, referred to as arterial lines and venous lines depending on whether they take blood to the kidney or back to the patient (Figure 4). They are made of PVC and although many varieties are available, they have basic characteristics. The arterial line usually carries an insert made of silastic which allows some form of peristaltic pump to be used. There also are various devices which permit a heparinised saline solution, which provides anti-coagulation for the system to be infused into the haemodialysis circuit, the preferred site is after the blood pump, thus reducing

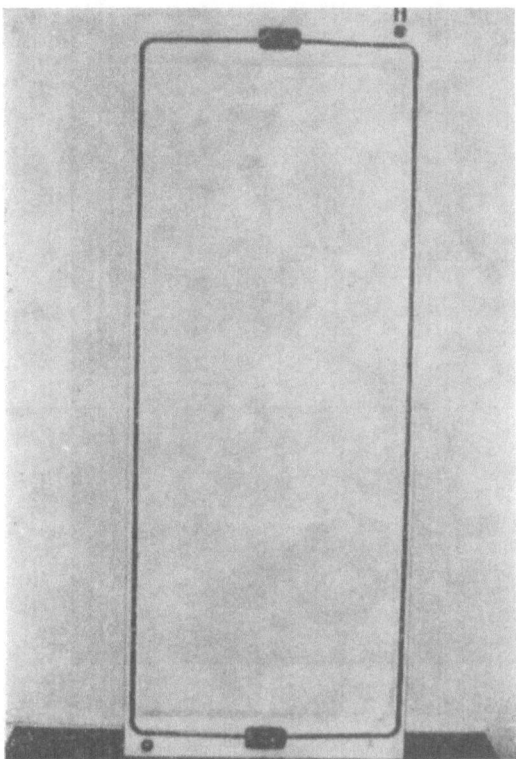

Figure 2. (B) One of the three polypropylene boards of the Kiil dialyser showing the peripheral gasket, with housings, for the ports of the blood compartment at either end.

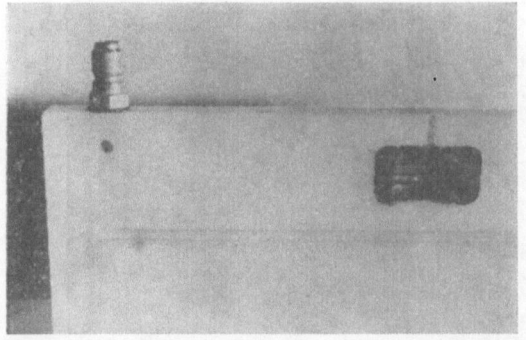

Figure 2. (C) Finer detail of a board showing the metal port for the dialysate compartment. The pattern of grooving can just be made out.

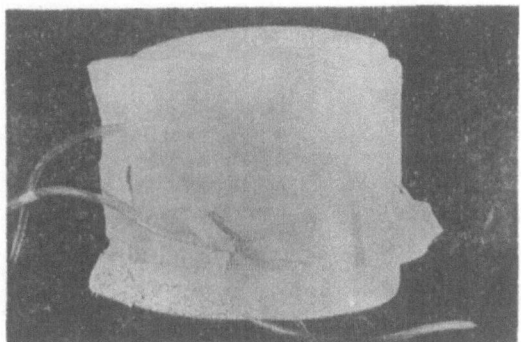

Figure 3. A twin coil dialyser with the plastic mesh support cut back to show one of the two 'sausage skin' type of cellophane membranes in place.

the risk of air entering the circuit owing to the positive pressure in the circuit beyond the pump. Invariably the venous line has a reservoir called the bubble trap, near to the dialyser, whose purpose is to provide a reservoir so that any air which might accumulate in the circuit can be removed if necessary. The level of the blood in this trap is usually monitored by some form of photoelectric device so that should the level fall the blood pump will stop and thus eliminating, as far as possible, the potential risk of air getting into the venous part of the circuit and causing air embolism.

Access to the circulation is gained either by using a Cimino–Brescia fistula or a Scribner silastic Teflon shunt. In the former, an anastomosis is made between the radial artery and the cephalic vein or one of its branches near the wrist. The arterio-venous fistula so created provides big veins carrying blood flows which enable needles from 16G to 14G to be inserted and blood flows of up to 200 ml/min can be obtained using a peristaltic type of pump. Usually two needles are inserted—one provides an 'arterial' and the other a 'venous' return site (Figure 5). Latterly, so called single-needle systems have been developed where a 14G needle with a Y junction permits an intermittent flow to operate through the arterial and venous lines by a system of valves.

In the Scribner shunt a Teflon insert into the posterior tibial artery is joined by a silastic segment and an internal bridge to a similar insert in one of the saphenous veins (Figure 6). The patient merely has to remove the internal bridge to provide an arterial site or a venous site. As a rule, a blood pump is not required.

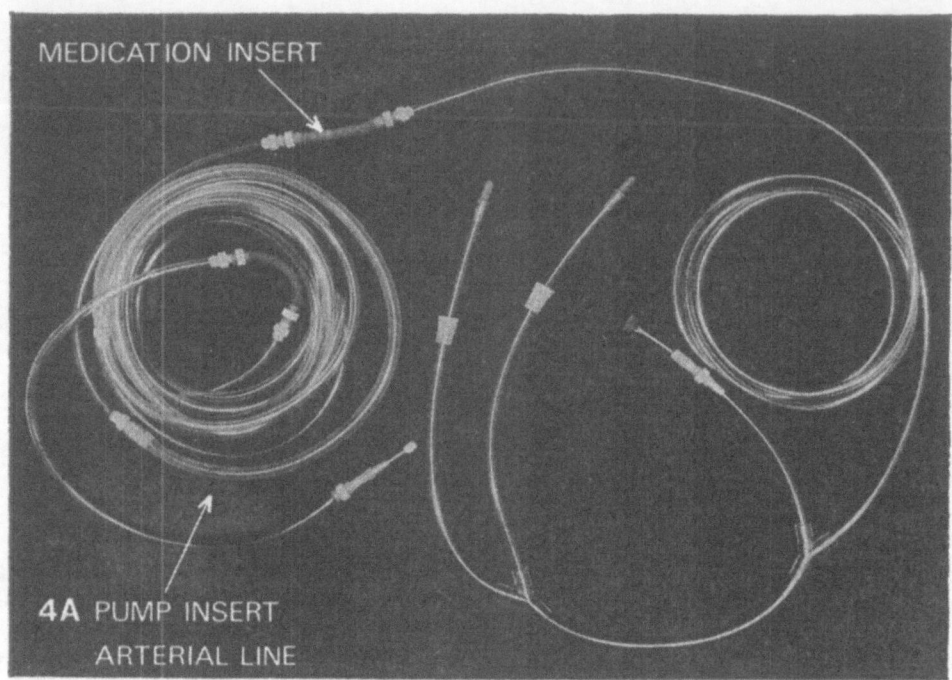

Figure 4. (A) Arterial line.

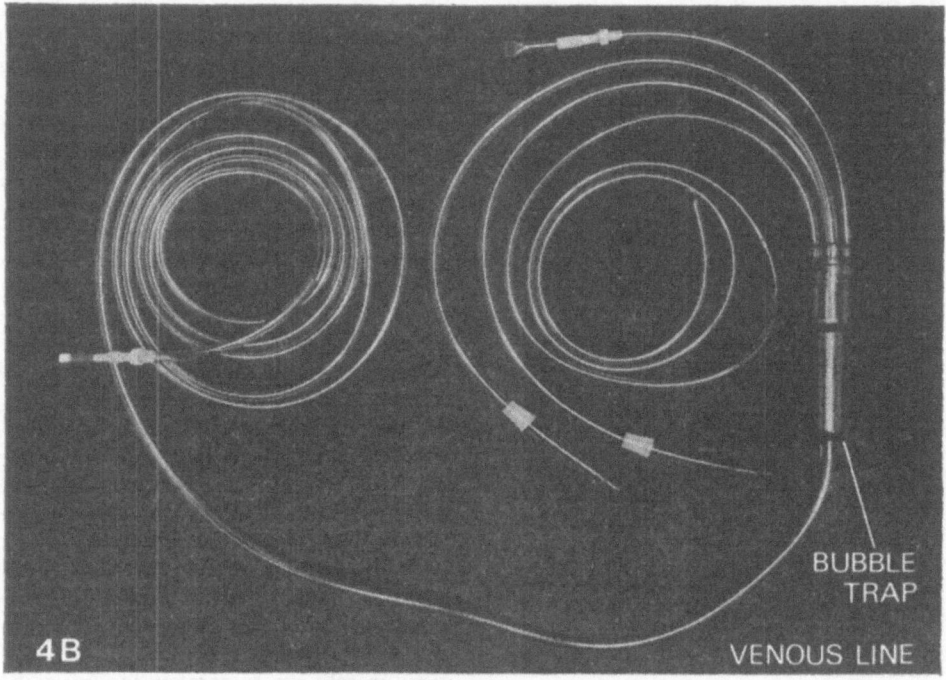

Figure 4. (B) Venous line.

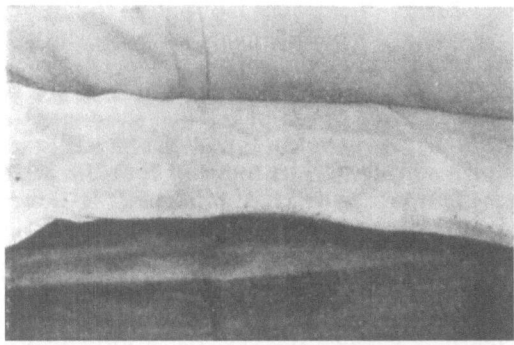

Figure 5. Brescia fistula. (A) Showing the dilated forearm veins.

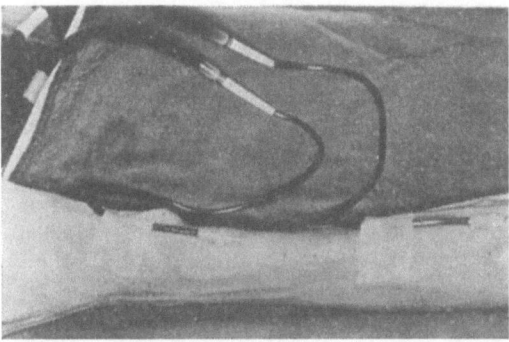

Figure 5. (B) Showing the needles *in situ* attached to the arterial and venous lines.

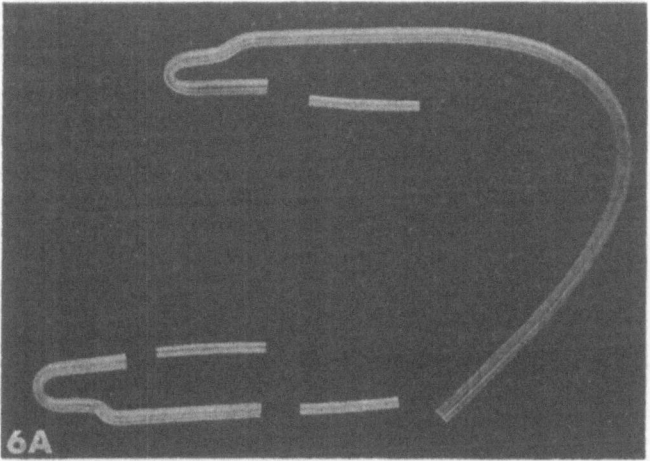

Figure 6. (A) View of the five components of a Scribner shunt showing the two Teflon blood vessel inserts, a long and short silastic segment with a Teflon bridge.

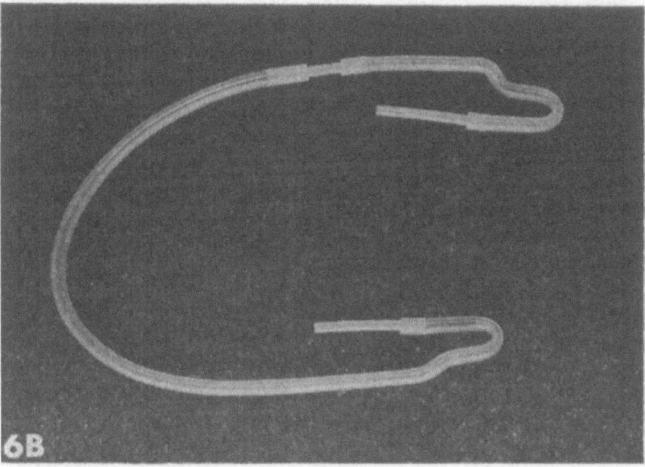

Figure 6. (B) The components joined together.

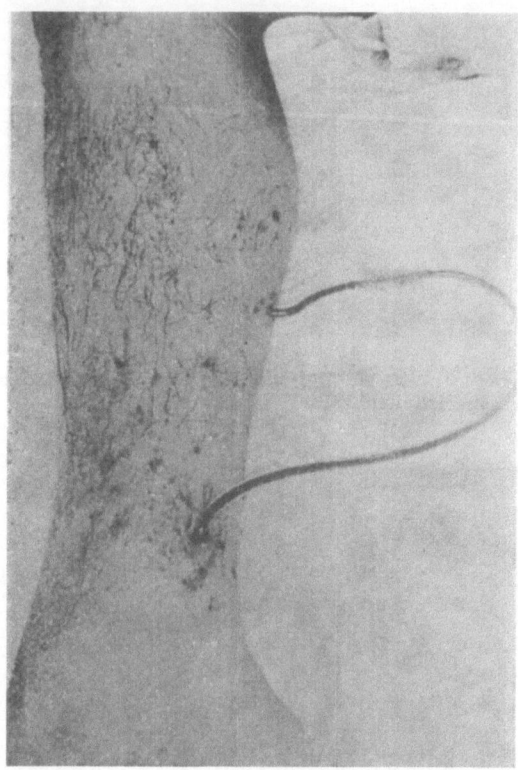

Figure 6. (C) Scribner shunt *in situ* in patient's leg.

TECHNIQUE

It is common practice with a dialyser, particularly the Kiil type, to use it for three dialyses before it is either rebuilt or discarded. The following account refers to the Kiil type of dialyser. The boards are unclamped, stripped down, and then commonly immersed for at least an hour in Milton as a disinfectant. The rubber gaskets which provide a seal should be removed and the three boards, particularly the gasket grooves, dried to eliminate the risk of persisting bacterial contamination. Then the two layers of the membrane are carefully laid over the board, one at a time, and holes cut in to allow the dialysate to circulate, the blood ports being put in between the two layers of the membrane. A pressure test to 250 mmHg is then performed. When the dialyser has been tested, the dialysate compartment and the blood compartment are both filled with formalin solution as a disinfectant and the kidney may be left until it is ready for use a day or so later. Before the kidney can be used, this formalin must be removed from the system and it is usual to wash out only the dialysate compartment connect-

ing this to the mains tap water, the formalin dialysing out from the blood compartment across the semi-permeable membrane. It is, however, important to check that all the formalin has been removed prior to use of the kidney, the water in the blood compartment is replaced by sterile saline thus removing the last traces of formalin prior to use. This process is called priming. It is, however, important that this priming process which, of course, also involves the arterial and venous lines is only undertaken an hour or so prior to dialysis. If the circuit is left in the primed state for too long it is possible for bacterial growth to occur. When dialysis is about to take place, the source of arterial blood is connected to the arterial line, the blood pump is used to circulate slowly, driving out the saline prime in front of the blood column until the whole of the kidney and the lines are virtually full of blood when the venous line is connected to the patient completing the circuit (Figure 7). The total volume of blood outside the body is of the order of 200–300 ml. The patient will, as a rule, feel no effect from this but if he is a little dehydrated then, of course, this relatively small loss may bring about a drop in blood pressure with a feeling of faintness, particularly on sitting up. At the end of dialysis the process is reversed in that saline is introduced at the arterial line, driving the blood back into the patient through the venous line either using a pump or by pressurising the saline container. When the saline has almost reached the patient the pump is turned off and the needles withdrawn or shunt disconnected. It is customary to dispose of the lines after each dialysis and use fresh on each occasion. The dialysate and blood compartments of the dialyser are filled with formalin until the next dialysis is about to start when the priming process is repeated. It is customary to undertake three dialyses per week of approximately 10 hours duration each, though the length of time is tending to fall. The dialyser is used for three dialyses being 'formalised' between each dialysis thus requiring rebuilding once a week.

One of the hazards of the actual dialysis procedure is that the membrane may puncture, letting blood escape down the dialysate compartment and this is in effect potentially a major arterial haemorrhage from the patient. Fortunately many of the leaks that occur start as very minor leaks with only tiny traces of blood escaping and it is for this purpose that a photo-electric device is incorporated in the proportionating machines which is sensitive to tiny amounts of blood and sets off an alarm so that the patient may examine the situation and decide whether he needs to discontinue the dialysis before a major blood loss

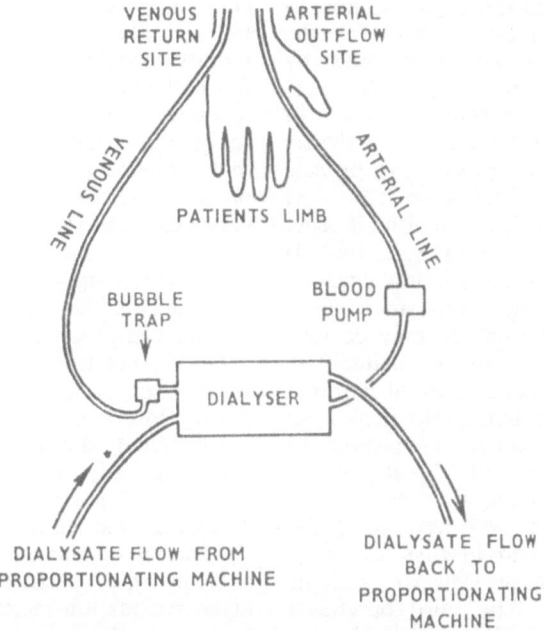

Figure 7.   Diagram of completed circuit.

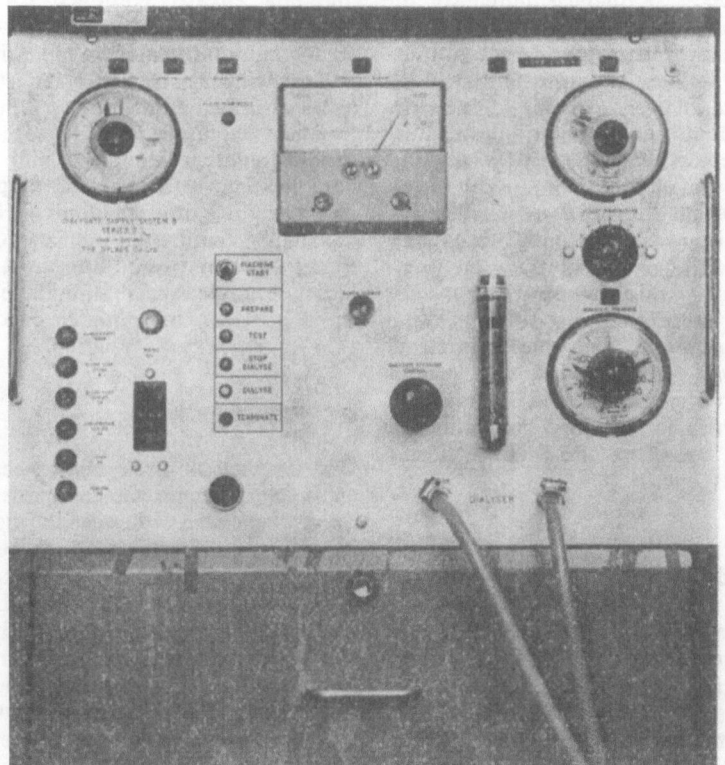

Figure 8. A view of the control panel of a proportionating machine.

occurs. There are several hazards, in addition to the loss of blood, which may occur during the dialysis but many of them are preventable by careful management and monitoring of the procedure. The proportionating machines (Figure 8) have the dual function of production of dialysate and monitoring not only the production process but the dialysis procedure itself. One feature of the production process which is monitored regularly is the temperature of the dialysis fluid. If it is too low not only is the dialysis less efficient, but the patient's body temperature may drop. Equally if it is too high the patient may develop hyperpyrexia. The concentration of sodium in the fluid which is clearly very important is monitored, if it becomes more hypotonic than ideal (Table 1) haemolysis may occur and indeed the patient may become gravely ill. Equally if the sodium content rises too high, then the patient may develop thirst which may provide grave difficulties in his management in that he drinks much more fluid than it is possible to eliminate by the dialysis procedure. The third parameter of the production process which is measured is the flow of dialysis fluid which is ideally kept at 500 ml/minute. The parameters of the dialysis procedure which are monitored, as opposed to the production process of dialysis fluid, are the so-called venous pressure which is really a misnomer for the pressure is measured at the bubble-trap and it is only really a measure of the blood pressure within the dialysis system. This varies according to the blood flow and the internal diameters of the needles used since they are the narrowest part of the circuit. Commonly, however, unless quite small bore dialysis needles are used, it is low. It is possible by partially closing a valve to increase the so-called dialysate pressure which is the negative pressure across the membrane which contributes to ultrafiltration and this too is monitored. The combination of the negative dialysis pressure and the venous bubble trap pressure gives the total transmembrane pressure which is the best indicator of ultrafiltration and therefore fluid loss during dialysis.

TRAINING PERIOD

The patients are admitted to the training unit following a variable period of conservative management. The shunt or fistula has usually been created a few days previously. The patients are first taught how to measure their own pulse, temperature and blood pressure, and the care of their shunt. Next they are taught about the prin-

ciples and techniques involved in haemodialysis. In the author's view this takes a minimum of 3 months, particularly if it is necessary to teach the patients to needle, and up to 5 or 6 months in some individuals before one can leave them to dialyse safely at home. Although it is common practice to train the patient with a spouse or other relative, our experience suggests it is better to make the patient responsible for his own treatment, and not to involve a relative apart from rebuilding the dialyser and teaching them how to take the patient off dialysis should they become completely incapacitated.

During the training period the patient and his wife, if appropriate, are given dietetic advice. The dietary intake of protein, sodium and potassium is restricted, the protein intake to between 60 and 70 g daily—only a little below normal. The sodium and potassium intake are more severely restricted—the latter to some 60 mEq/day and the former to between 20 and 50 mEq/day.

While the patient is undergoing training, arrangements are made for adapting the patient's home. Ideally a room in the house is adapted, it should be not less than 100 sq. feet, but not infrequently there is insufficient space and either rehousing is necessary or a portable type of building already equipped for dialysis is used. The adaptations necessary to a room consist of a hot and cold water supply with suitable drains, a large sink is necessary to enable the dialyser to be disinfected adequately. The electrical supply to the room must be adequate to cope with the proportionating machines and adequate lighting and heating—often a 30 amp socket may be necessary for the machine. The room requires adequate ventilation since formalin is used. Finally a waterproof floor is necessary and adequate storage space should be provided since supplies reach the patients every 1–2 months.

COMPLICATIONS

The first set of problems associated with the organic components of the patient's problems are those associated with vascular degeneration, which in turn is closely related to hypertension. Now, of course, hypertension is a common but not invariable feature of chronic renal disease. While it is perfectly possible to control the blood pressure of the great majority of patients on intermittent haemodialysis by adequate fluid and sodium restriction, a minority of patients require modest doses of hypotensive agents such as methyl dopa and β-blocking agents. A small proportion, in some cases, said to be as many as 10%, but in our experience much less, of patients' blood pressures are difficult to control using these measures and it is said that these patients have an intensely high secretion of renin and require bilateral nephrectomy. To be set against the benefits this operation may bring is the somewhat less well defined risk that the patients' anaemia may not be so well corrected when the patients' kidneys have been removed. Nevertheless the principal cause of mortality of patients on intermittent haemodialysis is degenerative vascular disease, particularly coronary artery disease and cerebrovascular disease, and it is clearly of crucial importance that the patients' blood pressure is controlled as well as possible.

The second major problem these patients face, and indeed perhaps one of the most important factors in determining the degree of rehabilitation they achieve, is anaemia. It is well known that the anaemia of chronic renal failure is a normochromic anaemia but during haemodialysis an extra component of repetitive small blood losses is introduced and it is important that any element of iron deficiency is detected and corrected as quickly as possible. Sternal marrow puncture with assessment of the iron stores is the most reliable way of detecting this. It is common to give these patients parenteral iron but the well dialysed patient is able at least to maintain his haemoglobin if he is given oral iron supplements. The blood losses from contemporary dialysers using careful wash-back techniques should not exceed more than 5 ml per dialysis but even this, of course, mounts up when the process is repeated three times weekly, week in and week out. Other haematinics have been used in this situation but there is no convincing evidence of B_{12} deficiency. There is some evidence that folate deficiency may occur, certainly serum folate levels are low in these patients, but the response to folic acid is in fact disappointing. Claims are also made for the usefulness of androgenic steroids, particularly testosterone, in this situation, but their use is probably of dubious value and this is particularly true in the female where the virilising side effects may become quite unacceptable.

The other principal hazard to these patients is metabolic bone disease, of which the aetiology is still to some extent obscure. It is due partly to a combination of both osteomalacia and secondary hyperparathryoidism, the proportion of each varying in individuals, one of the basic problems being the failure of synthesis of 1.25-dihydroxy-cholecalciferol in chronic renal disease, in addition to which there is a tendency for phosphate retention to occur bringing the third component of soft tissue calcification. It is extremely difficult in practical terms to control the serum phosphate level since the required dosage of aluminium hydroxide—7 g daily—is seldom taken over the long periods of time necessary in these patients. When long term dialysis was started the dialysate calcium content was usually kept at about 5 mg% but it is now usually accepted that a concentration between 6 and 7 mg% is to be preferred because the skeletal calcium loss does then appear to be smaller.

Another potent source of complication and indeed mortality in these patients is infection, both with *M. tuberculosis* and other bacteria. They may, of course, be dealt with by using antibiotics, and it is perhaps appropriate that a brief mention is made of the difficulties of controlling the dosages in patients on haemodialysis. On the whole the penicillins can be used without anxiety provided the patient is not penicillin sensitive. Drugs of the tetracycline group are probably best avoided in this situation since accumulation with resulting hepatotoxicity may occur while if gentamicin or streptomycin are used then the dosage requires very careful consideration and, where possible, control by repeated assay of blood levels. Nevertheless, despite the careful use of antibiotics, death from chest infections and meningitis does occur in these patients. Staphylococcal infections, often septicaemic, associated with the shunt infections, are not uncommon but fortunately usually respond well to anti-staphylococcal therapy.

There is no doubt that the treatment does impose considerable stresses upon patients, and, of course, part of the selection process is to try and offer the treatment to those patients one feels will stand up to these stresses best. However, one can identify two principal times of great stress, which are one, when the patient is first told about the need for haemodialysis and starts the period of training. He has to adjust to the knowledge of his severe disability and the limitations that his treatment will impose upon his life. Although many of these patients have been chronically ill for many months before the necessity for treatment arises they are often surprised that they require treatment of this type despite the publicity given to it.

The second period of great stress is when the patient first dialyses at home away from the relative security of the training unit. About one third of the patients in our experience require some form of anxiolytic or anti-depressant medication for a few weeks during the early months of their treatment.

Sleep on dialysis can be a problem at home

and the use of mild hypnotics usually copes adequately with this problem—diazepam is the preferred drug in doses of 5–10 mg each night.

RESULTS

Home dialysis is a remarkably successful form of treatment. The life expectancy of most patients when treatment starts is a few weeks or at best a few months. The mortality of treatment at 2 years is 15% rising to 25% at 5 years, at least a half of the deaths occurring in the first 6 months of treatment. The most common causes of death are those associated with vascular degeneration, followed by infection. The degree of rehabilitation as defined by the ability to work is remarkably high—over 90%. Perhaps surprisingly, both the degree of rehabilitation and survival figures for home dialysis slightly exceed those for live related donor transplantation, while the graft survival is, of course, lower than the patient survival —since most of the patients with failed transplants will have returned to home dialysis. The two forms of treatment are, however, complementary in any patient—apart from those with an obstructive uropathy where transplantation is usually contraindicated. Most patients on dialysis look forward to the day when they can have a successful transplant and be relieved of the restrictions imposed by dialysis which becomes more irksome as the months and years of treatment go by, if only for a year or two before they return to dialysis.

In conclusion, home dialysis offers a remarkably high chance of survival to patients suffering from end stage chronic renal failure whatever the aetiology. This is, however, bought at quite a high cost—not only financially—about £50 a week—but in terms of restrictions placed on the patient and stresses put on the patient and his family. Often too in the case of manual and semi-skilled individuals, there is a marked drop in earning capacity despite the high degree of rehabilitation this method of treatment achieves.

7

A GUIDE TO THE TREATMENT OF TROPICAL DISEASES IN NON-TROPICAL COUNTRIES

H. A. K. ROWLAND

Every year large numbers of people travel abroad to all parts of the world, for a variety of reasons and for varying lengths of stay. They often seek advice on what they should do to comply with health regulations and to prevent ill health while they are away. Large numbers of people also return from abroad each year after varying stays in different parts of the world; on or after entry they may seek medical advice because of symptoms; alternatively they may want to know whether they have 'picked up a bug' on their travels. This chapter is concerned with the management of such persons.

TRAVELLING OVERSEAS

Persons travelling overseas may encounter diseases which are either absent in their own country or less common there than in countries which they may visit; they will want to be protected against such infections as far as is possible. The particular infection will of course vary from country to country and will also depend on the circumstances under which the traveller lives and the duration of his stay; thus the risks are quite different in a crowded holiday resort in Europe, a rural area of West Africa, a desert area in the Middle East and a congested city in the Orient; they are different if the journey is made overland to Nepal and sleeping in a tent or by fast aircraft to an air conditioned hotel in Bangkok or Rio de Janeiro.

Protection against illness may be afforded by avoidance of infection such as by the use of a mosquito net or the boiling of water for drinking, or combating infection acquired by immunisation or suppression.

Malaria

Malaria has been eradicated from large areas in which is was previously endemic but there are still many parts of the world, especially in Africa

where it remains. Prophylaxis, meaning protection from infection cannot be achieved because there is no non-toxic drug capable of destroying sporozoites, the infective form of the parasite injected by the biting mosquito; protection therefore depends on causal prophylaxis and suppression. There are drugs available which destroy the pre-erythrocytic forms of *Plasmodium falciparum*, that species of parasite responsible for malignant tertian (MT) malaria, infection with which carries a mortality; they therefore destroy the source of the blood forms giving rise to the clinical attack and are referred to as 'causal prophylactics'; proguanil and pyrimethamine are such drugs. Schizontocides are those compounds having an effect on the asexual forms of the parasite developing within the red cells and regular treatment with such drugs may keep the level of infection in the blood below that at which clinical manifestations are present; they are known as 'suppressives' and include proguanil and pyrimethamine and the more powerful schizontocides, quinine, chloroquine, camoquine and mepacrine.

Persons returning from malarious areas frequently give a history of malaria while on suppressives. So often a blood film was not taken at the time of the febrile attack so that the diagnosis may be in question. Even if parasites are seen in the film it is possible that the suppressive was not taken regularly; finally it may be that the parasite is truly resistant to the blood concentration of drug resulting from the particular suppressive regimen. There is no doubt that *P. falciparum* parasites in certain parts of the world are resistant to blood levels of drug produced by standard courses of treatment; this is a quantitative phenomenon rather than an all-or-nothing one so that increased dosage may be successful. Since chloroquine sulphate (or diphosphate) is the most powerful schizontocide available it is advisable to reserve this drug for the treatment of an acute attack of malaria; proguanil and pyrimethamine therefore remain the drugs of choice for suppression. For an adult, proguanil 100 mg daily or pyrimethamine 25 mg weekly is the standard dosage; children should be given a proportionate dose and syrup is available for very small children. Suppression should be started on arrival in a malarious area, continued for the whole of the stay without fail and for 4 weeks after leaving the endemic region.

Protection against mosquito bites is afforded by netting over windows and doors provided it is intact which is so often not the case and probably mosquito nets over beds is the better method; even a still night under a net in humid West Africa is not unbearable. The best repellent, which is effective for some hours against mosquitoes and other insects, is dimethylphthalate, an oily liquid which is not unpleasant to apply, is inexpensive and makes an evening on a verandah even more pleasant.

Smallpox

The eradication programme started in 1967 under the auspices of the World Health Organisation has been most successful; for that year notifications were made by 38 countries. The figure steadily fell so that only India, Pakistan, Bangladesh and Ethiopia reported cases in 1974. Success of such a campaign depends on there being no animal reservoir and this seems to be unlikely; monkeypox is a disease of monkeys in captivity but 18 human cases have been reported; the opinion is that this will not interfere with the smallpox eradication scheme. Thus the need for vaccination by travellers has greatly decreased but the dangers of vaccination still exist.

Control of smallpox is being actively carried out in parts of the tropics but the disease is still endemic in some African countries, Brazil, India and Indonesia where the incidence may be greater than five cases per 100 000 population per annum. Recent vaccination against smallpox gives marked protection; there are however risks associated with the procedure so that the principle should be applied intelligently and the danger of smallpox weighed against that of vaccination.

Ill effects are especially seen in the young in whom the incidence of severe nervous system and skin complications is greater than in older persons. Encephalomyelitis occurs in about 15 of every million children vaccinated during the first year of life and carries a 40% mortality with the possibility of permanent disability in those who survive. During the second year of life the incidence falls to three per million still with high mortality; thereafter the incidence rises again but with no mortality.

The important skin complication is eczema vaccinatum – a vesicular eruption at the site of skin lesions in a patient with existing eczema. Although occurring at all ages it is especially important under the age of one year because of the higher mortality at that time. An unvaccinated child with infantile eczema may also develop this complication by contact with a person who has been recently vaccinated against smallpox.

These observations suggest that smallpox vaccination should be carried out during the second year of life; in healthy children travelling to areas of the world endemic for smallpox, vaccination may be carried out between the ages of 6 and 12 months. If travelling to areas where smallpox is not endemic this should be delayed and a certificate issued giving the reason. Vaccination should not be carried out under the age of 6 months; the response tends to be less good at this time.

Existing eczema especially in a small child is an absolute contraindication; if there is a recent history of such skin lesions and vaccination is urgent, as in those in contact with the disease, it may be carried out and anti-vaccinial gamma-globulin given at the same time. Vaccination is also contraindicated during pregnancy because of the risk of fetal death from generalised vaccinia; the only possible circumstance under which this might be relaxed is close contact with a smallpox patient. In those whose immune response is less good than normal, vaccination may be followed by a progressive ulceration at the site of scarification; this may be seen in persons suffering from agammaglobulinaemia and in persons on steroid therapy. Again if vaccination is thought to be essential it should be accompanied by anti-vaccinial gamma-globulin.

Enteric fever (Typhoid)

Typhoid fever is unusual in this country and at least half of the 200 or so cases seen each year are in persons recently arrived from warmer climates where such infections are much more common. 'Enteric fever' covers all salmonella septicaemias and may therefore be due to *Salmonella typhi*, *S. paratyphi* or one of the many salmonella organisms acquired from animals and more often giving rise to food poisoning. All salmonellae other than *S. typhi* tend to produce a diarrheic illness which may be associated with constitutional upset; blood culture may be positive for the particular organism in such patients.

It is therefore advisable for travellers overseas to be protected as far as is possible from such infections. (See also Short visits overseas). Infection is via the gastrointestinal tract, water and food being the mode of transmission. Care in the boiling of water, the preparation of ice from boiled water, the proper cooking of food and the disinfection of vegetables to be eaten raw, provide considerable protection. Enthusiasm for such measures tends to wane with time even in persons in their own quarters and is often non-existent in hotels and restaurants.

The other protective measure is immunisation, first introduced by Pfeiffer and Kolle (1896) and by Wright in 1896. This appeared to be of benefit although it was not properly tested until comparatively recently. It is difficult to believe that typhoid immunisation was not of value under the appalling conditions in the trenches in the First World War, and the difference in incidence of enteric infections between British and Italian troops and the effect of adequate vaccination in the latter in North Africa during the Second World War, are strongly suggestive of protection conferred by inoculation.

Only during the past 20 years has the value of vaccine been demonstrated; well designed experiments carried out in Yugoslavia (Yugoslav Typhoid Commission, 1957, 1962, 1964), in Guyana (Typhoid Panel, 1964) and in Poland (Polish Typhoid Committee, 1965) showed that the attack rate of typhoid fever diagnosed by blood culture positive for S. typhi was lower in those vaccinated than in controls. Different vaccine preparations have seemed better than others in the different trials; formol-killed, phenol-preserved vaccine is probably as good as any other, 2 injections of 0.5 ml (1.0 × 10^9 organisms/ml) subcutaneously at a 4-week interval giving considerable protection for a period of 2 years; that protection is not complete is shown by the fact that some inoculated persons did develop culture-positive typhoid fever. There is some evidence that intradermal inoculation in which case the dose is 0.1 ml rather than 0.5 ml is followed by fewer general and local reactions; the antibody response following immunisation by this route is as good as that after subcutaneous injection. Alcoholised vaccine may not be given intradermally.

Vaccines available in this country are either monovalent (S. typhi only) or contain S. typhi (1.0 × 10^9 organisms/ml) and S. paratyphi A and B (0.5 × 10^9 organisms/ml), and may or may not be combined with tetanus toxoid. The value of including S. paratyphi in the vaccine has not been proven and it has been suggested that these organisms contribute to side effects. Current practice is to give 0.5 ml subcutaneously followed by 1 ml 4 weeks later, or as long afterwards as

is possible; booster doses of 0.5 ml are given at yearly or 2-yearly intervals thereafter although the optimum follow-up regimen has not yet been determined by clinical trial. Using the intradermal route all doses are 0.1 ml. Enteric fever is relatively uncommon in the very young so that immunisation need not be carried out under the age of 1 year; inoculation carries no risk to the fetus but because of the possible side effects it is perhaps better avoided during pregnancy if possible.

Cholera

Since the pandemics of cholera which occurred from the early 1800s until the early part of this century, cholera remained confined to the Far East, Bengal being its home – that is until recently when it has spread to the Middle East, Africa and Europe. Originally the responsible organism was the classical Vibrio cholerae; during the past 10 years its biotype V. cholerae El Tor has steadily ousted it so that the latter organism is now primarily responsible for infections throughout the world. It was originally thought that V. cholerae El Tor was less pathogenic but this is now known not to be true, the clinical course being indistinguishable from that produced by the classical vibrio. In addition it seems that the El Tor infection perhaps affects younger children and that the carrier state may be longer.

The portal of entry is the gastrointestinal tract, water being the important mode of transmission; the source of infection is man only and the susceptible recipient is anyone not well protected. Protection may be provided by immunisation but there is some evidence that repeated contact with the organism in endemic areas provides some degree of naturally acquired immunity; this is to some extent supported by studies on vibriocidal antibody in such areas. This naturally acquired immunity may have played some part in preventing a catastrophic epidemic in Calcutta and neighbouring areas during the disasters in the summer of 1971; the circumstances – refugees living under appalling conditions of sanitation and overcrowding, the presence of a substantial number of cases of cholera and the rain starting—seemed just those required to produce a devastating epidemic, but they did not.

Inoculation against cholera is not efficient, providing partial protection for perhaps 3 or 4 months; the killed vaccine currently employed in this country contains 8.0 × 10^9 organisms/ml of the Inaba and Ogawa strains, doses of 0.5 and 1.0 ml being given subcutaneously at a 4-week interval. Vaccines made from the *El Tor* strain are in use in some countries and might be expected to be more effective in the face of this infection than vaccines made from the classical vibrio. Cholera vaccination is seldom followed by side effects; it need not be given to very small children.

Vaccination should not be allowed to give a false sense of security; it is no substitute for good hygiene practice – the boiling of all water, the proper cooking of vegetables and in an endemic area, probably the avoidance of raw vegetables, are of the greatest importance. One wonders too whether the time, money and effort expended in mass vaccination of a population probably partially protected by repeated natural infections, would not be better employed in the emergency provision of clean water and better excreta disposal. However the traveller leaving this country for anywhere overseas at this time (August 1975) would be advised to be inoculated although this is no longer required by international regulation.

Yellow fever

Although causing a large number of deaths in the past in the 'White Man's Grave' of West Africa and in Panama, and although there are occasional epidemics today, yellow fever would seem to be a relatively unimportant disease at the present time. How much of this reduction in incidence is attributable to man's efforts and how much for other reasons is difficult to say. The infection is transmitted by the mosquito *Aedes aegypti* so that measures directed against these insects are important and the remarks made regarding personal protection against the bites of malaria-transmitting anopheline mosquitoes are valid here also. Man is not the only source of infection to mosquitoes, monkeys constituting an important reservoir. The susceptible recipient is anyone not protected; clearly natural immunity or naturally acquired immunity is of importance in endemic areas because subclinical infections, as gauged by the mouse protection test, are common.

Artificially induced immunity using the 17D virus is extremely efficient, giving solid protection for at least 10 years; it is given as a single dose of 0.5 ml subcutaneously, and by international regulation is valid as from 10 days following a primary inoculation but immediately following a revaccination within 10 years of the previous immunisation. The procedure is complicated by no side effects; it should not be carried out within 3 weeks of a primary smallpox vaccination or within 4 days of a revaccination; the reverse

however is not so – smallpox vaccination may follow yellow fever inoculation without such an interval and in fact the practice in some West African countries in the past was to give the two together. Yellow fever immunisation need not be carried out in children under the age of 9 months; the preparation is available only at certain centres because it must be used within 30 minutes of exposure to room temperature.

Poliomyelitis

Poliomyelitis is common in tropical countries and conforms more to 'infantile paralysis' than it has done in this country of recent years. Most children going overseas from Britain will have been given poliomyelitis vaccine and a certain number of adults also; if required it is given orally in a dose of 3 drops at monthly intervals for 3 doses.

Tetanus

Tetanus is also much more common in warm climates than in the UK; again most children leaving this country will have been given triple vaccine (diphtheria, whooping cough, tetanus), and adults, especially those going to work in rural areas or outside modern cities might be advised to be inoculated or reinoculated with tetanus toxoid. In fact it would seem that tetanus is extremely uncommon wherever immunisation has been carried out, no matter how long ago.

Viral hepatitis

There is evidence that the administration of gamma-globulin, even in the face of an existing epidemic affords protection against a clinical attack of viral hepatitis. Its effect which is that of passive immunity, is however short lived extending for perhaps 2 months only. There is the suggestion that under cover of such passive protection, naturally acquired immunity may develop in a subclinical attack and that this is more likely if two doses of gamma-globulin are given at a 6-month interval. Viral hepatitis is extremely common in tropical countries at the present time; gamma-globulin is given at the rate of 0.2–0.4 ml/kg body weight corresponding to about 0.5 g and should be given shortly before leaving this country to those requiring it. Who such persons should be is difficult to say; often it is the traveller who requests it.

Schedule for travel overseas

To comply with these recommendations for vaccination is clearly a formidable procedure and if only because of the time available the schedule must often be altered. A convenient basic course is one modified from that suggested by Dr L. Roodyn, Inoculation Centre, Hospital for Tropical Diseases, London, and is set out in Table 1; it may be adjusted or supplemented by poliomyelitis or tetanus immunisation to meet the requirements of the individual which will vary depending on the time available, the region to be visited and by previous inoculations.

tropical countries, the reasons for this being poorly understood. Equally inexplicable is the apparent relief afforded by Enterovioform (iodochlorhydroxyquinoline) which seems to 'keep going' so many travellers on such visits. Some people go further and take with them sulphonamide preparations or a tetracycline. Enterovioform and sulphaguanidine will do no harm and

Table 1. Basic immunisation schedule for overseas travel.

Attendance	Immunisation	Dose
First	Monovalent typhoid vaccine	0.1 ml intradermally
	Cholera vaccine	0.5 ml subcutaneously
	Yellow fever vaccine	0.5 ml subcutaneously
Second (4 weeks after first)	Typhoid vaccine	0.1 ml intradermally
	Cholera vaccine	1.0 ml subcutaneously
	Smallpox vaccine	single scarification
Third (just before departure)	Gamma-globulin	0.2–0.4 ml/kg intramuscularly

MISCELLANEOUS DISORDERS

Persons visiting warm climates not infrequently suffer from skin disorders of which the commonest are insect bites, prickly heat and fungus infections. The majority of people experience discomfort at the site of mosquito, sandfly or other insect bites; in some however the reaction is more violent with considerable extension of the original lesion. An antihistamine cream may give some relief; the value of dimethylphthalate as an insect repellent has already been mentioned. Prickly heat is especially seen in the moist parts of the tropics and may be very uncomfortable affecting all ages including babies: it is not painful and does not itch – it 'pricks' as its name describes. Astringent lotions of which 1:1000 mercury perchloride is a very cheap example, give some relief. Fungus infections again are especially common in the warm damp parts of the world, the lesions being found in the warm moist parts of the body – the crutch, groins, axillae and feet; the old remedy, Whitfield's ointment (Ung. ac. benz. co.) is quite as effective as the more recent preparations such as undecenoate and much cheaper. Personal hygiene and attempts to keep affected parts dry by for example, frequent changes of socks into which talcum powder has been sprinkled, also help; no socks at all is even better.

Diarrhea greatly troubles many persons visiting

are to be valued if they make a stay overseas more enjoyable but the use of tetracycline should be discouraged.

SHORT VISITS OVERSEAS

The most common complaint made by patients after a short stay overseas is undoubtedly diarrhea; a high proportion of persons making such visits seem to suffer from some change in bowel habit, many accepting this as an inevitable accompaniment of their stay. Some may be troubled throughout the whole of their visit but surprisingly may not be greatly incapacitated or have to alter their plans. "Travellers' diarrhea" as this is often termed is variously attributed to 'change in food', 'change in water' or 'change in bowel flora' but it is not at all clear what actually happens. Where facilities for investigation exist which is not the rule, pathogens are isolated from only a small proportion of such diarrheic stools.

On return to this country the diarrhea often improves or does not recur but in some it continues and calls for investigation; although there are some patients whose attack remains undiagnosed, in the majority a cause is found.

Some help may be obtained from the history; fellow travellers or other members of the party may have been similarly afflicted and a common time of onset might suggest a salmonella infection; it should be remembered that diarrhea apparently due to such an organism may persist for weeks. On the other hand they may be present in the stools without producing symptoms. Salmonellae other than *S. typhi* and *S. paratyphi* are largely infections of animals in which, in this country at any rate, the prevalence has increased of recent years, as has the proportion showing drug resistance which may be transferable to other organisms. This situation which has caused some anxiety because of the possibility that resistance may be transferred to say *S. typhi*, has been attributed to intensive farming methods, the mixing of animals in markets, transport vehicles and abattoirs, the incorporation of antibiotics in feeding stuffs and the widespread and often indiscriminate use of these drugs in both veterinary and medical practice.

The diagnosis of salmonella infections depends on the isolation of the organism from the stools, or from the blood in those whose infection becomes systemic; a positive culture can rarely be obtained in less than 4 days, typing of the organism taking even longer. Serological tests are of little help in the diagnosis of salmonella infections.

Entamoeba histolytica

This parasite, especially common in the warm humid parts of the world, more commonly produces an asymptomatic than a symptomatic infection and one which is endemic rather than epidemic; in the sort of patient being considered here diarrhea is a more common symptom than dysentery and may appear for the first time (even years) after return to this country, and be confined to a single attack. Although frank or severe dysentery is unusual in this sort of patient, liver abscess does occur so that it is important to establish the diagnosis and institute appropriate treatment. Diagnosis depends on the recognition of the parasite, either as the vegetative amoeba or as the infective cyst in the stools where it must be differentiated from the harmless *Entamoeba coli*.

Giardia lamblia

This intestinal flagellate is also common in warm climates and is a frequent cause of diarrhea which persists after return to this country. Symptoms may be intermittent and in the absence of reinfection the infection dies out spontaneously within a few months. Diarrhea may be troublesome and associated with weight loss, malaise and steatorrhea; the diagnosis again depends on the recognition of the parasite in the stools and treatment is effective.

Shigella infection

Infections with shigella species occur in all parts of the world including the UK but are especially prevalent where standards of hygiene are low. As with salmonellae, shigella organisms may be present in the stools of asymptomatic persons; they may however produce diarrhea or frank dysentery and no doubt are responsible for a proportion of bowel upsets experienced by those on a visit overseas. Since the attack even untreated last only up to 2 weeks or so this organism is unlikely to be the cause of diarrhea which persists after return to this country. The carrier state is also short lived so that a negative stool culture does not exclude a shigella organism as the cause of recent diarrhea. In the tropics *S. flexneri* is the species responsible for most cases of bacillary dysentery.

Tropical sprue

Tropical sprue, that curious condition about the aetiology of which so little is still known, has a strict geographical distribution; although occurring in the Caribbean it is usually in persons who have visited India and the Far East that the diagnosis is made in this country. There are however no rules regarding the period of stay in an endemic area before the disease manifests itself; symptoms may begin 2 weeks after arrival or be delayed for 20 years. Although the character of the stools and times of bowel action may suggest the diagnosis, the onset may be acute with watery diarrhea not characteristic of sprue. Return to the temperate climate may or may not be followed by some amelioration of symptoms. Diagnosis depends on the demonstration of malabsorption and can conveniently only be made in hospital. In the sort of patient under consideration here in whom symptoms have been short-lived treatment is almost invariably followed by complete recovery. Such an attack need not preclude a further visit to an area endemic for sprue.

A few patients remain in whom no cause can be found for their diarrhea; spontaneous remission is fortunately the rule. Persons presenting with diarrhea after a short visit to a warm climate must have their stools examined microscopically and bacteriologically. Many otherwise excellent laboratories however are inexperienced in the examination of stools for parasites, one facilitated by a concentration technique such as the formol-ether method. If the patient's symptoms persist and if laboratory investigations are negative, it is suggested that he be referred to one of the hospitals specialising in tropical disorders or that permission be sought for a stool specimen to be examined there.

With the great increase in high-speed air travel and the extension of cholera to Africa and Europe during 1971 it is inevitable that persons will arrive in this country with *V. cholerae* in their stools. They may be asymptomatic or have diarrhea ranging from the mild to the very severe and the possibility must always be borne in mind in those with diarrhea and recently arrived from abroad. *V. cholerae* is not a difficult organism to isolate from stools so that a diagnosis can be made quickly, provided of course that it is considered. It would be very unlikely if such introduction into this country had not already occurred; circumstances here are however such that further transmission is unlikely.

Pyrexia

Fever is a much less common complaint of short stay visitors than is diarrhea but may appear after their return to this country. The fact that they recently visited a warm climate does not mean that those causes of pyrexia affecting persons who have not been out of the country, should be forgotten; additional investigations should however be carried out. The patient with pyrexia but not seriously ill and without abnormal physical signs is customarily treated symptomatically and observed; should the high temperature persist investigations are carried out by the patient's doctor or the hospital to which he may have been referred – a white count is requested, the urine is examined microscopically and cultured and a radiograph of the chest obtained; later blood culture and serological reactions may be instituted.

In persons not recently returned from overseas and without an obviously treatable condition this delay is justifiable; in those arriving from abroad especially from a malarious area and particularly one endemic for *P. falciparum* infections such a delay may be important. Recently a man developed cerebral malaria and died deeply jaundiced and in renal failure 10 days after the onset of pyrexia which started a few days after return to this country following a short visit to West Africa. It is likely that malaria suppressives taken had been intermittent; the importance of continuing suppressive measures for a month after return to this country should be stressed. A blood film for malaria parasites, preferably a thick and thin film, should therefore be included in the *early* investigation of a febrile patient recently arrived from overseas. These should be examined by someone experienced in the work and it helps

if 'recently arrived from . . . ?, malaria, is specifically stated on the request form. They are best examined at the tropical disease hospitals where such material is routinely handled; a telephone call followed by the slides by post is a wise precaution.

Blood culture for enteric organisms should also be instituted earlier in recently arrived febrile patients; typhoid fever is more common in warm climates than in Britain, at least half the diagnoses made in this country being in persons entering from overseas for one reason or another. It is perhaps not generally appreciated that blood, stool and urine culture increase the likelihood of making the diagnosis no matter how long the patient has been ill; those eventually found to have enteric fever are often not severely ill when first seen.

Dengue seems to be very uncommon in persons recently returned from tropical areas where it is prevalent; it may be that a diagnosis of influenza is made in this influenza-like illness, the added features of glandular enlargement and measly rash being mild or unrecognised. The diagnosis is difficult to prove but although the limb pains make this a most uncomfortable illness, recovery is the rule.

Pyrexia may herald viral hepatitis, a condition so common in tropical countries at the present time. Its management differs in no way from that arising in this country. Liver abscess, toxoplasmosis and tryanosomiasis, although uncommon, are causes of pyrexia in persons making only a short visit overseas. Expert advice is required in both diagnosis and management.

Rash

Some persons visiting especially the humid tropics are greatly troubled by prickly heat but this improves rapidly on return to a temperate climate. Similarly insect bites, which in some persons may be followed by an allergic-like local reaction or complicated by secondary infection resulting from scratching, subside on return to this country. It is also in the warm humid parts of the world that fungus infections especially of the crutch and feet are especially common. They also tend to improve on return to a cooler climate and their management does not differ from that in persons who have not been out of the country. Any vesicular eruption in a person having recently entered this country must clearly be treated with the greatest suspicion. It must be remembered that previous vaccination may modify the rash of smallpox; expert opinion should be obtained without delay.

LONG TERM VISITORS OVERSEAS

Those whose home is in this country and who present after tours of duty in the tropics constitute a different group from short stay visitors overseas. Their period of residence is longer and many have spent this in rural areas of the tropics; the possibilities are therefore greater. In these persons cosmopolitan disorders must not be forgotten but in addition must be considered disorders common to tropical areas in general and specific for the particular region where the patient has worked. These embracing the whole of medicine in the tropics cannot be dealt with in this chapter. The remarks made concerning the management of short term visitors are equally applicable to those who have resided for longer in the tropics. Many such persons make routine visits to one of the specialised hospitals on return to this country at the end of tours of duty. Some have no complaints while others have vague symptoms such as lassitude, weight loss or looseness of the bowels. Often some abnormality is detected and these routine visits are to be encouraged. Where the cause of symptoms in such patients is not apparent, the practitioner is recommended to seek advice from one of the tropical disease hospitals.

IMMIGRANTS FROM TROPICAL AREAS

Included in this group are those entering this country for the first time and those who have been home on a visit to their country of origin; long visits of this kind are common. Such persons may reach this country by air during the incubation period of some serious infective disorders of which malaria, typhoid fever and smallpox are the most common; many patients seen suffering from these disorders have recently left their country of origin.

The management of acute illness is the same as for short stay visitors for less acute illness. It is advisable to obtain a further opinion from a general or specialised hospital. While it is understandable that general hospitals should like to keep an 'interesting patient' this is not always in the best interest of the individual who might be better served if expert opinion is obtained early rather than late when all other investigations have proved negative. Just as there are good and bad ways of handling a placental praevia, an acute abdomen and a spontaneous pneumothorax, so there are good and bad ways of handling a *P. falciparum* infection and an amoebic liver abscess.

To discover that a patient has been overseas is possibly the greatest hurdle to overcome, such information not always being volunteered. The management of acute illness should be as outlined here; failure to make a diagnosis calling for assistance from a specialised hospital. The investigation of less acute illness should be as for permanent residents of this country, expert opinion being obtained when a satisfactory diagnosis is not obtained. This should be sought early rather than late – by general hospitals as well as by general practitioners.

8

CONTRACEPTION

MALCOLM POTTS

CONTRACEPTION AND THE CLINICIAN

Birth control is a private and individual affair but professional assistance, when properly trained and fully informed, can be of great benefit both to individual health and social advancement, as well as to making an essential contribution to the well being of the community as a whole. Economic progress is virtually halted when demographic growth rates exceed 2% per year and a formidable challenge to the global resources and environment is obviously presented by rates in this order. Our present situation is difficult for anyone to imagine accurately, but some perspective may be gained by realising that there will be an increase of more people in the next decade than those who presently live in North and South America combined, or (to put it in historical terms) by a number exceeding the estimated population of the planet 200 years ago.

From the medical viewpoint family planning is made up of a limited series of well tried and relatively simple techniques. But in social and human terms the problem is more complicated and the clinician is often wise to build upon the foundations of what couples already do, rather than to try and impose a series of sophisticated methods in a foreign and insensitive way. Over the past hundred years the need for family planning has become more apparent than previously and the goals set by couples in the control of their own fertility have become more exact. There has been moderate improvement in methods and an increasing involvement and interest by physicians in meeting the universal need for birth control.

But some degree of family limitation can be identified in most historical communities and most contemporary cultures. In fact, the artificial limitation of human fertility is so widespread that it is difficult to estimate the full potential of the human reproductive system over a fertile life time. The Huttarites, who are an eccentric religious group in the USA, are exposed on the one hand to efficient modern preventive and curative medicine but reject, on the other, artificial contraception and abortion. Girls marrying under 20 produce, *on average*, 10 live children before the menopause. But even in this community the rules of monogamy and of chastity before marriage ensures that fertility is less than the maximum possible. Nevertheless the Huttarites remain an exception and average family sizes in both developed and developing countries demonstrate that fertility is always curtailed by one or more man-made limiting factors.

SOCIAL FACTORS AND FERTILITY

During the twentieth century the average age of the menarch in developed countries has fallen below the teens and almost into the first decade of life. Most Western girls will run through seven or eight years of fertile life and many will experience ten years or more before marriage.

The medical profession has little direct influence in altering the pattern of relations that determine the ages of marriage, but the profession sometimes plays the role of an impassioned bystander and should always be an interested observer. Early marriage is associated with a higher divorce rate than later on in life and pregnancy early in life carries higher risks to the mother and baby. Among other important social variables in the limitation of human fertility are the rate of divorce and remarriage, the level of celibacy (which tends to be positively correlated with late marriage, for example in Eire) and the prevalence of primary or secondary infertility, due to venereal and other diseases.

Sexual intercourse prior to marriage has been a feature of many Western communities for generations, but currently three additional trends have started to emerge: the age of first intercourse has fallen; the length of time before marriage (and therefore the number of partners involved) has increased; and a proportion of young women are turning to doctors for contraceptive advice whereas previously only the male partner used contraceptives and obtained them anonymously. The events which are taking place seem to be mainly the result of economic and educational changes among young people and do not appear to be directly related to the availability, or non-availability, of birth control advice. For example, Japan has had a liberal abortion law for over twenty years but only 10–12% of those who have legal terminations are unmarried. In Britain however half those having terminations are unmarried, and similarly, the British illegitimacy rate is five times that of Japan. In other words, broad cultural influences, rather than an ability to deal with an unwanted pregnancy, determine premarital sexual behaviour. The illegitimate pregnancy is, after all, something that happens to *other* girls.

Illegitimate babies have a higher neonatal death rate than those born in wedlock and the mother can also be shown to be at greater risk during pregnancy and delivery. There is therefore a great deal of scope for improvement in family planning services among the unmarried. Among a series of over 1000 single girls seeking advice on abortions in Birmingham between 1968 and 1970 approximately half never used any form of contraception and two-thirds omitted any protection on the occasion they became pregnant.

Oral contraceptives, because of their high degree of predictability and their freedom from coitally-dependent manoeuvring, are first choice for single women seeking a physician's advice. Condoms, because of their fair reliability and the opportunity to obtain them without unsavoury interrogation are first choice among men. But some unmarried individuals or couples present with additional sexual or emotional problems and may be in need of wise counsel as well as reliable contraceptives.

BIOLOGICAL FACTORS AND FERTILITY

The age of the menarch is related to body weight, menstruation first occurring when a girl weighs something over 47 kg. If the proportion of total body weight present as fat falls below approximately 17% then anovulatory cycles may ensue. The age of the cessation of periods tends to be inversely correlated with their onset. Within the fertile years primary and secondary infertility (infertility after one or more conceptions), due for example to endocrine disorders or infectious disease, cut down the number of women who run the risk of conception.

When a healthy woman, not using any form of contraception, begins to have regular intercourse a cycle of reproductive activity will be set in motion which has two distinct components.

1. Regular intercourse, on average, takes place for three to six ovulatory cycles before pregnancy occurs. But this mean figure conceals a skewed distribution curve in which most women fall pregnant rapidly but a minority may go on for a year or more of unprotected intercourse before conception occurs. It can be demonstrated that the frequency of intercourse is a determinant in the length of time taken to get pregnant, but it is not an outstandingly important one.

2. Pregnancy itself, and the anovulatory interval which will succeed the end of pregnancy. In the case of term delivery, followed by a stillbirth or without breast feeding, this latter interval may last for two to three months, but if lactation is established it can continue for a year or more. When the pregnancy ends in a spontaneous or induced abortion fertility may return within two cycles. In the absence of contraceptive protection more abortions can be fitted into a given interval of a woman's fertile life than term deliveries, and if term delivery is associated with lactation then two, or possibly three, induced abortions might be needed to avert one live birth. But the use of contraceptives greatly extends the time taken to conceive. In these circumstances, even with the use of a relatively ineffective method of contraception, the interval between pregnancies may be greatly extended.

CONTRACEPTIVE METHODS

Today, the use of reversible contraceptive methods is divided in approximately three equal ways. In the UK the sale of condoms and spermicides, through a variety of retail outlets, accounts for one body of contraceptive users. Coitus interruptus and the rhythm method, account for approximately another third of users. The remaining third of the population plans its families with advice from doctors and very occasionally nurses and midwives. In this group the oral contraceptives are now used by over one fifth of the population and their use exceeds that of all other methods distributed by physicians. In the rest of Europe coitus interruptus is relatively more important, while in North America physicians play a larger role in contraception than is the case in Britain. This general division of usage establishes realistic perspectives by which to judge standards of clinical care for physical–medical methods and marks out the very large area of potential improvement which remains in family planning services. The single most important contribution of any physician to family planning is to keep the topic in mind; to use his influence to help a couple establish rational contraceptive measures; and, above all, to create opportunitnies when help may be sought. All women who have had a baby or an abortion, as well as a great many others (and many husbands) should be *offered* the opportunity to discuss family planning methods. The discussion should not have to be initiated by the user herself, or himself.

Contraceptive methods have in the past been classified in a large number of different ways. However there is little point in over complicating what is in fact a very simple set of distinctions. It is proposed here to discuss the methods under three separate headings—methods that depend upon the user alone; methods that involve the use of some equipment which is readily and commercially available; and methods which necessitate the involvement of the physician.

User-dependent methods

(i) *Coitus interruptus.* At a world level male withdrawal before ejaculation is almost certainly the commonest form of reversible contraception. It is so widely used in the Western world that it can easily be overlooked. The question 'Do you use any method of contraception?' may elicit the answer 'No', while the same woman may tell you 'My husband is always careful'. The method is known by various colloquial terms and one quoted in East Yorkshire is 'Going to Beverley and getting off at Cottingham'.

Demographically, the use of coitus interruptus is very significant and partly accounts for the fact that, when Western Europe entered the historical period of industrialisation, birth rates were considerably lower than those found in many contemporary developing countries.

Like many common activities whose significance is often underestimated, coitus interruptus has been the subject of myth making rather than scientific observation. It has been said to be ineffective because the pre-ejaculatory fluid is supposedly capable of fertilisation—a contention which has never been proved. The method is widely claimed by doctors to be psychologically harmful for one or both partners, a thesis which is certainly not substantiated by a review of the literature on mental illness in Britain. The unreliability of the method is also over-emphasised.

When presented with a couple who have habitually practised the method but who feel in need of advice, the attitude of the helpful clinician towards withdrawal should not be to deter them from its use by unsubstantiated criticism, but to suggest, at least in suitable cases, that there are probably better ways of planning one's family.

(ii) *The rhythm method.* There are several distinct 'safe period' methods, one of which, since it requires a thermometer, might properly be placed in the 'equipment' category. Any safe period variation of course depends upon being able to predict (or at least detect) the time of ovulation and hence avoid intercourse at or around this time.

The least reliable of the two rhythm variants is that depending on the use of the calendar. The patient notes the length of six to twelve menstrual cycles, and on the basis of this information attempts to assess what her 'normal' cycle length might be. In so doing she makes the assumption that she *does* show some degree of menstrual regularity and also that variations in cycle length are largely due to differences in the proliferative rather than the secretory phase of the cycle.

The two sets of rules which have been adopted for determining on which days to avoid intercourse were elaborated independently by Knaus in Austria and Ogino in Japan over 30 years ago. Using the Knaus criteria, 18 days are subtracted from the duration of the shortest cycle of the twelve and 11 from the duration of the longest. This calculation gives the 'outer limits' of the safe period between for the cycle in question. For example, the limits range from days 7 to 21 for a woman whose cycle length ranges from 25 to 32 days and during this time intercourse is not permitted. It takes little mathematical skill to realise that for a woman who shows such a range of variation (and such women are by no means uncommon) intercourse must be restricted to rather less than half of the cycle if these criteria are rigorously followed.

The temperature method depends upon the fact that following ovulation in some women there is a rise in basal body temperature of some one half of one degree Fahrenheit. The woman attempts to detect the shift by taking daily readings of her rectal temperature immediately on waking and plotting them on an appropriate chart. Ideally, the chart should show a biphasic aspect, having a higher mean value in the second half of the cycle than in the first. Intercourse is avoided before the temperature rise and for 3 days after it. Some charts, even when well recorded are difficult to interpret. The cervical mucus, like the basal body temperature, also responds to the hormone changes that take place at ovulation. At ovulation the cervical discharge increases in amount and becomes more watery. Women can learn to recognise these changes. If any regime is adhered to strictly the opportunities for intercourse during the cycle are very severely restricted.

The value of the rhythm method has been hotly debated in the medical literature but a number of reports exist which suggest that it shows a relatively high level of effectiveness especially when it is the temperature version that is being practised. Certainly, every clinician knows at least one couple either as patients or as friends who have used the method successfully for years. But it would be most unwise to attempt to generalise from a small sample of highly motivated individuals to a far larger group of relatively indifferent ones. Although rhythm can work effectively if all the rules are strictly observed it is unlikely to work well in the population as a whole, despite well publicised statements to the contrary.

Commercially available methods

(i) *Condom*. The sheath, or French letter, has a long but uncertain history since its invention in the sixteenth century as a protection against syphilis. It is an obvious, safe and sensible method of contraception and for many it has the added appeal of not requiring the advice or involvement of a third party.

Condoms are made plain or teat-ended and are generally coated with some form of lubricant. Users tend to buy the most expensive available, although price is not necessarily the best criterion of quality. Much attention is paid to adequate standards of manufacture and it should always be remembered that rubber goods have a limited shelf life and are therefore marked with an expiry date on the packet.

The effectiveness may be increased by the use of a spermicide, but it should rarely be necessary to use such a material. It is now possible to coat condoms with a spermicidal lubricant. It should be clearly stated that condoms seldom burst and that defects in manufacture (pinhole flaws and similar deficiencies) very rarely occur, despite ideas which have entered the folk lore and which are based on condom surveys carried out many years ago. It follows that it is not necessary to blow them up, fill them with water or cigarette smoke prior to use. Indeed, these unrolling and handling processes are likely to do more harm than good to the tough but thin latex membrane.

It also follows that pregnancies which occur amongst users are largely the result of misuse rather than of deficiencies in the sheath itself. Probably the greatest cause of conception in this situation is allowing the penis to become flaccid whilst it is still within the vagina. Semen can then leak past the ring at the distal end (rather than through any holes in the proximal region) and hence gain access to the cervix. An opportunity should always therefore be taken to encourage any men who enquire about the matter to withdraw from the vagina soon after orgasm and to grip the ring of the condom with their fingers whilst they are doing so.

Condoms should be available in all family planning clinics. For some couples who have sought professional advice they may still be the best single choice of method. They are useful during lactation or when intercourse is being resumed after a pregnancy; for covering the initial interval until an oral contraceptive can be relied upon, or a vasectomy becomes effective; or indeed at any time of change or uncertainty. Classically, they have the advantage of reducing the risks of infection for those men exposed to venereal diseases and there is reasonable evidence that prolonged use of the condom in a partnership reduces the woman's risk of developing cancer of the cervix.

They have the disadvantage of interrupting the sequence of play which precedes intercourse and some men object that they seriously diminish sensation. There has been a certain shyness on the part of the professional family planners in trying to create an erotic image for this form of contraception. Although difficult, such an approach does not seem impossible, as the trade in coloured condoms and patterns with comic devices at the closed end testifies.

Spermicidal preparations. There are a number of different spermicidal preparations available on the market which are intended to be used alone rather than in combination with a diaphragm, cap or condom. At least four different physical forms exist—creams, jellies, aerosol foams and suppositories and newer methods of delivering spermicides into the vagina are being developed.

Because of their large bulk, their relative messiness and the fact that they tend to produce a certain amount of leakage from the vagina, pessaries and suppositories are probably losing a certain amount of their popularity in the face of such preparations as the aerosol foam. Nonetheless they are still bought in substantial quantities. Jellies and creams suffer from the practical drawback that they have to be applied to the vagina through some form of applicator nozzle, which involves a degree of premeditation on the woman's part.

Some of the published figures for creams, aerosols and jellies show that when properly used they can give adequate levels of contraceptive protection, probably almost as good as those afforded by the condom among some groups of users. They are not suitable for the unmarried, but can be happily used during family building by some couples.

Physician involved methods

(i) *Vaginal barriers.* Rubber or plastic barriers that cover the anterior wall of the vagina and cervix, or simply fit over the cervix itself, have been known for over a century. At one time they were almost the only reasonable option open to a woman who wanted to control her fertility and their use has played a very significant role in the evolution of the family planning movement and in the involvement of physicians, especially female, in contraceptive matters.

Today by far the commonest of the barrier methods is the diaphragm or Dutch Cap, a rubber domed device varying from 5 to 10 cm in diameter with a coiled or flat spring in the circumference. To some women, who are unfamiliar with the capacity of their own vaginas, the diaphragm when first seen appears more like a rubber dustbin lid than a contraceptive. However, when properly fitted both partners should be virtually unaware of its presence. A good fit is essential and to ensure it the potential user should be examined vaginally to determine the tone of the perineal muscles, whether there is any degree of prolapse and if the cervix is likely to be accessible on self examination.

The diaphragm should never be used without a spermicide and its principal function is as much to hold a sufficiently high concentration of spermicide close to the cervix as to act as a mechanical barrier. Because of the need to apply the spermicide to the diaphragm prior to its insertion, the need to leave it in place for eight hours after the last intercourse and the need to apply a second quantity of spermicide to the vagina if a morning intercourse occurs, some women find the method tedious.

The diaphragm is rarely suitable for women engaging in premarital relationships as the failure rate is high enough to cause concern. The freedom from side effects and relative simplicity of the method make it a much more attractive choice during family building. The ability, unconsciously, to misuse the method is said sometimes to be turned to advantage by women who emotionally want a child, but feel on rational (usually monetary) grounds that it would be wise to wait a little longer.

Observation shows that with practice the use effectiveness of the method improves and after the desired family size has been achieved some women use the method well and find it satisfactory over many years. Perhaps even more than most methods, the use of vaginal barriers is greatly influenced by the enthusiasm of the adviser. While not often a method of choice among socially underprivileged groups, it has been well used even in those cases, when the woman has been looked after by someone (usually a nurse or midwife) who strongly favours the method and who is also a good teacher.

(ii) *Steroidal contraceptives.* The possibility of evolving a contraceptive method using exogenous ovarian hormones to inhibit ovulation was first explored by the Austrian physiologist, Ludwig Harberlant in the 1920s, but he was unable to interest the medical profession in such a possibility. When the first synthetic steroids were used, among other things for the treatment of dysmenorrhea, it was noted that one of the side effects of therapy was an inhibition of ovulation. But still the contraceptive potential of the method was not exploited. It took the forcefulness of Margaret Sanger and the foresightedness of the Planned Parenthood Federation of the USA, which gave a small grant to Gregory Pincus at the Worcester Foundation in Massachusetts, to initiate the work which was to lead in 1956 to the first trials of what was to become known all over the world as 'the Pill'.

In developed countries oral contraceptives are now by far the commonest method of contraception used by couples who seek the advice of a physician on family planning. In the developing world today, over 50 million women use oral contraceptives, but outside China their adoption in the developing world has been slower than it need have been because supervision by a doctor has usually been made a prerequisite for use.

The pill has one singular advantage over all other contraceptive methods—its effectiveness is virtually 100% when it is properly used. It has given women a degree of freedom from the fear of pregnancy that they never previously imagined to be possible. In Western countries contraception has become a subject which can be discussed far more freely than before. A question like 'are you on the pill?' can be both asked and answered without embarrassment and the revolution that goes with pilltaking is as much social as biological.

The use of oral contraceptives presents physicians with two main problems: what is the role of the medical profession in supplying the individual and what should be their advice to the community as a whole?

The only strict contraindications to use of the pill are certain rare hereditary liver diseases. It is not usual to give oral contraceptives to women with a history of venous thrombosis, but it can be justified if no other method of preventing pregnancy is applicable. The effect of ovarian hormones on established or treated cancer (especially of the breast) is complex. In a well ordered world the specialist advising the woman about her malignancy should supervise her contraception, rather than the family, or family planning, doctor, attempting to become a specialist in endocrinology.

A large number of different formulations of combined estrogen and progestin pills are marketed—for manufacturers' patent reasons as much as to meet human physiological variation. Recorded deaths due to thromboembolic disease in England have declined since formulations containing 50 μg or less of estrogen became widely used and they may be offered as first choice to women beginning oral contraception. Women over 40 are at a reasonably greater risk of thrombosis and heart disease, and it may be wise to use alternative methods.

Some clinicians attempt to select a pill that complements what they diagnose to be the woman's endogenous endocrine state, but when double blind cross over trials or two or more preparations of placebos have been used in parallel with active tablets, a great many variables in reported side effects have been proven to be independent of detailed pharmacology. If clinical skills are to be put into choosing a formulation to fit an individual it should probably be reserved for those relatively few cases that cannot be settled on a single, majority-use brand.

In fact, it is becoming accepted practice to use physicians as a second line of defence to solve problems among users, rather than as first line routine prescribers.

If the risks are small and few can be predicted, then how should oral contraceptives be made available to the community as a whole? The physician will be asked questions by individuals who are uncertain about adopting pill use and specialists will be concerned in important policy decisions about availability.

It is of the nature of a drug, such as oral contraceptives, that it is impossible to eliminate all unpredictable adverse, or beneficial, effects until it has been used by millions of women for a generation—and indeed until their children are themselves mature. What can be said about the pill at the present moment is that the demonstrable advantages greatly outweigh the known risks and that there is increasing confidence in its use so that simple non-doctor methods of distribution are becoming responsible and possible.

In addition to its contraceptive effectiveness, retrospective case control studies in Britain and the USA and the prospective study of the Royal College of General Practitioners in Britain have all shown that the use of combined oral contraceptives *protects* against breast cancer. There is a step-wise decline in the probability of a woman being admitted to hospital with a diagnosis of 'lump' in the breast, for every year of the pill use. So far, the numbers under study are insufficient to prove if this effect includes a reduction in cancer, but there are biological reasons for hoping it may: breast cancer is least likely if a woman has a pregnancy early in life and the hormonal balance in pill users is more like that of pregnancy or lactation than regular menstruation. However, it should be emphasised that the relations involved are complex and poorly understood.

The Royal College of General Practitioners study is the most comprehensive available in the world and followed more than 20 000 users and matched controls. It confirmed (for British women) the thrombotic risk, a raised incidence of gall bladder disease and blood pressure changes, but it failed to discover any serious unsuspected adverse effects and was reassuring in relation to future fertility.

The International Planned Parenthood Federation, and some other expert bodies, now argue that a medical prescription need not be a prerequisite of pill distribution. Innovative village distribution schemes are proving very successful in Colombia, Brazil, Thailand and other places and professional opinion in Britain is moving towards nurse, midwife and health visitor distribution with the doctor as advisor and problem solver.

(iii) *The intrauterine device*. Just as the pill was hailed in the mid-nineteen sixties as being the answer to all our contraceptive problems, so too, after a slightly more cautious period of evaluation, was the intrauterine device. The virtual rediscovery of the IUD in 1959, after it had fallen from popularity in the nineteen-thirties, forms a fascinating chapter in medical history. Within a short time, a spate of different designs appeared, each with some hoped-for advantage over other designs, and each of them was hopefully patentable.

The results of trials with such devices as the Lippes loop and the Margulies spiral, trials carried out under strict medical supervision, were remarkably encouraging. The pregnancy rate appeared to be lower than that found with any other contraceptive method except the pill. In addition, of course, a method which would give such protection after only one single application and a method which required a positive effort of will to have it removed and hence to remove its (totally reversible) contraceptive effects obviously had a great deal to be said for it.

Much debate has always centred around the problem of whether the introduction of a foreign body into the uterus predisposes to pelvic infection. The evidence now suggests that inflammatory conditions of this type need not be a problem. It has been demonstrated that IUDs can be inserted post abortion, even in the presence of mild infection when there has been illegal interference. The only really uncertain area concerns the outcome of pregnancies occurring with the IUD still in place. Some fatalities have occurred following second trimester abortions in such cases. If a woman becomes pregnant with an IUD in place the device should be removed. Some doctors recommend therapeutic abortion in such cases.

Perforation can occur at insertion (and possibly later), but may be treated conservatively if there are no symptoms, unless the device involved is a closed, ring shaped device which can give rise to an internal hernia.

Despite very considerable research efforts, it is still not established precisely why devices exert a contraceptive action at all. There have been almost as many theories as there have investigators. Most of them now agree that the device's action is exerted within the uterine cavity, perhaps by destroying the egg (or even the sperm), perhaps by altering the uterine environment.

The results of large-scale field use of IUDs in Korea and elsewhere have shown that to ensure that the device does remain within the uterine cavity is a major problem in any population where almost continual access to the physician is not easily attained. The problem is two-fold. In the first place the difficulty is that IUDs tend to be rejected spontaneously by the uterus—a rejection that depends upon the design of the product, age, parity, etc. In addition, requests for removal of a device because its presence produces pain and bleeding during the first post-insertion cycles are common. For these reasons it now seems unlikely that certain IUD programmes will ever attain the goals that were originally set.

In Western countries the continuation rate is higher because a woman who thinks she has lost her IUD can have its presence immediately checked by her doctor and a woman who feels that she is having trouble with the method can go to him for guidance—assuming of course that he is sufficiently knowledgeable about the topic to be able to provide it and also assuming that he himself believes in the value of intrauterine contraception.

It may well be that in the next 5 years the situation will improve. New designs of device which have been intensively studied appear to be free from some of these drawbacks, and a new generation of IUDs is currently under investigation. For some reason, the presence of copper appears to lessen the expulsion rate, the bleeding rate and the pregnancy rate. Although the actual fiitting and removal of an IUD requires only a modicum of skill and can be responsibly delegated to auxiliary workers, the ability to inspire confidence in the method does demand a particular set of attitudes on the part of the doctor involved.

STERILISATION AND ABORTION

All reversible methods of contraception have a measurable failure rate. It has to be recognised that no currently available method, with the possible exception of the use of oral contraceptives over many years, is sufficiently practical to permit a population of users to achieve the fertility goals which are common in developed countries.

Sterilisation should be available as a free choice to men and women who have the number of children they feel they want. Male sterilisation is less demanding in surgical skill, less hazardous and more open to reversibility than female sterilisation. Voluntary sterilisation has now become the commonest method of family planning in parts of the USA and on the West Coast vasectomy is the most popular of the two options.

Abortion is now available on request, or on broad medico-social grounds, for well over half the world's population, from Catholic Austria to Communist China and from poor India to the wealthy United States. However, gross and unnecessary differences remain in the medical profession's attitude to abortion decision making and the provision of abortion services. Just, workable, objective, external criteria for granting abortion requests are impossible to devise: if it is allowed for all tubal pregnancies (as in the Catholic ethic) although these can very occasionally go to term, why not for some intrauterine pregnancies which sometimes, but by no means always go to term? If for heart disease, why not depression? If for rubella why not for the socially deforming environment of potential illegitimacy?

Fortunately, the physician is not required to diagnose indications for abortion. The individual knowing most about the situation and best placed to make a responsible judgement, balancing the emotional and biological investments in the pregnancy to date against the social and emotional costs of having the child is the woman in whose uterus the embryo is growing. Unless she is a minor or mentally retarded, the doctors responsibility is to ensure her decision is freely made, that she has soberly reviewed the other options open to her and that she clearly understands the nature and possible consequences of the operation.

In surgical, emotional and ethical terms, termination of pregnancy can be divided into three profoundly different categories. Menstrual regulation is the technique of emptying the uterus within 10–14 days of the first missed period, if necessary before the diagnosis of pregnancy can be fully established. It can be completed in a few minutes under a paracervical block or with no anaesthetic at all. The procedure is spreading rapidly in several countries : 15 000 cases have been analysed in detail and results are encouraging.

Excellent epidemiological data are now available on established abortion procedures. Termination before 12 weeks is fundamentally different from termination after 12 weeks. The former procedure is simple, can be done by a relatively inexperienced surgeon, can be done as an out-patient procedure and the operation can be performed in a matter of minutes and the total contact with professional care need not extend over a few hours. Termination after 12 weeks is more hazardous, it usually requires a general anaesthetic and in-patient treatment. For early abortion vacuum aspiration is slightly better than dilatation and curettage. The mortality rate for early abortion in New York has been in the order of 1–2/100 000. For late abortion hysterotomy is the most hazardous procedure and is to be condemned. Prostaglandins are a useful late option. One of the prime responsibilities of the medical profession *is to make sure abortions are performed as early as possible in pregnancy*.

The follow-up of abortion cases shows a great deal of satisfaction with the operation. Contraceptive practice commonly improves after an abortion. There is no evidence that the availability of legal abortion affects patterns of social behaviour: for example, the law in Britain and Singapore is identical, but the ratio of unmarried girls requiring abortion is ten times higher in Britain, suggesting it is broad cultural factors that control the frequency of premarital intercourse.

One of the few universal findings of social biology is that it is those with Y chromosomes who make up the most violent half of the human race, and destroy most life. Male physicians most commonly fall into the trap of treating abortion as a disease requiring a diagnosis—which it is not, rather than as a human problem requiring a rapid decision by the person best placed to decide— which it is.

THE ROLE OF THE PHYSICIAN

What should be the role of the physician, as far as the spread of family planning practices? The answer is three-fold: he must be a clinician in the obvious sense of the word but he must also be both a psychologist and a salesman if he is to make a significant contribution to the contraceptive practices of his patients.

He must be a clinician for obvious reasons. He must be competent to deal with the medical aspects of the contraceptives which he is distributing. He must be able, for example, to detect a woman with dubious liver function for whom the pill should not be prescribed, or to detect a very occasional patient presenting with abdominal symptoms due to uterine perforation by an IUD. But in general these strictly 'medical' aspects of the subject will not take up the greater part of his time. Far more of it will be spent discussing the forms of contraception (if any) that his patients are currently using and perhaps suggesting that more effective or acceptable alternatives exist.

The doctor himself must fully realise that no one method will suit any one couple for their entire reproductive lives. The newly wed pair, desperately anxious to avoid the birth of their first child until they are properly established, differs from the couple who may wish to *delay* the appearance of the second although they would not be unduly alarmed if it followed the first fairly quickly; and they in turn differ from the situation where the family is perceived as complete.

As the couple's contraceptive needs change, so the doctor's own attitudes must remain flexible to accommodate them. But in one respect he has to be inflexible and that is in his role as a contraceptive salesman. Even today, relatively few couples approach their medical advisers for help in this highly personal and sometimes embarrassing area. Even today in Britain, America and much of Western Europe a distressingly large number of unplanned pregnancies occur. It is one of the roles of the physician to take the notion of birth control to his patients rather than waiting for them to come to him. He must do it tactfully and helpfully but above all he must do it. And in order to do so, he himself must believe in the message that he is broadcasting.

(*It is a pleasure to acknowledge the help of my friend Dr. Clive Wood in the preparation of this chapter.*)

9

REHABILITATION

P. J. R. NICHOLS

GENERAL PRINCIPLES OF REHABILITATION

Introduction

Rehabilitation implies the promotion of maximum possible recovery and although these sections are concerned with physical impairments recovery depends on the patient's mental concentration and attitudes (his motivation) almost as much as his physical capability. Rehabilitation should start as soon as the immediate definite treatment is underway and aims at returning the patient to his original work and way of life. If there is a residual disability the rehabilitation aim is to overcome this as far as possible and reduce the handicap to a minimum. The best rehabilitation is return to home and work even though there may be permanent disability.

In 1958 the Piercy Committee published its report (Cmnd 9883 HMS0) on all aspects of the existing provision for rehabilitation, training and resettlement of disabled persons. In the report it emphasised that rehabilitation should be a continuing process beginning with the onset of the illness or injury. It defined rehabilitation as 'the whole process of restoring a disabled person to a condition in which he is able as soon as possible to resume a normal life', and it recommended that one consultant should be based in a department of physical medicine, also that resettlement clinics should be set up to assess disability and recommend appropriate rehabilitation. It further emphasised the need for co-operation between all services concerned in rehabilitation.

In effect, very little happened. In 1972 two more major reports on rehabilitation were published known as the Tunbridge Report 'Rehabilitation—Report of a Sub-committee of the Standing Medical Advisory Committee' and the Mair Report 'Medical Rehabilitation: the pattern for the future'. Once again the medical profession was exhorted to become more aware of rehabilitation principles and both reports recommended the establishment of a large formal organisation for providing rehabilitation.

It is, however, somewhat misleading to use the term 'rehabilitation' as though it referred to a separate speciality. If we accept the definitions already given it cannot be a separate speciality, it is a philosophy of total patient care. Rehabilitation should be discussed in specific clinical terms, e.g. stroke rehabilitation, rehabilitation of the elderly amputee, rehabilitation of the rheumatoid arthritic, rehabilitation of the severe head injury, or in specific organisational terms, e.g. rehabilitation of the severely disabled or industrial rehabilitation. Only when the rehabilitation problem is clarified can real scientific contributions be made. Inevitably, accurate clinical diagnosis and the early definitive treatments are the most significant factors in determining the end results of rehabilitation.

Organisation

Physical rehabilitation began as part of orthopaedic after care and received considerable impetus during the world wars when it was an urgent economic need. Most early rehabilitation units were under the direct control of orthopaedic surgeons, and the spa physicians were particularly concerned with physical treatments. In World War II the interests came together and a number of rehabilitation units were established with physical medicine specialists supervising orthopaedic rehabilitation.

The lessons learnt in World War II were simple but very effective. The emphasis was on group therapy for patients with similar disabilities with a graduated progression through the classes as the patients improved. Each class had an activity programme based on a few simple remedial exercises and the group therapy was augmented by specific physiotherapy and occupational therapy when necessary.

Although a few rehabilitation units have survived, the armed forces style of residential accommodation has not been widely copied in civilian practice in this country. There is a tendency for such centres to become geographically and organisationally isolated and rehabilitation units developed in major hospitals tend to become overloaded with acute care patients (the demand upon beds being so heavy) or with long stay geriatric patients.

There have been various experimental day rehabilitation centres and combined medical and industrial centres. Some rehabilitation units have been outstandingly successful and have clearly demonstrated that the extrovert technique of the orthopaedic approach is applicable to medical disorders of the locomotor system with appropriate adaptation according to age and general medical conditions. In some countries the development of rehabilitation centres has extended to such a degree that there is considerable pressure for the use of the term 'rehabilitation medicine'. This concept of a therapeutic speciality with a tendency for the segregation of the patients in rehabilitation centres is contrary to the trends in this country. In general, in the United Kingdom, rehabilitation is regarded as being part of the general after care of patients and tends to be a relatively unorganised outpatient activity.

Rehabilitation and resettlement of a disabled patient, whether to work or to domestic responsibility, depends on many factors besides the severity of the disability. Among these factors are the age of the patient, the nature of the work, the patient's educational and domestic background, and social and economic factors. A particularly relevant factor determining the success of resettlement is the time elapsing from the onset of the disability until definite plans for return to work or retraining can be launched. At the present time the responsibility for industrial assessment and training lies with the Department of Employment and Productivity. However, a combined medical and industrial rehabilitation unit at Garston Manor is already proving that medical and industrial rehabilitation can be phased into each other, each complementing and helping the other although each are the responsibility of different departments. If industrial assessment and retraining, whether for industry or home life, is available alongside medical rehabilitation the total disability period can be reduced.

Rehabilitation should be a continuous process from hospital to workbench and this path cannot be smooth and efficient if administrative barriers are allowed to persist.

Types of rehabilitation

At this point is is necessary to review the general need for rehabilitation and the probable pattern of activity in any rehabilitation department. There are four categories of patient described:

Those patients for whom full recovery is to be expected.

Those with permanent but stable disabilities such as an amputation or paralysis following a nerve injury.

Those with unstable disabilities such as rheumatoid arthritis.

Those with chronic and degenerative disorders such as osteoarthrosis or multiple sclerosis.

However, it is unwise to regard any disability as stable. The effect of ageing or intermittent illness will have greater impact on a person with a disability. Many amputees have generalised vascular disease and paraplegics have frequent urinary infections and renal involvement.

Thus it is more realistic to classify rehabilitation into (a) the management of patients with a temporary disability, and (b) those with a chronic permanent disability. Those with a temporary disability require intensive rehabilitation immediately following the initial definitive treatment. In these circumstances early decisions regarding prognosis, aims of treatment, and early institution of rehabilitation and resettlement programmes are the key to rapid return to work and home independence.

Thus rehabilitation should be part of the management of acute illness or injury and be concerned with reablement, functional activities, and resettlement in home and work. In these circumstances it should be the responsibility of the specialist clinician (e.g. cardiologist or neurologist) concerned.

Rehabilitation of the chronically disabled has a different aim. Maintenance and support are the keystones. Repeated assessment is necessary to pick up problems early and prevent unnecessary morbidity and the main aim is the patient's social resettlement. This type of rehabilitation in the future may be more properly planned as a domiciliary or community based service.

Principles of rehabilitation of temporary disability

The majority of illnesses and injuries which have had efficient primary definitive treatment can be rehabilitated within the organisation of the District General Hospital as inpatients or as outpatients on a Day Hospital basis, or as residents in a hostel. With adequate rehabilitation the incidence of prolonged morbidity can be significantly reduced and the duration of disability can be shortened providing patients start their rehabilitation soon after the onset of disability.

Indeed, the delay in making decisions and delay in communicating decisions are potent causes of morbidity and delay return to work. Often it is only necessary for the doctor to tell the patient to return to work. If the patient has a residual disability it is often only a case of a doctor (either GP or hospital doctor) contacting the employer. But too often the appropriate decisions are not taken or decisions depend too much upon personal idiosyncracies or variations in organisation of the local medical services. For example, although uncomplicated appendicitis is characterised by rapid and smooth recovery, traditions, the patient's domestic convenience, and the whim of the individual surgeon are the factors which determine the time of removal of the sutures and the length of the patient's stay in hospital. The time off work varies from 10 days for housewives, to 2 weeks for schoolchildren, and up to 10 weeks for some insured persons. There is a similar wide range of morbidity after fracture of the wrist and hand—a relatively minor injury—requiring only a short period of immobilisation of the hand and wrist and with little interference with function and rarely with complication. Patients in manual work naturally have to have more time off work than those in sedentary occupations. Litigation is involved in about one third of these cases, but there is little evidence in this group of injuries of impairment of motivation to return to work. But although many patients could manage their usual work while in plaster of Paris they do not return to work as they, not unreasonably, feel that the wearing of the plaster might interfere with work and render them unacceptable to an employer. It is within this field of minor or temporary disabilities that about half the patients referred for physiotherapy can be considered. These represent the continuing commitment to 'orthopaedic' rehabilitation, together with other 'temporary' surgical or medical disabilities.

The advantage of organised rehabilitation lies in its ability to combine an integrated medical and functional assessment with the co-ordination of activities of the many agencies concerned with the patient's return to work and integrate the several aspects of rehabilitation, medical, social and industrial.

Rehabilitation of chronic or unstable conditions

Although physical rehabilitation is traditionally orthopaedically orientated, experience has shown that the techniques devised for accidents can be applied to many medical disabilities.

Rheumatoid arthritis, hemiplegia, and degenerative neurological disorders comprise a high proportion of all the patients with physical disability. The physical management of these patients is not very different from the rehabilitation of injuries, but the tempo and the pattern of activity are very different. Because the numbers are so large there has been a marked change in emphasis towards these patients in all physiotherapy and rehabilitation departments.

In rheumatoid arthritis with early diagnosis, treatment, intensive care in exacerbations and regular follow up during remissions, a high proportion of patients can be kept independent at home and at work. With increasing advances in surgical techniques for management of rheumatoid arthritis, the percentage of patients remaining at work will increase, but the use of such techniques imposes an increasing demand on the rehabilitation services, both for assessment and after-care. The majority of patients with rheumatoid arthritis can be improved functionally by planned rehabilitation although the men are often unable to continue in either heavy or manual work or very skilled work. Strokes are numerically one of the commonest disabilities of the locomotor system and with good rehabilitation about 20% of the survivors will return to full work and a further 30% will make a useful contribution about the house. It is the impairment of intellectual function and speech defects which usually are the stumbling block to resettlement and these are related, as with head injuries, to the extent of the original lesion and the subsequent brain damage.

Intensive rehabilitation

Most patients benefit considerably from periods of intensive rehabilitation and closely supervised convalescence. Special centres, structurally and functionally orientated towards recovery, have a purposive atmosphere and instill confidence. The individual skills of the rehabilitation team are integrated and co-ordinated to assist each patient to achieve maximal functional efficiency. Patients who do particularly well with these special rehabilitation facilities are those with multiple injuries, those with complex lesions (such as crush injuries of the hand or injuries of the head or spine), and those requiring a high standard of physical fitness before return to work is possible, such as members of the armed forces or sportsmen. The intensive full time regime and the integration of retraining for work with the exercise programme are of the utmost benefit.

The crucial period is usually the early weeks of incapacity—the period before the individual has had time to adjust to the role of the invalid. Early rehabilitation — active convalescence — bridges the gap between hospital bed and work-bench or kitchen sink.

Probably one in three patients discharged from hospital would benefit considerably from a period of rehabilitation to speed recovery and confidence, and to allow for realistic planning of return to work. The benefits to the individual patients from such a rehabilitative period are complemented by the economic advantage to the community.

But there are many factors mitigating against the inherent will to recover. For example, the victim of a road accident may reasonably choose to draw available disability benefits and call upon available services, e.g. home helps, rather than accept an intensive rehabilitation programme followed by a vocational training programme.

There is considerable evidence that the will to work is affected by the work content, and the working conditions more than the cost advantages. Furthermore, employers and fellow employees are sometimes reluctant to accept workers back without guarantee of complete fitness and there is considerable need for encouraging more flexible arrangements for return to work with a residual disability.

As far as the chronic, unstable or permanent disabilities are concerned it is important to distinguish between the value of a short period of intensive rehabilitation and the long term care of the patient with a chronic disability. Patients who suffer from a residual or permanent disability need to understand and accept their disability before there is any chance of their undertaking the necessary steps to circumvent it. Because of the inability to accept the physical disability and a persistent demand for treatment directed towards a 'cure' much physical treatment is expended in the misguided belief that it is actually contributing to physical improvement, whereas it is probably only sufficing to maintain the morale of both the patient and the doctor. For those patients who need to face the long term or chronic disability or a permanent handicap, more specialised facilities for adequate assessment are required. In the final analysis it is often the patient's own personality which determines the level of handicap.

The real problem is to clarify the aims of rehabilitation, to define the goals and the techniques whereby each goal may be achieved. The main aim must be to return all patients in hospital to the community and to maintain them there, and whenever possible to prevent them being admitted or readmitted to hospital except for the specific treatment which can only be provided in hospital.

The role of the remedial professions

Both physiotherapists and occupational therapists have a mixed role. They have specific therapeutic skills similarly directed towards improvement of locomotor function. They have training in the assessment of patients' physical conditions. They are concerned with evaluating the patients' recovery and likely future capability. There are three obvious components of the therapist's role: assessment, instruction, and therapeutic procedures. In any clinical situation, the importance of the individual components will vary and they will vary from patient to patient and from time to time. Therapeutic procedures are more important in treating temporary disabilities whereas instruction and assessment assume greater importance in the management of chronic disabilities.

Part of the therapist's skill lies in adapting her approach and technique to the patient's ever changing clinical and psychological need. Indeed, it is because of the flexibility of approach and the breadth of the skills and techniques which makes a critical evaluation of physical therapy so difficult. Furthermore, much of the patient's response may be due to non-specific factors, e.g. the patient's expectations and attitudes, his mood, personality and response to the therapist, and his ability to comprehend instructions and learn new skills. The therapist's ability to exploit the situation makes it difficult to distinguish between the patient's response to specific effects of physical treatment and the situation of general care.

In collaboration with general practitioners it is hoped that the remedial professions will be able to identify the real needs of patients. Some can be treated at home, thus saving admission to hospital, others can be provided with appropriate help with activities of daily living rather than being referred to hospital for intermittent inconsequent physiotherapy. In collaboration with the Social Services many patients could be treated, assessed and maintained in the community: thus reserving hospital facilities for those situations and conditions which really require hospital care and attention.

The role of the general practitioner

A sample survey of the handicapped and impaired in Great Britain was carried out on behalf of the Department of Health and Social Security, and published in 1971. This sample suggested that between 3% and 6% of the population had some physical disability. Apart from those people who are recovering from a temporary disability due to illness or injury and therefore in need of therapeutic rehabilitation services, each general practitioner is likely to have 10–20 patients in his practice who are severely or significantly handicapped and needing considerable support. These patients are likely to fall into one of the following groups:

The arthritics
Chronic bronchitics
Cardiovascular lesions
Cerebral palsy
Spinal lesions (including spina bifida)
Lower limb amputations
Multiple sclerosis
Muscular dystrophy or other neuromuscular lesions.

The magnitude of the problem of the chronically disabled has increased over the past few decades with the introduction of antibiotics and the improvement in general care provided for the elderly and disabled.

It is also significant that the survey indicates that the great majority (about 60–70%) of disabled people are over the age of 65 years. It is for this reason that the care of the severely disabled and care of the elderly tends to become inextricably intermingled although the problems of the young disabled are very different and should be tackled differently and in different places. The general practitioner role is complicated because he will often have to decide, or help the family to decide, upon the most appropriate management. Many general practitioners are reluctant to undertake responsibility for care of chronically disabled people, whereas they would probably be better if they were maintained within the family. Full and realistic assessment of the clinical and functional problems must be made in the context of the family, the home and the community facilities. Collaborative care between hospital and community is as appropriate for the young disabled as it is for the elderly. For these reasons, rehabilitation services must have close community links with doctors and remedial therapists having both hospital and community experience and responsibility.

Although most active rehabilitation of temporary disability is due to accident or illness and will be carried out in hospital departments, a closer collaboration with general practitioners, works doctors, school doctors and the community services could reduce invalidism.

Too frequently return to work or functional activity is delayed because of the time-lag in authoritative clinical decisions or inadequate appraisal of the real implications of the disability.

During the early recovery stage, the rehabilitation services should provide;

(a) intensive physical therapy for selected patients requiring, and able to respond to, rehabilitation
(b) assessment of patients' physical, psychological and social capabilities and potential
(c) opportunity for patients to prove physical fitness and functional capabilities.

There is considerable evidence that the rate of recovery (return to work after many common disabilities such as fractures of the lower limb) could be speeded up if the rehabilitation of such patients was better arranged.

If the community services and general practitioner services could undertake a greater responsibility for the chronically disabled and the pressure for palliative and unevaluative physical treatment reduced, then those facilities could be used in a more intensive fashion for conditions more likely to respond.

Disablement resettlement officer

Resettlement is the process of returning the patient to the most appropriate social situation and aims at returning the patient to his original work and way of life, overcoming residual disability and reducing the handicap to a minimum. Resettling patients at home is the main aim, and for those who are in the younger age group, resettling in work is the next aim.

Resettling a disabled person in work depends on the severity of the disability, his age, the nature of the work, his educational and domestic background, and social and economic factors. One of the most important factors affecting the success of resettlement is the time lapse from the onset of disability until plans for return to work or training are brought into effect.

When return to his original work is not possible, a detailed analysis of his working capability is necessary as a preliminary to retraining and re-employment. At the present time, the responsibility for industrial assessment and training lies with the Department of Employment and Productivity. A special service was set up for the disabled under the Disabled Persons (Employment) Act (1944). At each of the local offices there is a disablement resettlement officer whose responsibility is to assist disabled persons to find appropriate employment where and when this is possible. Such an officer may devote all or part of his time to these duties depending upon the volume of work. His job is largely to implement the compilation of the Register of Disabled Persons, the Quota Scheme for employment of disabled people and admission to Industrial Rehabilitation Units for assessment of the work potential of disabled people. The Quota Scheme places an obligation upon every substantial employer to give employment to a quota of registered disabled people. This scheme has advantages and disadvantages and is currently under review.

The Register of Disabled Persons was set up in 1944 but there are many disabled who do not register, and many are registered who suffer little handicap. Industrial rehabilitation units tend, because of their very nature, to be separate from the health service rehabilitation facilities. This means that the patient has to complete his 'medical rehabilitation' before starting industrial rehabilitation. There are several experimental attempts to organise industrial assessment and retraining alongside medical rehabilitation thus reducing the total disability time and making rehabilitation a continuous process from hospital to workbench. Hospital rehabilitation departments usually try to initiate industrial rehabilitation. Until such time as hospital rehabilitation services have direct access to the excellent assessment and training facilities of the industrial units while still supervising the patient's overall management, there is continuing need to organise local collaborative schemes.

Recently the Department of Employment and Productivity has appointed some Hospital Disablement Resettlement Officers to help to assess patients' resettlement problems, and to provide the critical link between hospital, work and industrial retraining facilities. A Hospital DRO should be a man well-versed in local industry, with personal contacts, who can talk to patients soon after their admission, in their own language, help to allay their fears, act as a go-between from hospital to employer, and advise both sides on the patient's likely working capabilities. He is able to identify resettlement problems early and to plan for return to work and retraining.

This pilot scheme has been very successful and provides an important extension of the rehabilitation services.

REHABILITATION PERSONNEL AND SERVICES

Rehabilitation personnel

Rehabilitation is the concern of all clinicians (consultants and general practitioners). In practice, nurses, physiotherapists, occupational therapists and remedial gymnasts are those most closely concerned with physical recovery. Social workers and community health workers have a major contribution in continuing care at home. Disablement Resettlement Officers (DROs) and industrial training staff are concerned with resettlement in work.

Certainly the rehabilitation of temporary disability will tend to remain the responsibility of the hospital for it is there that most of the severe temporary disabilities are treated (fractures, etc.). The responsibility for the chronically disabled is increasingly being placed upon the community services.

Rehabilitation services

A co-ordinated scheme ensuring early identification of the rehabilitation and resettlement problem, providing comprehensive physical therapy in an intensive competitive atmosphere, and adequate training and follow up services could help to reduce the level of invalidism and morbidity, and contribute to the financial welfare of the country. Whatever the disability, formal intensive rehabilitation, instituted as soon as possible after the onset of disability, can improve the rate of return of function and the quality of the end result. But rehabilitation cannot provide what was not present before illness or accident. There is plenty of good evidence that a period of organised rehabilitation improves the functional capability of the disabled and promotes the return to home and to work. This is true for temporary *and* chronic disability.

The effectiveness of rehabilitation, whether the disability is a minor one, or whether the patient is severely disabled, depends upon many factors including his personality, economic necessity, and physical disability. The rehabilitation services can provide an assessment of the disability and an assessment of the likely outcome. It can help the patient to regain function and it can help him to accept and adapt to his permanent disability. It can plan his return to work and help him to retrain for other work if he cannot return to his former job, or to cope with life if he is unable to work. The rehabilitation services include hospital consultants, remedial professions, disablement resettlement officers, social workers and the general practitioner and community services.

Responsibility for rehabilitation services

Full rehabilitation implies clinical, functional, social and welfare assessment and a co-ordinated approach to the patient's total management. A consultant with responsibilities for directing the rehabilitation services of a District General Hospital will usually have his own particular clinical interests such as rheumatology, neurology or orthopaedics. He may also collaborate very closely with colleagues in geriatric medicine and mental subnormality where there is a pressing need for rehabilitation services. His responsibilities for rehabilitation may be administrative only or he may develop rehabilitation medicine as his major interest.

In the integrated Health Service there is now a trend for physical therapists to develop a deeper understanding of their subject and so to become more able to assume greater responsibility for the day to day variations in therapy, and for the management of the departments in which they work. The training and experience of physical therapists varies considerably, and the training given in different countries also varies considerably, particularly in the proportion of practical to theoretical knowledge imparted.

In the United Kingdom the training is orientated towards the practical aspects of physical therapy, and the qualifications to practise this are granted in a Diploma. In many other countries, although the therapists complete a Degree course, their practical experience is much less.

As a general principle, physical therapists should be primarily practical in their approach and their training, and their work should be directed towards practical assessment and practical treatment. The therapist's knowledge of available treatments and the expected response to them from any patient should be dependent upon the individual response that she evokes from that patient. The clinician's function is to establish the overall guidance and direction of the patient's management.

Thus, in the field of rehabilitation the doctor's role is one of giving the therapists the chance of achieving the best results by:

(a) giving an accurate diagnosis
(b) giving clear indications of the aims of treatment
(c) giving a clear indication of the likely outcome
(d) specifying where therapy or disease characteristics may necessitate particular care in the administration of various treatments.

In general, it is emphasised that short intensive periods of therapy are more likely to have a therapeutic value than the prolonged intermittent attendances for palliative treatment which rapidly become more of a social outing than a therapeutic activity. Therapists are nowadays taught and encouraged to record details of the nature and effect of treatment so that feed-back information from her trained observations may substantially influence future management and enable her to contribute fully to its outcome.

The remedial professions

The three professions conventionally grouped under the heading 'remedial professions' are physiotherapy, occupational therapy and remedial gymnastics. Many other professions are contributing to the rehabilitation and care of the physically disabled in greater and lesser degrees depending upon the disability. They also make a significant contribution in other spheres, particularly the psychiatric field, educational and social services, but membership of these other professions is small, and it is only physiotherapists and occupational therapists with whom general practitioners are likely to come into close and frequent contact.

Physiotherapy

The Report on Rheumatic Diseases by the Arthritis and Rheumatism Council (1971) entitled 'Physiotherapy in Rheumatic Disease' delineates the place of physiotherapy in a clear and unequivocal fashion. The Report ends on a salutory note:

'The uncritical prescription of (for example) short wave diathermy for undiagnosed musculoskeletal pains may satisfy the patient that "something is being done" while a self-limiting condition runs its natural course; but it is undoubtedly indefensible because a valuable service (in short supply) is being wasted and both doctor and physiotherapist may come to believe eventually that they are providing a scientifically rational treatment.'

It also comments that:

'The physiotherapist although highly trained, nevertheless relies upon the doctor to make a precise diagnosis and to specify the objectives of treatment in anatomical and functional terms. Through contact with the patient, the experienced physiotherapist can provide a valuable physical and/or psychological assessment of the patient.'

Thus, when asking for physiotherapy, it is necessary to decide:

(1) What is the expected benefit?
(2) Is there an easier way of achieving the benefit such as injecting the site of pain with with corticosteroids?

(3) How often and for how long should physio-therapy be given? (the clinician should regularly review the progress of the patients for this will prevent waste of treatment and act as an incentive).

(4) Will it seriously interfere with the patient's job and will special transport be necessary? Can the benefit expected be justified by the inconvenience and time required?

(5) Could the physiotherapist train the patient so that physiotherapy could be continued at home?

Many traditional treatments have a limited value; for example:

(1) Electrical methods of heating the tissues (short wave diathermy, infrared and ultrasound radiation) provide only temporary relief of pain as a hot water bottle may relieve abdominal discomfort. Simple forms of heat and cold thus sometimes enable painful structures to be more effectively exercised. They have no other action.

(2) Electrical methods of stimulating the muscles to contract have no direct therapeutic value, but may help in overcoming muscle inhibition and with retraining muscles after surgical procedures.

(3) Ultraviolet radiation is only needed to treat dermatological complaints.

(4) Massage is time consuming and need seldom be prescribed. It has specific value in very few situations such as reducing edema, and in the treatment of scar tissue.

(5) Infrequent physiotherapy given on an out-patient basis can have little physiological value; such time is only of use to train the patient in a regular routine of exercises to carry out in his own home, and as a system of intermittent reassessment.

The uncritical continuation of ineffective treatment is inexcusable, and as the largest numbers of patients referred by general practitioners for physiotherapy are suffering from degenerative disorders, the apparent efficacy of the placebo and the enthusiastic acceptance and demand for comforting palliative treatments often masks the ineffectiveness of the treatment.

The traditional image of physiotherapy as a form of treatment depending upon electrical gadgetry has obscured the real advances which have been made.

However the physiotherapist should have freedom to use these palliative measures to prepare the patient for more active measures.

The main contribution of the physiotherapist in rehabilitation lies in the maintenance or increase of joint movement and correction of instability, achieved by:

> Exercises
> Splintage (if necessary)
> Functional retraining.

The majority of physiotherapists are employed in hospital departments but there is a trend towards employing physiotherapists in community situations, either based upon community hospitals or day wards and local authority day centres. A few experiments in providing domiciliary physiotherapy have demonstrated the value of integrating the service with general practitioner services. The efficacy of such services will need very careful evaluation, for any form of domiciliary service is bound to be 'labour intensive', satisfying for the therapist because it brings her into very close contact with people, and comforting for the patient. Whether it really contributes significantly to the patient's clinical situation will depend upon the general practitioner's skill at selecting cases as well as the therapist's understanding and experience.

So much physical therapy is empirical but does it matter whether treatment is unscientific? 'Rheumatism' is a useful term which patients think they understand and can usually find for themselves a cause. They will wish to attribute their symptoms to specific causes such as draughts, dampness, overwork or minor accidents. This is more satisfying than ascribing the aches and pains to increasing age or physical deterioration. But patients seek medical confirmation for their erroneous beliefs, and it is questionable whether correcting the beliefs is of value. When there is a question of litigation the situation is, however, very different.

As far as treatment is concerned, much physiotherapy is acceptable because it provides physical treatment for what the patient believes is a definite physical condition. But frequently the physiotherapist becomes part of the treatment. If the physiotherapist has confidence she inspires confidence. Her effectiveness depends on her sincerity, whether or not she is right in her diagnosis, and treatment; if she inspires confidence and a right-minded attitude towards recovery in her patients, she will get good results.

Physiotherapy treatment is conventionally divided broadly into passive (or palliative) treatments for the alleviation of symptoms and active treatments for the preservation and restoration of function.

Passive palliative physical treatment is widely

used for the alleviation of pain, the common treatments being used are heat, cold and massage. Although these treatments are often advocated for the immediate painful response to injury and thus liable to rapid resolution, many of the conditions treated are degenerative, chronic and episodic, and subject to their own characteristic patterns of exacerbation and remission. Thus in all cases it is difficult to evaluate the effect of treatment on the natural history of the condition under treatment. Furthermore, there is little scientific evaluation of the comparative effect of different treatments. The majority of conditions treated are changing and much of the response is non-specific.

Active physical treatment is based upon exercises which may range from the assisted activity of very weak muscles to hard physical activity akin to an athlete's circuit training programme. The exercises may be individually given or patients may be treated in groups. The exercises can be given in the patient's hospital bed, in water (hydrotherapy) or in a gymnasium. The physiotherapist will frequently precede exercise routines with a period of passive palliative treatment, hence the common prescription 'heat and exercises'. The skill of the therapist lies in achieving the response the clinician wishes to achieve within the constraints of the disability. To achieve maximal effect she may need to vary her approach and the techniques she uses from patient to patient and from time to time in any one patient. A fixed prescription such as 'short wave diathermy and quadriceps exercise' for a painful, swollen, osteoarthritic knee may therefore unnecessarily and unwisely restrict the therapist. She may find the patient responds better to ice packs. As far as the quadriceps exercise, the therapist needs guidance as to the severity of the disability but will naturally take the patient through a programme of static exercises (quadriceps setting) through to non-weightbearing exercises as the quadriceps muscle bulks up and the effusion regresses. Unless she is given this clinical freedom for which she is trained she cannot achieve the best possible results.

Heat can be provided in many forms, e.g. hot water, radiant heat, short wave diathermy, ultrasonics or wax baths. The choice may depend upon convenience of application, availability of apparatus or the personal preference of the therapist, patient or doctor. The form in which it is applied probably has little significance.

Electrical stimulation of muscle may sometimes be of use in regaining function after injury or surgery or in situations of muscle inhibition (e.g.

quadriceps inhibition). Once again, various techniques are available to the physiotherapist and an experienced therapist should be given a wide range of freedom to employ the techniques she has mastered to achieve the clinically acquired end result.

Manipulative procedures are being more widely taught in physiotherapy schools. These include various massage techniques for manipulating soft tissue. These have a place in the management of some results of trauma—soft tissue adhesions and scar tissue. Formal manipulation of peripheral joints is usually a procedure carried out by orthopaedic surgeons with the patient under anaesthetic, but some stiffened joints respond well to passive stretching associated with active movement regimes carried out by the physiotherapist.

Manipulation of the neck and spine for 'disc lesion' is an area of clinical management which generates much discussion and much emotion. Although there are many undoubted occasions of dramatic response, acceptable comparative studies are rare and inconclusive. Proponents of manipulation are enthusiastic and often uncritical in their claims. It is a technique which appeals to some general practitioners and although some achieve good short term results there is little evidence that there is any beneficial effect on the natural history of disc degeneration or disc prolapse.

Exercise can be assisted or resisted, and the quantity and quality of the assistance or resistance can be almost infinitely varied. Isometric (static) exercises are particularly indicated for painful or immobilised joints. Mobilising exercises can be done with or without weightbearing transmitted through the moving joint. Clearly clinical situations will dictate the most appropriate technique. Aside from these considerations the exact technique may not be of particular importance. The main principle is that in order to increase a muscle's power it is necessary to exercise it hard. Indeed, the principles employed by athletes in training are relevant, providing they are tempered by the clinical situation. As there are numerous athletic training routines so are there numerous therapeutic exercise routines.

Some physiotherapists working with the neurologically disabled have developed a technique for exploiting the patterns of movement in normal and abnormal neurological situations or by facilitating muscle contraction by employing proprioceptive stimuli. Such techniques appear to have particular application in the training of children with cerebral palsy and in some patients with brain injury.

Physiotherapists are increasingly prepared to undertake responsibility for the measurement of response to treatment and to build an evaluative technique to monitor improvement. Such approaches are the basis of specific clinical research projects and also teach therapists and doctors to understand the variability of response.

Occupational therapy

Occupational therapy is a much smaller profession than physiotherapy but it is also much misunderstood and inadequately used in the management of physical disability.

The Board of Occupational Therapists in their booklet 'Future Education and Training of Occupational Therapists' (Council of Professions Supplementary to Medicine, 1972) outlines the role of the occupational therapist in a most clear and concise fashion:

'(a) At the initial stage to make a contribution through practical and social situations to the diagnosis and assessment of psychological and physical disabilities of patients of all ages.

(b) At the continuous treatment stage of the patient to contribute to the development of functional ability to the maximum level of physical and psychological competence, through the use of therapist/patient relationship and of appropriate activities in appropriate settings.

(c) At the resettlement stage to prepare the patient for the home and social and economic situation to which he will return. This can most usefully be done in the realistic setting of the occupational therapy workshop and the home rehabilitation unit.

These functions may be performed:

(a) In hospitals with short term patients who may have long term problems, and in special units calling for specialised care of the longer term patients.

(b) In the community where the therapist will continue to treat discharged hospital patients, and to care for the permanently handicapped and the elderly, either in the patients' own homes or in treatment or work centres.'

The traditional diversional activity of occupational therapy is now only a minimal requirement of the hospital environment. The occupational therapist contributes to rehabilitation by:

(a) Early appraisal (assessment) of functional capabilities and potential in the social situation (i.e. functional assessment in terms of home or work environment).

(b) Active therapeutic rehabilitation in terms of co-ordinated functional activities (i.e. hand injuries).

(c) Prevocational training whether domestic or work, forming a bridge between hospital and home.

Occupational therapists have been working in the community and domiciliary situation for some years. Although some local authorities employ them mainly to occupy patients attending day centres, the greater contribution lies in identifying and assessing individual needs for disabled persons in the home. Selecting and providing aids and appliances, and training the patient and the family to use the aids and appliances is an activity which has expanded rapidly and widely since the passing of the Chronic Sick and Disabled Persons Act (1970 (3). Under this Act the local authority is required to identify and to assess the requirements of handicapped people. To do this they require personnel with skills such as those of occupational therapists. With increasing interest in rehabilitation services in hospitals, there are not enough occupational therapists, nor physiotherapists and it is hoped that part of the reorganisation and integration of the Health Service will eventually lead to a more rational 'sharing' of therapists between hospital and community.

Occupational therapists contribute to the assessment of disability and capability of patients of all ages. They provide therapeutic activities in terms of practical situations. As recovery proceeds they help prepare the patient for return home and for the social and economic situation to which they will return. The therapeutic activities are particularly valuable in the rehabilitation of injuries and disabilities of the hands and arms. By the use of specific crafts it is possible to encourage function and increase movement and power. Dexterity and manipulative skills are redeveloped. As recovery progresses light crafts give way to heavy activities involving the use of tools. For example, carpentry is excellent for building up the power of grip, increasing elbow and shoulder movement and encouraging co-ordination and stamina.

Retraining in housework and domestic activities can be part of the day to day function of a hospital OT department. Practising these activities can be as useful in encouraging functional recovery as exercises in a gymnasium. Finally, for those with persistent disability realistic assessment can help plan return home and return to work or lead to the appropriate activities in domestic and work situations, the supply of essential aids and appliances and the relevant training in their use. Close collaboration between occupational therapists and physiotherapists is essential and there will be many situations where there is planned overlap and others where duplication of effort should be avoided. Similarly there is an essential collaboration between hospital occupational therapy departments and domiciliary services (where these are not integrated) to ensure smooth transfer from hospital to home.

Collaboration between hospital occupational therapists, domiciliary occupational therapists, the social services and the Disablement Resettlement Officer is also essential for the patient in need of these services. All these various members of the rehabilitation team need to understand each other's contributions and learn how they can complement each other in achieving the united objective of obtaining maximal recovery for the individual patient.

MANAGEMENT OF SOME COMMON DISABILITIES

This section includes some general comments on some of the common causes of physical disability with which general practitioners may have to cope. All these conditions are generally considered as requiring physical therapy yet there is no evidence that the natural history is in any way influenced by such treatment.

All these disabilities are affected by age and changing circumstances if nothing else, thus it is always remiss to cease reviewing even the apparently most stable of disabilities. What is more important is to be continually prepared to make critical and pragmatic decisions about the absolute and relative value of physical treatment.

Pain in the neck and arm
Cervical spondylosis
Pain in the neck and/or shoulder is one of the commonest of all symptoms which lead to people seeking medical advice.

Frequently the pain is considered to accompany degenerative changes in the cervical spine although the radiological signs of cervical spondylosis are so common that the connection may well be fortuitous. In order to incriminate the cervical spine it is necessary to demonstrate definite involvement of the cervical spine in the presence of partial root distribution. A full root distribution of symptoms can be accepted as evidence of involvement at the level of the cervical spine even in the absence of overt signs in the neck.

There are two main groups of patients with pain in the neck and arm, or pain in the arm deriving from the neck.

The first group are usually young people who have suffered sudden trauma such as an athletic injury or a 'whiplash' injury sustained in a road traffic accident. The second group are usually middle-aged or elderly presenting with a recurrent history of neck pain, limitation of movement, and some root pain. The pins and needles are usually worse at night. Women are affected more than men and the symptoms are frequently precipitated by many common activities, e.g. gardening and shopping, which involve heavy lifting.

The first group are notoriously difficult to treat. Although most whiplash injuries eventually resolve many may require persistent immobilisation with a firm cervical collar for many months. This period of immobilisation may need to be followed by a period of gradual supervised mobilisation by gentle exercises and occasionally by manipulation. These patients are often difficult to manage, the circumstances of the trauma may involve litigation and consequently they are usually the concern of orthopaedic or accident departments.

The second group of patients is very numerous and many can often be adequately managed by the general practitioner. Neck and arm pain associated with degenerative changes in the neck is so common that it is almost the rule for a high proportion of the population.

The symptoms are qualitatively unrelated to severity of the radiological change. The symptoms are usually self-limiting and only about one quarter of the patients have pain which persists for longer than 3 months. If such patients are treated with an adequate collar worn continuously night and day the symptoms will remit in the majority of cases within 3–4 weeks. Indeed, lack of response to an adequate collar may be regarded as a good reason for seeking further opinion. The use of a collar can be supplemented by the use of a 'butterfly' pillow, advice about reducing heavy lifting, prolonged driving and avoiding all activities which exacerbate symptoms. Palliative physiotherapy, traction, manipulation and many other 'treatments' have their enthusiastic advocates. Undoubtedly patients respond to many treatments but there is no sustained evidence that any treatment has any long term effect on the natural history. Certainly the immediate use of a collar made of double thickness orthopaedic felt and covered with stockingette is simple and effective. The collar may be shaped to accommodate the chin. Its application should always relieve and not exacerbate symptoms. Sometimes more effective and prolonged immobilisation is required and this can be achieved with a collar made of various materials such as Plastazote, plaster of Paris, or moulded leather, These will only be supplied through hospital appliance services.

For the chronic sufferer many simple techniques can help. The use of a firm mattress in a bed together with a 'butterfly' pillow is often helpful in preventing exacerbation of symptoms at night. Avoidance of heavy lifting, e.g. carrying shopping, is advocated. For those who work at desks, raising the desk and tilting its surface is helpful, thus obviating the need to work continuously with the neck flexed. Housewives can be helped to reorganise some of the more difficult aspects of housework by a domiciliary occupational therapist who can visit the home and see the difficulties at first hand.

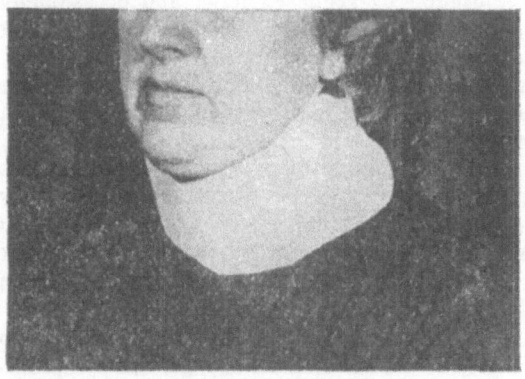

Figure 1. A simple collar made of orthopaedic felt.

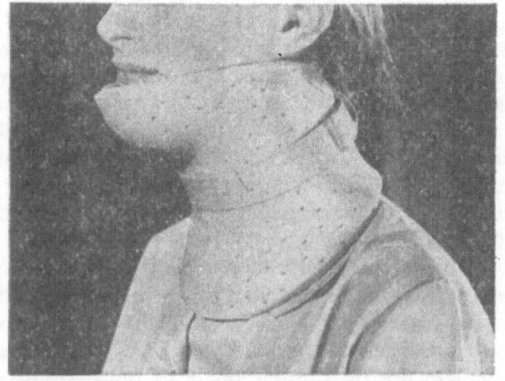

Figure 2. A plastazote collar extended to enclose the chin and to prevent extension of the neck.

Thus the early use of a simple cervical collar, the avoidance of provocative factors, and the judicious use of analgesics and relaxants (diazepam is useful during this condition), the GP will be able to manage many patients with symptoms arising from degenerative arthritis of the neck, but if symptoms persist the referral for further investigation is advisable.

The painful stiff shoulder

There are a number of patients who develop a painful stiff shoulder correlated to cervical spondylosis. The shoulder movement may be restricted in a specific movement, particularly adducted and either internal and external rotation (rotator cuff lesions), or it may be a true 'frozen' shoulder, involving restriction of all movements of the gleno-humeral joint.

Most of these conditions are self-limiting, but the painful stiff shoulder may be associated with other more sinister conditions such as myocardial infarction, hemiplegia, or underlying lung disease. Traditionally these conditions are treated by injection of steroid, analgesics, manipulation, or physiotherapy—usually a mix of palliative treatment with exercise. Once again, there is no evidence that any one treatment is clearly more effective than another. The judicious use of analgesics, if pain is severe, rest in a sling, and elimination of any sinister underlying pathology should be the first approach. As the symptoms begin to resolve it is important to encourage movement within the painless range. As symptoms continue to improve to the available painless range increases. Full recovery may take many months but can be confidently predicted.

Backache

Backache is another very common symptom which plagues patients, general practitioners and hospital consultants. The majority of the patients with these symptoms are suffering from mechanical or degenerative disorders of the lumbar spine.

The acute disc lesion is not so much of a problem in diagnosis and will often respond to immediate rest in bed with a firm mattress and adequate analgesics and sedation. If the pain does not settle or neurological signs persist further investigation is indicated. But patients with persistent low back pain associated with degenerative change in the lumbar spine at some time respond to palliative heat, rest in a firm bed, use of a surgical corset or active mobilisation of the spine with exercise. The problem often lies in finding the appropriate treatment at the time.

Acute severe disabling pain warrants immediate

investigation; chronic recurrent pain failing to respond to rest and restricted activity should also be referred for further investigation.

Backache, with or without sciatica, may well be the presenting symptom for a number of conditions which should be excluded. Haemoglobin, ESR, and X-ray of the lumbar spine and pelvis are the usual investigations required to supplement clinical examination. Presuming the underlying pathology has been eliminated, many patients frequent the GP's surgery, orthopaedic clinics and physiotherapy departments. Some patients will manage themselves, using a corset when they have an exacerbation of symptoms, maintaining muscle power and mobility with appropriate exercises, avoiding activities which are likely to provoke pain.

Other patients become part of the hard core of the unemployed. Such patients are often referred to Industrial Rehabilitation Units but the success rate, in terms of permanent return to employment, is not very high.

The general practitioner can help considerably by instituting immediate rest for the acute backache including providing an 'instant' corset; by helping to evaluate the personality and motivation of the chronic backache sufferer; and they can help to maintain the average patient with intermittent symptoms with advice, analgesics, and by avoiding unnecessary introspective invalidism on the one hand and yet insisting on regular exercise, avoidance of obesity and modifications of their way of life to prevent unnecessary provocation of their symptoms on the other hand.

Rheumatoid arthritis

There are over a million people in the United Kingdom who suffer from rheumatoid arthritis. It commonly starts in early adult life affecting rather more women than men, and running a remittant or intermittent course. There is a considered belief that the diagnosis is incompatible with continued independence and working, but this is quite untrue. The majority of patients with rheumatoid arthritis can retain a good functional level, remaining at work and independent at home for many years. The majority of those at work can continue at least until a stage of planned retirement. The man who is a manual worker may well have to change his employment, but office or sedentary workers with rheumatoid arthritis are more troubled by the problems of commuting than those of work. Some patients with severe hand involvement might have difficulty with work involving skilled manipulative procedures and housewives with young families may have problems with the heavier aspects of housekeeping.

Prolonged standing, difficult journeys and heavy repetitive work are the major problems.

With careful clinical management maintaining patients on the optimum drug regime and regular care from a special rheumatology centre where periods of intensive inpatient care can induce remission of symptoms with rest, drugs, splintage and physiotherapy, will be enough to maintain many patients for a number of years. Surgery is playing an increasing part in the management of the disease and more units are developing where rheumatologists and orthopaedic surgeons can collaborate in preventive as well as corrective surgical management. The increasing use of joint replacement will have considerable impact on the management of the more severe problems.

Within the modern rheumatology unit there is increasing use of the skills of physiotherapists and occupational therapists to teach the patients to manage their own disease.

Firstly, the patient needs to understand the disease and the need to avoid the unnecessary manoeuvres which precipitate pain, the tricks which enable the patient to overcome common difficulties in dressing, toileting, travel, housework and leisure activities are as much part of the treatment as regular drug regime. The use of simple aids such as 'tap turners' or 'pick-up sticks' are as important as the use of night splints to rest painful joints. The patient needs to be taught to 'preserve' his joints without *unnecessarily* restricting his life. Such prophylactic measures are more important than attending for intermittent physiotherapy.

Much clothing and household equipment can be adapted to make it easier for the arthritic housewife. Here the hospital and the domiciliary occupational therapists need to collaborate in provision of aids and regular monitoring of the patient's capability. Marked change in activities of daily living may herald a change in the disease status and as such warrant review at the rheumatology unit long before overt clinical signs or laboratory tests alert the doctor.

For both men and women mobility out of doors is often a critical function. The use of sticks, or crutches, or elbow crutches can facilitate walking when the lower limbs are markedly involved. But unfortunately, over-use of the upper limbs can lead to severe changes in the joints which have to take unnatural weight over many years. It is essential to avoid precipitating trouble in upper limb joints and care must be taken to explain this to patients. The use of gutter crutches, carrying trolleys, and even the prophylactic use of an appropriate wheelchair may help to preserve the joints at risk. Those with more severe disease who require help with transport to get to work may be entitled to their own personal transport supplied through the Department of Health and Social Security, or some financial help in lieu. Cases of doubt should be referred to the Appliance Medical Officer at the nearest DHSS Artificial Limb and Appliance Centre. The provision of appropriate transport may be the most important factor in keeping an arthritic man at work, or enabling an arthritic housewife to continue running her house.

Finally, it is important to note the sexual aspects of the disease. The disease affects men and women in their prime, but because of painful stiffness of joints, there may well arise difficulties and frustrations in relation to sex. For women, pregnancy often brings relief from symptoms, but motherhood imposes increasing strain. Frank advice on contraception is often needed and marriage counselling with the problems of arthritis in mind can be helpful to the couple frustrated by pain and limitation of one partner.

Strokes

Strokes probably represent the commonest problems of rehabilitation both in the community and in hospital practice. The elderly (over 65) occupy 40–45% of all hospital beds and cerebrovascular disease is the commonest single cause of bed occupancy in this group.

Each year about 90 000 to 100 000 people in the United Kingdom will have a stroke and although about half will fail to survive more than 3–4 weeks, this disability places a high demand upon rehabilitation facilities.

Of those surviving, about 20% of stroke patients can return to full activity and a further 30% will make a useful contribution in the home. Thus approximately 50% of those affected can achieve a working status. It is the impairment of intellectual function and speech defects which are usually the stumbling blocks to resettlement, and these are related, as with head injuries, to the extent of the original lesion and the subsequent brain damage.

Strokes are the third most common condition referred to physiotherapy departments and occupy about 10% of available physiotherapy time.

The incidence of stroke is about 2 per 1000. In other terms, in a population of 200 000 such as an average District General Hospital might serve, there are likely to be about 400 strokes each year. Of these, about 180 die within three months, 80 will recover without residual disability, 130 will survive with residual hemiplegia and 20 with other sequelae of brainstem lesions.

It is conventional to treat residual hemiplegia with active exercises, calipers, walking aids, wheelchairs and speech therapy, in various mixtures according to the severity of the residual disability. However, there is little evidence deriving from adequate comparative studies to give real guidance as to the management of an individual patient.

There is mounting evidence relating to survival and general levels of independence which might be achieved but there is little detailed guidance which can be used to improve the quality of life of survivors. Little is known about the proportion of stroke patients who are not admitted to hospitals and their pattern of survival and recovery.

Although there is considerable pressure to provide physical therapy for the majority of patients with residual hemiplegia, improvements may continue over many years both in limbs and in speech function.

So many factors are involved, age, sex, neurological deficit and complicating clinical conditions, such as previous stroke, heart disease, hypertension, the side of stroke, etc.

Recovery of function, the use of aids and adaptation to the disability will depend upon social background, educational status and more particularly whether the lesion is predominantly motor loss or was accompanied by a major perceptual cognitive or language deficit. Indeed, there is considerable evidence to the effect that it is the extent of the neurological deficit associated with age and vascular change which is the determining factor.

No amount of physical rehabilitation can compensate for extensive brain damage although long term management can help to retrain a number of patients. Communication difficulties are as important in the social situation as physical ones. Language disorder is greatest at the onset of stroke and may resolve spontaneously. The greatest spontaneous recovery occurs between 2 and 6 months from the onset of the disorder.

The greatest spontaneous physical recovery occurs between 2 weeks and 2 months from onset.

There is some evidence that physical rehabilitation should be at the greatest intensity during the early stages of recovery, and speech therapy, if it is available, should probably continue for at least 6 months.

In both cases, it is relevant to consider the contribution to be made by therapists. It is probably more important for the therapist to adequately train the patient, relatives and attendants to encourage near 'normal' activities rather than encourage the patient, family or medical adviser to concentrate their attention on 'treatment periods'.

The best treatment of the residual hemiplegia is to practise walking, and the best treatment for speech defect is to practise talking.

The walk of the hemiplegic will never be perfect, and speech may never recover completely. It is therefore important that all concerned accept a pragmatic approach and encourage activity rather than seek a 'cure' and its achievement by means of regular frequent 'treatment'.

Sympathetic neighbours, friends and relatives who will sit with the patient with a speech defect and encourage speech and communication in relaxed familiar surroundings are likely to be of more value than intermittent ambulance journeys to clinical situations for the brief attention of an over-worked speech therapist. Once the physiotherapist has helped the patient to overcome the early difficulties of balance and manipulating an appropriate walking aid, repeated walking practice at home will become part of the resettlement programme.

Severe distortion of body image will make it difficult to retrain walking and also for retraining in activities of daily living. Physiotherapists and occupational therapists are continually seeking new methods of overcoming the deficits in patients' understanding of their own disabilities which preclude their ability to overcome the disability.

Then there is a need for skilled nursing during the early stages to maintain clear airways, adequate fluid intake, prevention of skin damage, and avoidance of urinary retention and faecal impaction. The physiotherapist will help to maintain a full range of motion of the affected limbs, particularly to prevent the development of 'frozen shoulder'. At this stage, about 20% will require intensive care and a few will need specialised neurological investigation and care. As recovery takes place passive care of the paralysed limbs changes to encouragement and active movement and re-establishment of the pattern of sitting, standing and walking.

Once recovery begins to show itself, the major problem is to establish the realistic prognosis and the likely functional outcome. Once the critical early weeks have passed, the likely outcome clarifies and it is then that plans can be made for the patient's return home. This will depend more upon the competence of the family,

their desire to look after the patient, and their social situation, rather than the clinical condition. Economic status, possible adaptation of housing and the availability of local support are the keystones. Periodic hospital admission, some remedial therapy at a day hospital, or day centre, are of more value as assessment sessions than therapeutic sessions. One encouraging development is the establishment of voluntary self-help groups for patients and relatives, promoting social integration, in co-ordinating transport and providing continued encouragement and mutual support.

REHABILITATION OF LOWER LIMB AMPUTEES

The young amputee rarely presents problems of rehabilitation but nowadays, over 60% of all amputees are over the age of 60 years and are suffering from peripheral vascular disease and unfortunately amputation is often carried out as an ablative procedure after many other procedures directed towards saving a gradually dying limb. The patient, being elderly, often responds poorly, and is resigned to severe physical handicap. It is important to try to convince the patient to accept amputation as the means of getting rid of a source of severe pain and discomfort, and is the first stage in regaining active function.

The use of conventional pylons or 'early walking aids' enables many lower limb amputees to be mobilised early, often while still in the surgical ward. With such aids, many patients can be returned home walking a few weeks after amputation.

A well organised integrated limb fitting service, backed by rehabilitation services, can ensure the provision of the appropriate appliance or prosthesis at the right place at the right time.

However, a high proportion of elderly amputees have additional complicating conditions. Frequently, the circulation of the remaining limb is impaired, indeed, of the survivors of amputation a high proportion come to second amputation within a few years of the first. Many other amputees have cardiovascular disease and the general expected level of post-amputation activity is very limited. Indeed, fewer than half of all elderly ischaemic limb amputees and almost none of the elderly double amputees achieve competent independent walking with prostheses.

It is more important in the early post operative phase to pay attention to the general physical fitness and training in self-independence of the patient by using a wheelchair. Psychological preparation for the amputation and treatment of the almost inevitable depression after the operation are essential parts of the total rehabilitation of the elderly amputee.

The increasing availability of a simple easy to fit early walking aid should facilitate an early return home. Those who improve sufficiently can proceed with the fitting of a more definitive prosthesis when it is clear that their physical, psychological and social status warrants the additional time and effort on the patient's part which the necessary procedures demand.

Realistic resettlement requires some adaptations at home so that bathroom, toilet and dressing independence can be achieved using a wheelchair. Social integration also may depend upon the wheelchair and appropriate help. Once again, it is important that all concerned regard the wheelchair not as a sign of decrepitude but as a very real aid to increased, or otherwise unavailable, mobility. Even for those who achieve walking with an artificial limb or limbs, there must be times when they will be better served by an appropriate wheelchair, especially for outdoor activities.

MULTIPLE SCLEROSIS

The physical features of multiple sclerosis which are particularly pertinent to the problem of rehabilitation are:

(a) the onset is usually between 20 and 40 years of age

(b) the disease is usually progressive

(c) the high incidence of spasticity, spasms and tremor

(d) the high incidence of incontinence.

Spasticity

The spasms and spasticity are disabling in their own right and often predispose to even more disabling contractures. Drugs such as diazepam and chlordiazepoxide and more recently lioresal have been widely used to reduce the spasm and are a useful supplement to physical therapy. Ice packs will often reduce spasm and enable the physiotherapist to obtain a greater degree of mobility and by passive and active movements to help the patient gain a more active control of movements and prevent the development of contractures.

The injection of 2–5 ml of 42% alcohol into the motor point of a muscle may be of considerable value particularly in the adductors of the thighs enabling the legs to be abducted for toilet purposes. The injection of very small quantities of 1 or 2% phenol is a more difficult procedure usually monitored by electromyography and achieving a long lasting result.

Although patients with multiple sclerosis often react badly to surgical procedures for contractures such as adductor tenotomy, or abturator neurectomy these procedures may be considered if response to simple management is inadequate.

Tremor

Tremor of the upper limbs can be very disabling interfering with feeding and writing in particular. Aids such as special spoons, felt-tipped pens, etc., may be of value and some patients are helped with weighted cuffs, but there is little that can be done to damp down severe tremor. Head tremor can also be very distressing. A surgical collar, padded headrest on the wheelchair, or a head-restraining strap may help to control the tremor enough for a patient to be fed more easily or to enable him to read or write. The effect of nystagmus and head tremor can sometimes be reduced by the use of an eye-patch or 'blinkers' restricting sideways vision. The combined tremor of head and upper limbs is almost unmanageable. Although a weighted walking frame may give stability tremor and spasm of the legs can prevent a patient from walking.

Physiotherapy

Exercise therapy has been advocated as a valuable form of treatment but few patients can be persuaded to persevere with vigorous muscle exercise which is as demanding as that for an athlete, and very demanding for physiotherapy staff.

The need for continued exercise as a therapeutic activity and as diversional morale boosting activity can be aided by the installaton of simple do-it-yourself bars at home. The patient can undertake daily standing and walking exercises and thus help to prevent contracture of the lower limbs and trunk. If these bars are in the bathroom then independence for toilet activities can be maintained. For other patients it may be of value to train the domestic partner to undertake regular stretching and passive mobilisation of the affected joints. The use of a wheelchair, hoists, and electric beds, are also aids for the relatives as much as for the patient, and as such are an important part of rehabilitation.

Incontinence

Frequency and urgency of micturition are symptoms which the patient may volunteer but the patient with multiple sclerosis is particularly reluctant to admit to incontinence. Residential care however may reveal previously denied incontinence. The female patient in particular, although denying incontinence will frequently accept the need for and appreciate the effect of an indwelling catheter.

Management of the incontinence by continous catheterisation in the female or drainage urinal in the male, reduces some of the extra housework occasioned by the patient.

Psychological features

The rehabilitation of most severely disabled patients depends on the patient's personality, financial incentives, and the degree of the disability, in that order.

The patient with multiple sclerosis seems to have a distinct personality. In general, they do not respond well to conventional rehabilitation programmes and they usually demonstrate a singular inability to adapt to their disability. These patients do not develop trick movements, and they rarely become skilful with any appliances beyond a standard wheelchair, sticks or crutches. It is this lack of adaptability to develop trick movements and use appliances which gives the key to the difficulties of rehabilitation in multiple sclerosis. Their euphoria, often regarded as evidence of high morale, is a pathological phenomenon strongly associated with intellectual impairment. It seems likely that the presence and severity of intellectual deterioration is the crucial factor in determining the outcome of rehabilitation.

Careful psychometric testing of MS patients may show up intellectual deficits even when these are not manifest on routine clinical enquiry and these must be taken into account whenever therapeutic advice of any complexity is given. The onset of the intellectual damage is insidious and often undetected and may precede obvious gross physical disability. Two thirds of patients with multiple sclerosis suffer from typical patchy dementia with impairment of conceptual thinking and perseveration that is sometimes known as the chronic amnestic syndrome or the chronic brain syndrome. Intellectual loss may not be the whole answer to the problems of motivation of the MS patient, but when the deficit is considerable, as it often is, it is not necessary to invite explanation in other terms.

It can be shown that many of these patients are depressed, even in the presence of euphoria. It is important to try to uncover the depression so often underlying the euphoria because it can be improved by the use of drugs such as chlordiazepoxide. In our experience chlordiazepoxide is a valuable drug because it has an anti-depressant and an anti-spasmodic effect and this is more useful than diazepam.

As the patient becomes more euphoric, periods spent at or in hospital give the family some welcome and necessary relief and help.

Summary

Thus, as for other conditions, rehabilitation must be based upon careful total assessment of the patient in the context of their physical disability, psychological make-up, their family and social circumstances, and the physical organisation of their life. The assessment and management must be continuous as the situation may change gradually or suddenly without warning. Mobility must be maintained by the use of a wheelchair, hand propelled or electrically propelled. Their family must be given practical help for they have to bear the brunt of both the physical and intellectual deterioration over many years. It is very important that help should be given to help cope with incontinence.

Appliances, aids, physiotherapy and the usual accoutrements of physical therapy are only adjuncts and are often rejected by the patient with multiple sclerosis. The major weapon is an understanding of the problems so that these problems can be interpreted by all who are concerned with the welfare of these patients.

SPINAL INJURIES

Spinal injury units were established because of the need to assess, treat and rehabilitate and initiate resettlement of patients suffering from paraplegia. The clinical and rehabilitation needs of these patients were such that an integrated spinal injury organisation was a natural solution.

Since the institution of spinal injury centres, the results of treatment and rehabilitation have steadily improved and now some centres claim that 40% to 60% of paraplegics return to work or domestic independence. Achieving these results depends on a high standard of initial definitive treatment and a co-ordinated and intensive period of rehabilitation; this involves training in bladder care, skin care, and a wheelchair existence, and usually extends over a period of 6 to 9 months.

Ideally, these centres are sited at District General Hospitals with adequate supportive facilities, and form a focus for much of the rehabilitation services of that particular hospital. Once the paraplegic has developed a high level of independence in a spinal injuries unit he can usually plan to leave the shelter of hospital or hostel.

The predominant problems facing these patients and their general practitioners are mainly associated with skin care, and urinary infection. Most spinal injury centres arrange regular admission particularly to check renal function.

Such patients present few problems to their GPs.

Higher lesions however with tetraplegia are much more disabled, and more prone to both renal and chest infections, and to skin breakdowns. The increased risk and their greater dependence place a greater responsibility upon the general practitioner. Although these conditions are increasing in number mainly associated with road traffic accidents they are not, as yet, a significant problem for the majority of doctors in general practice.

HEAD INJURIES

The majority of patients with head injury suffer a minor injury requiring only simple treatment. Good initial assessment followed quickly by a period of rehabilitation in the department of the District General Hospital is all that post-concussion syndrome requires.

The more severe head injury patient requires a sophisticated system of progressive care, involving physical rehabilitation together with educational, speech and behaviour therapy. Intellectual impairment with loss of memory, loss of concentration, loss of sense of responsibility, and emotional lability and depression are the main adverse features.

There is considerable pressure for the provision of special Head Injury Rehabilitation Centres in association with neurological and neurosurgery centres. Such centres require residential accommodation and a high ratio of staff to patients.

Some patients with head injury tend to become agressive and require close collaboration between neurological, psychiatric and rehabilitation staff. In severe cases, the process of rehabilitation may extend over many years, but with good facilities for physical, psychiatric and industrial rehabilitation and follow up, many patients with head injury can be returned to work in the community.

THE SEVERELY DISABLED

Each patient is an individual and each severely disabled patient needs individual care. For optimal results, the patients must be gently led and guided along appropriate lines by unhurried exploration of possibilities.

Many severely disabled patients have lived with their handicap for many years, many suffer pain, and all suffer frustration. They are not always amenable to new ideas and conversely they may well set their sights beyond that which is practical or possible. Practical trials, whether successes or failures, are part of the assessment providing factual evidence for the therapist, patient and relatives. It is often difficult to deny an appliance or line of management but a practical demonstration of its lack of value is much more acceptable than either an ex-cathedra refusal, or a compliance which leads to a wrong decision. It is this slow practical appraisal that is so time-consuming and needs specialised units and staff.

The long term management of severely disabled people must be based on a detailed assessment of the patient's physical disability and a pragmatic appraisal of their possible capability. This assessment must be made in the context of the natural history of the disability, the severity of the handicap, the patient's psychological make-up and intellectual capabilities in the context of their possible ultimate environment, social and financial.

Successful management in their own home depends on maximal patient co-operation and considerable involvement of the general practitioner, and this is only forthcoming when both patient and general practitioner understand enough to become members of the rehabilitation team.

AIDS AND APPLIANCES

In the longer term a patient with a physical disability may often be best served by helping him to accept his handicap—this training is part of his rehabilitation, for unless he understands and accepts his limitations he cannot collaborate in procedures designed to improve or circumvent that handicap. This is where the provision, prescription and design of aids and appliances has a relevant part to play.

There is too often an impression that sophisticated aids are likely to bring untold advantages to the disabled and elderly. Unfortunately, this is not so. Certainly many aids and appliances currently provided are crude, ineffective, uncomfortable and costly. But the majority of rehabilitation and resettlement problems are social, medical or psychological and as such are not soluble by mechanical means.

Too frequently, aids are prescribed, made or demanded without a full assessment of the patient's potential, and his clinical, social and psychological needs. Aids, to be effective, should be simple, safe to operate, and quickly available and should provide the patient with an immediate and acceptable functional improvement. More complex appliances may be demonstrated to be of value to the patient or his relatives but the provision of appliances such as these imposes a further responsibility upon the prescriber to ensure that adequate training is given to ensure efficient use of the appliance.

Aids

Aids are simple, cheap, stock-in-trade devices of most departments caring for the physically disabled. They are usually provided in the hope that they will increase a patient's independence in activities of daily living. They are most frequently supplied for personal care and household activities. 'Pick up sticks', long handled combs, and adapted crockery and cutlery are among the common aides supplied by occupational therapists.

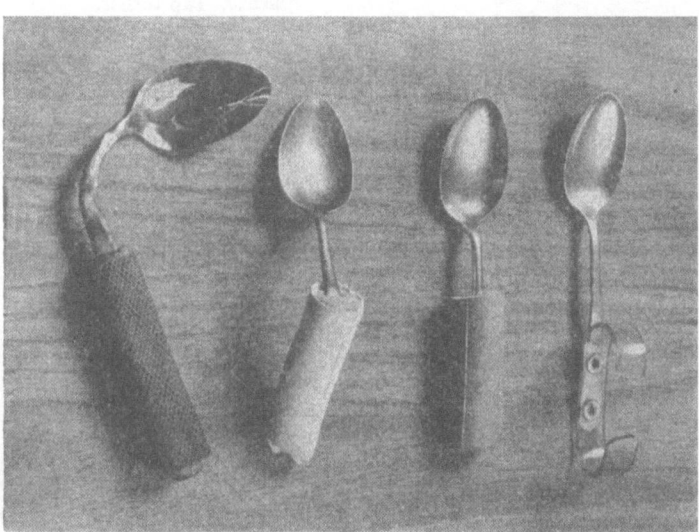

Figure 3. Cutlery with adapted handles.

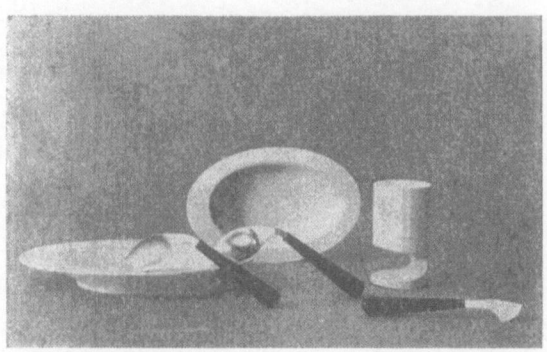

Figure 4. Tableware specially designed for the rheumatoid arthritic.

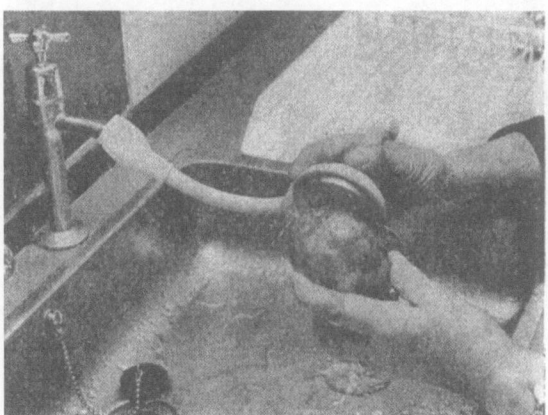

Figure 5. Vegetable scraper.

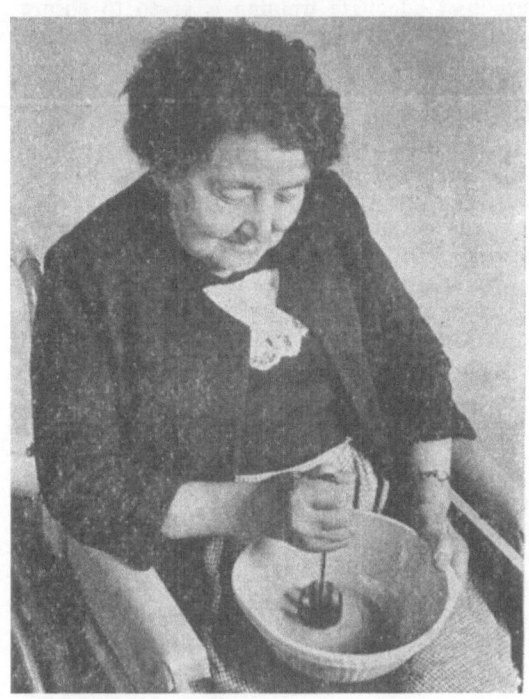

Figure 6. One handed beater.

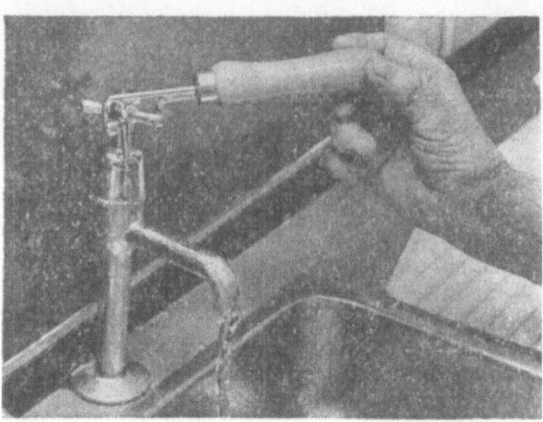

Figure 7. Tap-turner.

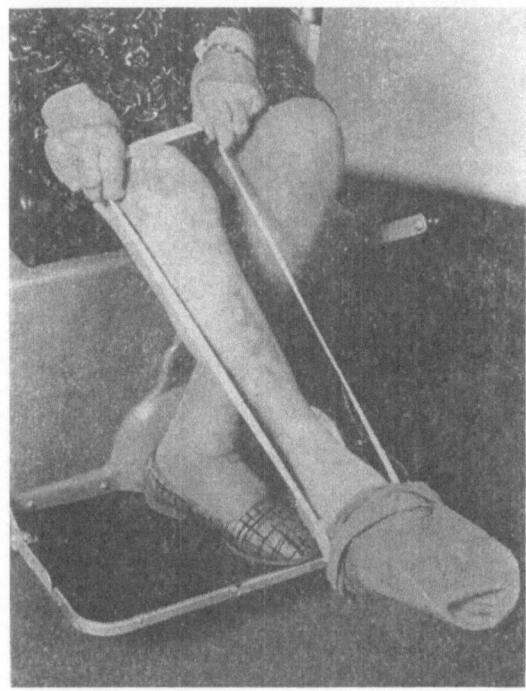

Figure 8. Stocking-aid.

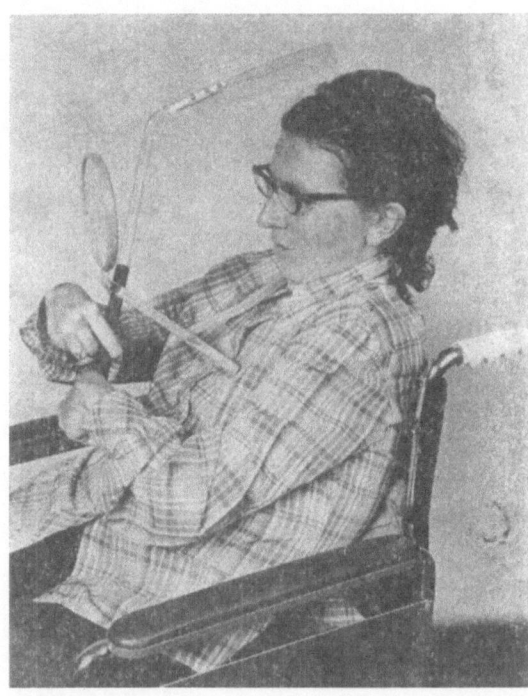

Figure 9. Patient with very restricted arm movements using long-handled comb and a neck hung mirror.

Equipment

Large devices to help the disabled are classified as 'equipment'. Hoists, commodes, bath seats, special armchairs, and beds come into this category. Such equipment is usually provided by the local authority.

Appliances

Aids and equipment are distinguished from 'appliances' which are medical devices made for and usually fitted to an individual patient—for example: calipers, splints and prostheses. Walking aids and wheelchairs, although often individually prescribed and technically appliances, are usually regarded as mobility aids. Whether the device is a simple aid such as a 'tap turner' or a complex appliance such as an electric hoist, it must serve a specific need and add to the patient's independence if it is to be fully accepted and used.

Inappropriate provision of aids and appliances is common. Many devices occupy space in wardrobes and cupboards and are seldom used. Often this is due to the unwillingness of the patient or the family to change existing routines. Although a need for an aid may be demonstrated during assessment, the patient and family may not want to use it. Although the device may give the patient some independence, the family may find it quicker and less complicated to avoid using the equipment. For example, many families will continue to lift the patient themselves rather than use a hoist.

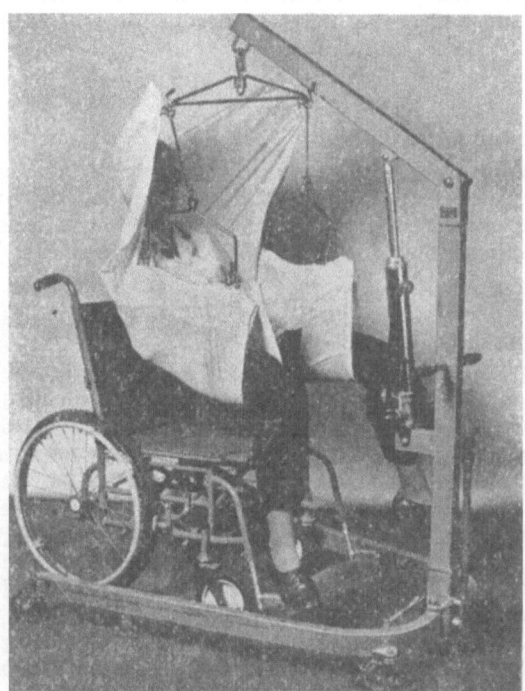

Figure 10. Portable hoist being used with a "hammock" sling with a commode aperture and individual leg pieces.

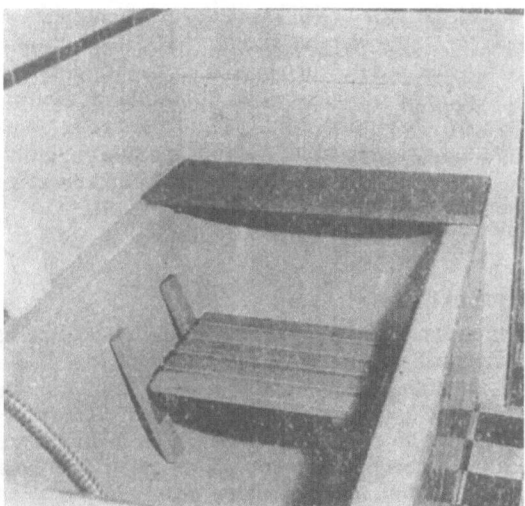

Figure 11. Bath seat and bath board.

Sometimes a period of time elapses between initial recommendation and the implementation into home routines. During this critical period, training can be forgotten unless reinforced and the recommended equipment may not be maximally effective when it is eventually provided.

Some patients will prefer to remain dependent and no matter how effective aids and appliances may be they cannot be persuaded to use them.

Functional assessment

Clinical assessment is based on a stylised system of 'history taking', clinical examination, muscle power charting, and so on, without which significant details may be missed. Functional assessment can be systemised and formalised, based on activities of daily living and graded activities, as follows:

Personal Care: Washing
Feeding
Toilet
Dressing

Mobility: Walking aids
Wheelchairs
Transfers

Household: Cooking
Housework

Hobbies and leisure activities
Work

The physical procedures of assessing daily living activities in near real-life situations often achieves a considerable understanding of the important and immeasurable variables such as the patient's willingness to co-operate, his tolerance of failure, levels of aspiration, ability to understand new situations, awareness of limitations and capabilities, his level of intelligence, and education; in short, his motivation.

Personal toilet

Independence for micturition and defaecation is an integral part of a person's self-respect. Both activities are complex and can be difficult for the elderly and disabled. Many people in these categories tend to deny or play down their difficulties because of embarrassment, self-respect, or a fear that admission of difficulties will lead to their total loss of independence and a denial of their wish to remain living where they want to live.

Incontinence and excretory incompetence are potent causes of permanent admission to hospital care. Lack of independence in these areas often precludes independent or partially dependent life at home or in appropriate unsupervised or even supervised accommodation. For the younger disabled such lack of independence may mitigate against acceptance in normal school, for training or work when otherwise even a severely disabled person could cope with the situation. Toilet and bathing aids are the commonest to be supplied by local authorities for the disabled at home. These are usually in the form of aids to raise the height of toilet seats, to provide additional grab rails to help the person get on and off the toilet, and a simple form of seat to enable him to get in and out of the bath. Additional rails in toilet, bath, corridors and staircase are simple to fit and of great value. In general, they should be about 1¼ inches (30mm) diameter, fixed with

well fitted wall plugs and held by adequate (say 2 inch) screws to the wall. It is to be remembered that when they use grab rails a disabled person's full weight may have to be taken by the rail. Usually they should be horizontal or vertical rails unless trials indicate that an angled rail is needed. In the bathroom and toilet such rails should have a non-slip surface.

Washing, shaving and grooming can be helped by simple aids which are the stock-in-trade of most occupational therapy departments. More individual are the needs of disabled people to adapt their clothes to make dressing and undressing easier. Appropriate styles and material can help. The use of velcro instead of buttons and other small fastenings and re-design of the usual openings and fastenings are other ways of increasing independence which an occupational therapist can devise and demonstrate.

Eating and drinking

Eating and drinking can be helped by the use of specially designed crockery and cutlery, or by relatively simple adaptations to conventional equipment.

Mobility

It has been estimated that there are nearly half a million people in this country whose mobility is reduced by disability not due to old age. Often mobility is the key to the whole programme of rehabilitation of the severely physically disabled.

The ability to walk is often precariously balanced upon the patient's remaining strength and his determination. He may be able to walk albeit with a considerable struggle, and often with considerable risk, but often it is necessary to decide between continuing this activity or accepting other means of mobility to achieve more efficient means of progression. Walking aids of various kinds may help. Sticks, quadruped sticks, crutches, elbow crutches and walking frames are all available. But assessment in home surroundings by physiotherapist or occupational therapist will determine the most suitable.

There are some patients for whom walking remains a marginal activity but the ability to take a few steps enables them to continue to transfer independently, or to perform limited activities out of their wheelchairs. Once walking becomes a struggle and is only achieved at the exclusion of other more contributory activities, whether leisure or work, wheelchair mobility is usually recommended.

Many of the more severely disabled can

achieve some degree of independence of mobility with the appropriate wheelchair, whether self-propelled, propelled by their feet, or powered by an electric motor.

The majority of wheelchairs provided through the Department of Heath and Social Security are used to take the moderately and mildly disabled, young and old, out of the house. Thus it is as important to determine the type of use as well as studying the disabled person when prescribing a wheelchair. If it is only to be used (as 60% are) to push them along the road, to church, around the shops, or to a local club, and all of these in conjunction with transport in a motor car, then it is important to provide a wheelchair which will fold small enough to go into a car (or in the car boot). This means that it must be light enough to be lifted by the attendant—also often elderly or frail. A lightweight car transit chair is probably nowadays the most commonly required chair. With small wheels it is not designed to be self-propelled, the larger wheels for self-propelling add considerably to the chair's weight and make it very awkward for transporting.

For those who will use the chair indoors as well, it will depend as much on the size and design of the house as much as anything else, as to the type of chair provided. Frequently it is necessary to provide a chair too small for real comfort in order to achieve necessary indoor mobility. General practitioners can prescribe standard wheelchairs which should be adequate for most circumstances, but prescriber and patient may have to accept that wheelchair existence is almost always a compromise and a chair suitable for comfort may not be suitable for manoeuvring in a confined space. Similar but greater constraints apply to the powered indoor wheelchairs, where comfort may have to be sacrificed for manoeuvrability or vice versa. It is possible to enable even the very severely disabled to achieve independence of mobility providing they have the space to accommodate the vehicle. As with non-powered chairs, there may be problems of differing requirements and constraints in the house and outside the house, and it may be impossible in any one set of circumstances to provide one chair suitable for both situations. Increasingly there are specialised clinics for prescribing, testing, adapting and training in the use of a wheelchair. These may be held at hospitals, rehabilitation units, or at DHSS Appliance Centres. Furthermore, the available designs of chairs are changing and the facilities for the severely disabled increasing year by year.

Transferring

An important part of the management of disabled persons is the amount of manhandling which they may require. Helping someone to stand, sit, get on and off a wheelchair can put severe physical strain upon those having to help. Once again the occupational therapist and the physiotherapist are trained to help to overcome these problems. The use of a hoist for example is a great saving in physical effort, but unfortunately, too often, hoists are asked for and supplied but there is inadequate skilled training of the family in the use of the equipment. The majority of hoists supplied through the local authority and social services are not in full use because the patient's relatives have not been adequately assessed and trained. The selection of the correct slings may be critical, the hoist supplied may be inappropriate to the domestic situation, and should be a different design. But above all, the attendant and the patient need to have the confidence which can only be gained by training. A wide range of hydraulic, hand-operated and electrically powered hoists are available and a wider understanding of the use of this versatile equipment could undoubtedly make much domiciliary nursing much easier.

Household activities

There is an infinite range of gadgets to help the disabled housewife, ranging from one handed tin openers, and tap turners to expensive installations such as split level cookers which obviate the need to bend down while cooking. For the young disabled housewife complete kitchen design may be a considerable contribution to the independence of the entire family. For the elderly and frail it may be more appropriate to arrange for 'meals on wheels' and regular help from neighbours, relatives and volunteer agencies. A detailed domestic assessment by the domiciliary occupational therapist in collaboration with the doctor's appraisal of the situation will be required in each individual case.

In many situations emergency call systems and regular visits are of prime importance.

For the very severely disabled there are a variety of sophisticated devices under the general heading of Environmental Control Systems (e.g. possum–patient operated selector mechanism) which are provided through the Regional Health Authorities. These systems enable the patient to use a telephone call system, operate a radio, television, lights, doors and other necessary outlets.

10

PROSPECTS IN MEDICAL TREATMENT

JOHN M. EVANSON

In the history of therapeutics, serendipity has contributed so significantly to some of the major advances that any attempts to look ahead may be out of date by the time such predictions appear in print. But fortunately this risk is small and it is satisfyingly true that current progress in medical treatment owes more to advancement of basic scientific knowledge than perhaps at any time in the past. There remain great areas of morbidity—where previously, treatment at best has been empirical, ineffective but harmless, and at worst provided the seeds of iatrogenic disease —which now show promise of yielding to the rational scientific approach. The identification of multifactorial 'risk' factors in conditions such as chronic bronchitis, pulmonary neoplasia and myocardial infarction provides preventive medicine with a challenging opportunity to transform the spectrum of disease, and the developing biochemical and cytological techniques for the antenatal diagnosis of congenital disorders may allow the eradication of some of the more hideous conditions to which man has been heir.

An illustrative area of progress and promise at the more directly therapeutic level is in diseases of bone, where already the very real advances in understanding of physiology are being exploited in treatment methods. The link between calcium homeostasis in the dog and the rat, and the alleviation of pain in Paget's disease of bone may at first sight seem a tenuous one, but the discovery of the calcium-lowering hormone, calcitonin, in animals, and its subsequent characterisation, has provided the first effective approach to management of this disorder of bone.

Calcitonin, a polypeptide hormone of approximately 4000 molecular weight, is elaborated and secreted by the parafollicular cells of the thyroid gland but, paradoxically, has not yet been assigned a defined physiological role in man. Its therapeutic efficacy, however, in reversing biochemical abnormalities and inducing symptomatic relief in Paget's disease of bone now seems in little doubt. The hormone effectively diminishes the breakdown of bone, independent of parathyroid hormone, and the urinary excretion of hydroxyproline peptides, the end product of bone collagen breakdown, is correspondingly diminished. The theoretical basis for the trial of calcitonin in Paget's disease has already been amply vindicated in its successful use in those patients, albeit a minority, whose disease produces disabling pain. What remains to be proved is the long term effect of the hormone in arresting pathological bone resorption and restoring more normal osteoblastic bone formation. Preliminary observations in so-called juvenile Paget's disease might suggest that this is a therapeutic possibility and, if this is so in the older age group, where Paget's disease is increasingly common, the prevention of grotesque and disabling deformities becomes a realisable aim.

One disadvantage of calcitonin as a therapeutic agent is the need for it to be given parenterally —because of its peptidic nature. Thus an alternative and more attractive form of treatment in Paget's disease—and one which promises to have wider application—is the orally administered compound sodium edidronate. This substance is a member of that group of compounds known as phosphonates which resemble the naturally occurring pyrophosphates (of characteristic composition $-P-O-P-$) except for the substitution of a central oxygen atom by carbon (giving a typical chemical bond $-P-C-P-$). The phosphonates represent a synthetic group of compounds with exciting actions both on the synthesis of bone, where they may inhibit bone crystal formation, and on resorption, where they may block degradation of existing mineralised bone. Trials of EHDP (sodium edidronate) in Paget's disease have already indicated, as with calcitonin, that biochemical and symptomatic improvement can be achieved by prolonged treatment, without significant side effects. The hope for the future relates to the development of further synthetic analogues with more specific action on the synthetic or resorptive sides of bone metabolism such that the treatment or prevention of the common condition of involutional osteoporosis might become a distinct therapeutic possibility. Quantitatively, the problem of osteoporosis in the elderly presents the greatest challenge, but its insidious onset and frequently late presentation with fractures makes it a particularly difficult one to solve.

In the narrower sphere of bone disease produced by disordered vitamin D metabolism, recent advances have already led to more effective therapy in some conditions and predict the elucidation in the near future of a variety of inherited anomalies of bone metabolism. It is now accepted that the biological action of naturally occurring vitamin D, cholecalciferol, is dependent upon its conversion to the active metabolite 1,25-dihydroxycholecalciferol, and that the transformation of vitamin D to this compound occurs in two stages, the first in the liver (to 25-hydroxy vitamin D) and the second—(to 1,26-dihydroxy vitamin D)—in the kidney. 'Renal rickets' is then, theoretically, eminently treatable with the dihydroxy compound and preliminary studies suggest that this is indeed so. The concept of 'vitamin D resistance' in chronic renal failure has thus been placed on a firm scientific basis and the management of the bony complications of chronic haemodialysis, now being used with increasing frequency and success, can be approached more rationally. Here again, the production in the laboratory, of related compounds, more easily synthesised but having similar biological effects, has already begun.

This story of progress involving the discovery of a natural hormone, the laboratory synthesis of a biologically active compound and the clarification of the intermediary metabolism of a traditionally accepted vitamin, has improved substantially the prospects of effective medical treatment in a whole range of bone diseases.

Another quite different area where we may expect the development of effective therapeutic agents has arisen from current interest in the prostaglandins. These ubiquitous compounds are basically short-chain fatty acids with individual members having different substituted end groupings, side groupings and chemical bonds, endowing them with a bewildering range of biological actions on various target organs. Some have already been subjected to clinical trials as for instance in inducing abortion or induction of labour at full term. The physician's ambition to find a means of achieving medical vagotomy and render much of the gastric surgeon's work redundant might ultimately find its fulfilment in the application of these compounds to peptic ulcer therapy. An ancient Chinese belief that semen, (which we now know contains at least 13 different prostaglandins), was of value in the

treatment of peptic ulceration may have its explanation in the recently demonstrated effect of one synthetic analogue, designated 15-methyl-prostaglandin E_2, in suppressing gastric acid and pepsin secretion and promoting gastric mucus production when given orally. Such actions might be expected to provide optimal conditions for peptic ulcer healing and there are some early clinical observations to support this view. In the same way that the discovery of the natural steroids of the cortisone group gave rise to a wealth of natural and synthetic analogues of broad therapeutic application, it is likely that the prostaglandins will provide a range of physiological and artificial compounds of similar clinical value.

To date, the taking over of the function of a failing organ by extracorporeal means, either on a temporary or semi-permanent basis, has found its fullest expression in the development of haemodialysis for renal failure. In attempts to evolve similar life-support systems for acute liver insufficiency caused by acute hepatitis or hepatic necrosis, the ingenuity and enthusiasm applied to the devising of techniques such as pig liver perfusion and allied procedures has not always been matched by success in their clinical application. But we are now perhaps at a stage when optimism is more justified, for the most recent studies using coated activated charcoal perfusion to maintain life in acute hepatic coma have given results better than any heretofore. Even without a full understanding of the nature of the toxic substances responsible for the clinical picture in acute liver failure, it now seems that their removal by an extracorporeal perfusion technique may be achieved and life maintained until spontaneous recovery of hepatic function takes place. In irrecoverable chronic hepatic failure, the prospects of long term maintenance, along the lines of chronic haemodialysis for renal failure, remain extremely remote in view of the crucial synthetic activities of the liver in addition to its detoxicating role.

There are several clinical fields where future progress in treatment may be anticipated not so much from the discovery of new agents or techniques, but rather from the better application of the wealth of drugs already available. The significant advances made in recent years in the management of the leukaemias, particularly of childhood, owe much to meticulous study of timing, combination and route of administration of known cytotoxic drugs. Other varieties of malignant disease will undoubtedly be approached in a similar manner. In the therapy of hypertension our need is not only, or primarily, for

o

the development of more effective agents but rather for a clearer definition of the indications for the exhibition of the diverse variety of anti-hypertensive drugs we already have at our disposal. In the management of patients, drug therapy is only a part, and the avoidance of iatrogenic disease must be a consideration in all clinical decisions. To treat or not to treat may frequently pose a greater clinical problem than what to treat with!

INDEX

Nalorphine 176
Nandrolone 257
Naphthylamine 316
Napkin rash 47
Naproxen 183
Narcotic analgesics 174–179, 272, 276, 278, 281
Nasolacrimal duct (lacrimal sac infection) 154
Necator americanus 10
Neck, acute 290
Neisseria meningitidis 76
Neocinchophen 182
Neomycin 15, 50, 154, 155, 226, 271, 278, 279, 353, 356
Neonatal hypoglycaemia 63
Neoplasia: see Carcinoma
Neostigmine 86, 189
Nepenthe 328
Nephrectomy (hypertension) 118
Nephritis, acute 19–20
Nephrohathy, analgesic 180
Nephrotic syndrome 20–22
  diabetes 31
Nephrotoxins 22, 25–26
Neuralgia 80, 155, 169
Naphritis, optic 159
Neurologically disabled (physiotherapy) 391
Neuromuscular-blocking agents 190–191
Neuropathy
  obstructive arterial disease 121
  toxic peripheral 84
  uraemic 25
Neurosyphilis 68, 69
Neurotoxicity (Hodgkin's disease) 102–103
Niacin: see Nicotinic acid
Niclosamide 10, 235
Nicotinamide 262
  deficiency 84
Nicotinic acid (niacin) 68, 262, 355
Nicoumalone 219
Nifenazone 181–182
Nifuratel 73
Night blindness 261
Nikethamide 140, 141, 247
Niridazole 146, 147, 233
Nitrazepam 79, 172–173, 272, 276, 279, 329
Nitrimidazine 73
Nitrofurantoin 27, 28, 29, 30, 229, 275, 281
Nitrogen
  balance (chronic renal failure) 24
  liquid 51
  mustards 238–240
Nodal bradycardia 129
Noisy belching 6
Noradrenaline 185, 205–207

Northisterone 258
Nose
  boils 50
  epistaxis (haemophilia) 105
Novobiocin 275, 281
Nystagmus 398
Nystantin 47, 73, 103, 230, 331

Oat-cell carcinoma of the bronchus 86, 319
Obesity, nutritional 57–58
  cardiac failure 111
  diabetes mellitus 59
  hypertension 118, 120
Obstructive arterial disease 120–121
Occupational therapy 386, 392
  domicillary 405
  terminal care 327
Occupation, change of (disc prolapse) 45
Occular myasthenia 86
Oestradiol 259
Oleandomycin 275
Oligaemia (low venous pressure) 124–125
Oliguric renal failure 22
Onchocerca volvulus 236
Onchocerciasis 236–237
Oophorectomy 319
Open-engle glaucoma 158
Ophthalmology
  antimalarial therapy 183
  basilar artery insufficiency 159
  blepharitis 54
  burns 156
  central retinal artery occlusion 159
  central retinal venous thrombosis 159
  chalazion 154
  conjunctivitis 154–155
  corticosteroid side effects 256
  cranial arteritis 82, 159
  detachment, retinal 160
  diabetic retinopathy 62
  exophthalmos 64
  ganglion blockers 203
  gastro-enteritis 149
  glaucoma 158
  gonococcal ophthalmia neonatorum 72
  hordeolum 154
  hyperthyroidism 64
  ischaemic optic atrophy 159
  keratitis, *Herpes simplex* 155
  lacrimal sac infection 154
  lid laceration 157
  migraine 159
  myasthenia, ocular 86
  neuritis, cranial 159–160
  ophthalmicus, *Herpes zoster* 155

orbital injuries 157
pipilledema 159
practolol therapy 144
rapid eye movement (sleep) 170
red eye 157
refractive error 158
Reiter's disease 72–73
sickle-cell disease 93
strabismic amblyopia 158–159
trauma 155–158
visual field loss 159
vitamin A therapy 261
vitamin B$_{12}$ deficiency 85
vitreous haemorrhages 160
Ophthalmoplegia, progressive supranuclear (Steele–Richardson syndrome) 84
Opiates 174–176
  terminal care 328
Oral contraceptives
  gonadal dysgenesis 66
  hirsuitism 66
  hypertension 118
  liver disease 279
  migraine 79
  pulmonary heart disease 113
Orbital
  decompression (exophthalmos) 64
  rim fracture 157
Orchidectomy
  adenocarcinoma 320
  testes, carcinoma of the 320
Orchitis (mumps) 152
Orciprenaline 135, 185, 306, 330
Orphenadrin 83, 168
Orphenadrine hydrochloride 168
Osmotic diuretics 213
Osteoarthritis 43–44
Osteodystrophy, renal (uraemia) 24–25
Osteomalacia
  calciferol therapy 254
  cirrhosis 14
  phenytoin therapy 78
  post-gastric surgery 9
  renal dialysis 365
Osteomyelitis 42–43, 225
Osteoporosis 406
Otitis media, acute 152, 312
Ovary
  carcinoma of the 319
  ovulation 251, 377
  polycystic syndrome 66
Overdose 296
  anticoagulants 106
  aspirin 296
  barbiturate 170, 171, 296, 297
  glutethimide 171
  iron tablets (desferrioxamine) 245, 246
  paracetamol 14, 180